Nunn's Applied Respiratory Physiology

Nunn's Applied Respiratory Physiology

Fourth edition

J.F. Nunn
MD, DSc, PhD, FRCS, FRCA, FANZCA(Hon), FFARCSI(Hon)
Formerly Head of Division of Anaesthesia, Medical Research Council Clinical Research Centre; Honorary Consultant Anaesthetist, Northwick Park Hospital, Middlesex; Previously, Professor of Anaesthesia, University of Leeds; Dean of Faculty of Anaesthesia, Royal College of Surgeons of England

Foreword by John W. Severinghaus
Cardiovascular Research Institute, San Francisco; Department of Anaesthetics, University of California

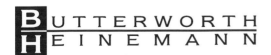

Butterworth-Heinemann Ltd
Linacre House, Jordan Hill, Oxford OX2 8DP

ℛ A member of the Reed Elsevier group

OXFORD   LONDON   BOSTON
MUNICH   NEW DELHI   SINGAPORE   SYDNEY
TOKYO   TORONTO   WELLINGTON

First published 1969
Reprinted 1971 (twice), 1972, 1975
Second edition 1977
Reprinted 1978, 1981
Third edition 1987
Reprinted 1989
Fourth edition 1993

© Butterworth-Heinemann Ltd 1993

British Library Cataloguing in Publication Data
A catalogue record for this book is
available from the British Library

Library of Congress Cataloguing in Publication Data
A catalogue record for this book is
available from the Library of Congress

ISBN 0 7506 1336 X

Printed and bound in Great Britain by The University Press, Cambridge

Contents

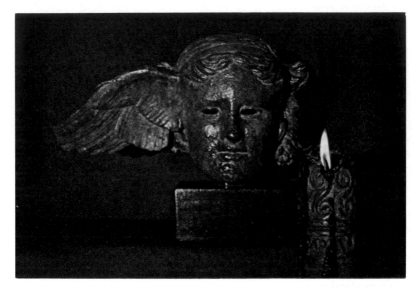

Hypnos and the Flame
(original photograph courtesy of Dr John W. Severinghaus)

Foreword to the fourth edition

In every era, whether the Reformation or the genetic revolution, fad captures the crowd. Protestant theologian Rheinhold Niebuhr depicted the role of the remnant to be preservation of culture and tradition (his neo-orthodoxy), as the Western world largely turned to secular humanism. During the quarter century since John Nunn's book first appeared, the drama of clones, codons, channels and genomes has swept blood and gas under the rug in medical schools, cornered the funds and co-opted a generation of inquiry. Respiratory research, proceeding in relative obscurity, seldom seen in *Science, Nature* or *The Times,* nevertheless accounts for much of the 5000 pages a year now published by the *Journal of Applied Physiology*.

For students entering anaesthesia, ill-prepared to manage pulmonary problems, *Applied Respiratory Physiology* fulfils the role of the remnant. What a rarity! A single-authored medical text, thrice updated, the essence needed by newcomers and old-timers alike, extracted from the world's literature without assistance, barely increasing its bulk, while keeping it clear, concise and comprehensive. Who else would be the only one to catch his own minor Latin translation error in an earlier edition?

With John Nunn's update of lung science, let me refresh the 'Flame for Hypnos' metaphor, in which Flame stood for learning, facts and science. C.P. Snow's two-cultures, humanities and sciences, arose, in Robert Pirsig's view*, when the primacy of Quality, as defended in the dialogues of Plato by Phaedrus a sophist, collapsed under Socrates' weighty support of Truth and Fact, the roots of science. Until it conceived nuclear fission, Science could largely ignore Ethics. Now the two cultures must be rejoined if we would survive. So too, as the tools of Hypnos matured, a vigilant remnant unmasked slights of Quality that had been too long condoned. New emphases emerged in anaesthesiology: Safety, Quality Control and Continuing Medical Education. The gain with each new device or drug wants new skill and care, that the offspring of Hypnos might excel in every action and remove each risk to life and health. These two views of reality, Sophists' Quality and Socratic Truth, have come to be recognized as co-essential. Thus may Hypnos restore the Hellenic cloak of Phaedrus.

John W. Severinghaus

Zen and the Art of Motorcycle Maintenance.

Preface to the first edition

Clinicians in many branches of medicine find that their work demands an extensive knowledge of respiratory physiology. This applies particularly to anaesthetists working in the operating theatre or in the intensive care unit. It is unfortunately common experience that respiratory physiology learned in the preclinical years proves to be an incomplete preparation for the clinical field. Indeed, the emphasis of the preclinical course seems, in many cases, to be out of tune with the practical problems to be faced after qualification and specialization. Much that is taught does not apply to man in the clinical environment while, on the other hand, a great many physiological problems highly relevant to the survival of patients find no place in the curriculum. It is to be hoped that new approaches to the teaching of medicine may overcome this dichotomy and that, in particular, much will be gained from the integration of physiology with clinical teaching.

This book is designed to bridge the gap between pure respiratory physiology and the treatment of patients. It is neither a primer of respiratory physiology nor is it a practical manual for use in the wards and operating theatres. It has two aims. Firstly, I have tried to explain those aspects of respiratory physiology which seem most relevant to patient care, particularly in the field of anaesthesia. Secondly, I have brought together in review those studies which seem to me to be most relevant to clinical work. Inevitably there has been a preference for studies of man and particular stress has been laid on those functions in which man appears to differ from laboratory animals. There is an unashamed emphasis on anaesthesia because I am an anaesthetist. However, the work in this speciality spreads freely into the territory of our neighbours.

References have been a problem. It is clearly impracticable to quote every work which deserves mention. In general I have cited the most informative and the most accessible works, but this rule has been broken on numerous occasions when the distinction of prior discovery calls for recognition. Reviews are freely cited since a book of this length can include only a fraction of the relevant material. I must apologize to the writers of multi-author papers. No one likes to be cited as a colleague, but considerations of space have precluded naming more than three authors for any paper.

Chapters are designed to be read separately and this has required some repetition. There are also frequent cross-references between the chapters. The principles of methods of measurement are considered together at the end of each chapter or section.

In spite of optimistic hopes, the book has taken six years to write. Its form, however, has evolved over the last twelve years from a series of lectures and tutorials given at the Royal College of Surgeons, the Royal Postgraduate Medical School, the University of Leeds and in numerous institutions in Europe and the United States which I have been privileged to visit. Blackboard sketches have gradually taken the form of the figures which appear in this book.

The greater part of this book is distilled from the work of teachers and colleagues. Professor W. Melville Arnott and Professor K. W. Donald introduced me to the study of clinical respiratory physiology and I worked under the late Professor Ronald Woolmer for a further six years. My debt to them is very great. I have also had the good fortune to work in close contact with many gifted colleagues who have not hesitated to share the fruits of their experience. The list of references will indicate how much I have learned from Dr John Severinghaus, Professor Moran Campbell, Dr John Butler and Dr John West. For my own studies, I acknowledge with gratitude the part played by a long series of research fellows and assistants. Some fifteen are cited herein and they come from eleven different countries. Figures 2, 3, 6, 11 and 15 [Figures 5.3, 3.4 and 3.1 in the fourth edition] which are clearly not my blackboard sketches, were drawn by Mr H. Grayshon Lumby. I have had unstinted help from librarians, Miss M. P. Russell, Mr W. R. LeFanu and Miss E. M. Reed. Numerous colleagues have given invaluable help in reading and criticizing the manuscript.

Finally I must thank my wife who has not only borne the inevitable preoccupation of a husband writing a book but has also carried the burden of the paper work and prepared the manuscript.

J.F.N.

Preface to the fourth edition

Respiratory physiology as taught to my generation of medical students in the 1940s bore little relevance to clinical practice. The situation was transformed by the major war-time advances achieved by the American workers Fenn, Rahn, Otis and Riley, and then presented in spectacular fashion to the medical public in *The Lung* by Comroe and his co-authors. The first edition of *Applied Respiratory Physiology* was written at the time when measurement of arterial P_{CO_2} and P_{O_2} had just become practicable in the clinical field. The new understanding of the factors which control these important quantities in health and disease could now be applied, and those who practised acute medicine in the 1950s will remember what an immense advance this was. The first edition was written to transmit this new knowledge to a wider clinical sphere. It was an exciting time and clinical respiratory physiology was then in the forefront of progress, enjoying the glamour which is now the preserve of molecular biology.

Respiratory research did not stand still but moved into new and exciting areas, which required a second edition, written in the mid 1970s. Among the new developments were the identification of the central chemoreceptors, improved understanding of mechanisms of pulmonary oedema, recognition of the role of free radicals in oxygen toxicity and elucidation of further non-respiratory functions of the lungs. It had become clear that reduction in functional residual capacity underlay many of the abnormalities of pulmonary function during anaesthesia and it had been shown that changes in levels of 2,3-diphosphoglycerate could displace the oxyhaemoglobin dissociation curve. Respiratory physiologists were moving into novel fields which often paralleled those in other disciplines of medicine.

New fields of research continued to emerge and the third edition, written in the mid 1980s, required a change in format with the first part of the book devoted to basic principles, now with a full chapter on the non-respiratory functions of the lung. There were major advances in our understanding of the medullary neurons concerned with breathing, and in the distribution of ventilation and perfusion to respiratory units of different ventilation/perfusion ratios. The second part of the book was devoted to applications and permitted a much more detailed and systematic discussion of new advances in understanding of applied situations. In every section of the applications there were major advances to review. They included an explosion of knowledge in the role of pharyngeal obstruction in the respiratory disorders of sleep, and in our understanding of exercise at extreme altitude. There were many new developments in artificial ventilation, recognition of the histology of pulmonary barotrauma and a novel approach to extracorporeal removal of carbon dioxide. There was a great expansion in understanding the role of free radicals in oxygen toxicity, and this was associated with important studies of the mechanisms of pulmonary tissue damage in the adult respiratory distress syndrome.

Since the third edition, the pace of respiratory research has quickened and diversified to an extent, much of which could not have been anticipated. In particular, how many of us would have guessed that nitric oxide would play such a crucial role in pulmonary vasomotor control and that this highly reactive free-radical gas would appear to have an important role in therapy of the adult respiratory distress syndrome? The relationship between oxygen consumption and delivery in disease has become a valuable field of research, and there have been further important developments in the mechanisms and significance of pharyngeal obstruction in sleep and anaesthesia. The pulse oximeter has ushered in a new era of continuous clinical monitoring of oxygenation. The simulated laboratory ascent of Everest has provided much detail of high altitude physiology and confirmed the earlier field studies of West, Pugh and others. We now have the earliest intimations of respiratory studies by West during prolonged weightlessness in space. Understanding of the pulmonary effects of anaesthesia have been revolutionized by the outstanding tomographic studies by Hedenstierna and his colleagues in Stockholm. Milic-Emili has again broken new ground, this time in the time-dependence of lung mechanics due to viscoelastic flow in lung tissue. Finally, I thought the time was ripe to present a chapter on the atmosphere, which is basic to respiration and can no longer be taken for granted as an unchanging entity.

The formidable task of assimilation of this new knowledge has been helped by an unprecedented explosion in major books on respiration, including the *Handbooks of the American Physiological Society*, the immense *Scientific Foundation* (Crystal and West) and the many volumes on specific topics produced by Marcel Dekker. The total shelf length of these volumes is measured in metres, and condensation of the essential information into a book of this length has been a daunting task.

I wish to express my personal gratitude to all those who have helped me in my understanding of the many new concepts, and in particular to Michael Halsey, David and Barbara Royston, Warren Zapol, Goran Hedenstierna, John Severinghaus, Bryan Marshall, Milic-Emili, John West and Gordon Drummond. British Airways kindly reviewed the information on commercial flying. Erwald Weibel has again provided wonderful electron micrographs and Louise Perks has translated concepts into intelligible diagrams. I am specially indebted to John Severinghaus for contributing his arresting Foreword to the fourth edition to cap his Foreword to the first edition of twenty-four years ago. Finally and not least my dear wife has once again borne the burden of a preoccupied husband immersed in papers and word-processors for an inordinate length of time.

J.F.N.

Part 1

Basic Principles

Chapter 1

The atmosphere

The atmosphere of the earth has a composition and pressure which is unique in the solar system. It has evolved by a complex chain of circumstances in which biological influences have been of major importance. In turn many species, including *Homo sapiens*, have evolved to derive maximal benefit from the present state of the gaseous environment. However, major changes in the atmosphere now appear to be taking place, largely as a result of human intervention. If these changes continue into the future, there will inevitably be a deterioration of quality of life and survival for some but not all species.

Pressure and composition of the atmosphere

Sea level pressure is 101.3 kPa (760 mmHg or 1033 cmH$_2$O). The pressure declines with increasing altitude and Table 15.1 shows the standardized relationship between pressure and altitude, from which there are some important exceptions (page 339). The troposphere has a relatively constant composition and extends from sea level to the tropopause, which is at an altitude of 17 km at the equator and 6–8 km at the poles. The mean altitude is about 11 km, where the pressure is 23 kPa (173 mmHg). Temperature also falls progressively with altitude in the troposphere to reach a minumum of −56°C at the tropopause. This provides the cold trap beyond which the escape of water vapour is greatly curtailed. Above the tropopause is the stratosphere, the lower part of which includes the operating altitudes of jet airliners. Temperature rises with altitude in the stratosphere to reach a temperature close to 0°C at the stratopause (50 km). The stratosphere is exposed to both ionizing radiation and intense ultraviolet radiation which causes photodissociation of gases. This results in many chemical changes that cannot occur in the troposphere, including, for example, the formation of ozone.

The composition of the earth's atmosphere is quite unlike that of any other body in the solar system (Table 1.1). Small bodies, such as Mercury and most of the planets' satellites, have a gravitational field which is too weak for the retention of any atmosphere at all (Figure 1.1). The large planets (Jupiter, Saturn, Uranus and Neptune) have a gravitational field which is sufficiently strong to retain all gases, including helium and hydrogen, thereby ensuring the retention of a reducing

Table 1.1 Composition of the atmosphere of the earth (by volume in dry gas)

Nitrogen	78.084%	Neon	18.18 p.p.m.
Oxygen	20.946%	Helium	5.24 p.p.m.
Argon	0.934%	Methane	1.70 p.p.m.
Carbon dioxide	0.035%	Krypton	1.14 p.p.m.
		Hydrogen	0.50 p.p.m.
		Nitrous oxide	0.28 p.p.m.
		Ozone	0.10* p.p.m.
		Xenon	0.086 p.p.m.
		CFCs	0.003 p.p.m.

*Very variable

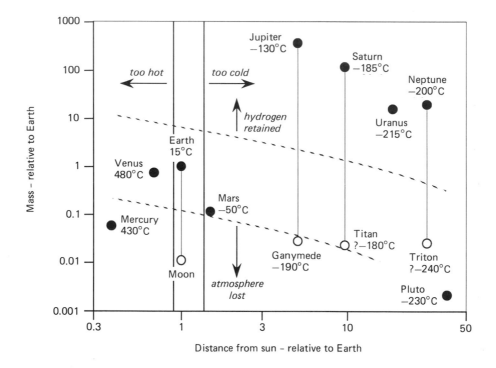

Figure 1.1 The planets and some of their larger satellites, plotted according to distance from the sun (abscissa) and mass (ordinate), both scales being logarithmic and relative to Earth. Mean surface temperatures are shown. Potential for life as we know it exists only within the parallelogram surrounding the earth.

atmosphere. The gravitational field of Earth is intermediate, resulting in a differential retention of the heavier gases (oxygen, carbon dioxide and nitrogen), while permitting the escape of hydrogen and helium. This is crucial to the development of an oxidizing atmosphere. Water vapour (molecular weight only 18) would be lost from the atmosphere were it not for the cold trap at the tropopause.

Surface temperature

Surface temperature of a planetary body is of crucial importance to the composition of the atmosphere and therefore the potential for life. To a first approximation, temperature is dependent on the distance of a planet from the sun and the intensity of solar radiation (Figure 1.1). The major secondary factor is the greenhouse effect of any atmosphere which the planet may possess. Mercury and Venus have surface temperatures far above the boiling point of water. All planets (and their satellites) which are further away from the sun than the earth have a surface temperature too cold for liquid water to exist. In the solar system, only Earth is of a size and distance from the sun at which liquid water can exist on the surface. It is difficult to see how life as we know it could exist anywhere else in the solar system.

Origin of the atmosphere

The primary and secondary reducing atmospheres

The earth was probably formed by the gravitational accretion of cold material 4600 million years ago. This is shown in relation to the life of the sun in Figure 1.2, where it will be seen that the sun is currently about the middle of its main sequence, with energy derived from thermonuclear fusion of hydrogen to form helium. The resulting solar radiation is steadily increasing as the sun progresses towards becoming a red giant, when it is expected to envelop the inner planets. The newly formed earth heated as a result of the kinetic energy of the accreting masses, radioactive decay and solar radiation. The heat so formed was sufficient to melt the entire earth, including the surface, and the outer core and mantle have remained liquid or semi-solid up to the present. The crust of the earth is currently solid to a mean depth of only a few kilometres beneath the oceans, and tens of kilometres under the continents.

Initially there was probably a tenuous primary atmosphere of hydrogen and helium, which was lost because of the weak gravitational field. However, the primary atmosphere was replaced by a secondary atmosphere formed by thermal and radioactive decomposition of various constituents of the earth with outgassing to the surface, later via volcanoes and fumaroles. This is a process which is widespread in the solar system, and active volcanoes have been observed on Mars and on Io, a satellite of Jupiter. In the case of Earth, loss of water of crystallization has yielded enormous quantities of water vapour, carbonates have been decomposed to give carbon dioxide, and nitrides and ammonium compounds have produced nitrogen and ammonia. Radioactive decay has released hydrogen, helium and argon (the latter from potassium-40). Sulphur compounds have yielded hydrogen sulphide and sulphur dioxide. Analysis of the effluent gases from Hawaiian volcanoes (Table 1.2) has confirmed the likely presence of these gases in the secondary atmosphere.

Important physicochemical changes occurred in the primitive atmosphere. Helium and hydrogen tended to be lost from the earth's gravitational field. Ammonia dissociated to nitrogen and hydrogen, the former retained and the latter lost from the atmosphere. Some carbon dioxide was reduced by hydrogen to methane, but very large quantities reacted with surface silicates to became trapped as carbonates while forming silica. Carbon dioxide has probably remained in the

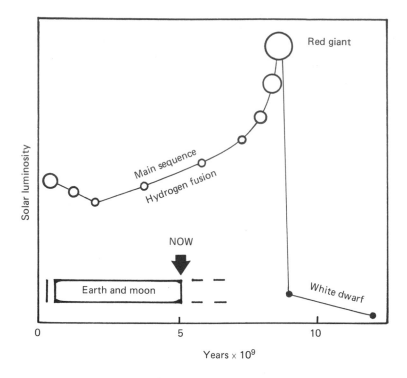

Figure 1.2 Solar luminosity plotted against the age of the sun, the open circles giving a qualitative impression of the diameter of the sun. Superimposed is an indication of the life of the earth and moon, which is now about half way through the main sequence of the sun deriving its energy from hydrogen fusion to helium. The times can only be very approximate. (After Chapman and Morrison, 1989)

Table 1.2 Average composition of gas evolved from Hawaiian volcanoes

Water vapour	70.75%	Carbon monoxide	0.40%
Carbon dioxide	14.07%	Hydrogen	0.33%
Sulphur dioxide	6.40%	Argon	0.18%
Nitrogen	5.45%	Sulphur	0.10%
Sulphur trioxide	1.92%	Chlorine	0.05%

14 samples collected by T.A. Jaggar from Halemaumau lava lake in 1919, and analysed by E.S. Shepherd. Concentrations are expressed as per cent by volume at 1200°C. The earth's secondary reducing atmosphere may have been broadly similar in composition.

atmosphere throughout the life of the earth, and it now forms more than 90% of the atmospheres of Venus and Mars. Immense quantities of water vapour condensed to form surface water when the crust of the earth had cooled sufficiently, but traces underwent photodissociation to hydrogen and oxygen. However, oxygen from this source was present in only minimal quantities and the atmosphere remained reducing for at least the first thousand million years of the life of the earth.

The evolution of life in the secondary reducing atmosphere

The surface of the earth cooled rapidly by radiation, and solidification of the crust of the earth is thought to have occurred some 600 million years after the formation of the earth. Some metamorphic rocks beneath the Greenland ice cap have been dated as early as 3800 million years ago (Cloud, 1988). Further cooling permitted condensation of surface water with the formation of oceans (approx. 1400 million km^3). Rain clouds resulted in recirculation of water, producing rivers, freshwater lakes and lagoons. This produced an environment compatible with the evolution of life, an event of immense complexity about which only speculation is possible. In 1953, Miller published his classic study in which he demonstrated the production of a range of organic compounds from likely components of the secondary reducing atmosphere, by electrical spark discharge, but without the intervention of any living organism. This work, and the many studies which it triggered, have proved beyond reasonable doubt that the constituents of the primitive atmosphere, when dissolved in surface water, could react in the presence of ultraviolet radiation and electrical discharge (both of which were abundant) to produce a wide range of organic compounds including sugars, amino acids, lipids and nucleotides, albeit in racemic mixtures and polymerized in random sequences. Certain meteorites (carbonaceous chondrites) contain organic compounds, which can no longer be considered the exclusive product of living organisms. Encapsulation of organic compounds in lipid membranes has been achieved in the laboratory, and it is now possible to envisage the formation of lifeless 'protocells' as a probable, if not inevitable, consequence of conditions in the earth some 3500–3800 million years ago.

The next stage in the evolution of life is less easy to understand and has not been tested in the laboratory. However, time, space and variety of environment were all available in abundance, and it has been postulated that random sequencing of ribonucleic acid (RNA) eventually produced by chance a template for the formation of an enzyme which conferred some biochemical advantage on a particular 'protocell'. This enabled it to compete effectively with its neighbours, as well as to replicate the RNA. It is conceivable that this process progressed, with a steadily increasing repertoire of useful proteins being encoded by self-replicating RNA, until transmission of the genetic code was eventually taken over by deoxyribonucleic acid (DNA) in organisms with the greatest potential. The problem has always been to understand how useful proteins could be formed without the appropriate sequences in RNA or DNA, and how RNA and DNA could be polymerized without the appropriate enzymes. Nevertheless, life did evolve, and the earliest geological evidence of life is the appearance of stromatolites (microbial deposits), dated to 3400–3500 million years ago in Australia (Walter, Buick and Dunlop, 1980).

The origin of oxygen in the atmosphere

There was only limited potential for the anaerobic life which is presumed to have evolved in the soup of abiogenically preformed organic compounds. The original input of energy into the ecosystem was the conversion of inorganic into organic compounds under the influence of solar ultraviolet radiation and electrical discharge (e.g. from lightning). It is likely that the explosion of living organisms eventually outstripped their energetic basis, and a new energy source was needed. A radical change was initiated approximately 3000–3500 million years ago, when there was the first evidence of the utilization of visible light as an energy source, with production of oxygen by photosynthesis. The essential reaction was as follows:

$$6CO_2 + 6H_2O + \text{energy} = C_6H_{12}O_6 + 6O_2$$

This required the incorporation of chloroplasts into cells, but solar visible light, unlike ultraviolet radiation, could not be filtered off by the formation of oxygen and ozone. Thus the energy supply was firmly guaranteed. The crucial feature of the reaction was the utilization of this new source of energy for biosynthesis, and it seems very likely that oxygen was produced simply as a waste product.

The evidence for this early production of oxygen is strong and can be approximately dated. There are numerous reports of stromatolites in the period 2700–3500 million years ago, and some are likely to be deposits from algae or cyanobacteria capable of photosynthesis. The earliest true fossils of algae are in the gun flint cherts on the north shore of Lake Superior, and are dated to 1900 million years ago (Tyler and Barghoorn, 1954). In the earliest rock, iron was deposited in reduced form, such as the banded iron deposits dated 3800 million years ago (Cloud, 1988). During the last 2600 million years, iron has been deposited in ferric form, as in the 'red beds', and this is taken to indicate an oxidizing environment.

It now seems likely that appreciable quantities of oxygen began to accumulate in the atmosphere about 2200 million years ago. It is impossible to say how quickly its concentration increased, but it is generally assumed to have risen steeply just before the beginning of the overt fossil record in the Cambrian period (570 million years ago). There may well have been a further rise in the Devonian when ultraviolet screening permitted the land to be colonized (see below). There is some evidence that the atmospheric oxygen concentration cannot have changed very much since the beginning of the Carboniferous period (345 million years ago). From that time to the present, there is a continuous record of carbon left by forest fires in sedimentary deposits. Fires would be unlikely to start with an oxygen concentration of less than 18% and would have raged out of control if the concentration exceeded about 25% (Lovelock, 1979).

The consequences of an oxidizing atmosphere

At first, oxygen produced by photosynthesis was absorbed into the ferrous iron beds on the surface of the earth which provided a vast sink for oxygen. Eventually, however, free oxygen accumulated in solution in the surface water and also in the atmosphere which then became oxidizing, a process facilitated by the loss of hydrogen from the earth's gravitational field. It seems likely that anaerobic organisms would have been less than amused by the appearance of molecular oxygen in their environment. Chapter 32 describes the toxicity of oxygen and its derived free radicals, against which primitive anaerobes would probably have had no defences. Three lines of response can be identified. Firstly, some anaerobes without defences against oxygen sought an anaerobic microenvironment in which to remain and survive. Secondly, the vast majority of organisms developed defences in depth against oxygen and its derived free radicals, as described in Chapter 32. Thirdly, the whole of the animal kingdom adopted aerobic metabolism which gave them enormous energetic advantages over organisms relying on anaerobic metabolism as described in Chapter 11. This required the incorporation of mitochondria, but the increased availability of biological energy was essential for the evolution of all forms of life more complex than micro-organisms.

Photosynthesis and aerobic metabolism also established a cycle of energy exchange between plants and animals (Figure 1.3), with an ultimate energy input in the form of solar visible light which could be interrupted only under exceptional circumstances. Such circumstances probably occurred in some of the great extinctions, which marked the end of certain geological eras, the best known being the extinction of the dinosaurs at the end of the Mesozoic era, 65 million years ago. There is good evidence that this resulted from the impact of an asteroid, probably in the Yucatan, causing a persistent world-wide dust cloud, comparable to the postulated 'nuclear winter', and leaving a 1 cm thick, iridium-rich deposit at the cretaceous/tertiary junction throughout the world. The alternative theory is a major volcanic eruption but, whatever the cause, it is thought that the dust cloud cut off solar visible light for many consecutive months. This cooled the earth, stopped photosynthesis, interrupted the food chain and resulted in the extinction of an estimated 40% of marine genera. An even greater extinction occurred at the end of the Palaeozoic era (230 million years ago), with the estimated loss of 75% of marine genera (Chapman and Morrison, 1989).

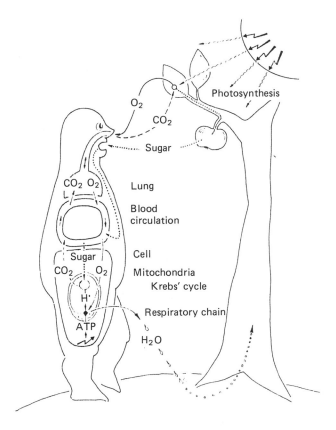

Figure 1.3 The closed circle of oxygen/carbon dioxide exchange between animals and plants. (Reproduced from Weibel (1984) by permission of the author and publishers; © Harvard University Press)

Oxygen and ultraviolet screening

In addition to its toxicity and potential for more efficient metabolism, oxygen had a profound effect on evolution by ultraviolet screening. Oxygen itself absorbs ultraviolet radiation to a certain extent, but ozone (O_3) is far more effective. It is formed in the stratosphere from oxygen which undergoes photodissociation producing free oxygen atoms. The oxygen atoms then rapidly combine with oxygen molecules to form ozone thus:

$$O_2 \rightleftharpoons 2O$$
$$\downarrow$$
$$O + O_2 \rightleftharpoons O_3$$

The absolute quantity is very small, being the equivalent of a layer of pure ozone only a few millimetres thick. A Dobson unit of ozone is defined as the equivalent of a layer of pure ozone 0.01 mm thick. About 10% of the total atmospheric ozone is in the troposphere, mainly as a pollutant. This also acts as an ultraviolet screen and may become relatively more important in the years to come.

Life evolved in water which provided adequate screening from ultraviolet radiation. The first extensive colonization of dry land by plants and animals was in the Devonian period (345–395 million years ago), and it is postulated that this coincided with oxygen and ozone reaching concentrations at which the degree of ultraviolet shielding first permitted organisms to leave the shelter of an aqueous environment.

Ozone is in a state of dynamic equilibrium in the stratosphere and its concentration varies markedly from year to year, in addition to displaying a pronounced annual cycle. Ozone can be removed by the action of many free radicals including chlorine and nitric oxide (Stephenson and Scourfield, 1991). Highly reactive chlorine radicals cannot normally pass through the troposphere to reach the stratosphere, but the situation has recently been disturbed by the widespread manufacture of chlorofluorocarbons (e.g. CF_2Cl_2) for use as propellants and refrigerants. These compounds are highly stable in the troposphere with a half-life of the order of 100 years. This permits their diffusion through the troposphere to reach the stratosphere, where they undergo photodissociation to release chlorine radicals, which then react with ozone as follows:

$$Cl + O_3 \rightarrow ClO + O_2$$
$$\uparrow \qquad\qquad \downarrow$$
$$Cl + O_2 \leftarrow ClO + O$$

Chlorine is recycled and it has been estimated that a single chlorine radical will destroy 10 000 molecules of ozone before it combines with hydrogen to form the relatively harmless hydrochloric acid. The annual changes in stratospheric ozone concentration, and the variation from one year to another, make it extremely difficult to predict future trends. The Antarctic 'hole' in the ozone layer forms in October of each year, when spring sunlight initiates photochemical reactions. From normal levels of 200–400 Dobson units, values fell as low as 121 Dobson units in 1987 and 124 in 1989.

Carbon dioxide and the greenhouse effect

The balance of heat gain from solar radiation is the difference between incoming radiation, mainly in the visible wavelengths, and outgoing radiation which is largely infrared. The latter is partially trapped in the troposphere, mainly by water vapour and carbon dioxide. The chilling effect of a clear starlit night is familiar to all, and there is a clear analogy in a greenhouse. The glass transmits incoming visible light but impedes the loss of infrared radiation from the contents of the greenhouse, which have converted visible light to heat and so emit infrared radiation. It is estimated that the present greenhouse effect raises the mean surface temperature of the earth by some 25°C.

The atmospheric concentration of carbon dioxide is a major determinant of the greenhouse effect and must contribute greatly to the very high surface temperature of Venus (480°C). There is therefore grave concern that excessive burning of fossil fuels may increase atmospheric carbon dioxide concentrations to a level which will result in global warming. Not the least serious consequence would be melting of polar ice which would increase the volume of the oceans by some 2% and cause flooding of low-lying lands. Major changes in sea level have repeatedly occurred in recent geological history, but it is feared the pace of change may now be faster. Long-term studies in Hawaii have shown predictable diurnal and annual variations in atmospheric carbon dioxide concentration amounting to some 7 p.p.m. (parts per million). However, against this background it has been possible to demonstrate a linear increase in mean concentration of 1.42 p.p.m. between 1973 and 1986 (Thoning, Tans and Komhyr, 1989). Against a current mean concentration of 350 p.p.m., this is a precipitous rise in terms of geological history. The burning of fossil fuels contributes some 2% of the total turnover of atmospheric carbon, which is approximately 200×10^9 metric tonnes/year, excluding any formation or decomposition of carbonates. Nevertheless, it is rather larger than the estimated net gain of 3×10^9 metric tonnes/year. These changes in atmospheric carbon dioxide concentration, and any corresponding changes in oxygen concentrations, are several orders of magnitude less than those which might have any direct biological significance for the respiratory system of an aerobic organism.

The relationship between carbon dioxide concentration and world temperature is extremely difficult to evaluate in view of the very wide variations in mean global temperatures and the relatively short time for which accurate records have been kept. A longer time span can be studied by sampling ice cores in which the composition of the gas bubbles give an indication of both temperature and carbon dioxide concentrations. With cores dated back to 150 000 years ago, there is a remarkably good correlation between the estimated temperatures and the concentrations of both carbon dioxide and methane (Lorius et al., 1990). Carbon dioxide concentrations were found to be in the range 200–300 p.p.m. However, it is not entirely certain whether the carbon dioxide governed the temperature or vice versa.

Other greenhouse gases

Methane is present in the atmosphere at a concentration of only 1.7 p.p.m. However, it absorbs infrared some 25 times as effectively as carbon dioxide and therefore makes a small but not insignificant contribution to the greenhouse effect. The chlorofluorocarbons are of special interest. There are no infrared absorption bands for water vapour and carbon dioxide between 7 and 13 μm wavelength, and heat loss in this band is disproportionate. It follows that any gas or vapour, such as the chlorofluorocarbons, with strong infrared absorption in this range will have a disproportionate greenhouse effect. Such a gas could be considered not so much as thickening the panes in the greenhouse as replacing a missing pane. It is therefore not surprising that chlorofluorocarbons have an effect some 10 000 times greater than carbon dioxide. Present atmospheric concentrations are only of the order of 0.003 p.p.m., so their overall effect is barely one-tenth that of carbon dioxide at present. However, with their long half-life, they cannot be ignored.

Evolution and adaptation

This chapter has outlined the environmental conditions under which evolution has proceeded to the present, with special reference to the atmosphere. As in the past, nothing is permanent and we can expect a continuation of the interaction between organisms and their environment. What is new is that one species now has the power to change the environment in a way which will affect all organisms.

Chapter 2

Functional anatomy of the respiratory tract

A clear understanding of structure is a sure foundation on which to base a study of function. This chapter is not a comprehensive account of the structure of the respiratory tract but concentrates on those aspects which are most relevant to an understanding of function. The respiratory muscles are considered in Chapter 6.

Mouth, nose and pharynx

Breathing is normally possible through either nose or mouth, the two alternative air passages converging in the oropharynx. Nasal breathing is the norm and has two major advantages over mouth breathing. Firstly, particulate matter is filtered by the vibrissae hairs. Secondly, humidification of inspired gas by the nose is highly efficient, because the nasal septum and turbinates greatly increase the surface area of mucosa available for evaporation. However, the nose may offer more resistance to air flow than the mouth, particularly when obstructed by polyps, adenoids or congestion of the venous sinuses. Nasal resistance may make oral breathing obligatory and many children and adults breathe only or partly through their mouths at rest (Rodenstein and Stanescu, 1986). With increasing levels of exercise, the respiratory minute volume eventually reaches a level at which the oral airway is brought into play. This normally occurs above a minute volume of about 35 l/min.

Deflection of gas into either the nasal or the oral route is under voluntary control and accomplished with the soft palate, tongue and lips. These functions are best considered in relation to a paramedian sagittal section (Figure 2.1). Part (a) shows the normal position for nose breathing, with the mouth closed by occlusion of the lips, and the tongue lying against the hard palate. The soft palate is clear of the posterior pharyngeal wall. At least in the supine position, this cannot be explained by gravity and it requires tonic action of certain muscles, probably palatoglossus, palatopharyngeus and tensor palati. Electrical activity has been demonstrated in tensor palati during normal inspiration (Hairston and Sauerland, 1981).

Part (b) shows forced mouth breathing, as for instance when blowing through the mouth, without pinching the nose. The soft palate is arched upwards and backwards by contraction of tensor palati and lies against a band of the superior constrictor of the pharynx known as Passavant's ridge which, together with the soft palate, forms the palatopharyngeal sphincter (Passavant, 1869; Whillis, 1930). These fibres of the superior constrictor are hypertrophied in cases of cleft palate.

13

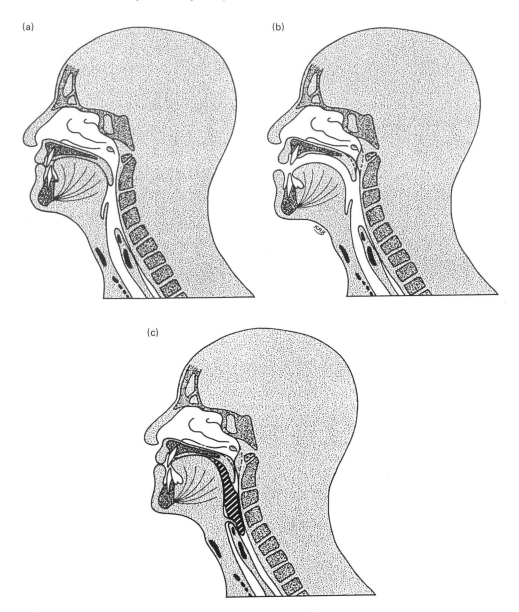

Figure 2.1 Median sagittal section of the pharynx showing: (a) normal nasal breathing with the oral airway occluded by the lips and tongue; (b) deliberate oral breathing with the nasal airway occluded by the palatopharyngeal sphincter; and (c) swallowing with occlusion of larynx and nasopharynx. Note down-folding of the epiglottis.

Note also that the orifice of the pharyngotympanic (eustachian) tube lies above the palatopharyngeal sphincter and the tubes can be inflated by the subject himself only when the nose is pinched. As the mouth pressure is raised, this tends to force the soft palate against the posterior pharyngeal to act as a valve. The combined palatopharyngeal sphincter and valvular action of the soft palate is very strong and can easily withstand mouth pressures in excess of 10 kPa (100 cmH₂O). Figure 2.2 shows the cross-sectional configuration of the upper airway during quiet breathing through the mouth (G.B. Drummond, 1991, personal communication).

Part (c) shows the occlusion of the respiratory tract during the second, involuntary, stage of swallowing, when the bolus is just passing over the back of the tongue. The nasopharynx is occluded by contraction of both tensor and levator palati. The larynx is elevated 2–3 cm by contraction of the infrahyoid muscles, stylopharyngeus and palatopharyngeus, coming to lie under the epiglottis. In addition, the aryepiglottic folds are approximated causing total occlusion of the entrance to the larynx (Fink and Demarest, 1978). This extremely effective protection of the larynx is capable of withstanding pharyngeal pressures as high as 80 kPa (600 mmHg) which may be generated during swallowing.

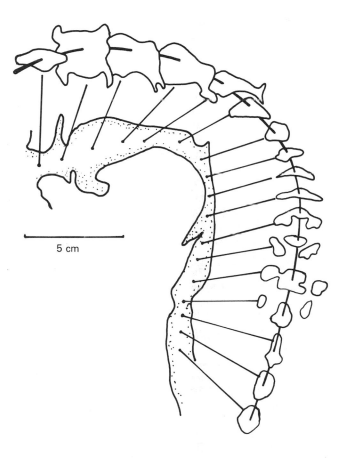

5 cm

Figure 2.2 Cross-sections of the oral, pharyngeal, laryngeal and tracheal airway, related to a median sagittal section (compare with Figure 2.1b. Sections were obtained by magnetic resonance imaging and kindly supplied by Dr G.B. Drummond and Dr I. Marshall.

Patency of the pharyngeal airway

The effect of downstream pressure and pharyngeal compliance. During inspiration through the nose, the pressure in the pharynx must fall below atmospheric by an amount equal to the product of inspiratory gas flow rate and the flow resistance afforded by the nose (see Figure 4.1). This inevitable development of a sub-atmospheric downstream pressure in the pharynx tends to pull the tongue backwards and cause the pharynx to collapse, which requires only a few kilo-pascals. There is more danger of pharyngeal collapse when pharyngeal compliance is high. Large fat deposits around the pharynx increase compliance and so favour collapse and pharyngeal airway obstruction (Horner et al., 1989a).

Pharyngeal dilator muscles. Pharyngeal obstruction in response to subatmospheric downstream pressure during inspiration is opposed by reflex contraction of pharyngeal dilator muscles, of which the best known is genioglossus. The afferent side of the reflex arises from mechanoreceptors in the pharynx and larynx, which respond in a graded manner to subatmospheric pressure. This mechanism is blocked by topical anaesthesia of the pharynx (Horner et al., 1991), and upper airway obstruction occurs more frequently during sleep after selective topical oropharyngeal anaesthesia (McNicholas et al., 1987). The mechanism is extremely efficient. Airway diameters are well maintained down to pressures 1.5 kPa (15 cmH_2O) below atmospheric, during active but not passive breathing manoeuvres (Wheatley et al., 1991). Anteroposterior diameters of the pharynx are not significantly different during inspiration and expiration, even with loaded breathing (Nunn, Charlesworth, Lumb, Taylor and Nandi, 1992, unpublished observations). There are no significant changes with posture in the normal subject (Yildrim et al., 1991). Cross-sectional areas may now be measured by acoustic reflectometry (Marshall, Rogers and Drummond, 1991).

Genioglossus is the easiest pharyngeal dilator muscle to study and both tonic and phasic inspiratory electromyographic (EMG) activity have been demonstrated in man (Remmers et al., 1978; Sauerland et al., 1981). In the rabbit, electrical activity of the genioglossus has been related to the pharyngeal pressure (Mathew, Abu-Osba and Thach, 1982a, b), each 0.1 kPa (1 cmH_2O) below atmospheric pressure causing 100% increase in activity. EMG activity is increased in the supine position, presumably to counteract the effect of gravity on the tongue (Douglas et al., 1992). In goats, genioglossal EMG is activated by hypoxia (saturation less than 80%) (Parisi, Santiago and Edelman, 1988). There is normally phasic inspiratory activity in geniohyoid (Wiegand, Zwillich and White, 1989), which also brings the tongue forward.

Anatomical considerations suggest that patency of the nasopharynx is maintained by tensor palati, palatoglossus and palatopharyngeus. Tonic but not phasic respiratory activity has been detected in levator palati (Tangel, Mezzanotte and White, 1991). The soft palate tends to fall back against the posterior pharyngeal wall in the supine position without contraction of these muscles.

Pharyngeal obstruction is clearly multifactorial (Horner and Guz, 1991). Failure of the various mechanisms to preserve the pharyngeal airway may occur in sleep or anaesthesia, and their occurrence and prevention are discussed in Chapters 14 and 20.

The larynx
(for detailed description see Fink and Demarest, 1978)

The larynx evolved in the lungfish at an early date for the protection of the airway during such activities as feeding and perfusion of the gills with water. While protection of the airway remains its most important function, the larynx has developed further as the organ of speech, and its ability to lock the thorax has given greatly increased power to the muscles of the upper limbs. In addition, as the narrowest part of the airway, it provides a choke for fine control of airway resistance. During quiet breathing, this resistance is governed by movement of the vocal cords and is greater during expiration than inspiration. Phasic expiratory electrical activity is normally present in the thyroarytenoid muscles (Kuna, Insalco and Woodson, 1988). This may help to prevent collapse of the lower airways (page 77).

The larynx may be occluded at various levels. The aryepiglottic muscles and their continuation, the oblique and transverse arytenoids, act as a powerful sphincter cabable of closing the inlet of the larynx, by bringing the aryepiglottic folds together and pulling the epiglottis backwards and downwards towards the arytenoid cartileges. This action is opposed by the thyroepiglottic muscles. The vocal processes of the arytenoid cartileges form the posterior attachments of the vocal cords, and are approximated by inward rotation of the arytenoid cartileges. This is achieved mainly by the contraction of the lateral cricoarytenoid muscles and opposed by the posterior cricoarytenoid muscles. The latter show respiratory phasic activity during inspiration (Brancatisano, Dodd and Engel, 1984) and this accords with the phasic change in laryngeal resistance mentioned in the previous paragraph. The cricothyroid muscles tilt the cricoid and arytenoid cartilages backwards and also move them posteriorly in relation to the thyroid cartilage. This produces elongation and therefore tensioning of the vocal cords. This action is opposed by the thyroarytenoid muscles which draw the arytenoid cartilages forwards towards the thyroid and so shorten and relax the vocal cords. They also rotate the arytenoids medially (acting with the lateral cricoarytenoids) approximating the vocal cords. The deeper fibres of the thyroarytenoids comprise the vocales muscles which exert fine control over pitch of the voice. All the laryngeal muscles are supplied by the recurrent laryngeal nerves except for the cricothyroid which is supplied by the external laryngeal nerves.

Occlusion of the larynx is achieved in various degrees ranging from whispering to swallowing. Speech requires approximation of the vocal cords by contraction of the lateral cricoarytenoids, with tensioning of the folds by the cricothyroid muscles, opposed by the thyroarytenoids. Tighter occlusion of the larynx, known as effort closure, is required for making expulsive efforts. It is also needed to lock the thoracic cage and so to secure the origin of the muscles of the upper arm arising from the rib cage, thus increasing the power which can be transmitted to the arm. Effort closure is also a part of the mechanism involved in the protection of the larynx during swallowing. In addition to simple apposition of the vocal folds and arytenoid cartilages as described above, effort closure involves apposition of the cuneiform cartilages and vestibular folds. The next stage involves approximation of the thyroid cartilage and hyoid bone, with infolding of the aryepiglottic folds and apposition of the median thyrohyoid fold to the lower part of the abducted vestibular folds (Fink and Demarest, 1978). The full process enables the larynx to withstand the highest pressures which can be generated in the thorax, usually at least 12 kPa (120 cmH$_2$O) and often more (Bartlett, 1989). Sudden release of the obstruction is essential for effective coughing, when the linear velocity of air through the larynx is said to approach the speed of sound.

The most important sensory innervation of the larynx is from the internal branch of the superior laryngeal nerve which supplies the area above the vocal cords. The recurrent laryngeal nerve supplies the area below the cords. The larynx is well supplied with mechano- and chemoreceptors. The normal response is laryngeal spasm which may be intense and life-threatening. The larynx is particularly sensitive to water though not to isotonic saline (Bartlett, 1989).

The tracheobronchial tree

Classic accounts of the structure of the lung have been presented by Miller (1947) and von Hayek (1960). The most useful approach to understanding the tracheo-bronchial tree is that of Weibel (1963, 1991a) who numbered successive generations of air passages from the trachea (generation 0) down to alveolar sacs (generation 23). Table 2.1 traces their essential characteristics progressively down the respiratory tract. As a rough approximation it may be assumed that the number of passages in each generation is double that in the previous generation, and the number of air passages in each generation is approximately indicated by the number 2 raised to the power of the generation number. This formula indicates one trachea, two main bronchi, four lobar bronchi, sixteen segmental bronchi, etc.

Trachea (generation 0)

The trachea has a mean diameter of 1.8 cm and length of 11 cm. It is supported by U-shaped cartilages which are joined posteriorly by smooth muscle bands. The part of the trachea in the neck is not subjected to intrathoracic pressure changes, but it is very vulnerable to pressures arising in the neck due, for example, to haematoma formation after thyroidectomy. An external pressure of the order of 4 kPa (40 cmH$_2$O) is sufficient to occlude the trachea. Within the chest, the trachea can be compressed by raised intrathoracic pressure during, for example, a cough, when the decreased diameter increases the linear velocity of gas flow and therefore the efficiency of removal of secretions.

The mucosa is columnar ciliated epithelium containing numerous mucus-secreting goblet cells. The cilia beat in a co-ordinated manner, causing an upward stream of mucus and foreign bodies. Cilial beat is rendered ineffective by clinical concentrations of anaesthetics (Nunn et al., 1974) and also by drying which is prone to occur when patients breathe dry gas through a tracheostomy.

Main, lobar and segmental bronchi (generations 1–4)

The trachea bifurcates asymmetrically, with the right bronchus being wider and making a smaller angle with the long axis of the trachea. Foreign bodies therefore tend to enter the right bronchus in preference to the left. Main, lobar and segmental bronchi have firm cartilaginous support in their walls, U-shaped in the main bronchi, but in the form of irregularly shaped and helical plates lower down. Where the cartilage is in the form of irregular plates, the bronchial muscle takes the

Table 2.1 Structural characteristics of the air passages

	Generation (mean)	Number	Mean diameter (mm)	Area supplied	Cartilage	Muscle	Nutrition	Emplacement	Epithelium
Trachea	0	1	18	Both lungs	U-shaped	Links open end of cartilage			
Main bronchi	1	2	13	Individual lungs					
Lobar bronchi	2 → 3	4 → 8	7 → 5	Lobes	Irregular shaped and helical plates	Helical bands	From the bronchial circulation	Within connective tissue sheath alongside arterial vessels	Columnar cilated
Segmental bronchi	4	16	4	Segments					
Small bronchi	5 → 11	32 → 2 000	3 → 1	Secondary lobules					
Bronchioles Terminal bronchioles	12 → 16	4 000 → 65 000	1 → 0.5			Strong helical muscle bands		Embedded directly in the lung parenchyma	Cuboidal
Respiratory bronchioles	17 → 19	130 000 → 500 000	0.4	Primary lobules	Absent	Muscle bands between alveoli	From the pulmonary circulation		Cuboidal to flat between the alveoli
Alveolar ducts	20 → 22	1 000 000 → 4 000 000	0.3	Alveoli		Thin bands in alveolar septa		Form the lung parenchyma	Alveolar epithelium
Alveolar sacs	23	8 000 000	0.3						

(After Weibel, 1963)

form of helical bands which form a geodesic network. The bronchial epithelium is similar to that in the trachea although the height of the cells gradually diminishes in the more peripheral passages until it becomes cuboidal in the bronchioles. Bronchi in this group (down to generation 4) are sufficiently regular to be individually named (Figure 2.3). Total cross-sectional area of the respiratory tract is minimal at the third generation (Figure 2.4).

These bronchi are subjected to the full effect of changes in intrathoracic pressure and will collapse when the intrathoracic pressure exceeds the intraluminar pressure by about 5 kPa (50 cmH$_2$O). This occurs in the larger bronchi during a forced expiration, so limiting peak expiratory flow rate (see Figures 4.8 and 4.9). This occurs at lower flow rates in patients with chronic obstructive airway disease (Macklem, Fraser and Bates, 1963; Macklem and Wilson, 1965).

Small bronchi (generations 5–11)

The small bronchi extend through about seven generations with their diameter progressively falling from 3.5 to 1 mm. Since their number approximately doubles with each generation, the total cross-sectional area increases markedly with each generation to a value (at generation 11) which is about 10 times the total cross-sectional area at the level of the lobar bronchi.

Down to the level of the smallest true bronchi, air passages lie in close proximity to branches of the pulmonary artery in a sheath containing pulmonary lymphatics, which can be distended with oedema fluid giving rise to the characteristic 'cuffing' (Plates 1 and 2). This is responsible for the earliest radiographical changes in pulmonary oedema.

Since these air passages are not directly attached to the lung parenchyma, they are not subject to direct traction and rely for their patency on cartilage within their walls and on the transmural pressure gradient which is normally positive from lumen to intrathoracic space. In the normal subject, this pressure gradient is seldom reversed and, even during a forced expiration, the intraluminar pressure in the small bronchi rapidly rises to more than 80% of the alveolar pressure, which is more than the extramural (intrathoracic) pressure.

Secondary lobule. The area supplied by a small bronchus immediately before the change to a bronchiole is sometimes referred to as a secondary lobule, each of which has a volume of about 2 ml and is defined by connective tissue septa.

Bronchioles (generations 12–16)

An important change occurs at about the eleventh generation where the internal diameter is about 1 mm. Cartilage disappears from the wall below this level and ceases to be a factor in maintaining patency. However, beyond this level the air passages are directly embedded in the lung parenchyma, the elastic recoil of which holds the air passages open like the guy ropes of a tent. Therefore the calibre of the airways below the eleventh generation is mainly influenced by lung volume, since the forces holding their lumina open are stronger at higher lung volumes. The converse of this factor causes airway closure at reduced long volume (see page 79).

In succeeding generations, the number of bronchioles increases far more rapidly than the calibre diminishes (Table 2.1). Therefore the total cross-sectional area

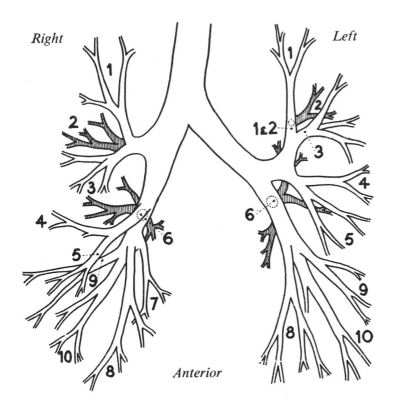

Right

Left

Anterior

UPPER LOBE

1. Apical bronchus
2. Posterior bronchus
3. Anterior bronchus

Right   *Left*

MIDDLE LOBE   LINGULA

4. Lateral bronchus   4. Superior bronchus
5. Medial bronchus   5. Inferior bronchus

LOWER LOBE

6. Apical bronchus   6. Apical bronchus
7. Medial basal (cardiac)   8. Anterior basal bronchus
8. Anterior basal bronchus
9. Lateral basal bronchus   9. Lateral basal bronchus
10. Posterior basal bronchus   10. Posterior basal bronchus

Figure 2.3 Named branches of the tracheobronchial tree, viewed from the front. (Reproduced by permission of the Editors of Thorax)

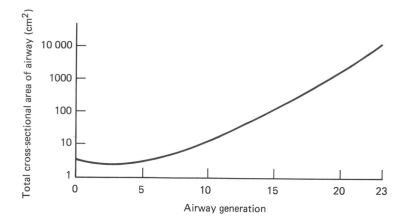

Figure 2.4 The total cross-sectional area of the air passages at different generations of the airways. Note that the minimal cross-sectional area is at generations 3 (lobar to segmental bronchi). The total cross-sectional area becomes very large in the smaller air passages. It approaches a square metre in the alveolar ducts. (Redrawn from data of Weibel, 1964)

increases until, in the terminal bronchioles, it is about 100 times the area at the level of the large bronchi (Figure 2.4). Thus the flow resistance of these smaller air passages (less than 2 mm diameter) is negligible under *normal* conditions (Macklem and Mead, 1967). However, the resistance of the bronchioles can increase to very high values when their strong helical muscular bands are contracted by the mechanisms illustrated in Figure 4.7. This can wrinkle the cuboidal mucosa into longitudinal folds and may result in total airway obstruction.

Down to the terminal bronchiole, the air passages derive their nutrition from the bronchial circulation and are thus influenced by systemic arterial blood gas levels. Beyond this point the smaller air passages rely upon the pulmonary circulation for their nutrition.

Respiratory bronchioles (generations 17–19)

Down to the smallest bronchioles, the functions of the air passages are solely conduction and humidification. Beyond this point there is a gradual transition from conduction to gas exchange. In the three generations of respiratory bronchioles there is a gradual increase in the number of alveoli in their walls (Figure 2.5 and Plate 3). The epithelium is cuboidal between the mouths of the mural alveoli in the earlier generations of respiratory bronchioles but becomes progressively flatter until it is entirely alveolar epithelium in the alveolar ducts. Like the bronchioles, the respiratory bronchioles are embedded in lung parenchyma. However, they have a well marked muscle layer, with bands which loop over the opening of the alveolar ducts and the mouths of the mural alveoli. There is no significant change in calibre of advancing generations of respiratory bronchioles (approx. 0.4 mm diameter), and the total cross-sectional area at this level is of the order of hundreds of square centimetres.

Primary lobule or terminal respiratory unit. This is probably the equivalent of the alveolus when it is considered from the functional standpoint. The primary lobule is

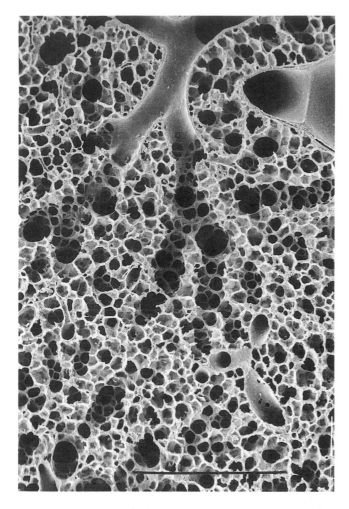

Figure 2.5 Thick section showing three generations of respiratory bronchioles in the plane of the section. The section is from a rabbit and the horizontal bar is 1 mm. Human alveoli would be considerably larger. (Photograph kindly supplied by Professor E. M. Weibel)

usually defined as the zone supplied by a first order respiratory bronchiole. According to this definition, there are about 130 000 primary lobules, each with a diameter of about 3.5 mm and containing about 2000 alveoli (Table 2.2). They probably correspond to the small zones which are seen to pop open when a collapsed lung is inflated at thoracotomy.

Alveolar ducts (generations 20–22)

Alveolar ducts arise from the terminal respiratory bronchiole, from which they differ by having no walls other than the mouths of mural alveoli (about 20 in number). The alveolar septa form a series of rings forming the walls of the alveolar

Table 2.2 Distribution of alveoli in a primary lobule or acinus (syn. terminal respiratory unit)

	Generation (as in Table 2.1)	Number of alveoli per unit (mean)	Number of units per generation (mean)	Number of alveoli per generation (mean)
Respiratory bronchioles:				
1st order	17	5	1	5
2nd order	18	8	2	16
3rd order	19	12	4	48
Alveolar ducts:				
1st order	20	20	8	160
2nd order	21	20	16	320
3rd order	22	20	32	640
Alveolar sacs	23	17	64	1088
Total number of alveoli in primary lobule				2277

Diameter of primary lobule at FRC, 3.5 mm; volume of primary lobule at FRC, 23 μl; number of primary lobules in average lung, 130 000; total number of alveoli in average lung, 300 000 000; diameter of alveolus at FRC, 0.2 mm.
(After Weibel, 1963)

ducts and containing smooth muscle. About half of the alveoli arise from ducts, and some 35 per cent of the alveolar gas resides in the alveolar ducts and the alveoli which arise directly from them.

Alveolar sacs (generation 23)

The last generation of the air passages differ from alveolar ducts solely in the fact that they are blind. About 17 alveoli arise from each alveolar sac and account for about half of the total number of alveoli (Table 2.2).

The alveoli

Number and size. The mean total number of alveoli is usually given as 300 million but ranges from about 200 million to 600 million, correlating with the height of the subject (Angus and Thurlbeck, 1972). The size of the alveoli is proportional to lung volume but they are larger in the upper part of the lung except at maximal inflation when the vertical gradient in size disappears (Glazier et al., 1967). The vertical gradient is dependent on gravity and presumably disappears under conditions of zero gravity in space. The reduction in size of alveoli and the corresponding reduction in calibre of the smaller airways in the dependent parts of the lung have most important implications in gas exchange which are considered later (pages 79, 157, 165). At functional residual capacity the mean diameter is 0.2 mm, astonishingly close to the estimate of 1/100 inch (0.25 mm) made by the Reverend Stephen Hales in 1731.

The alveolar septa

The septa are under tension generated partly by elastic fibres, but more by surface tension at the air/fluid interface (page 37). They are therefore generally flat (Figure 2.6), making the alveoli polyhedral rather than spherical. The septa are perforated by small fenestrations known as the pores of Kohn (Figures 2.6 and 2.7, and Plate 4). These pores provide collateral ventilation which can be demonstrated between air spaces supplied by fairly large bronchi (Liebow, 1962). Direct communications have also been found between small bronchioles and neighbouring alveoli (Lambert, 1955).

The interstitial space is asymmetrically disposed in relation to the capillaries (Figures 2.6 and 2.8). On one side the capillary endothelium and the alveolar epithelium are closely apposed and the total thickness from gas to blood is about 0.3 μm (Figure 2.9). This may be considered the 'active' side of the capillary and gas exchange must be more efficient on this side. The other side of the capillary, which may be considered the 'service' side, is usually more than 1–2 μm thick and contains elastin and collagen fibres, nerve endings and occasional migrant poly-

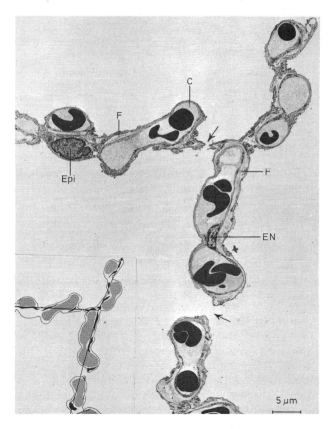

Figure 2.6 Electron micrograph of the junction of three alveolar septa of inflated lung of dog, showing the form of the continuous network of collagen fibrils, into which the capillary network is interwoven. C, capillary; EN, endothelial nucleus: Epi, epithelial nucleus (type I); F, collagen fibrils; arrows point to pores of Kohn. (Reproduced from Weibel (1973) by permission of the author and the Editors of Physiological Reviews)

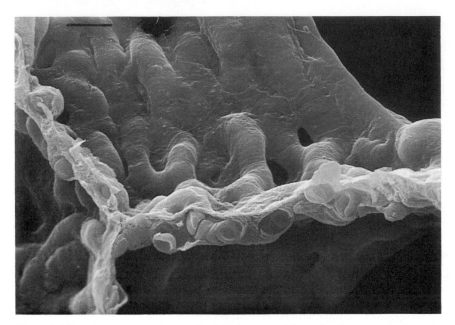

Figure 2.7 Scanning electron micrograph of the junction of three alveolar septa which are shown in both surface view and section. Two pores of Kohn are seen to the right of centre. Erythrocytes are seen in the cut ends of the capillaries. The scale bar (top left) is 10 μm. (Reproduced from Weibel (1984) by permission of the author and the publishers; © Harvard University Press)

morphs and macrophages. The distinction between the two sides of the capillary has considerable physiological significance. The active side tends to be spared in the accumulation of both oedema fluid (Figure 2.10 and page 485) and fibrous tissue in fibrosing alveolitis or Hamman–Rich syndrome (page 208).

The fibre scaffold. The alveolar septum contains a network of fibre which forms a continuum between the peripheral fibres and the axial spiral fibres of the bronchioles (Weibel and Bachofen, 1991). The septal fibre is in the form of a network, through which are threaded the pulmonary capillaries, which are themselves a network. Thus the capillaries pass repeatedly from one side of the fibre scaffold to the other (see Figures 2.6 and 2.7). The fibre lies on the thick (or 'service') side of the capillary, while the other is free to bulge into the lumen of the capillary. The left side of the capillary in Figure 2.8 is the side with the fibres.

At the cellular level, the scaffolding for the endothelial and epithelial cells is provided by the basement membrane (Crouch, Martin and Brody, 1991). This comprises collagen IV, laminin, heparan sulphate proteoglycan and entactin/ nidogen. Collagen provides a diamond-shaped matrix of great strength relative to its bulk. The other constituents are concerned with cell attachment and regulate the permeability to proteins. These aspects of the function of the basement membrane are important. It has been shown that increase in the capillary transmural pressure gradient above about 3 kPa (30 cmH$_2$O) may cause disruption of endothelium and/or epithelium, while the basement membrane tends to remain intact, sometimes as the only remaining separation between blood and gas (Tsukimoto et al., 1991).

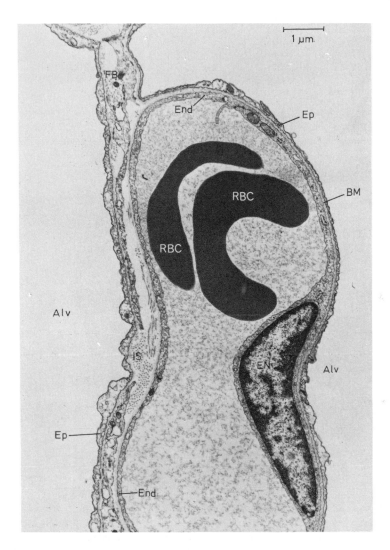

Figure 2.8 Details of the interstitial space, the capillary endothelium and alveolar epithelium. Note that the thickening of the interstitial space is confined to the left of the capillary) (the 'service side') while the total alveolar/capillary membrane remains thin on the right (the 'active side') except where it is thickened by the endothelial nucleus. Alv, alveolus; BM, basement membrane; EN, endothelial nucleus; End, endothelium; Ep, epithelium; IS, interstitial space; RBC, erythrocyte; FB, fibroblast process. (Electron micrograph kindly supplied by Professor E.R. Weibel)

Special cell types

A number of structurally distinct cells may be identified as follows (see general reviews by Ryan, 1982; Gail and Lenfant, 1983; Weibel, 1984, 1985).

Capillary endothelial cells (see review by Simionescu, 1991). These cells are continuous with the endothelium of the general circulation and, in the pulmonary

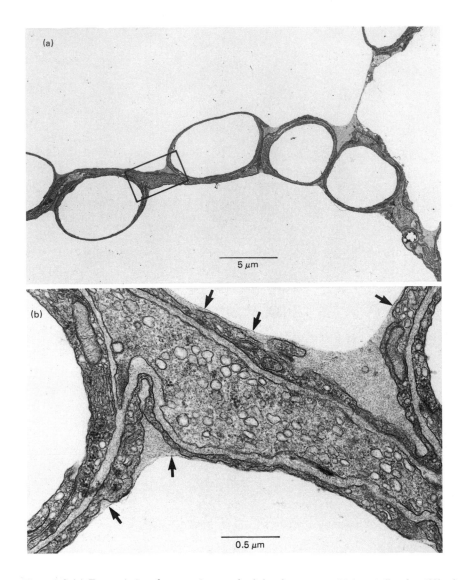

Figure 2.9 (a) Transmission electron micrograph of alveolar septum with lung inflated to 40% of total lung capacity (compare with Figure 2.6). The section in the box is enlarged in (b) to show alveolar lining fluid, which has pooled in two concavities of the alveolar epithelium and has also spanned the pore of Kohn in (a). There is a thin film of osmophilic material (arrows), probably surfactant, at the interface between air and the alveolar lining fluid. (Reproduced from Gil et al. (1979) by permission of the authors and the Editors of Journal of Applied Physiology)

capillary bed, have a thickness of only 0.1 μm except where expanded to contain nuclei (see Figures 2.6 and 2.8). Scanning electron microscopy shows the surface to be covered with projections resembling coral (Ryan, 1982). Transmission electron microscopy shows the flat parts of the cytoplasm to be devoid of all organelles except for small vacuoles (caveolae or plasmalemmal vesicles) which may open

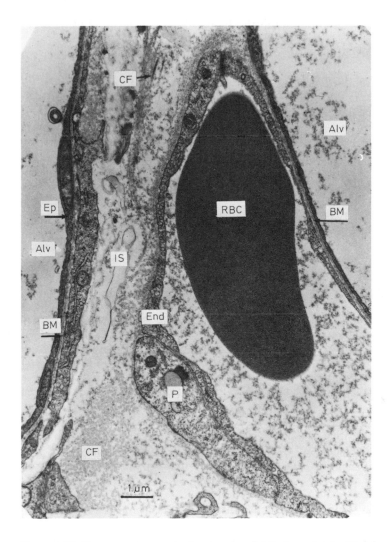

Figure 2.10 Electron micrograph showing the distribution of interstitial haemodynamic pulmonary oedema. Note that the interstitial space on the 'service side' of the pulmonary capillary has been considerably thickened by oedema fluid while the 'active side' remains unchanged in thickness. Alv, alveolus; BM, basement membrane; CF, collagen fibres; End, endothelium; Ep, epithelium; IS, interstitial space; P, pericyte; RBC, red blood corpuscle. (Reproduced from Fishman (1972) by permission of the author and the American Heart Association)

onto the basement membrane or the lumen of the capillary or be entirely contained within the cytoplasm (see Figure 2.9). It is not clear whether they are engaged in pinocytosis or whether they are static. The lining of the caveolae acts as an extension of the cell membrane beyond its already vast size of about 126 m^2 (Weibel, 1983). Surface enzymes are located on the lining of the caveolae as well as on membrane lining the capillaries (Ryan, 1982). The pulmonary capillary endothelium has a metabolic activity approaching that of the liver (Chapter 12). The total volume of capillary endothelium in the human lung is estimated to be 49 ml (Weibel, 1984).

The endothelial cells abut against one another at fairly loose junctions which are of the order of 5 nm wide (DeFouw, 1983). These junctions permit the passage of quite large molecules, and the pulmonary lymph contains albumin at about half the concentration in plasma (Rippe and Crone, 1991). Macrophages pass freely through these junctions under normal conditions, and polymorphs can also pass in response to chemotaxis.

Endothelial cells can be grown in culture, but it is only possible to harvest cells derived from larger vessels and not from the pulmonary capillaries. Nevertheless, cultures of cells derived from the larger blood vessels possess most of the metabolic activities known to be present in the pulmonary microcirculation (Ryan, 1982).

Alveolar epithelial cells – type I. These cells line the alveoli and also exist as a thin sheet approximately 0.1 μm in thickness, except where expanded to contain nuclei (see Figures 2.6 and 2.8). Like the endothelium, the flat part of the cytoplasm is devoid of organelles except for small vacuoles.

Epithelial cells cover several alveoli as a continuous sheet and meet at tight junctions with a gap of only about 1 nm (DeFouw, 1983). These junctions may be seen as narrow lines snaking across the septa in Figure 2.7. The tightness of these junctions is crucial for prevention of the escape of large molecules, such as albumin, into the alveoli, thus preserving the oncotic pressure gradient essential for the avoidance of pulmonary oedema (see page 487). Nevertheless, these junctions permit the free passage of macrophages. Polymorphs may also pass in response to a chemotactic stimulus. Figure 2.9 shows the type I cell covered with a film of alveolar lining fluid although it has been proposed that the surface is normally dry (Hills, 1982).

The total volume in the human lung is estimated to be 23 ml (Weibel, 1984). They are particularly sensitive to damage from high concentrations of oxygen (page 552). Type I cells are end cells and do not divide *in vivo*. However, they have been co-cultured *in vitro* with type II cells on a matrix secreted by the latter (see review by Schneeberger, 1991).

Alveolar epithelial cells – type II. These are the stem cells from which type I cells arise. They do not function as gas exchange membranes, and are rounded in shape and situated at the junction of septa. They have large nuclei and microvilli (Figure 2.11). The cytoplasm contains characteristic striated osmiophilic organelles which contain stored surfactant (Mason and Williams, 1991). Type II cells are easily grown in culture and tend to proliferate in lung explant tissue cultures. They are resistant to oxygen toxicity, tending to replace type I cells after prolonged exposure to high concentrations of oxygen (page 552).

Alveolar brush cells – type III. Brush cells are seen only rarely and their function is not established. It is possible that they may have a receptor function but neuronal connections have not been demonstrated.

Alveolar macrophages. The lung is richly endowed with these phagocytes which pass freely from the circulation, through the interstitial space and thence through the gaps between alveolar epithelial cells to lie on their surface within the alveolar lining fluid (Figure 2.12). They can re-enter the body but are remarkable for their

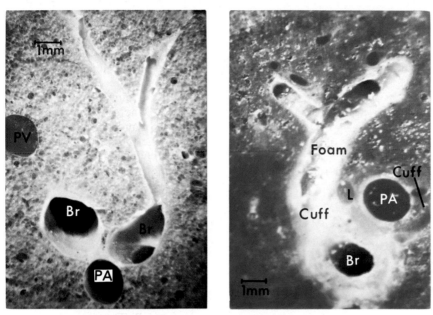

Plate 1   Plate 2

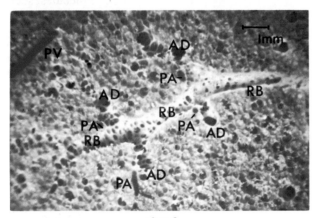

Plate 3

Plate 1. Branchings of cartilaginous bronchi (BR), together with associated pulmonary artery (PA). The corresponding pulmonary vein (PV) is separate. Rapidly frozen normal cat lung showing natural colours. (Photograph by courtesy of Dr N. A. Staub)

Plate 2. Severe pulmonary oedema in freshly frozen dog lung. The bronchi (BR) contain oedema fluid foam and are surrounded by free fluid cuffs. The pulmonary artery and its branches (PA) are also surrounded by cuffs. Note the presence of a distended lymph vessel (L). Lung parenchyma in the background is severely waterlogged. (Reproduced from Staub (1963b) by courtesy of the author and the Editor of Anesthesiology)

Plate 3. Branchings of respiratory bronchioles (RB) showing transition to alveolar ducts (AD). Each airway branch is accompanied by its associated branch of the pulmonary artery (PA). The pulmonary vein (PV) lies separate. Fresh frozen cat lung. (Photograph by courtesy of Dr N. A. Staub)

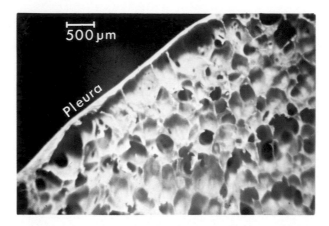

Plate 4

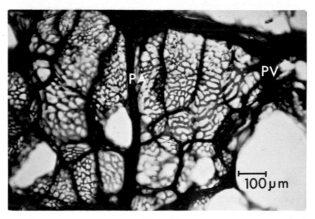

Plate 5

Plate 4. *Fresh frozen human lung showing size and shape of alveoli close to the pleura. Note numerous fenestrations between adjacent alveoli. (Photograph by courtesy of Dr N. A. Staub)*

Plate 5. *Maximally congested pulmonary capillary network in alveolar septum of fresh frozen dog lung. Average length of capillaries from pulmonary artery (PA) to pulmonary vein (PV) is 600–800 μm and crosses several adjacent alveoli. Note capillaries leaving and entering larger blood vessels at right angles. (Photograph by courtesy of Dr N. A. Staub)*

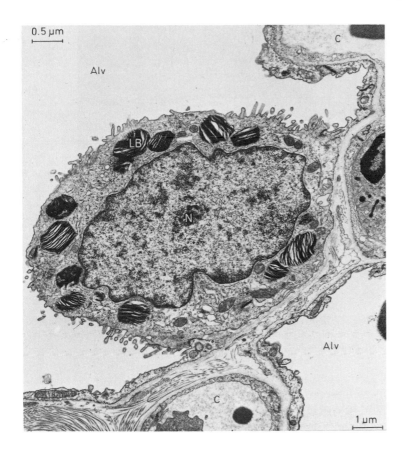

0.5 µm

Alv

C

LB

N

Alv

C

1 µm

Figure 2.11 Electron micrograph of an alveolar epithelial cell of type II of dog. Note the large nucleus, the microvilli and the osmiophilic lamellar bodies thought to release the surfactant. Alv, alveolus; C, capillary; LB, lamellar bodies; N, nucleus. (Reproduced from Weibel (1973) by permission of the author and the Editors of Physiological Reviews)

ability to live and function outside the body. The macrophages are active in combating infection and scavenging foreign bodies such as dust particles. They contain a variety of destructive enzymes but are also capable of generating oxygen-derived free radicals (page 548). These are highly effective bactericidal agents but the processes used may also rebound to damage the host. Dead macrophages may release the enzyme trypsin which may cause tissue damage in patients who are deficient in the protein α_1-antitrypsin (page 308).

Neutrophils. These cells are not normally present within the alveoli but may appear in response to a neutrophil chemotactic factor released from the alveolar macrophages. They are usually present in the alveoli of smokers (page 382).

Mast cells. In common with other organs, the lungs contain numerous mast cells which are located in the alveolar septa and also below the mucosa of the airways.

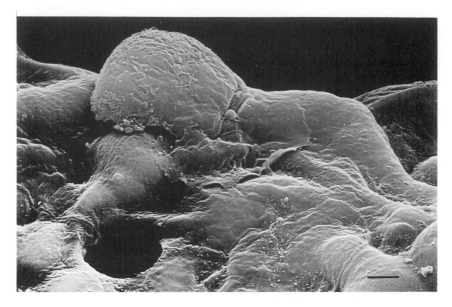

Figure 2.12 Scanning electron micrograph of an alveolar macrophage advancing to the right over epithelial type I cells, preceded by its lamella. The scale bar is 3 μm. (Reproduced from Weibel (1984) by permission of the author and the publishers; © Harvard University Press)

Some also lie free in the lumen of the airways and may be recovered by bronchial lavage. Their important role in bronchoconstriction is described on pages 73 et seq. seq.

Non-ciliated bronchiolar epithelial (Clara) cells. These cells are found in the mucosa of the terminal bronchioles. They are metabolically active and secrete at least three proteins including antiproteases and a surfactant apoprotein (Plopper, Hyde and Buckpitt, 1991). It is unlikely that they secrete surfactant as was once believed.

APUD cells. These cells occur in bronchial epithelium and, from morphological considerations, are believed to be a part of the APUD series, so named because of their ability to undertake amine and amine-precursor uptake and decarboxylation. APUD cells elsewhere are known to produce a range of hormones including ACTH, insulin, calcitonin and gastrin.

The pleura
(see review by Sahn, 1988)

The pleural space is 10–20 μm wide and lined with mesothelium of the parietal and visceral pleurae. The mesothelium comprises a single layer of cells which may be flattened, cuboidal or columnar, thickness varying from 1 to 4 μm. The surface is covered with microvilli. The parietal pleura has stomata (2–12 μm diameter) which communicate directly with lymphatics. Below the visceral pleura there are lymphatic collecting vessels which communicate with the hilum by lymphatics running along the boundaries between segments and lobes.

The pleural fluid is estimated indirectly to be of the order of 10 ml, and has a protein content of about 1.5 g/dl. It contains some 1500 cells/µl, which are mainly monocytes. Pleural fluid arises mainly from the pulmonary circulation and the microvascular endothelium is the main barrier to transudation. Factors governing its formation and the development of a pleural effusion are generally similar to the factors in the Starling equation which governs the formation of pulmonary extracellular fluid and the development of pulmonary oedema (page 487). However, there are two additional factors which do not apply to pulmonary oedema. A pleural effusion may result from translocation of ascitic fluid through lymphatics and diaphragmatic defects. In addition a pleural effusion may result from a reduced pleural pressure caused, for example, by pulmonary collapse.

The pulmonary vasculature

Pulmonary arteries

Although the pulmonary circulation carries roughly the same flow as the systemic circulation, the arterial pressure and the vascular resistance are normally only one-sixth as great. The media of the pulmonary arteries is about half as thick as in systemic arteries of corresponding size. In the larger vessels it consists mainly of elastic tissue but in the smaller vessels it is mainly muscular, the transition being in vessels of about 1 mm diameter. Pulmonary arteries lie close to the corresponding air passages in connective tissue sheaths. Table 2.3 shows a scheme for considera-

Table 2.3 Dimensions of the branches of the human pulmonary artery

Orders	Number	Mean diameter (mm)	Cumulative volume (ml)
17	1	30	64
16	3	15	81
15	8	8.1	85
14	20	5.8	96
13	66	3.7	108
12	203	2.1	116
11	675	1.3	122
10	2 300	0.85	128
9	5 900	0.53	132
8	18 000	0.35	136
7	53 000	0.22	138
6	160 000	0.14	141
5	470 000	0.086	142
4	1 400 000	0.054	144
3	4 200 000	0.034	145
2	13 000 000	0.021	146
1	300 000 000	0.013	151

Data are from Singhal et al. (1973). In contrast to the airways (Table 2.1), the branching is asymmetrical and not dichotomous. Singhal et al. therefore grouped the vessels according to orders and not generation as in Table 2.1. Pulmonary capillaries arise directly from vessels designated Order 1 (see Plate 5).

tion of the branching of the pulmonary arterial tree (Singhal et al., 1973). This may be compared with Weibel's scheme for the airways (Table 2.1).

Pulmonary arterioles

The transition to arterioles occurs at an internal diameter of 100 μm. These vessels differ radically from their counterparts in the systemic circulation, being virtually devoid of muscular tissue. There is a thin media of elastic tissue separated from the blood by endothelium. Structurally there is no real difference between pulmonary arterioles and venules.

Pulmonary capillaries

Pulmonary capillaries tend to rise abruptly from much larger vessels, the pulmonary metarterioles (Staub, 1963b). The capillaries form a dense network over the walls of one or more alveoli and the spaces between the capillaries are similar in size to the capillaries themselves (Plate 5). In the resting state, about 75% of the capillary bed is filled but the percentage is higher in the dependent parts of the lungs. This gravity-dependent effect is the basis of the vertical gradient of ventilation/perfusion ratios in the lung (page 165). Inflation of the alveoli reduces the cross-sectional area of the capillary bed and increases resistance to blood flow. One capillary network is not confined to one alveolus but passes from one alveolus to another (see Figure 2.7) and blood traverses a number of alveolar septa before reaching a venule. This clearly has a bearing on the efficiency of gas exchange (page 202).

From the functional standpoint it is often more convenient to consider the pulmonary microcirculation rather than just the capillaries. The microcirculation is defined as the vessels which are devoid of a muscular layer and it commences with arterioles of diameter 75 μm and continues through the capillary bed as far as venules of diameter 200 μm. Special roles of the microcirculation are considered in Chapters 12 and 26.

Pulmonary venules and veins

Pulmonary capillary blood is collected into venules which are structurally almost identical to the arterioles. In fact, Duke (1954) obtained satisfactory gas exchange when an isolated cat lung was perfused in reverse. The pulmonary veins do not run alongside the pulmonary arteries but lie some distance away, close to the septa which separate the segments of the lung (see Plate 1).

Bronchial circulation

Down to the terminal bronchioles, the air passages and the accompanying blood vessels receive their nutrition from the bronchial vessels which arise from the systemic circulation. Part of the bronchial circulation returns to the systemic venous system but part mingles with the pulmonary venous drainage, thereby constituting a shunt (pages 137 and 180).

Bronchopulmonary arterial anastomoses

It is well known that in pulmonary arterial stenosis, blood flows through a precapillary anastomosis from the bronchial circulation to reach the pulmonary capillaries. It is less certain whether this can occur in normal lungs (page 137).

Pulmonary arteriovenous anastomoses

It has been established that, when the pulmonary arterial pressure of the dog is raised by massive pulmonary embolization, pulmonary arterial blood is able to reach the pulmonary veins without apparently having traversed a capillary bed (page 181). The nature of this communication and whether it occurs in man are discussed in Chapter 8.

Pulmonary lymphatics
(see review by Staub, 1974)

There are no lymphatics visible in the interalveolar septa, but small lymph vessels commence at the junction between alveolar and extra-alveolar spaces. There is a well developed lymphatic system around the bronchi and pulmonary vessels, capable of containing up to 500 ml, and draining towards the hilum. Down to airway generation 11 the lymphatics lie in a potential space around the air passages and vessels, separating them from the lung parenchyma. This space becomes distended with lymph in pulmonary oedema (see Plate 2) and accounts for the characteristic butterfly shadow of the chest radiograph. In the hilum of the lung, the lymphatic drainage passes through several groups of tracheobronchial lymph glands, where they receive tributaries from the superficial subpleural plexus. Most of the lymph from the left lung usually enters the thoracic duct, where it can be conveniently sampled in the sheep. The right side drains into the right lymphatic duct. However, the pulmonary lymphatics often cross the midline and pass independently into the junction of the internal jugular and subclavian veins on the corresponding sides of the body. Studies in dogs have indicated that approximately 15% of the flow in the thoracic duct derives from the lungs (Meyer and Ottaviano, 1972).

Pulmonary lymphatics are intimately concerned in the pathogenesis of pulmonary oedema (page 487) and in the transport system for inactivated proteases (page 309).

Chapter 3

Elastic forces and lung volumes

The movements of the lungs are entirely passive and respond to forces external to the lungs. In the case of spontaneous breathing the external forces are the respiratory muscles, whilst artificial ventilation is usually in response to a pressure gradient which is developed between the airway and the environment. In each case, the pattern of response by the lung is governed by the physical impedance of the respiratory system. This impedance, or hindrance, falls mainly into two categories:

1. Elastic resistance of tissue and alveolar gas/liquid interface.
2. Frictional resistance to gas flow.

Additional minor sources of impedance are the inertia of gas and tissue and the friction of tissue deformation. Work performed in overcoming frictional resistance is dissipated as heat and lost. Work performed in overcoming elastic resistance is stored as potential energy, and elastic deformation during inspiration is the usual source of energy for expiration during both spontaneous and artificial breathing.

This chapter is concerned with the elastic resistance afforded by lungs and chest wall, which will be considered separately and then together. When the respiratory muscles are totally relaxed, these factors govern the resting end-expiratory lung volume or functional residual capacity (FRC), and therefore lung volumes will be considered later in this chapter.

Elastic recoil of the lungs

The lungs can be considered as an elastic structure, with transmural pressure gradient corresponding to stress, and lung volume corresponding to strain. Over a limited range of lung volume these variables obey Hooke's law, and the change in lung volume per unit change in transmural pressure gradient (the compliance) corresponds to Young's modulus. Elastance is the reciprocal of compliance. Compliance is usually expressed in litres (or millilitres) per kilopascal (or centimetre of water). Stiff lungs have a low compliance. Elastance is expressed in kilopascals (or centimetres of water) per litre. Stiff lungs have a high elastance.

The nature of the forces causing recoil of the lung

For many years it was thought that the recoil of the lung was due entirely to stretching of the yellow elastin fibres present in the lung parenchyma. However, as is so often the case, the workings of the body are far more complex than first impressions suggest. In 1929, von Neergaard showed that a lung completely filled with and immersed in water had an elastance which was much less than the normal value obtained when the lung was filled with air. He correctly concluded that much of the 'elastic recoil' was due to surface tension acting throughout the vast air/water interface lining the alveoli.

Surface tension at an air/water interface produces forces which tend to reduce the area of the interface. Thus the gas pressure within a bubble is always higher than the surrounding gas pressure because the surface of the bubble is in a state of tension. Alveoli resemble bubbles in this respect, although the alveolar gas is connected to the exterior by the air passages. The pressure inside a bubble is higher than the surrounding pressure by an amount depending on the surface tension of the liquid and the radius of curvature of the bubble according to the Laplace equation:

$$P = 2T/R$$

where P is the pressure within the bubble (dyn/cm^2), T is the surface tension of the liquid (dyn/cm) and R is the radius of the bubble (cm).

In coherent SI units (see Appendix A), the appropriate units would be pressure in pascals (Pa), surface tension in newtons/metre (N/m) and radius in metres (m). Note that mN/m is identical to the old dyn/cm.

On the left of Figure 3.la is shown a typical alveolus of radius 0.1 mm. Assuming that the alveolar lining fluid has a normal surface tension of 20 mN/m (or dyn/cm), the pressure within the alveolus will be 0.4 kPa (4 cmH$_2$O), which is rather less than the normal transmural pressure at FRC. If the alveolar lining fluid had the same surface tension as water (72 mN/m), the lungs would be very stiff.

The alveolus on the right of Figure 3.la has a radius of only 0.05 mmHg and the Laplace equation indicates that, if the surface tension of the alveolus is the same, its pressure should be double the pressure in the left-hand alveolus. Thus gas would tend to flow from smaller alveoli into larger alveoli and that lung would be unstable which, of course, is not the case. Similarly, the retractive forces of the alveolar lining fluid would increase at low lung volumes and decrease at high lung volumes, which is exactly the reverse of what is observed.

These paradoxes were clear to von Neergaard in 1929 and he concluded that the surface tension of the alveolar lining fluid must be considerably less than would be expected from the properties of simple liquids and, furthermore, that its value must be variable. Observations on bubbles in lung froth (Pattle, 1955) and later on alveolar extracts (Brown, Johnson and Clements, 1959) have demonstrated that the surface tension of alveolar lining fluid is indeed much lower than water. Furthermore, its value is not constant but changes in proportion to the area of the interface. Figure 3.lb shows an experiment in which a floating bar is moved in a trough containing an alveolar extract. As the bar is moved to the right, the surface film is concentrated and the surface tension changes as shown in the graph on the right of the Figure. During expansion, the surface tension increases to 40 mN/m, a value which is close to that of plasma but, during contraction, the surface tension falls to 19 mN/m, a lower value than any other body fluid. The course of the relationship between pressure and area is different during expansion and contraction, and a loop is described.

The consequences of these changes are very important. In contrast to a bubble of soap solution, the pressure within an alveolus tends to decrease as the radius of

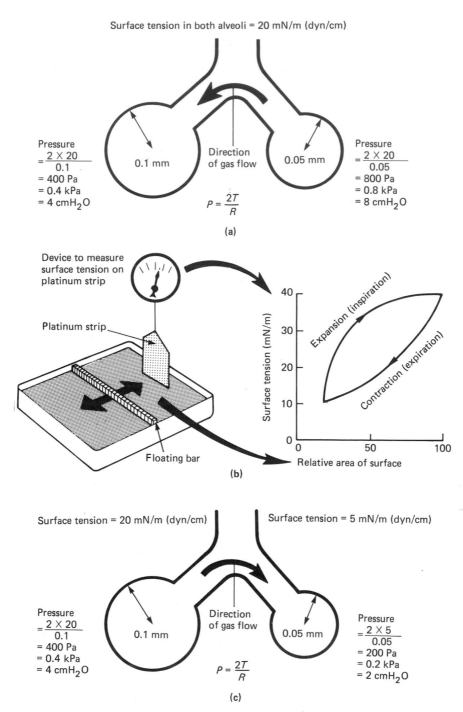

Figure 3.1 Surface tension and alveolar transmural pressure. (a) The pressure relations in two alveoli of different size but with the same surface tension of their lining fluids. (b) The changes in surface tension in relation to the area of the alveolar lining film. (c) The pressure relations of two alveoli of different size when allowance is made for the probable changes in surface tension.

curvature is decreased. This is illustrated in Figure 3.lc where the right-hand alveolus has a smaller diameter and a much lower surface tension than the left-hand alveolus. Gas tends to flow from the larger to the smaller alveolus and stability is maintained. Similarly, the recoil pressure of the lung decreases with decreasing lung volume, thus giving the entirely illusory appearance of being an elastic body obeying Hooke's law.

The alveolar surfactant

The low surface tension of the alveolar lining fluid and its dependence on its area (Figure 3.1 b) are due to the presence of a surface active material. Generally known as the surfactant, it consists of phospholipids which have the general structure shown in Figure 3.2. The fatty acids are hydrophobic and project into the gas phase. The other end of the molecule is hydrophilic and lies within the alveolar lining fluid. The molecule is thus confined to the surface where, being detergents, they lower surface tension in proportion to the concentration at the interface. During expiration, as the area of the alveoli diminishes, the surfactant molecules are packed more densely and so exert a greater effect on the surface tension, which then decreases as shown in Figure 3.1b.

The lung is known to be active in the synthesis of fatty acids, esterification of lipids, hydrolysis of lipid–ester bonds and oxidation of fatty acids (King and Clements, 1985). The main site of release of surfactants is the type II alveolar cell (page 30), and the lamellar bodies (see Figure 2.11) are believed to be stored surfactant.

Composition of surfactant. There is still uncertainty about the precise chemical composition of all constituents of surfactant, which is generally studied in fluid obtained from bronchoalveolar lavage. Some 90% of surfactant consists of lipids, the remainder including several specific proteins and small amounts of carbohydrate (van Golde, Batenburg and Robertson, 1988). Most of the lipid is phospholipid, of which some 70–80% is dipalmitoyl phosphatidyl choline. The remaining phospholipid is mainly phosphatidyl glycerol, which is not found in such concentrations elsewhere in the body. Trace phospholipids include phosphatidyl inositol, phosphatidyl ethanolamine and phosphatidyl serine. The fatty acid chains are mainly saturated and therefore straight. Harlan and Said (1969) advanced the attractive theory that straight fatty acids will pack together in a more satisfactory manner during expiration than would unsaturated fatty acids such as oleic acid which are bent at the double bond. Apart from the phospholipids, cholesterol is the

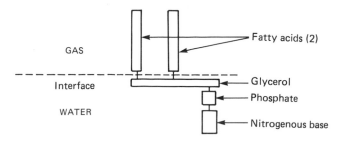

Figure 3.2 General structure of phospholipids.

main neutral lipid present. Proportions in lavage fluid are not necessarily the same as in the lung tissue, but it appears likely that dipalmitoyl phosphatidyl choline is mainly responsible for the effect on surface tension. The role of the other lipids is less certain.

Some 10% of surfactant is protein. Surface activity can occur in the absence of the proteins, but they increase the speed with which the surface film is established and this is very important. Apart from albumin and globulin, presumably leaked from plasma, the active proteins are in the range of molecular weights 26–38 kDa and they tend to associate with the surfactant lipids. In addition there are several proteins of molecular weight about 11 kDa which are strongly hydrophobic.

Surfactant levels increase in the late stages of gestation and are low in babies with the respiratory distress syndrome (RDS) (Avery and Mead, 1959; Pattle et al., 1962). Synthesis of surfactant is considered in Chapter 12, and the use of synthetic surfactant in Chapter 18.

Other effects of surfactant. Pulmonary transudation is also affected by surface forces. Surface tension causes the pressure within the alveolar lining fluid to be less than the alveolar pressure. Since the pulmonary capillary pressure in most of the lung is greater than the alveolar pressure (page 140), both factors encourage transudation, a tendency which is checked by the oncotic pressure of the plasma proteins (page 487). Thus the surfactant, by reducing surface tension, diminishes one component of the pressure gradient and helps to prevent transudation. Thus, a deficiency of surfactant might tip the balance in favour of the development of pulmonary oedema.

Surface forces also influence the rate of alveolar collapse. The disappearance of very small bubbles in water is accelerated by the rapidly increasing pressure gradient as the bubbles get smaller, due to the Laplace relationship. This may be observed in bubbles in water under the coverslip of a microscope. The rate of shrinkage of the bubbles increases progressively until they vanish abruptly when the radius of curvature has reached a critical value. At this stage, the pressure within the bubble has become so high that the gas within the bubble is rapidly driven into solution. This does not occur if surfactant is present, when there is an indefinite delay in the final disappearance of very small gas bubbles. The same effect would delay the absorption of gas from obstructed alveoli of small size.

There has been a suggestion that the alveolar lining is, in fact, largely dry with the surfactant acting as an anti-wetting agent (Hills, 1982). This would have implications which would run counter to much that has been written above.

The transmural pressure gradient and intrathoracic pressure

The transmural pressure gradient is the difference between intrathoracic (or 'intrapleural') and alveolar pressure. The pressure within an alveolus is always greater than the pressure to the surrounding interstitial tissue except when the volume has been reduced to zero. With increasing lung volume, the transmural pressure gradient steadily increases as shown for the whole lung in Figure 3.3. If an appreciable pneumothorax is present, the pressure gradient from alveolus to pleural cavity provides a measure of the overall transmural pressure gradient. Otherwise, the oesophageal pressure may be used to indicate the pleural pressure but there are conceptual and technical difficulties. The technical difficulties are

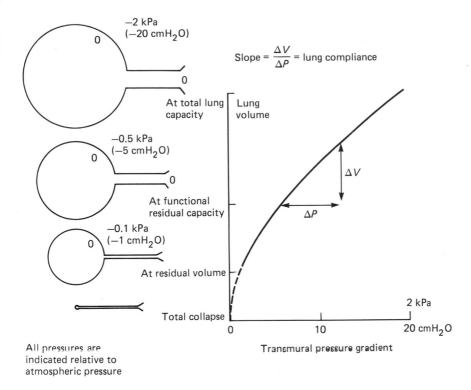

Figure 3.3 Relationship between lung volume and the difference in pressure between the alveoli and the intrathoracic space (transmural pressure gradient). The relationship approximates to linear over the normal tidal volume range. The calibre of the small air passage decreases in parallel with alveolar volume. Airways begin to close at the closing capacity (Figure 3.13) and there is widespread airway closure at residual volume, particularly in older subjects. Values in the diagram relate to the upright position and to decreasing pressure. Therefore the opening pressure of a closed alveolus is not shown.

considered at the end of the chapter while some of the conceptual difficulties are indicated in Figure 3.4.

The alveoli in the upper part of the lung have a larger volume than those in the dependent parts except at total lung capacity. The greater degree of expansion of the alveoli in the upper parts results in a greater transmural pressure gradient which decreases steadily down the lung at about 0.1 kPa (or 1 cmH$_2$O) per 3 cm of vertical height; such a difference is indicated in Figure 3.4a. Since the pleural cavity is normally empty, it is not strictly correct to speak of an intrapleural pressure and, furthermore, it would not be constant throughout the pleural 'cavity'. One should think rather of the relationship shown in Figure 3.3 as applying to various horizontal strata of the lung, each with its own volume and therefore its own transmural pressure gradient on which its own 'intrapleural' pressure would depend. The transmural pressure gradient has an important influence on many aspects of pulmonary function and so its horizontal stratification confers a regional difference on many features of pulmonary function, including airway closure, ventilation/perfusion ratios and therefore gas exchange. These matters are considered in detail in the appropriate chapters of this book.

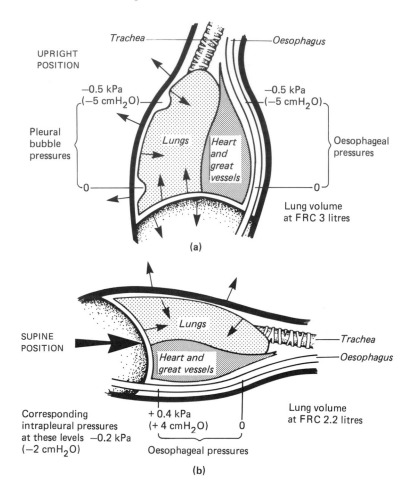

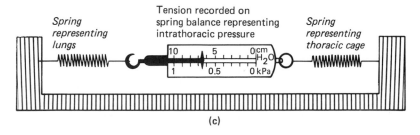

Figure 3.4 Intrathoracic pressures: static relationships in the resting end-expiratory position. The lung volume corresponds to the functional residual capacity (FRC). The figures in (a) and (b) indicate the pressure relative to ambient (atmospheric). The arrows show the direction of elastic forces. The heavy arrow in (b) indicates displacement of the abdominal viscera. In (c) the tension in the two springs is the same and will be indicated on the spring balance. In the supine position: (1) the FRC is reduced; (2) the intrathoracic pressure is raised; (3) the weight of the heart raises the oesophageal pressure above the intrapleural pressure.

At first sight it might be thought that the subatmospheric intrapleural pressure would result in the accumulation of gas evolved from solution in blood and tissues. In fact the total of the partial pressures of gases dissolved in blood, and therefore tissues, is always less than atmospheric (see Table 32.2), and this factor keeps the pleural cavity free of gas.

Time dependence of pulmonary elastic behaviour

In common with other bodies which obey Hooke's law, the lungs exhibit hysteresis. If an excised lung is rapidly inflated and then held at the new volume, the inflation pressure falls exponentially from its initial value to reach a lower level which is attained after a few seconds. This also occurs in the intact subject. Following inflation to a sustained lung volume, the pulmonary transmural pressure falls from its initial value to a new value some 20–30% less than the original pressure, over the course of about a minute (Marshall and Widdicombe, 1961). It is broadly true to say that the volume change divided by the initial change in transmural pressure gradient corresponds to the dynamic compliance while the volume change divided by the ultimate change in transmural pressure gradient (i.e. measured after it has become steady) corresponds to the static compliance. Static compliance will thus be greater than the dynamic compliance by an amount determined by the degree of time dependence in the elastic behaviour of a particular lung.

In practice static compliance is measured after a lung volume has been held for as long as is practicable, while dynamic compliance is usually measured in the course of normal rhythmic breathing. The respiratory frequency has been shown to influence dynamic pulmonary compliance in the normal subject (Mills, Cumming and Harris, 1963) but frequency dependence is much more pronounced in the presence of pulmonary disease (Otis et al., 1956; Channin and Tyler, 1962; Woolcock, Vincent and Macklem, 1969). The effect may be demonstrated during artificial ventilation of patients with respiratory paralysis, and Watson (1962a) found a marked increase in compliance when inspiration was prolonged from 0.5 to 1.7 seconds, but with a less marked increase on further extension to 3 seconds. Changes in the waveform of inflation pressure, on the other hand, had no detectable effect on compliance.

Hysteresis. If the lungs are slowly inflated and then slowly deflated, the pressure/volume curve for static points during inflation differs from that obtained during deflation. The two curves form a loop which becomes progressively broader as the tidal volume is increased (Figure 3.5). Expressed in words, the loop in Figure 3.5 means that rather more than the expected pressure is required during inflation and rather less than the expected recoil pressure is available during deflation. This resembles the behaviour of perished rubber or polyvinyl chloride, both of which are reluctant to accept deformation under stress but, once deformed, are again reluctant to assume their original shape. This phenomenon is present to a greater or less extent in all elastic bodies and is known as elastic hysteresis.

Effect of recent ventilatory history. The compliance of the lung is maintained by recent rhythmic cycling with the effect being dependent on the tidal volume. Thus a period of hypoventilation without periodic deep breaths may lead to a reduction of compliance, particularly in pathological states; compliance may then be restored by

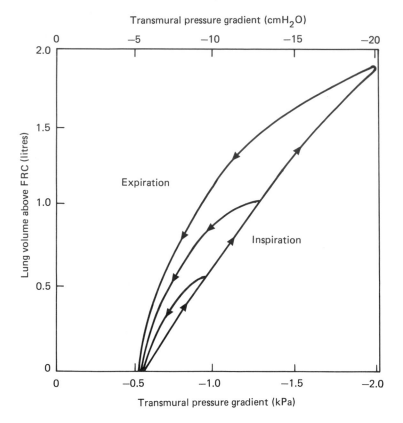

Figure 3.5 Static plot of lung volume against transmural pressure gradient (intraoesophageal pressure relative to atmosphere at zero air flow). Note that inspiratory and expiratory curves form a loop which gets wider the greater the tidal volume. These loops are typical of elastic hysteresis. For a particular lung volume, the elastic recoil of the lung during expiration is always less than the distending transmural pressure gradient required during inspiration at the same lung volume.

one or more large breaths corresponding to sighs. This was first observed during artificial ventilation of patients with respiratory paralysis (Butler and Smith, 1957), and later during anaesthesia with artificial ventilation at rather low tidal volumes (Bendixen, Hedley-Whyte and Laver, 1963). These observations led to the introduction of artificial ventilators which periodically administer 'sighs'. There can be no doubt of the importance of periodic expansion of the lungs during prolonged artificial ventilation of diseased lungs, but the case for 'sighs' during anaesthesia is less convincing, since it has no demonstrable effect on arterial PO_2 in an uncomplicated anaesthetic.

There is good evidence that compliance is reduced if the lung volume is restricted. Caro, Butler and DuBois, in 1960, demonstrated a reduction in compliance following a period of breathing within the expiratory reserve as a result of elastic strapping of the rib cage.

Causes of time dependence of pulmonary elastic behaviour

There are many possible explanations of the time dependence of pulmonary elastic behaviour, the relative importance of which may vary in different circumstances.

Redistribution of gas. In a lung consisting of functional units with identical time constants of inflation*, the distribution of gas should be independent of the rate of inflation, and there should be no redistribution when inflation is held. However, if different parts of the lungs have different time constants, the distribution of inspired gas will be dependent on the rate of inflation and redistribution will occur when inflation is held. This problem is discussed in greater detail on page 160 but for the time being we can distinguish 'fast' and 'slow' alveoli (the term 'alveoli' here referring to functional units rather than the anatomical entity). The 'fast' alveolus has a low airway resistance or low compliance (or both) while the 'slow' alveolus has a high airway resistance and/or a high compliance (Figure 3.6b). These properties give the fast alveolus a shorter time constant (as explained in Appendix F) and are preferentially filled during a short inflation. This preferential filling of alveoli with low compliance gives an overall higher pulmonary transmural pressure gradient. A slow or sustained inflation permits increased distribution of gas to slow alveoli and so tends to distribute gas in accord with the compliance of the different functional units. There should then be a lower overall transmural pressure and no redistribution of gas when inflation is held. The extreme difference between fast and slow alveoli shown in Figure 3.6b applies to diseased lungs and no such differences exist in normal lungs. Gas redistribution is therefore unlikely to be a major factor in healthy subjects, but it can be important in patients with increased airway obstruction, particularly in emphysema, asthma and chronic bronchitis. In such patients, the demonstration of frequency-dependent compliance is one of the earliest signs of an abnormality of gas distribution (Woolcock, Vincent and Macklem, 1969).

Recruitment of alveoli. Below a certain lung volume, some alveoli tend to close and only reopen at a considerably greater lung volume, in response to a much higher transmural pressure gradient than that at which they closed (Mead, 1961). Reopening of collapsed functional units (probably primary lobules) may be seen during re-expansion of the lung at thoracotomy.

Recruitment of closed alveoli appears at first sight to be a plausible explanation of all the time-dependent phenomena described above, but there are two reasons why this is unlikely. Firstly, the pressure required for reopening a closed unit is very high and is unlikely to be achieved during normal breathing. Secondly, there is no histological evidence for collapsed alveoli in normal lungs at functional residual capacity. In the presence of pathological lung collapse, a sustained deep inflation may well cause re-expansion and an increased compliance. This is likely to occur during 'bagging' of patients on prolonged artificial ventilation, but opening and closing of alveoli during a respiratory cycle is now considered unlikely.

Changes in surfactant activity. It has been explained above that the surface tension of the alveolar lining fluid is greater at larger lung volume and also during

---

*Time constants are explained in Appendix F.

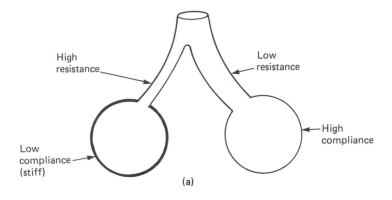

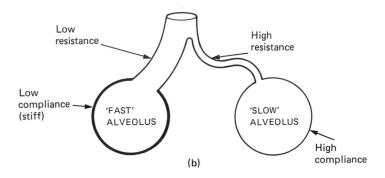

Figure 3.6 Schematic diagrams of alveoli to illustrate conditions under which static and dynamic compliances may differ. (a) Represents an idealized state which is probably not realized even in the normal subject, the reciprocal relationship between resistance and compliance results in gas flow being preferentially delivered to the most compliant regions, regardless of the rate of inflation. Static and dynamic compliance are equal. (b) Illustrates a state which is typical of many patients with respiratory disease. The alveoli can conveniently be divided into fast and slow groups. The direct relationship between compliance and resistance results in inspired gas being preferentially delivered to the stiff alveoli if the rate of inflation is rapid. An end-inspiratory pause then permits redistribution from the fast alveoli to the slow alveoli.

inspiration than at the same lung volume during expiration (Figure 3.1b). This is probably the most important cause of the observed hysteresis in the intact lung (Figure 3.5).

Stress relaxation. If a spring is pulled out to a fixed increase in its length, the resultant tension is maximal at first and then declines exponentially to a constant value. This is an inherent property of elastic bodies, known as stress relaxation. Like hysteresis, it is minimal with metals, detectable with rubber (particularly aged rubber) and very marked with many synthetic materials such as polyvinyl chloride. Stress relaxation is also dependent on the form of the material and is, for example, present in woven nylon but scarcely detectable in monofilament nylon thread. The crinkled structure of collagen in the lung is likely to favour stress relaxation and excised strips of human lung show stress relaxation when stretched (Sugihara, Hildebrandt and Martin, 1972). The time course is of the same order as the observed changes in pressure when lungs are held inflated at constant volume, and Marshall and Widdicombe (1961) concluded that the effect was due to stress relaxation. Viscoelastic tissue resistance is considered on pages 68 et seq.

Influence of alveolar muscle. It is possible that sustained inflation might cause reduction in the tone of muscle fibres within the terminal airways and alveolar wall, resulting in changes similar to those of stress relaxation. Alveolar muscle is present in the alveolar wall of the cat but there is difference of opinion as to the importance of alveolar muscle in man.

Displacement of pulmonary blood. A sustained inflation might be expected to displace blood from the lungs and so to increase compliance by reducing the splinting effect of the pulmonary vasculature. The importance of this factor is not known, but experiments with excised lung indicate that all the major time-dependent phenomena are present when the pulmonary vasculature is empty.

Factors affecting lung compliance

Lung volume. It is important to remember that compliance is related to lung volume (Marshall, 1957). An elephant has a much higher compliance than a mouse. This factor may be excluded by relating compliance to FRC to yield the specific compliance (i.e. compliance/FRC), which is almost constant for both sexes and all ages down to neonatal.

Posture. Lung volume changes with posture (page 53) and there are also problems in the measurement of intrapleural pressure in the supine position (see Figure 3.4). When these factors are taken into account, it seems unlikely that changes of posture have any significant effect on the specific compliance.

Pulmonary blood volume. The pulmonary blood vessels probably make an appreciable contribution to the stiffness of the lung. Pulmonary venous congestion from whatever cause is associated with reduced compliance.

Age. One would have expected age to influence the elasticity of the lung as of other tissues in the body. However, Butler, White and Arnott (1957) were unable to detect any correlation between age and compliance, even after allowing for predicted changes in lung volume. This accords with the concept of lung 'elasticity' being largely determined by surface forces.

Restriction of chest expansion. Elastic strapping of the chest reduces both lung volume and compliance. However, when lung volume is returned to normal, either by removal of the restriction or by a more forceful inspiration, the compliance remains reduced. Normal compliance can be restored by taking a single deep breath (Caro, Butler and DuBois, 1960).

Recent ventilatory history. This important factor has been considered above (page 43) in relation to the time dependence of pulmonary elastic behaviour.

Bronchial smooth muscle tone. A recent study in sheep showed that an infusion of methacholine, sufficient to result in a doubling of airway resistance, also decreased *dynamic* compliance by 50% (Mitzner et al., 1992). The airways might contribute to overall compliance or, alternatively, bronchoconstriction could enhance time dependence and so reduce dynamic, but perhaps not static, compliance (Figure 3.6).

Disease. Important changes in lung pressure/volume relationships are found in certain lung diseases. Emphysema is unique in that *static* pulmonary compliance is increased, as a result of destruction of pulmonary tissue and loss of both elastin and surface retraction. Although FRC is increased, distribution of inspired gas may be grossly disordered, as shown in Figure 3.6, and therefore the *dynamic* compliance is commonly reduced. In asthma the pressure/volume curve is displaced upwards without a change in compliance (Finucane and Colebatch, 1969). The elastic recoil is therefore reduced at normal transmural pressure and so the FRC is increased (see Figure 3.12 below).

Most other types of pulmonary pathology result in decreased lung compliance, both static and dynamic. In particular, all forms of pulmonary fibrosis (e.g. fibrosing alveolitis), consolidation, collapse, vascular engorgement, fibrous pleurisy and especially adult respiratory distress syndrome will all reduce compliance and FRC.

Elastic recoil of the thoracic cage

An excised lung will always tend to contract until all the contained air is expelled. In contrast, when the thoracic cage is opened it tends to expand to a volume about 1 litre greater than FRC. The FRC in a paralysed patient is the volume at which the inward elastic recoil of the lungs is balanced by the outward recoil of the thoracic cage.

The thoracic cage comprises the rib cage and the diaphragm. Each is a muscular structure and can be considered as an elastic structure only when the muscles are relaxed, and that is not easy to achieve except under the conditions of paralysis. Relaxation curves have been prepared relating pressure and volumes in the supposedly relaxed subject, but it is now doubted whether total relaxation was ever achieved. For example, it seems that the diaphragm is not fully relaxed at the end of expiration *in the supine position* but maintains a resting tone which is abolished by anaesthesia (Muller et al., 1979). This maintains the FRC about 400 ml above the value in the paralysed or anaesthetized patient (Chapter 20).

Compliance of the thoracic cage is defined as change in lung volume per unit change in the pressure gradient between atmosphere and the intrapleural space. The units are the same as for pulmonary compliance. The measurement is seldom made but the value is of the order of 2 l/kPa (200 ml/cmH$_2$O).

Factors influencing compliance of the thoracic cage

Anatomical factors. These factors include the ribs and the state of ossification of the costal cartilages. Obesity and even pathological skin conditions may have an appreciable effect. In particular, scarring of the skin overlying the front of the chest may result from scalding in children and this may actually embarrass the breathing.

In terms of compliance, a relaxed diaphragm simply transmits pressure from the abdomen which may be increased in obesity, abdominal distension and venous congestion. Posture clearly has a major effect and this is considered below in relation to FRC. Ferris et al. (1952) suggested that thoracic cage compliance was 30 per cent greater in the seated subject. Lynch, Brand and Levy (1959) found the total static compliance of the respiratory system to be 60% less when the subject was turned from the supine into the prone position: much of this difference is likely to be due to the diminished elasticity of the rib cage and diaphragm in the prone position.

Pressure/volume relationships of the lung plus thoracic cage

Compliance is analogous to electrical capacitance, and in the respiratory system the compliances of lungs and thoracic cage are in series. Therefore the total compliance of the system obeys the same relationship as for capacitances in series, in which reciprocals are added to obtain the reciprocal of the total value, thus:

$$\frac{1}{\text{total compliance}} = \frac{1}{\text{lung compliance}} + \frac{1}{\text{thoracic cage compliance}}$$

typical static values (l/kPa) for the supine paralysed patient being:

$$\frac{1}{0.85} = \frac{1}{1.5} + \frac{1}{2}$$

Instead of compliance, we may consider its reciprocal, elastance, for which the electrical analogue is conductance. The relationship is then much simpler:

$$\text{total elastance} = \text{lung elastance} + \text{thoracic cage elastance}$$

corresponding values (kPa/l) are then:

$$1.17 = 0.67 + 0.5$$

Relationship between alveolar, intrathoracic and ambient pressures

At all times the alveolar/ambient pressure gradient is the algebraic sum of the alveolar/intrathoracic (or transmural) and intrathoracic/ambient pressure gradients. This relationship is independent of whether the patient is breathing spontaneously or he is being ventilated by intermittent positive pressure. Actual values depend upon compliances, lung volume and posture, and typical values are shown for the upright conscious relaxed subject in Figure 3.7, and for the supine anaesthetized and paralysed patient in Figure 3.8. The values in these two illustrations are static and relate to conditions when no gas is flowing.

Lung volumes

Certain lung volumes, particularly the functional residual capacity, are determined by elastic forces and this is therefore a convenient point at which to consider the various lung volumes and their subdivision (Figure 3.9).

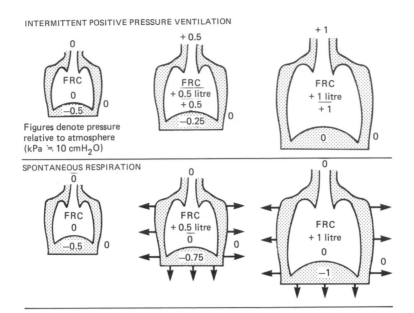

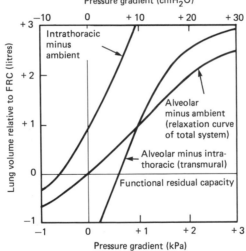

Figure 3.7 Static pressure/volume relations for the intact thorax for the conscious subject in the upright position. The transmural pressure gradient bears the same relationship to lung volume during both intermittent positive pressure ventilation and spontaneous breathing. The intrathoracic-to-ambient pressure difference, however, differs in the two types of ventilation due to muscle action during spontaneous respiration. At all times:

$$\frac{\text{alveolar/ambient}}{\text{pressure difference}} = \frac{\text{alveolar/intrathoracic}}{\text{pressure difference}} + \frac{\text{intrathoracic/ambient}}{\text{pressure difference}}$$

(due attention being paid to the sign of the pressure difference).
*   Lung compliance, 2 l/kPa (200 ml/cmH$_2$O); thoracic cage compliance, 2 l/kPa (200 ml/cmH$_2$O); total compliance, 1 l/kPa (100 ml/cmH$_2$O).*

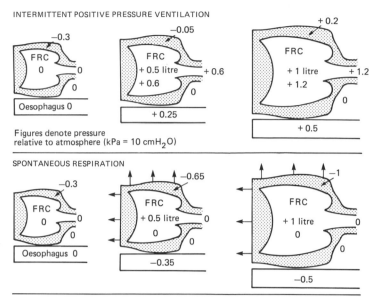

INTERMITTENT POSITIVE PRESSURE VENTILATION

Figures denote pressure
relative to atmosphere (kPa = 10 cmH₂O)

SPONTANEOUS RESPIRATION

PRESSURE/VOLUME CURVES FOR THE PARALYSED SUBJECT

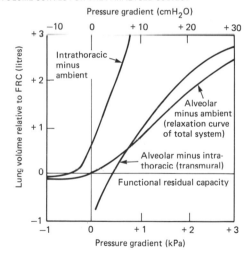

Figure 3.8 Static pressure/volume relations for the intact thorax for the anaesthetized patient in the supine position. The transmural pressure gradient bears the same relationship to lung volume during both intermittent positive pressure ventilation and spontaneous breathing. The intrathoracic-to-ambient pressure difference, however, differs in the two types of respiration due to muscle action during spontaneous respiration. At all times:

$$\frac{alveolar/ambient}{pressure\ difference} = \frac{alveolar/intrathoracic}{pressure\ difference} + \frac{intrathoracic/ambient}{pressure\ difference}$$

(due attention being paid to the sign of the pressure difference).

The oesophageal pressure is assumed to be 0.3 kPa (3 cmH₂O) higher than intrathoracic at all times. Lung compliance, 1.5 l/kPa (150 ml/cmH₂O); thoracic cage compliance, 2=l/kPa (200 ml/cmH₂O); total compliance, 0.85 l/kPa (85 ml/cmH₂O).

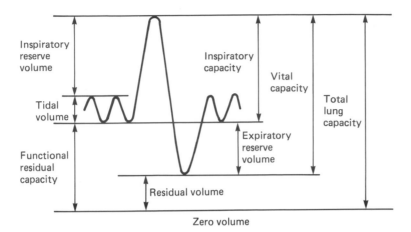

Figure 3.9 Static lung volumes. The 'spirometer curve' indicates the lung volumes which can be measured by simple spirometry. These are the tidal volume, inspiratory reserve volume, expiratory reserve volume, inspiratory capacity and vital capacity. The residual volume cannot be measured by observation of a simple spirometer trace and it is therefore impossible to measure the functional residual capacity or the total lung capacity without further elaboration of methods.

Total lung capacity (TLC). This is the volume of gas in the lungs at the end of a maximal inspiration. TLC is achieved when the maximal force generated by the inspiratory muscles is balanced by the forces opposing expansion. It is rather surprising that *expiratory* muscles are also contracting strongly at the end of a maximal inspiration.

Residual volume (RV). This is the volume remaining after a maximal expiration. In the young, RV is governed by the balance between the maximal force generated by expiratory muscles and the elastic forces opposing reduction of lung volume. However, in older subjects total closure of small airways may prevent further expiration.

Functional residual capacity (FRC). This is the lung volume at the end of a normal expiration. Within the framework of TLC, RV and FRC, other capacities and volumes shown in Figure 3.9 are self-explanatory.

Factors affecting the FRC

So many factors affect the FRC that they require a special section of this chapter. The actual volume of the FRC has particular importance because of its relationship to the closing capacity (page 53).

Body size. FRC is linearly related to height. Estimates range from an increase in FRC of 32 ml/cm (Cotes, 1975) to 51 ml/cm (Bates, Macklem and Christie, 1971). Obesity causes a marked reduction in FRC compared with lean subjects of the same height.

Sex. For the same body height, females have an FRC about 10% less than males (Bates, Macklem and Christie, 1971).

Age. Bates, Macklem and Christie (1971) found FRC to be independent of age in the adult, while Needham, Rogan and McDonald (1954) observed a slight increase in FRC with age. The nomogram of Cotes (1975) also allows for a slight increase with age. The author has pooled preoperative observations of FRC in the supine position derived from many studies (page 394) and these values showed no correlation with age.

Diaphragmatic muscle tone. FRC has in the past been considered to be the volume at which there is a balance between the elastic forces represented by the inward retraction of the lungs and the outward expansion of the thoracic cage (pages 48 et seq.). However, as explained above, it now appears that residual end-expiratory muscle tone is a major factor in the supine position, maintaining the FRC about 400 ml above the volume in the totally relaxed subject, which in practice means paralysed or anaesthetized (Figure 3.10).

Posture. Figures 3.4 and 3.11 show the reduction in FRC in the supine position, which may be attributed to the increased pressure of the abdominal contents on the diaphragm. Values of FRC in these Figures and Table 3.1 are typical for a subject of 168–170 cm height, and reported mean differences between supine and upright positions range from 500 to 1000 ml. Figure 3.11 shows that most of the change takes place between horizontal and 60 degrees head-up. Teleologically, end-expiratory diaphragmatic tone can be seen as a protection against the weight of the abdominal contents causing an unacceptable reduction of lung volume in the supine position. Values for FRC in other positions are shown in Table 3.1.

Lung disease. The FRC will be reduced by increased elastic recoil of the lungs, chest wall or both. Possible causes include fibrosing alveolitis, organized fibrinous pleurisy, kyphoscoliosis, obesity and scarring of the thorax following burns. Conversely, elastic recoil of the lungs is diminished in emphysema and asthma and the FRC is usually increased. This is beneficial since airway resistance decreases as the lung volume increases. In emphysema, there is an actual increase in static compliance due to loss of lung tissue. In asthma, the compliance is only marginally increased but there is an upward displacement of the transmural pressure/lung volume curve (Figure 3.12).

FRC in relation to closing capacity

In Chapter 4 (page 81) it is explained how reduction in lung volume below a certain level results in airway closure with relative or total underventilation in the dependent parts of the lung. The lung volume below which this effect becomes apparent is known as the closing capacity (CC). With increasing age, CC rises until it equals FRC at about 66 years in the upright position but only 44 in the supine position (Figure 3.13). This is a major factor in the decrease of arterial Po_2 with age (page 268).

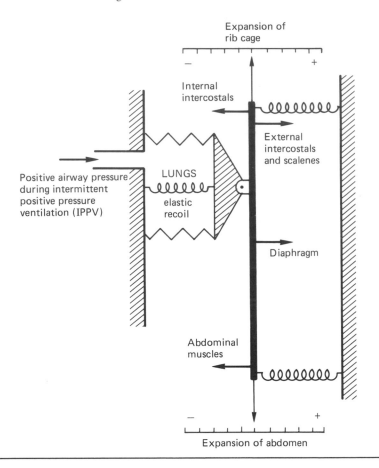

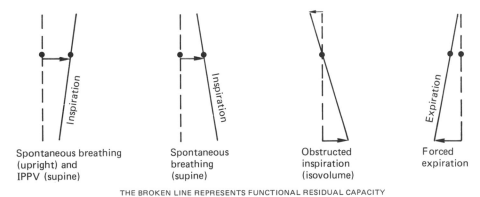

THE BROKEN LINE REPRESENTS FUNCTIONAL RESIDUAL CAPACITY

Figure 3.10 A model of the balance of static and dynamic forces acting on the respiratory system, derived from Hillman and Finucane (1987) and Drummond (1989b). The central bar, attached to the lungs, is floating freely, held in equilibrium by elastic forces at the end-expiratory position as shown. It may then be displaced either by passive inflation of the lungs or by the action of the various muscles shown in the diagram, during different respiratory manoeuvres as shown below. The arrows at the ends of the bar indicate changes in the cross-sectional areas of rib cage and abdomen.

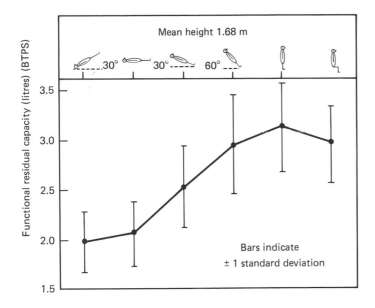

Figure 3.11 Studies by the author and his co-workers of the functional residual capacity in various body positions.

Table 3.1 Effect of posture on some aspects of respiratory function (Lumb and Nunn, 1991a)

Position	FRC litres (BTPS)	Rib cage breathing* (%)	Forced expiratory volume litres (BTPS) in 1 second
Sitting	2.91†	69.7†	3.79
Supine	2.10	32.3	3.70
Supine (arms up)	2.36‡	33.0	3.27
Prone	2.45†	32.6	3.49
Lateral	2.44†	36.5	3.67

Data for 13 healthy males aged 24–64.
*Proportion of breathing accounted for by movement of the rib cage.
The supine (arms up) position is that required for computed tomography.
Significance of difference relates to the supine position thus:
† $p < 0.001$
‡ $p < 0.01$

Principles of measurement of compliance

Compliance is measured as the change in lung volume divided by the corresponding change in the appropriate pressure gradient, there being no gas flow when the two measurements are made. For the lung the appropriate pressure gradient is alveolar/intrapleural (or intrathoracic) and for the total compliance alveolar/

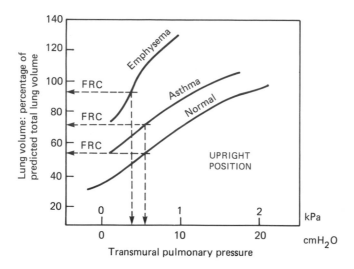

Figure 3.12 Pulmonary transmural pressure/volume plots for normal subjects, patients with asthma in bronchospasm and patients with emphysema. The broken horizontal lines indicate the FRC in each of the three groups and the corresponding point on the abscissa indicates the resting intrathoracic pressure at FRC. (Redrawn from Finucane and Colebatch, 1969)

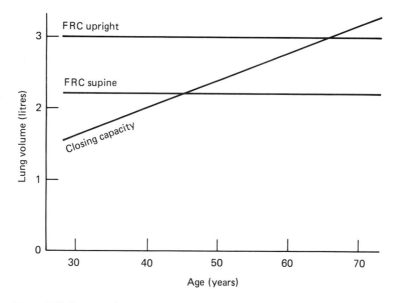

Figure 3.13 Functional residual capacity (FRC) and closing capacity as a function of age. (Redrawn from data of Leblanc, Ruff and Milic-Emili, 1970)

ambient. Measurement of compliance of the thoracic cage is seldom undertaken but the appropriate pressure gradient would then be intrapleural/ambient. This would be meaningless for measurement of compliance if there were any tone in the respiratory muscles.

Volume may be measured with a spirometer, a body plethysmograph or by integration of a pneumotachogram. Points of zero air flow are best indicated by a pneumotachogram. Static pressures can be measured with a simple water mano-meter but electrical transducers are more usual today. Intrathoracic pressure is usually measured as oesophageal pressure which, in the upright subject, is different at different levels. The pressure rises as the balloon descends, the change being roughly in accord with the specific gravity of the lung (0.3 g/ml). It is usual to measure the pressure 32–35 cm beyond the nares, the highest point at which the measurement is free from artefacts due to mouth pressure and tracheal and neck movements (Milic-Emili et al., 1964). In the supine position the weight of the heart may introduce an artefact (see Figure 3.4) but there is usually a zone some 32–40 cm beyond the nares where the oesophageal pressure is close to atmospheric and probably only about 0.2 kPa (2 cmH$_2$O) above the neighbouring intrathoracic pressure. Alveolar pressure equals mouth pressure when no gas is flowing: it cannot be measured directly.

Static compliance. In the conscious subject, a known volume of air is inhaled from FRC and the subject then relaxes against a closed airway. The various pressure gradients are then measured and compared with the resting values at FRC. It is, in fact, very difficult to ensure that the respiratory muscles are relaxed, but the measurement of lung compliance is valid since the static alveolar/intrathoracic pressure difference is unaffected by any muscle activity.

In the paralysed subject there are no difficulties about muscular relaxation and it is very easy to measure static compliance of the whole respiratory system. However, due to the uncertainties about interpretation of the oesophageal pressure in the supine position (see Figure 3.4), there is usually some uncertainty about the pulmonary compliance. Measurement of total respiratory static compliance in the paralysed patient may be made with nothing more complicated than a spirometer and a water manometer (Nims, Connor and Comroe, 1955), as shown in Figure 3.14. Note that it is easier to measure *lung* compliance in the upright position, and *total* compliance in the anaesthetized paralysed patient who will usually be in the supine position.

Dynamic compliance

These measurements are made during rhythmic breathing, but compliance is calculated from pressure and volume measurements made when no gas is flowing, usually at end-inspiratory and end-expiratory 'no-flow' points. Two methods are in general use.

Loops. The required pressure gradient and the respired volume are displayed simultaneously as X and Y coordinates. The resultant trace forms a loop as in Figure 3.15a, the 'no-flow' points being where the trace is horizontal. The dynamic lung compliance is the slope of the line joining these points when the pressure gradient is ambient/intrathoracic. The area of the loop is mainly a function of airway resistance (page 87).

Multichannel recording of volume, pressure gradient and flow rate. This method differs from the one described above only in the manner of display; the principles are the same. Volume and pressure are displayed separately (Figure 3.15b). The

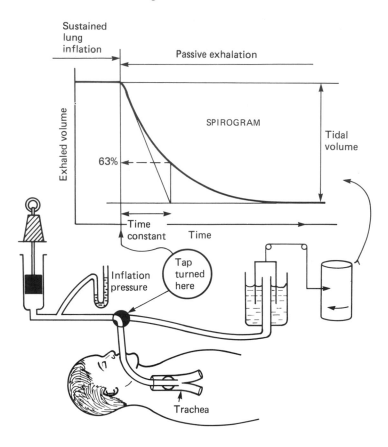

Figure 3.14 Measurement of resistance and compliance by analysis of the passive spirogram. This method is applicable only to the paralysed patient. Only a water manometer and a spirometer are required.

$$Static\ compliance = \frac{tidal\ volume}{inflation\ pressure}$$

$$Compliance \times resistance = time\ constant$$

$$Initial\ resistance = \frac{initial\ pressure\ gradient}{initial\ flow\ rate} = \frac{inflation\ pressure}{tidal\ vol./time\ constant}$$

volume change is derived from the volume trace and is divided by the difference in pressure at the two 'no-flow' points. In Figure 3.15b , these points are identified as the horizontal part of the volume trace but are more precisely indicated by a pneumotachogram which may be integrated to give volume and thereby dispense with a spirometer. This method was introduced in 1927 by von Neergaard and Wirz (1927a) and may be used for both spontaneous and artificial breathing. The calculations may conveniently be undertaken on-line with a microcomputer inter-faced to the volume and pressure transducers.

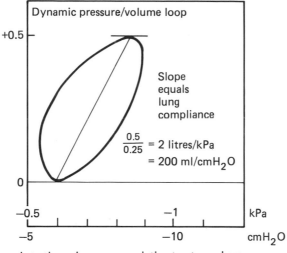

Dynamic pressure/volume loop

Slope
equals
lung
compliance

$\dfrac{0.5}{0.25}$ = 2 litres/kPa
   = 200 ml/cmH$_2$O

+0.5

0

−0.5   −1   kPa

−5   −10   cmH$_2$O

(a)   Intrathoracic pressure relative to atmosphere

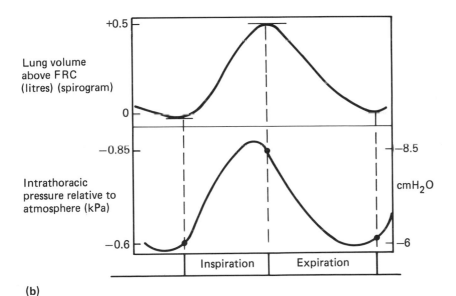

+0.5

Lung volume
above FRC
(litres) (spirogram)

0

−0.85   −8.5

Intrathoracic
pressure relative to
atmosphere (kPa)   cmH$_2$O

−0.6   −6

| Inspiration | Expiration |

(b)

Figure 3.15 Measurement of dynamic compliance of lung by simultaneous measurement of tidal excursion (lung volume relative to FRC) and intrathoracic pressure (relative to atmosphere). In (a) these variables are displayed as the Y and X co-ordinates on a two-dimensional plotting device (e.g. cathode ray oscillograph). In (b) they are displayed simultaneously against time on a two-channel oscillograph. In each case, lung compliance is derived as lung volume change divided by transmural pressure gradient change. The transmural pressure gradient is indicated by the intrathoracic pressure (relative to atmosphere) when the lung volume is not changing. At these times the alveolar pressure must equal the atmospheric pressure since no gas is flowing. End-expiratory and end-inspiratory 'no-flow' points are indicated in (b). They correspond to horizontal parts of the loop in (a).

Principles of measurement of lung volumes

Vital capacity, tidal volume, inspiratory reserve and expiratory reserve can all be measured with a simple spirometer (see Figure 3.9). Total lung capacity, functional residual capacity and residual volume all contain a fraction (the residual volume) which cannot be measured by simple spirometry. However, if one of these volumes is measured (most commonly the FRC), the others can easily be derived.

Measurement of FRC

Three techniques are available. The first employs nitrogen wash-out by breathing 100% oxygen. Total quantity of nitrogen eliminated is measured as the product of the expired volume collected and the concentration of nitrogen. If, for example, 4 litres of nitrogen are collected and the initial alveolar nitrogen concentration was 80%, then the initial lung volume was 5 litres.

The second method uses the wash-in of a tracer gas such as helium, the concentration of which may be conveniently measured by catharometry (Hewlett et al., 1974a). If, for example, 50 ml of helium is introduced into the lungs and the helium concentration is then found to be 1%, the lung volume is 5 litres.

The third method uses the body plethysmograph (DuBois et al., 1956). The subject is totally contained within a gas-tight box and he attempts to breathe against an occluded airway. Changes in alveolar pressure are recorded at the mouth and compared with the small changes in lung volume, derived from pressure changes within the plethysmograph. Application of Boyle's law then permits calculation of lung volume. This method would include trapped gas which might not be registered by the two previous methods.

Measurement of closing capacity is considered on page 88.

Chapter 4

Non-elastic resistance to gas flow

The previous chapter has considered elastic resistance to gas flow, which governs the relationship between pressure and lung volume under static conditions when no gas is flowing. Elastic resistance is only one component of the total impedance to gas flow, and this chapter will consider the remaining components, conveniently grouped together as 'non-elastic resistance'. Much the greater part of the residual forms of impedance are provided by resistance to air flow and tissue deformation. These are primarily related to gas flow rate, and together are termed 'pulmonary resistance'. Techniques are available to separate pulmonary resistance into airway resistance and pulmonary tissue resistance. The last and the smallest component of total pulmonary impedance is due to inertia of both gas and tissue. Unlike elastic resistance, work performed against non-elastic resistance is not stored as potential energy (and therefore recoverable), but is lost and dissipated as heat.

Excessive resistance to gas flow is the commonest and most important cause of ventilatory failure. Severe obstruction to breathing is life threatening and may arise anywhere from the smallest airways, through the tracheobronchial tree, larynx and pharynx to include external factors and any apparatus through which the patient may be breathing.

Gas flows from a region of high pressure to one of lower pressure. The rate at which it does so is a function of the pressure difference and the resistance to gas flow, thus being analogous to the flow of an electrical current (Figure 4.1). The precise relationship between pressure difference and flow rate depends on the nature of the flow which may be laminar, turbulent or a mixture of the two. It is useful to consider laminar and turbulent flow as two separate entities but mixed patterns of flow usually occur in the respiratory tract. With a number of important caveats, similar basic considerations apply to the flow of liquids through tubes, which is considered in Chapter 7.

Laminar flow

Characteristics of laminar flow

Below its critical flow rate, gas flows along a straight unbranched tube as a series of concentric cylinders which slide over one another, with the peripheral cylinder stationary and the central cylinder moving fastest (Figure 4.2). This is also termed

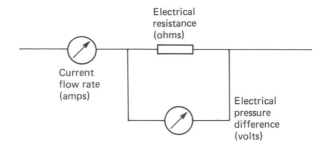

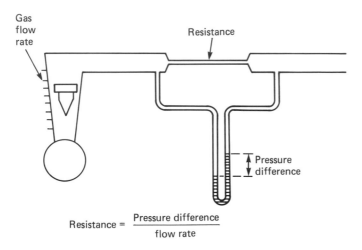

$$\text{Resistance} = \frac{\text{Pressure difference}}{\text{flow rate}}$$

Figure 4.1 Electrical analogy of gas flow. Resistance is pressure difference per unit flow rate. Resistance to gas flow is analogous to electrical resistance (provided that flow is laminar). Gas flow corresponds to electrical current (amps); gas pressure corresponds to potential (volts); gas flow resistance corresponds to electrical resistance (ohms); Poiseuille's law corresponds to Ohm's law.

streamline flow and is characteristically inaudible. Gas sampled from the periphery of a tube during laminar flow may not be representative of gas of a different composition advancing down the centre of the tube.

The advancing cone front means that some fresh gas will reach the end of a tube while the volume entering the tube is still less than the volume of the tube. In the context of the respiratory tract, this is to say that there may be a significant alveolar ventilation when the tidal volume is less than the anatomical dead space, a fact which was noted by Rohrer in 1915 and is very relevant to high frequency ventilation (page 444). For the same reason, laminar flow is relatively inefficient for purging the contents of a tube.

Quantitative relationships during laminar flow

With laminar flow, the gas flow rate is directly proportional to the driving pressure (Figure 4.2), the constant being thus defined as resistance to gas flow:

$$\text{pressure difference} = \text{flow rate} \times \text{resistance}$$

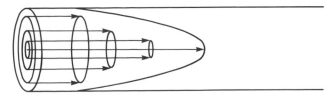

(a)

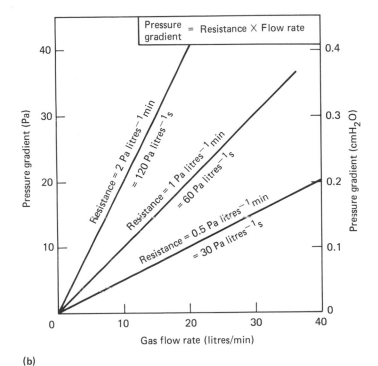

(b)

Figure 4.2 Laminar flow. (a) Laminar gas flow down a straight tube as a series of concentric cylinders of gas with the cental cylinder moving fastest. This gives rise to a 'cone front' when the composition of the gas is abruptly changed as it enters the tube. (b) The linear relationship between gas flow rate and pressure gradient. The slope of the lines indicates the resistance (1 Pa $\doteq$ 0.01 cmH$_2$O).

Note the parallel with Ohm's law (see Figure 4.1):

$$\text{potential difference} = \text{current} \times \text{resistance}$$

For gas flow in a straight unbranched tube, the value for resistance is:

$$\frac{8 \times \text{length} \times \text{viscosity}}{\pi \times (\text{radius})^4}$$

In this rearrangement of the Hagen–Poiseuille equation, the direct relationship between flow and the fourth power of the radius of the tube explains the critical importance of narrowing of air passages, as well as the choice of an appropriate cannula for an intravenous infusion.

Viscosity is the only property of a gas which is relevant under conditions of laminar flow. Helium has a low density but a viscosity close to that of air. Helium will not therefore improve gas flow if the flow is laminar. However, flow is usually turbulent when resistance to breathing becomes a problem.

In the Hagen–Poiseuille equation, the units must be coherent. In CGS units, dyn/cm^2 (pressure), ml/s (flow) and cm (length and radius) are compatible with the unit of poise for viscosity ($dyn \; sec \; cm^{-2}$). In SI units, with pressure in kilopascals, the unit of viscosity is newton second $metre^{-2}$ (see Appendix A). However, in practice it is still customary to express gas pressure in cmH_2O and flow in l/s. Resistance would then be cmH_2O per l/s.

It is sometimes convenient to refer to conductance, which is the reciprocal of resistance and is usually expressed as l/s per cmH_2O. Specific airway conductance (sG_{aw}) is the conductance of the lower airways divided by the lung volume (Lehane, Jordan and Jones, 1980). Since it takes into account the important effect of lung volume on airway resistance (page 79), it is a useful index of bronchomotor tone.

Turbulent flow

Characteristics of turbulent flow

High flow rates, particularly through branched or irregular tubes, result in a breakdown of the orderly flow of gas described above as laminar. An irregular movement is superimposed on the general progression along the tube (Figure 4.3), with a square front replacing the cone front of laminar flow. Turbulent flow is often audible and is almost invariably present when high resistance to gas flow is a problem.

The square front means that no fresh gas can reach the end of a tube until the amount of gas entering the tube is almost equal to the volume of the tube. Conversely, turbulent flow is more effective than laminar flow in purging the contents of a tube. Turbulent flow provides the best conditions for drawing a representative sample of gas from the periphery of a tube.

Quantitative relationships during turbulent flow

The relationship between driving pressure and flow rate differs from the relationship described above for laminar flow in three important respects:

1. The driving pressure is proportional to the square of the gas flow rate.
2. The driving pressure is proportional to the density of the gas and is independent of its viscosity.
3. The required driving pressure is, in theory, inversely proportional to the fifth power of the radius of the tube (Fanning equation).

The square law relating driving pressure and flow rate is shown in Figure 4.3. Resistance, defined as pressure gradient divided by flow rate, is not constant as in laminar flow but increases in proportion to the flow rate. It is thus meaningless to use the Ohm's law concept of resistance when flow is turbulent or partly turbulent, and units such as cmH_2O per l/s should be used only when flow is entirely laminar. The following methods of quantification of 'resistance' should be used when flow is totally or partially turbulent.

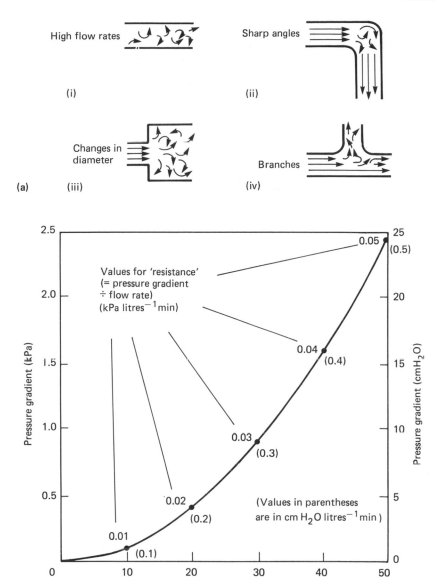

Figure 4.3 Turbulent flow. (a) Four circumstances under which gas flow tends to be turbulent. (b) The square law relationship between gas flow rate and pressure gradient when flow is turbulent. Note that the value for 'resistance', calculated as for laminar flow, is quite meaningless during turbulent flow.

Two constants. This method considers resistance as comprising two components, one for laminar flow and the other for turbulent flow. The simple relationship for laminar flow given above would then be extended as follows:

$$\text{pressure difference} = k_1 \,(\text{flow}) + k_2 \,(\text{flow})^2$$

k_1 contains the factors of the Hagen–Poiseuille equation while k_2 includes factors in the corresponding equation for turbulent flow. Mead and Agostoni (1964) summarized studies of normal human subjects in the following equation:

$$\text{pressure gradient (kPa)} = 0.24 \text{ (flow)} + 0.03 \text{ (flow)}^2$$

or

$$\text{pressure gradient (cmH}_2\text{O)} = 2.4 \text{ (flow)} + 0.3 \text{ (flow)}^2$$

The exponent ^{n}. Over a surprisingly wide range of flow rates, the equation above may be condensed into the following single-term expression with little loss of precision:

$$\text{pressure gradient} = K \text{ (flow)}^n$$

The exponent ^{n} has a value ranging from 1 with purely laminar flow to 2 with purely turbulent flow, the value of ^{n} being a useful indication of the nature of the flow. The constants for the normal human respiratory tract are:

$$\text{pressure gradient (kPa)} = 0.24 \text{ (flow)}^{1.3}$$

or

$$\text{pressure gradient (cmH}_2\text{O)} = 2.4 \text{ (flow)}^{1.3}$$

The graphical method. It is often convenient to represent 'resistance' as a graph of pressure difference against gas flow rate, on either linear or logarithmic coordinates. Logarithmic coordinates have the advantage that the plot is usually a straight line whether flow is laminar, turbulent or mixed, and the slope of the line indicates the value of ^{n} in the equation above.

Reynolds' number

In the case of long straight unbranched tubes, the nature of the gas flow may be predicted from the value of Reynolds' number, which is a non-dimensional quantity derived from the following expression:

$$\frac{\text{linear velocity of gas} \times \text{tube diameter} \times \text{gas density}}{\text{gas viscosity}}$$

When Reynolds' number is less than 1000, flow is laminar. Above a value of 1500, flow is entirely turbulent. Between these values, both types of flow coexist. Figure 4.4 shows the nature of the gas flow for three different gas mixtures in terms of gas flow rate and diameter of tube. It will be seen that mixed flow patterns will often be present under conditions which are likely to occur in the clinical situation.

The property of the gas which affects Reynolds' number is the ratio of density to viscosity. Values for some gas mixtures that a patient may inhale are shown relative to air in Table 4.1. Viscosities of respirable gases do not differ greatly but there may be very large differences in density. Note that use of a less dense gas such as helium not only reduces resistance during turbulent flow but also renders turbulent flow less likely to occur.

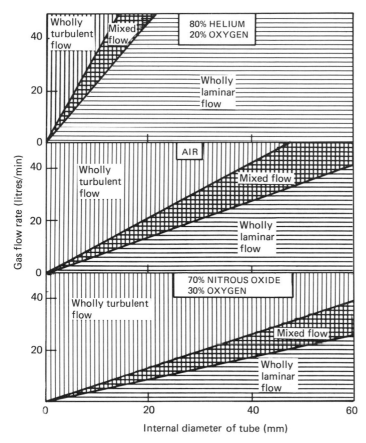

Figure 4.4 Graphs to show the nature of the gas flow through tubes of various diameters for three different gas mixtures; 25 l/min is a typical peak flow rate during spontaneous respiration. It will be seen that the nature of flow in the trachea and in endotracheal tubes will be markedly dependent on the composition of the gas mixture.

Table 4.1 Physical properties of anaesthetic gas mixtures relating to gas flow

	Viscosity relative to air	Vapour density relative to air	Vapour density / Viscosity relative to air
Oxygen	1.11	1.11	1.00
70% N_2O/30% O_2	0.89	1.41	1.59
80% He/20% O_2	1.08	0.33	0.31

Threshold resistors

Certain resistors are designed to allow no gas to pass until a threshold pressure is reached. Once that pressure is reached, gas passes freely with little further rise in pressure as the flow rate increases.

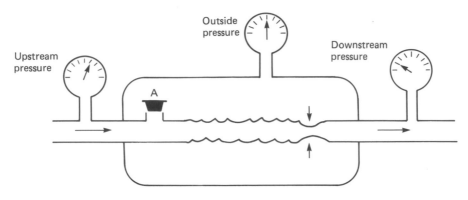

Figure 4.5 The Starling resistor consists of a length of flaccid collapsible tubing passing through a rigid box. When the pressure outside the collapsible tubing exceeds the upstream pressure, the tubing collapses where shown by the arrows. No gas can flow, whatever the level of the downstream pressure. If the orifice A is opened, the outside pressure rises with the upstream pressure and so limits flow rate to a level which is independent of the magnitude of the upstream pressure. The relevance of this to effort-independent expiratory flow rate is considered in page 77. The relevance of the Starling resistor to the pulmonary capillary circulation is considered on page 149.

The classic prototype threshold resistor is the Starling valve (Figure 4.5). Gas will flow only when the upstream pressure exceeds the pressure in the chamber surrounding the collapsible tubing. A similar effect may be obtained with a properly designed spring-loaded valve or by exhalation through a prescribed depth of water. Spring-loaded valves are now extensively used for application of positive end-expiratory pressure (PEEP) (page 451). The concept is not new and such devices have long been used as safety valves for boilers and pressure cookers.

Besides acting as a simple threshold resistor, the Starling valve has other special properties. Once gas is flowing, an increase in downstream pressure will distend the tubing and so decrease the resistance of the device. However, a decreased downstream pressure cannot initiate flow. These properties make the Starling resistor a useful model of blood flow through pulmonary vessels in relation to alveolar pressure (page 149), and also for the behaviour of collapsible air passages during expiration, considered later in this chapter.

Tissue resistance to gas flow

Mount (1955) identified a component of the work of breathing which he attributed to the resistance caused by tissue deformation. He provided hydrostatic and electrical analogues which clearly show that the effect is maximal at low respiratory frequencies. D'Angelo et al. (1989) and Milic-Emili, Robatto and Bates (1990) have described how the tissue resistance and its time-dependence may be measured (see also below), and have presented a 'spring and dashpot' model which describes this component of tissue resistance. The models of Mount and Milic-Emili's groups are shown in Figure 4.6, alongside the tracheal pressure changes which occur during an occlusion of the airway at the end of a passive inspiration produced by the application of positive airway pressure.

(a) Models that ignore time dependence of impedance

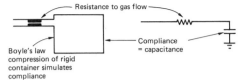

Resistance to gas flow

Compliance
= capacitance

Boyle's law
compression of rigid
container simulates
compliance

(b) Mount's model incorporating time-dependent tissue resistance

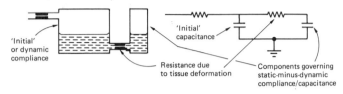

'Initial'
or dynamic
compliance

'Initial'
capacitance

Resistance due
to tissue deformation

Components governing
static-minus-dynamic
compliance/capacitance

(c) Spring and dashpot model of resistance to breathing

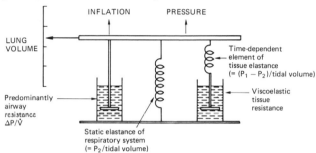

INFLATION   PRESSURE

LUNG
VOLUME

Time-dependent
element of
tissue elastance
$(= (P_1 - P_2)/\text{tidal volume})$

Predominantly
airway
resistance
$\Delta P/\dot{V}$

Viscoelastic
tissue
resistance

Static elastance of
respiratory system
$(= P_2/\text{tidal volume})$

(d) Occluded airway method of determining components in (c)

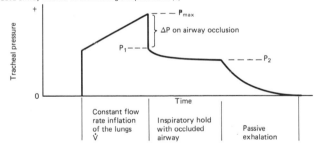

Tracheal pressure

P_{max}

ΔP on airway occlusion

P_1

P_2

Time

Constant flow
rate inflation
of the lungs
$\dot{V}$

Inspiratory hold
with occluded
airway

Passive
exhalation

Figure 4.6 (a) Simple pneumatic and electrical models of resistance and compliance (= capacitance). Time constant equals the product of compliance and resistance, and is not time dependent. (b) The models now have a second resistance and compliance (= capacitance), which imparts time dependence to the system. Time constant depends on the duration of inflation. (After Mount, 1955) (c) The spring and dashpot model of D'Angelo et al. (1989). Inflation of the lungs is represented by the bar moving upwards. The springs represent elastance (reciprocal of compliance) and the dashpots resistance. The spring and dashpot in series on the right confers time dependence which appears to be due to viscoelastic tissue resistance. (d) Effect of inflation followed by an end-inspiratory hold on tracheal pressure in a system comprising the components shown in (c).

Static compliance   = tidal volume/P_2
Dynamic compliance = tidal volume/P_1
Airway resistance   = $(P_{max} - P_1)$/inspiratory flow rate
The difference between P_1 and P_2 results from the behaviour of the spring and dashpot in series in (c), and appears to be caused by viscoelastic tissue resistance, which is thus the major cause of the difference between static and dynamic compliance (see text).

Figure 4.6a shows pneumatic and electrical analogues of a simple resistance/ capacitance (= compliance) network which provides an elementary but extremely useful model of the mechanical properties of the respiratory system. Note that in the pneumatic analogue, compression of gases according to Boyle's law is used to simulate compliance. In each analogue, time constant equals the product of resistance and capacitance (= compliance) (see Appendix F).

Figure 4.6b shows Mount's models which have secondary capacitances coupled by a second resistance (and with a different time constant). He produced convincing evidence that the additional component was uninfluenced by the viscosity or density of the gas inflating the lung and concluded that it represented tissue deformation which was time-dependent. Thus, with a very slow inflation, the additional capacitance (= compliance) becomes available, and this factor contributes to the excess of static over dynamic compliance.

Figure 4.6c shows the 'spring and dashpot model', described by D'Angelo et al. (1989), and to be compared with shock absorbers on motor cars. Dashpots here represent resistance, and springs elastance (reciprocal of compliance). Upward movement of the upper bar represents an increase in lung volume, caused by contraction of the inspiratory muscles or the application of inflation pressure as shown in the diagram. There is good evidence that, in humans, the left-hand dashpot represents predominantly airway resistance. The spring in the middle represents the static elastance of the respiratory system. On the right there is a spring and dashpot arranged in series. With a rapid change in lung volume, the spring is extended while the piston is more slowly rising in the dashpot. In due course (approx. 2–3 seconds) the spring returns to its original length and so ceases to exert any influence on pressure/volume relationships. This spring therefore represents the time-dependent element of elastance. While it is still under tension at end-inspiration, the combined effect of the two springs results in a high elastance of which the reciprocal is the dynamic compliance (see page 43). If inflation is held for a few seconds and movement of the piston through the right-hand dashpot is completed, the right-hand spring ceases to exert any tension and the total elastance is reduced to that caused by the spring in the middle. The reciprocal of this elastance is the static compliance which is therefore greater than the dynamic compliance.

The time-dependent change in compliance represented by the spring and dashpot in series could be due to many factors. D'Angelo et al. (1989) and Milic-Emili et al. (1990) advance reasons for believing that redistribution of gas (see Figure 3.6) makes only a negligible contribution in normal man and that the major component is due to viscoelastic flow resistance in tissue. These authors stress that the system shown in Figure 4.6c is only a simplified scheme to which many further components could be added; nevertheless the model accords well with experimental findings.

Figure 4.6d shows the changes in tracheal pressure during a constant flow rate of inflation of the lungs, followed by an inspiratory hold with airway occlusion. Immediately before occlusion, tracheal pressure reaches a value of P_{max} which is governed by both elastic and non-elastic resistance. Immediately after airway occlusion, the tracheal pressure falls to P_1, and $P_{max} - P_1$ is believed to reflect airway resistance according to the method of von Neergaard and Wirz (1927b) based on airway occlusion.

$$\text{Airway resistance} = (P_{max} - P_1)/\text{flow rate of inflation}$$

The decay of P_1 to P_2 represents the loss of the time-dependent element of tissue compliance (due to viscoelastic behaviour) and therefore represents the resistance afforded by tissue during inflation.

$$\text{Tissue resistance} = (P_1 - P_2)/\text{flow rate of inflation}$$

Note also that the static compliance equals the tidal volume divided by P_2, and the dynamic compliance equals the tidal volume divided by P_1.

Results in anaesthetized patients reported by D'Angelo et al. (1989) indicate that tissue resistance is of the order of half the total airway resistance, depending on lung volume and rate of inflation. The importance of this component has often been underestimated in the past and it is clearly important to distinguish airway resistance from that afforded by the total respiratory system (see methods section, later). Clearly there must be many pathological conditions, such as pulmonary fibrosis, oedema and the adult respiratory distress syndrome, in which the tissue component of resistance is greatly increased.

Inertance as a component of respiratory impedance

Respired gases, the lungs and the thoracic cage all have appreciable mass and therefore inertia, which must offer an impedance to change in direction of gas flow, analogous to electrical inductance. This component, termed inertance, is extremely difficult to measure, but inductance and inertance offer an impedance which increases with frequency. Therefore, although inertance is generally believed to be negligible at normal respiratory frequencies, it may become appreciable during high frequency ventilation (Dorbin, Lutchen and Jackson, 1988).

Increased airway resistance

Four grades of increased airway resistance may be identified.

Grade 1. Slight resistance is that against which the patient can indefinitely sustain a normal alveolar ventilation.

Grade 2. Moderate resistance is that against which a considerable increase in work of breathing is required to prevent a decrease in alveolar ventilation, with deterioration of arterial gas tensions. Patients vary in their response. Some increase their work of breathing, exhibiting obvious dyspnoea but maintaining normal arterial blood gas tensions. Others do not increase their work of breathing sufficiently to prevent an increase in arterial PCO_2 and a decrease in arterial PO_2. They may not appear dyspnoeic and their hypercapnia may be overlooked. In the case of chronic obstructive lung disease the former group are known as 'pink puffers' and the latter as 'blue bloaters' (page 423).

Grade 3. Severe resistance is that against which no patient is able to preserve his alveolar ventilation. Arterial PCO_2 is increased up to the level which interferes with the maintenance of consciousness, and there is is severe hypoxaemia unless the inspired gas is enriched with oxygen. Because of the very marked effect of changes in the inspired oxygen concentration, the increase in the arterial P_{CO_2} is the best indication of the gravity of the condition (see Chapter 21).

Grade 4. Respiratory obstruction may be defined as an increase in airway resistance which is incompatible with life if it is not relieved as a matter of urgency.

Provided patients remain calm, they can withstand surprisingly high resistance. However, once they are alarmed and start to struggle, they may enter a vicious cycle of raised oxygen consumption, increased ventilatory demand and increased work of breathing leading to a further increase in oxygen consumption which cannot be met.

Causes of increased airway resistance

As in obstruction of other biological systems, it is helpful to think in terms of conducting tubes being blocked by:

1. Material within the lumen.
2. Thickening or contraction of the wall of the passage.
3. Pressure from outside or suction within the air passage.

This classification applies to most of the locations considered below.

External apparatus

Even under ideal circumstances, tracheal tubes and tracheostomies have a greater resistance than the normal respiratory tract. Normally, this is of little consequence, but severe and potentially lethal increases of resistance can occur when these tubes are blocked, kinked or compressed.

The pharynx and larynx

The lumen may be blocked with foreign material such as gastric contents or blood. Laryngeal obstruction may result from carcinoma, diphtheria or oedema. The walls may contract as in laryngeal spasm, or the pharynx may collapse when inspiration is attempted against upstream resistance. The pharynx can withstand an inward transmural pressure gradient of only about 50 cmH$_2$O, and less in the sleeping or unconscious patient. Anatomical considerations are outlined in Chapter 2 and special consideration is given elsewhere to pharyngeal obstruction during sleep (page 334) and anaesthesia (page 384).

The lower respiratory tract

Intraluminar obstruction may result from oedema fluid, secretions, pus, tumour or foreign body. However, much the most important causes of increased resistance in the bronchial tree result from bronchospasm, mucosal oedema, flow-related collapse and volume-related collapse.

Bronchospasm

In this section it is convenient to include other aspects of bronchial hyper-reactivity, including mucosal oedema, mucus plugging and epithelial desquamation. Increased airway obstruction from these causes is a major feature of asthma and other conditions featuring airway hyper-reactivity as well as the response to various drugs, toxic substances and irritants. The section is summarized in Figure 4.7. Recent reviews include those by Hirshman and Bergman (1990) and Barnes (1991a, b).

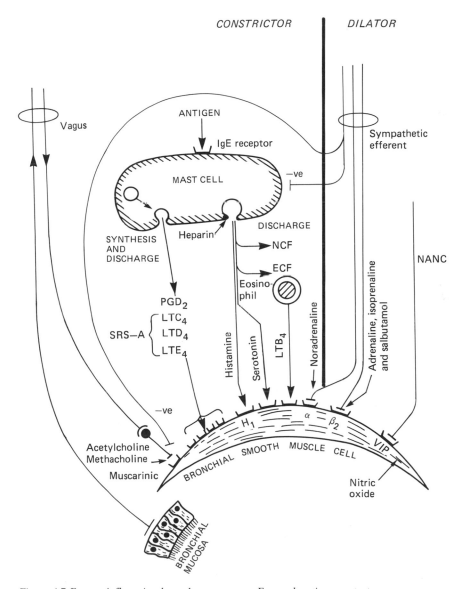

Figure 4.7 Factors influencing bronchomotor tone. For explanation, see text.

Parasympathetic system. This system is of major importance in the control of bronchomotor tone (see reviews by Boushey et al., 1980, and Barnes, 1991a). Afferents arise from receptors under the tight junctions of the bronchial epithelium and pass centrally in the vagus. The system responds to a great number of noxious stimuli, and histamine also acts directly on the parasympathetic afferents in addition to its direct action on airway smooth muscle. Efferent preganglionic fibres also run in the vagus to ganglia located in the walls of the small bronchi. Thence, short postganglionic fibres lead to nerve endings which release acetylcholine to act at muscarinic receptors in the bronchial smooth muscle. Stimulation of any part of the reflex arc results in bronchoconstriction, and some degree of resting tone is normally present. The muscarinic receptors can be stimulated with methacholine and blocked with atropine. The parasympathetic reflex arc plays a major part in the bronchoconstrictor response to inhaled irritants. Its action may be enhanced in a number of pathological states, including loss of bronchial epithelium (Vanhoutte, 1988), but is seldom primarily responsible for conditions of airway hypersensitivity.

Sympathetic system. In contrast to the parasympathetic system, the sympathetic system is poorly represented in the lung and not yet proven to be of major importance in man. Indeed it appears unlikely that there is any direct sympathetic innervation of the airway smooth muscle, although there may be an inhibitory effect on cholinergic neurotransmission in some species (Barnes, 1991a). Beta blockers may cause mild bronchoconstriction in healthy subjects, but there may be severe bronchoconstriction in some patients with asthma and bronchitis. In spite of the minimal significance of sympathetic innervation, bronchial smooth muscle has plentiful β_2-adrenergic receptors (Reinhardt, 1989), which are highly sensitive to adrenaline, a therapeutic standby for almost a century. Adrenaline also inhibits mediator release from mast cells. There are a few α-adrenergic receptors which are bronchoconstrictor but unlikely to be of much clinical significance.

Non-adrenergic non-cholinergic (NANC) system. The airways are provided with a third autonomic control which is neither adrenergic nor cholinergic. This is the only effective bronchodilator nervous pathway in man. The efferent fibres run in the vagus and pass to the smooth muscle of the airway where the neurotransmitters probably include vasoactive intestinal polypeptide (VIP) and peptide histamine methionine (PHM). Stimulation of NANC efferents or administration of VIP will both cause prolonged relaxation of bronchi. There is also a bronchoconstrictor part of the NANC system but its clinical significance is not yet clear.

Mast cells (type MC_T) are plentiful in the walls of airways and alveoli and also lie free in the lumen of the airways where they may be recovered by bronchial lavage (page 31). The surface of the mast cell contains a very large number of binding sites for the immunoglobulin IgE. Activation of the cell results from antigen bridging of only a small number of these receptors. The triggering mechanism is thus extremely sensitive. Activation may also be initiated by a wide range of compounds, including the complement fractions C3a, C4a and C5a, substance P, physical stimulation and many drugs and other organic molecules. In many respects basophils behave like mast cells, both in their activation and in the pattern of their response.

   The response of the mast cell to activation is probably mediated by an increase in cAMP and intracellular calcium ions (Robinson and Holgate, 1985). Within 30 seconds of activation, there is degranulation with discharge of a range of preformed mediators listed in Table 4.2. Histamine acts directly on H_1 receptors in the bronchial smooth muscle fibres to cause contraction, and on other H_1 receptors to increase vascular permeability. Histamine also acts on H_2 receptors to increase mucus secretion. In the granules, histamine is associated with heparin, which is probably not released but remains associated with the membrane of the mast cell. The granules also contain proteases, mainly tryptase, which detach epithelium from the basement membrane, resulting in desquamation and possibly activating an axonal reflex causing local release of substance P (Barnes, 1991a). Among other constituents are serotonin and chemotactic factors for both neutrophils and eosinophils.

The second major event after mast cell activation is the initiation of synthesis of arachidonic acid derivatives (page 315). The most important derivative of the cyclo-oxygenase pathway is prostaglandin PGD_2, which is a bronchoconstrictor, although its clinical significance is still not clear. The lipoxygenase pathway results in the formation of LTB_4 and the three sulphidopeptide leukotrienes, LTC_4, LTD_4 and LTE_4, formerly known collectively as slow-reacting substance (SRS-A), until the constituents were identified (Morris et al., 1980). The sulphidopeptide leukotrienes cause a slow but sustained contraction of bronchial muscle, which can be inhibited by indomethacin.

Neutrophils and eosinophils. Mast cell granules contain chemotactic factors for both these cells (NCF and ECF in Figure 4.7), and this effect is reinforced by histamine. Eosinophils are freely distributed alongside mast cells in the submucosa, and make their own contribution to bronchoconstriction, particularly by release of leukotrienes. Neutrophils contribute to proteolytic damage and may also release oxygen-derived free radicals (page 548).

Table 4.2 Mediators released from mast cells

Preformed mediators
Histamine
Heparin (probably not released)
Serotonin
Lysosomal enzymes:
  Tryptase
  Arylsulphatase
  Galactosidase
  Glucuronidase
  Hexosaminidase
  Carboxypeptidase
Neutrophil chemotactic factor
Eosinophil chemotactic factor

Mediators synthesized after activation
Prostaglandin D_2
Slow-reacting substance, comprising:
  LTC_4
  LTD_4
  LTE_4
Platelet-activating factor

Bronchial muscle receptors (see Figure 4.7). Muscarinic and β-adrenergic receptors may have directly competing effects on the activation of membrane-bound adenylate cyclase and thus the synthesis of cyclic adenosine monophosphate (cAMP) which controls the degree of relaxation of the bronchial smooth muscle (Hirshman and Bergman, 1990). Cyclic AMP is converted to 5′AMP by the enzyme phosphodiesterase which is inhibited by theophylline, the active component of the well tried preparation aminophylline. However, inhibition of phosphodiesterase occurs only at concentrations greatly in excess of those at which theophylline is an effective bronchodilator. Mackay, Baldwin and Tattersfield (1983) have presented evidence for believing that theophylline causes bronchodilatation by more than one mechanism, of which catecholamine release is one. In addition, it may block histamine release from the mast cell and it may also affect calcium entry. Furthermore, theophylline probably blocks the bronchoconstrictor effect of adenosine in asthmatics (Cushley, Tattersfield and Holgate, 1984) and also appears to drive the diaphragm, even in the long term (Murciano et al., 1984).

The sensitivity of the smooth muscle receptors to circulating substances and to drugs is probably of greater clinical relevance than their activation by the autonomic nervous system. The β2-adrenergic receptors are highly sensitive to adrenaline, salbutamol and isoprenaline but this is prevented by beta blockers. The muscarinic receptors are sensitive to methacholine and blocked by atropine. The H_1 receptor is sensitive to histamine but blocked by a wide range of antihistamines. Serotonin and α-adrenergic receptors are also bronchoconstrictor. The former can be blocked with ketanserin.

Physical and chemical factors. Physical factors capable of stimulating vagal afferents include mechanical stimulation of the upper air passages by laryngoscopy and the presence of foreign bodies in the trachea. Inhalation of cold air is a potent stimulus in the sensitive subject, and can be used as a provocation test (Heaton, Henderson and Costello, 1984). Inhalation of particulate matter or even an aerosol of water will cause bronchoconstriction. An aerosol of histamine produces part of its effect by stimulation of vagal afferents.

Many chemical stimuli result in bronchoconstriction. Gases include suphur dioxide, ozone and nitrogen dioxide. Liquids with a pH of less than about 2.5 provoke Mendelson's syndrome (1946), of which bronchoconstriction is a prominent feature in the early stages. Nitric oxide is a bronchodilator (W.M. Zapol, 1992, personal communication).

A great many drugs will activate the mast cell. This may follow sensitization of the cell but may also occur when a drug is first administered. Several drugs used by anaesthetists have this effect as a rare though frightening complication. Particular problems have occurred with *d*-tubocurarine, suxamethonium and Althesin (this last now withdrawn). In some cases the drug responsible for the reaction may be identified by skin testing, undertaken with care because this procedure may initiate bronchospasm. Splitting of complement C3 into C3a and C3b may be demonstrated soon after injection and the peripheral leucocyte count may decrease because of margination. The reaction usually occurs within a minute of administration and there is sometimes transient circulatory failure due to sudden vasodilatation. Alarming though this response may be, the mortality is apparently low.

Hyper-reactive airways. Asthmatics, some patients with chronic bronchitis and others exhibit exaggerated responses to a wide variety of the factors which can cause bronchoconstriction (Boushey et al., 1980). This may be demonstrated with provocation tests using histamine, methacholine or cold air. There is no single cause of the condition and possible factors include a reduction in resting airway calibre (considered below), increased sensitivity of the mast cell, loss of bronchial epithelium (Vanhoutte, 1988) and an increased responsiveness of the airway smooth muscle. Autonomic imbalance is now considered to be an uncommon cause. Hyper-reactive airways may be considered an essential precursor and feature of asthma.

Resting calibre of the airways. In the healthy subject, the small airways make only a small contribution to total airway resistance because their aggregate cross-sectional area increases to very large values after about the eighth generation (see Figure 2.4). However, they are the site of most of the important causes of obstruction in a range of pathological conditions, including chronic bronchitis, emphysema, bronchiectasis, cystic fibrosis, asthma and bronchiolitis (Macklem, 1971). These airways have been termed the 'quiet zone' because they must undergo a consider-able increase in their resistance before the change can be detected by tests of overall airway resistance which, in the healthy subject, is dominated by the resistance of the larger airways. Once their calibre is reduced sufficiently to exert a significant effect on airway resistance, further small changes in calibre have a major effect due to the relationship between flow and fourth or fifth power of the radius (pages 63 et seq.).

Flow-related airway collapse

All the airways can be compressed by reversal of the normal transmural pressure gradient to a sufficiently high level. The cartilaginous airways have considerable structural resistance to collapse but even the trachea may be compressed with an external pressure in the range 5−7 kPa (50−70 cmH$_2$0) which may result from neoplasm or haemorrhage. Airways beyond generation 11 have no structural rigidity (see Table 2.1) and rely instead on the traction on their walls from elastic recoil of the lung tissue in which they are embedded. They can be collapsed by a reversed transmural pressure gradient which is considerably less than that which closes the cartilaginous airways.

Reversal of the transmural pressure gradient may be caused by high levels of air flow during expiration (Figure 4.8). During all phases of normal breathing, the pressure in the lumen of the air passages should always remain well above the subatmospheric pressure in the thorax (Figure 4.8b and c), and the positive transmural pressure gradient ensures that the airways remain patent. During a maximal forced expiration (Figure 4.8d), the intrathoracic pressure will be well above atmospheric. This pressure will be transmitted to the alveoli which preserve their normal transmural pressure gradient due to their own elastic recoil. However, at high gas flow rates, the pressure drop down the airways is increased and there will be a point at which airway pressure equals the intrathoracic pressure. At that point (the equal pressure point) the smaller air passages are held open only by the elastic recoil of the lung parenchyma in which they are embedded or, if it occurs in the larger airways, by their structural rigidity. Downstream of the equal pressure point, the transmural pressure gradient is reversed and at some point may overcome the forces holding the airways open, resulting in airway collapse. This

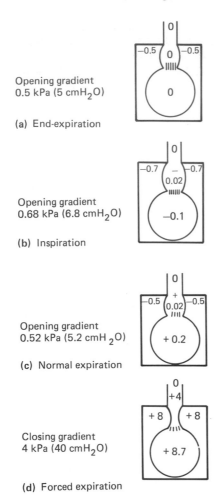

Opening gradient
0.5 kPa (5 cmH$_2$O)

(a) End-expiration

Opening gradient
0.68 kPa (6.8 cmH$_2$O)

(b) Inspiration

Opening gradient
0.52 kPa (5.2 cmH$_2$O)

(c) Normal expiration

Closing gradient
4 kPa (40 cmH$_2$O)

(d) Forced expiration

Figure 4.8 Typical transmural pressure gradients of the intrathoracic air passages under various conditions of ventilation. Note the pressure drop occurring in the smallest air passages, leading to a pressure difference between the alveoli and the larger air passages. (a) Static pressures at the end of expiration (upright, conscious subject). (b) Pressures at the middle of a normal inspiration. Note the increased favourable transmural pressure gradient of the intrathoracic airway. (c) Pressures at the middle of a normal expiration. Note the decreased (but still favourable) transmural pressure gradient of the intrathoracic airway. (d) Typical pressures during a forced expiration. Note the unfavourable transmural pressure gradient of the intrathoracic airway – leading to collapse.

effect is also influenced by lung volume (see below) and the equal pressure point moves progressively down towards the smaller airways as lung volume is decreased.

Flow-related collapse occurs in the larger bronchi during a forced expiration and limits the flow rate. It also accounts for the brassy note which is heard. During coughing, the reduction in calibre of the bronchi increases the linear velocity of air flow, thereby improving the scavenging of secretions from the walls of the air passages (Clarke, Jones and Oliver, 1970). Expiratory narrowing of the bronchi can often be seen at bronchoscopy.

Flow-related collapse of the smaller air passages occurs more easily in certain pathological states, particularly emphysema and asthma, in which it accounts for the phenomenon known as trapping. In emphysema, this is mainly due to destruction of lung parenchyma, resulting in loss of the elastic recoil which normally holds these airways open. In asthma, there is high bronchomotor tone and mucosal oedema which augments forces tending to collapse the air passages. Furthermore, the increased airway resistance augments the pressure drop along the airways, so facilitating the reversal of the transmural pressure gradient.

These effects are best demonstrated on a flow/volume plot. Figure 4.9 shows the normal relationship between lung volume on the abscissa and instantaneous respiratory flow rate on the ordinate. Time is not directly indicated. In part (a) of the Figure the small loop shows a normal tidal excursion above FRC and with air flow rate either side of zero. Arrows show the direction of the trace. At the end of a maximal expiration the black square indicates residual volume. The lower part of the large curve then shows the course of a maximal inspiration to TLC (black circle). There follow four expiratory curves, each with different expiratory effort and each attaining a different peak expiratory flow rate. Within limits, the greater the effort, the greater is the resultant peak flow rate. However, all the expiratory curves terminate in a final common pathway, which is independent of effort. In this part of the curves, the flow rate is limited by airway collapse and the maximal air flow rate is governed by the lung volume (abscissa). The greater the effort the greater the degree of airway collapse and the resultant gas flow rate remains the same. Figure 4.9b shows the importance of a maximal inspiration before measurement of peak expiratory flow rate.

Figure 4.10a shows the typical appearance of the flow/volume curve in a patient with obstructive airway disease. Residual volume is commonly increased, for reasons explained in the following section, and vital capacity is decreased. Inspiration is relatively normal but a forced expiration is characterized by a peak flow which is diminished in both rate and duration, giving rise to a typically boot-shaped curve. Various simple bedside tests indicate this state of affairs. The forced expiratory volume in 1 second ($FEV_{1.0}$) is the most reliable of the simple tests but the peak flow rate is more convenient. Large airway obstruction (due, for example, to carcinoma of the larynx) also results in a reduced $FEV_{1.0}$ and peak flow rate, the latter being relatively independent of lung volume (Figure 4.10b).

Volume-related airway collapse

Effect of lung volume on resistance to breathing. When the lung volume is reduced, there is a proportional reduction in the volume of all air-containing components, including the air passages. Thus, if other factors (such as bronchomotor tone) remain constant, airway resistance is an inverse function of lung volume (Figure 4.11) and there is a direct relationship between lung volume and the maximum expiratory flow rate which can be attained (see Figure 4.9). Furthermore, flow-related airway collapse (see above) occurs more readily at low lung volume when the initial airway calibre and the transmural pressure are less. Thus, in general, increasing lung volume will reduce airway resistance and helps to prevent trapping. This is most conveniently achieved by the application of continuous positive airway pressure (CPAP) to the spontaneously breathing subject or positive end-expiratory pressure (PEEP) to the paralysed ventilated patient (page 453). Many patients with obstructive airway disease acquire the habit of increasing their

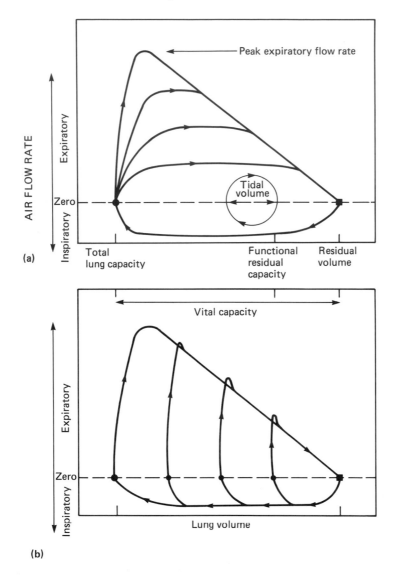

Figure 4.9 Normal flow/volume curves. Instantaneous air flow rate (ordinate) is plotted against lung volume (abscissa). (a) The normal tidal excursion is shown as the small loop. In addition, expirations from total lung capacity at four levels of expiratory effort are shown. Within limits, peak expiratory flow rate is dependent on effort but, during the latter part of expiration, all curves converge on an effort-independent section where flow rate is limited by airway collapse. (b) The effect of forced expirations from different lung volumes. The pips above the effort-independent section probably represent air expelled from collapsed airways.

expiratory resistance by exhaling through pursed lips. Alternatively, premature termination of expiration keeps the lung volume above FRC (auto-PEEP). Both manoeuvres have the effect of enhancing airway transmural pressure gradient and so reducing airway resistance and preventing trapping.

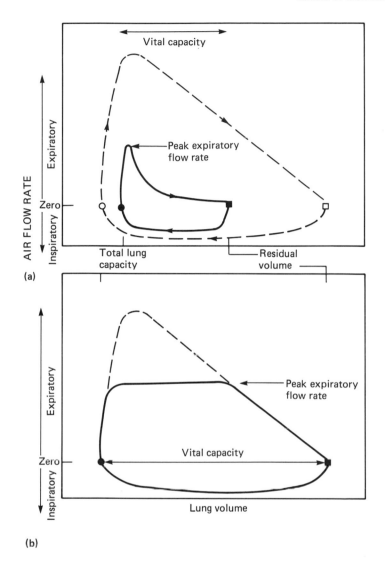

AIR FLOW RATE

Expiratory — Zero — Inspiratory

(a)

Vital capacity

Peak expiratory
flow rate

Total lung
capacity

Residual
volume

Expiratory — Zero — Inspiratory

Peak expiratory
flow rate

Vital capacity

Lung volume

(b)

Figure 4.10 (a) A flow/volume curve which is typical of a patient with obstructive airway disease of the smaller air passages. Note the diminished vital capacity and flattening of the effort-independent sector of the curve (compared with the broken curve which shows the normal). The expiratory curve is characteristically concave upwards. (b) The cut-off of high flow rates which is characteristic of upper airway obstruction (e.g. due to carcinoma of the larynx). The plateau is highly effort-dependent.

The closing capacity. In addition to the overall effect on airway resistance shown in Figure 4.11, there are most important regional differences. This is because the airways and alveoli in the dependent parts of the lungs are always smaller than those at the top of the lung, except at total lung capacity or at zero gravity when all are the same size. As the lung volume is reduced towards residual volume, there is a point at which dependent airways begin to close, and the lung volume at which

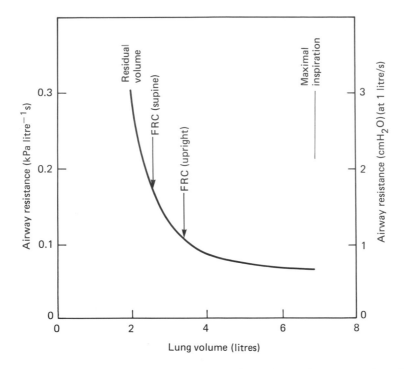

Figure 4.11 Airway resistance is a function of lung volume. This curve is a hyperbola and conductance (reciprocal of resistance) is linearly related to lung volume. (The curve is compounded of curves reported by Mead and Agostoni (1964) and Zamel et al. (1974).)

this occurs is known as the closing capacity (CC) (Figure 4.12). The alternative term, *closing volume* (CV), equals the closing capacity minus the residual volume (RV). Closing capacity increases with age and is less than FRC in young adults but increases to become equal to FRC at a mean age of 44 years in the supine position and 66 years in the upright position (see Figure 3.13). When the tidal range is wholly or partly within the closing capacity, some of the pulmonary blood flow will be distributed to inadequately ventilated parts of the lung. The closing capacity appears to be independent of body position but the FRC changes markedly with position (see Figure 3.11).

When the FRC is less than CC, some of the pulmonary blood flow will be distributed to alveoli with closed airways, usually in the dependent parts of the lungs. This will constitute a shunt (page 178), and must increase the alveolar/arterial PO_2 gradient. If the alveolar PO_2 remains the same then, the arterial PO_2 must be decreased. This can be seen when volunteers breathe below their FRC, and is particularly marked in older subjects who have a greater CC (Nunn et al., 1965b). Shunting of blood through areas of the lung with closed airways is an important cause of decreasing arterial PO_2 with increasing age (page 268) and changes of position (page 395). Reduction in FRC is closely related to the increased alveolar/arterial PO_2 gradient seen during anaesthesia (page 407).

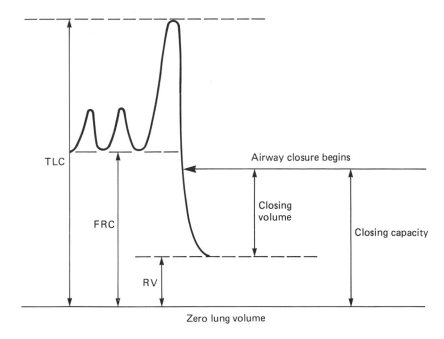

Figure 4.12 Spirogram to illustrate the relationship between closing volume and closing capacity. The example would be in a young adult with closing capacity less than functional residual capacity (FRC). RV, residual volume; TLC, total lung capacity.

Relationship between minute volume and instantaneous respiratory flow rates

The pressure required to overcome a particular resistance is related to the instantaneous gas flow rate. It is therefore important to appreciate the relationships between instantaneous flow rates and the minute volume of respiration which depends on the respiratory waveform (Figure 4.13). A triangular waveform gives the lowest ratio (2:1) between peak flow rates and minute volume. The sine waveform is approximated in spontaneous hyperventilation and the peak flow is π times the minute volume. In the more usual types of breathing the peak flow/minute volume ratios tend to be in the range 3.5:1–5:1.

Compensation for increased resistance to breathing

Inspiratory resistance

The normal response to increased inspiratory resistance is increased inspiratory muscle effort with little change in the FRC (Fink, Ngai and Holaday. 1958). Accessory muscles are brought into play according to the degree of resistance. Asthmatic patients show a remarkable capacity to compensate for increased resistance. Twenty patients in status asthmaticus studied by Palmer and Diament (1967) were found to have a mean arterial P_{CO_2} in the lower reaches of the normal

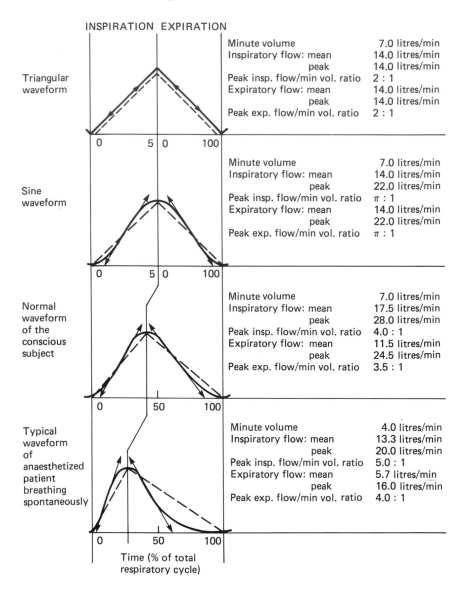

INSPIRATION EXPIRATION

Triangular waveform

Minute volume	7.0 litres/min
Inspiratory flow: mean	14.0 litres/min
peak	14.0 litres/min
Peak insp. flow/min vol. ratio	2 : 1
Expiratory flow: mean	14.0 litres/min
peak	14.0 litres/min
Peak exp. flow/min vol. ratio	2 : 1

0   5 0   100

Sine waveform

Minute volume	7.0 litres/min
Inspiratory flow: mean	14.0 litres/min
peak	22.0 litres/min
Peak insp. flow/min vol. ratio	π : 1
Expiratory flow: mean	14.0 litres/min
peak	22.0 litres/min
Peak exp. flow/min vol. ratio	π : 1

0   5 0   100

Normal waveform of the conscious subject

Minute volume	7.0 litres/min
Inspiratory flow: mean	17.5 litres/min
peak	28.0 litres/min
Peak insp. flow/min vol. ratio	4.0 : 1
Expiratory flow: mean	11.5 litres/min
peak	24.5 litres/min
Peak exp. flow/min vol. ratio	3.5 : 1

0   50   100

Typical waveform of anaesthetized patient breathing spontaneously

Minute volume	4.0 litres/min
Inspiratory flow: mean	13.3 litres/min
peak	20.0 litres/min
Peak insp. flow/min vol. ratio	5.0 : 1
Expiratory flow: mean	5.7 litres/min
peak	16.0 litres/min
Peak exp. flow/min vol. ratio	4.0 : 1

0   50   100

Time (% of total
respiratory cycle)

Figure 4.13 Respiratory waveforms showing the relationship between minute volume, mean flow rates (broken lines) and peak flow rates (indicated by arrows). The normal waveform of the conscious subject is taken from Cain and Otis (1949). The waveform of the anaesthetized patient is derived from 44 spirograms of patients during surgery.

range. An increased arterial PCO_2 because of increased airway resistance is always serious.

Mechanisms of compensation. There are two principal mechanisms of compensation for high inspiratory resistance. The first operates immediately and even during the first breath in which resistance is applied. It seems probable that the muscle spindles indicate that the inspiratory muscles have failed to shorten by the intended amount and their afferent discharge then augments the activity in the motor neuron pool of the anterior horn. This is the typical servo operation of the spindle system with which the intercostal muscles are richly endowed. The conscious subject can detect very small increments in inspiratory resistance (Campbell et al., 1961).

With moderate to severe increases in resistance, a second compensatory mechanism develops over about 90 seconds and overacts for a similar period when the resistance is removed (Nunn and Ezi-Ashi, 1961). The time course suggests that this mechanism is driven by elevation of arterial PCO_2. A similar two-phase response has been demonstrated in dogs (Bendixen and Bunker, 1962).

Expiratory resistance

Expiration against 1 kPa (10 cmH$_2$O) does not usually result in activation of the expiratory muscles in conscious or anaesthetized subjects. The additional work to overcome this resistance is, in fact, performed by the inspiratory muscles. The subject augments his inspiratory force until he achieves a lung volume at which the additional elastic recoil is sufficient to overcome the expiratory resistance (Campbell, 1957). The pattern of response in the anaesthetized patient (Figure 4.14) was demonstrated by Campbell, Howell and Peckett (1957) and Nunn and Ezi-Ashi (1961). The response is clearly counter to what might be expected from application of the Hering–Breuer reflex. The mechanism for resetting the FRC at a higher level probably requires accommodation of the intrafusal fibres of the spindles to allow for an altered length of diaphragmatic muscle fibres due to the obstructed

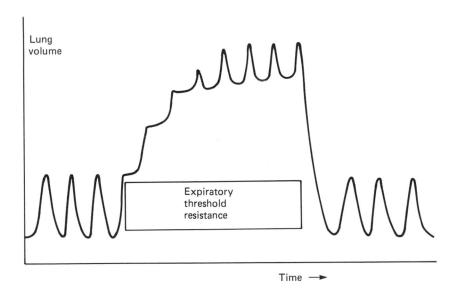

Lung volume

Expiratory threshold resistance

Time ⟶

Figure 4.14 Spirogram showing response of an anaesthetized patient to the sudden imposition of an expiratory threshold resistor. Note that there is immediate augmentation of the force of contraction of the inspiratory muscles. This continues with successive breaths until the elastic recoil is sufficient to overcome the expiratory resistor (Nunn and Ezi-Ashi, 1961).

expiration. This would reset the developed inspiratory tension in accord with the increased FRC (Nunn and Ezi-Ashi, 1961). The conscious subject normally uses his expiratory muscles to overcome expiratory pressures in excess of about 1 kPa (10 cmH$_2$O).

Studies of the response of the conscious subject to external resistance were reported by Cain and Otis (1949), McIlroy et al. (1956) and Zechman, Hall and Hull (1957). Immediate effects of excessive resistance may be less important than the long-term response of the patient. In common with other muscles, the respiratory muscles can become fatigued (see reviews by Moxham, 1984 and 1990). This is a major factor in the onset of respiratory failure (page 126).

It is difficult to predict the ventilatory response of patients with chronic obstructive airway disease. Some allow their arterial PCO$_2$ to increase (blue bloaters) while other strive to maintain a normal PCO$_2$ (pink puffers). In a study of patients presenting for surgery with FEV$_{1.0}$ values of less than 1 litre, there was no correlation between FEV$_{1.0}$ and arterial PCO$_2$, which was normal in many patients with an FEV$_{1.0}$ of less than 0.5 litre (Nunn et al., 1988).

Principles of measurement of flow resistance

Flow resistance is determined by the simultaneous measurement of gas flow rate and the driving pressure gradient. In the case of the respiratory tract, the difficulty centres around the measurement of alveolar pressure. Methods of presentation of results are discussed earlier in this chapter.

Apparatus resistance

Measurement of driving pressure during continuous flow of gas offers the simplest method and the approach shown in Figure 4.1 will usually suffice. Reciprocating gas flow has the advantage of testing under actual conditions of use and a sine wave pump may be used in conjunction with manometers having a rapid response.

Nasal resistance

Similar principles may be used for measuring nasal resistance. The subject breathes through his nose with his mouth closed round a tube leading to a manometer. Either continuous or reciprocating flow may be used, powered either by the subject himself or by some external device (Seebohm and Hamilton, 1958; Butler, 1960).

Airway and pulmonary resistance

Simultaneous measurement of air flow rate and intrathoracic-to-mouth pressure gradient. In Chapter 3 it was shown how simultaneous measurement of tidal volume and intrathoracic pressure yielded the dynamic compliance of the lung (see Figure 3.15). For this purpose, pressures were selected at the times of zero air flow when pressures were uninfluenced by air flow resistance. The same apparatus may be employed for the determination of flow resistance by subtracting the pressure component used in overcoming elastic forces (Figure 4.15). The shaded areas in the pressure trace indicate the components of the pressure required to overcome flow resistance and these may be related to the concurrent gas flow rates.

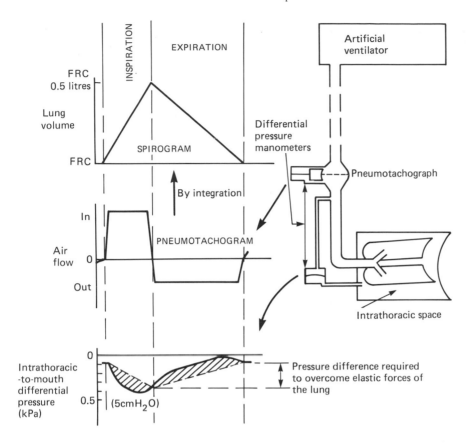

Figure 4.15 The measurement of pulmonary resistance and dynamic compliance by simultaneous measurement of air flow and intrathoracic-to-mouth differential pressure (von Neergaard and Wirz, 1927b). The spirogram is conveniently obtained by integration of the pneumotachogram. In the pressure trace, the dotted line shows the pressure changes which would be expected in a hypothetical patient with no pulmonary resistance. Compliance is derived as shown in Figure 3.15. Pulmonary resistance is derived as the difference between the measured pressure differential and that which is required for elastic forces (shaded area) compared with the flow rate shown in the pneumotachogram. Note that the pneumotachogram is a much more sensitive indicator of the no-flow points than the spirogram.

Alternatively, the intrathoracic-to-mouth pressure gradient and respired volume may be displayed as X and Y coordinates of a loop. Figure 3.15 showed how dynamic compliance could be derived from the no-flow points of such a loop. The area of the loop is a function of the work performed against flow resistance.

The interrupter technique. A single manometer may be used to measure both mouth and alveolar pressure if the air passages distal to the manometer are momentarily interrupted with a shutter. The method is based on the assumption that, while the airway is interrupted, the mouth pressure comes to equal the alveolar pressure. Resistance is then determined from the relationship between flow rate (measured before interruption) and the pressure difference between mouth (measured before interruption) and alveoli (measured during interruption). This measures airway resistance and excludes tissue resistance (D'Angelo et al., 1989). Both this and the preceding methods were first described by von Neergaard and Wirz (1927b).

Oscillating air flow. In this technique, a high frequency oscillating air flow is applied to the airways, with measurement of the resultant pressure and air flow changes. By application of alternating current theory it is possible to derive a continuous measurement of airway resistance (Goldman et al., 1970; Hyatt et al., 1970). The technique has been developed to function during a vital capacity manoeuvre and so to display airway resistance as a function of lung volume and derive specific airway conductance (Lehane, Jordan and Jones, 1980). More detailed information can be obtained by spectral analysis of random noise pressure waves (Michaelson, Grassman and Peters, 1975).

The body plethysmograph. During inspiration, alveolar pressure falls below ambient as a function of airway resistance and the alveolar gas expands in accord with Boyle's law. The increased displacement of the body is then recorded as an increase in pressure in the body plethysmograph. Airway (as opposed to respiratory) resistance may be derived directly from measurements of air flow and pressure changes (DuBois, Botelho and Comroe, 1956). The method is non-invasive and FRC may be measured at the same time.

Interrupted inflation. D'Angelo et al. (1989) and Milic-Emili, Robatto and Bates (1990) have redirected attention to this method, first described in 1965 by Don and Robson and described above (see Figure 4.6d). It has the advantage of distinguishing between airway and tissue resistance.

Analysis of the passive spirogram. Also suitable for the paralysed patient is the technique shown in Figure 3.14 and described by Nims, Connor and Comroe (1955). On page 57 it is explained how this technique is used to measure the static compliance. The time constant of expiration (easily derived) divided by the compliance will indicate the total resistance to expiration (see Appendix F).

Tests of ventilatory capacity as a measure of airway resistance

Formal measurement of airway resistance is seldom undertaken in the clinical situation, where the airway resistance is usually inferred from measurement of ventilatory capacity, which is most commonly reduced as a result of increased airway resistance. It must, however, be remembered that there are many other causes of reduction of ventilatory capacity which are nothing to do with airway resistance. Tests of ventilatory capacity and their interpretation are described at the end of Chapter 6.

Measurement of closing capacity

This is perhaps the most convenient place to outline the measurement of closing capacity. This is the maximal lung volume at which airway closure can be detected in the dependent parts of the lungs (page 79). The measurement is made during expiration and is based on having different concentrations of a tracer gas in the upper and lower parts of the lung. This may be achieved by inspiration of a bolus of tracer gas at the commencement of an inspiration from residual volume, at which

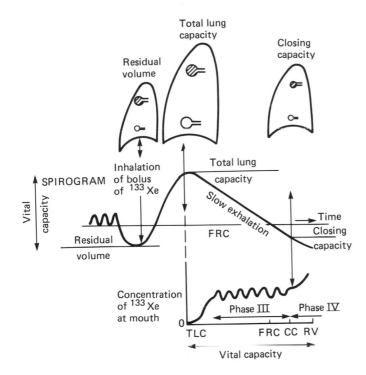

Figure 4.16 Measurement of closing capacity by the use of a tracer gas such as ^{133}Xe. The bolus of tracer gas is inhaled near residual volume and, due to airway closure, is distributed only to those alveoli whose air passages are still open (shown shaded in the diagram). During expiration, the concentration of the tracer gas becomes constant after the dead space is washed out. This plateau (phase III) gives way to a rising concentration of tracer gas (phase IV) when there is closure of airways leading to alveoli which did not receive the tracer gas.

time airways are closed in the dependent part of the lungs (Figure 4.16). The tracer gas will then be preferentially distributed to the upper parts of the lungs. After a maximal inspiration to total lung capacity, the patient slowly exhales while the concentration of the tracer gas is measured at the mouth. When lung volume reaches the closing capacity and airways begin to close in the dependent parts, the concentration of the tracer gas will rise (phase IV) above the alveolar plateau (phase III). Suitable tracers are ^{133}Xe (Dollfuss, Milic-Emili and Bates, 1967), 100% oxygen measured as a fall in nitrogen concentration (Anthonisen et al., 1969) or sulphur hexafluoride enhancement of the nitrogen method (Newberg and Jones, 1974). The technique can be undertaken in the conscious subject who performs the ventilatory manoeuvres spontaneously or in the paralysed subject in whom ventilation is artificially controlled.

Chapter 5

Control of breathing

Breathing results from rhythmic contraction and relaxation of striated muscles under automatic control. The subject is normally unaware of this action, which may, within limits, be over-ridden by voluntary cortical control or interrupted by swallowing and involuntary non-rhythmic acts such as sneezing or coughing. There is progressive realization of the immense complexity of the control system, with its automatic ability to adapt the action of the respiratory muscles to the changing demands of posture, speech, voluntary movement, exercise and innumerable other circumstances which alter the respiratory requirement or influence the performance of the respiratory muscles.

This chapter starts with a discussion of the origin of the rhythmicity of breathing in the neurons of the hindbrain which appear to subserve respiration ('respiratory centres'). The efferent path is then traced to the muscles of respiration with an account of the peripheral control systems. The next section is concerned with the chemical control of respiration and this is followed by a discussion of the influence of respiratory reflexes and mechanical factors.

The origin of the respiratory rhythm
(see review by von Euler, 1991)

In 1812, Legallois published reports showing that rhythmic inspiratory movements persisted after removal of the cerebellum and all parts of the brain above the medulla, but ceased when the medulla was removed. During the next 150 years a long series of distinguished investigators carried out more detailed localization of the neurons concerned in the control of respiration and studied their interaction. Marckwald and Kronecker (1880) differentiated between inspiratory and expiratory neurons, and Ramon y Cajal, as early as 1909, concluded from histological studies that the respiratory rhythm was generated in the nucleus of the tractus solitarius in the medulla. This view, which is so close to modern thinking, was eclipsed in the next few decades (see review by Mitchell and Berger, 1981).

Lumsden (1923a–d) described and named the pneumotaxic and apneustic pontine centres. He also advanced the concept of an internal feedback mechanism by which a tonic inspiration was inhibited at the end of inspiration by discharge of the pneumotaxic centre acting through the expiratory centre, the whole loop functioning as an internal pacemaker. These observations were based on ablation experiments which are now known to result in rather unpredictable functional loss in some remaining parts of the brain, due to trauma and interference with blood supply. Pitts, Magoun and Ranson (1939a) described the anatomical localization of the overlapping inspiratory and expiratory neurons in the medulla, dispelling the concept of discrete 'inspiratory and expiratory centres'. In a later paper (1939b), they advanced the concept of the inhibition of one centre by another, or by vagal afferents from stretch sensors in the lungs. In a third paper Pitts, Magoun and Ranson (1939c) concluded that respiratory rhythmicity is caused by two separate and alternative feedback loops, one based on the pneumotaxic centre and the other on the vagal reflex sensitive to lung stretch, the two mechanisms being similar and mutually replaceable. When removal of the pneumotaxic areas was combined with bilateral vagotomy, a sustained inspiration, or apneusis, was found to result. The suggestion of self-limitation of inspiration by vagal impulses arising from inflation of the lung was not new and had first been made in the classic studies of Breuer (1868), previously reported by his chief, Professor Hering (1868).

The next landmark in the long series of studies of the interaction of the various respiratory centres was the paper by Wang, Ngai and Frumin (1957), stressing the pontine apneustic centre as the site of the inspiratory tonicity and also as the site of rhythmic inhibition by both the pneumotaxic centre and the vagus. These concepts were widely accepted and taught for many years until challenged on the basis of new relatively non-traumatic experimental techniques, including recordings from single neurons and the production of focal cold lesions.

Eupnoea was demonstrated with an isolated medulla by Wang, Ngai and Frumin (1957) and following bilateral destruction of the pneumotaxic centre in vagotomized cat (St John, Glasser and King, 1972; Gautier and Bertrand, 1975). Further evidence for a medullary origin of the respiratory rhythm is provided by the studies of Hoff and Breckenridge (1949), Salmoiraghi and Burns (1960) and Salmoiraghi (1963). Guz et al. (1964, 1966b) demonstrated that bilateral vagal block had no obvious effect upon the pattern of respiration in man. There is now consensus that the respiratory rhythm can be generated within the medulla without input from the lungs or elsewhere in the body (Mitchell and Berger, 1981; Berger and Hornbein, 1987; von Euler, 1991). The new concept of the central role of the medulla is illustrated in the schematic diagram shown in Figure 5.1.

It is no longer sufficient to consider the generation of the respiratory rhythm to be simply oscillating networks of uniform populations of inspiratory and expiratory neurons. The respiratory pattern depends on a complex interaction of at least six types of neurons with identifiable firing patterns (von Euler, 1991). These include early inspiratory neurons, inspiratory ramp neurons, late-onset inspiratory interneurons (putative 'off-switch neurons'), early expiratory neurons, early peak whole expiratory neurons, expiratory ramp neurons. Furthermore, many such rhythm-generating networks are represented in parallel, so it is difficult to destroy the respiratory rhythm by isolated or electrical cold lesions (Speck and Beck, 1989). The system is thus very robust. The resultant respiratory cycle may be divided into three phases, as follows.

Inspiratory phase. A sudden onset is followed by ramp increase in motor discharge to the inspiratory muscles, including the pharyngeal dilator muscles. Pharyngeal dilator muscles start to contract shortly before the start of inspiration.

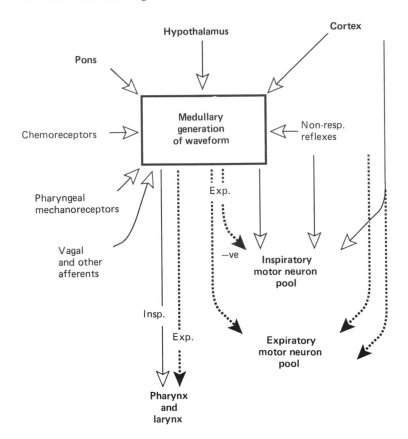

Figure 5.1 Afferent and efferent connections to and from the medullary generator of the respiratory waveform. The broken lines are expiratory pathways, but the expiratory motor neuron pool normally remains silent during quiet breathing. See text for details.

Post-inspiratory or expiratory phase I. This is characterized by declining discharge of the motor discharge to the inspiratory muscles, with a gradual let down of tone, resulting in an initial braking of the expiratory gas flow rate (page 120). This does not occur in anaesthesia or during artificial ventilation of the paralysed patient when the expiratory waveform is exponential.

Expiratory phase II. The inspiratory muscles are now silent. During quiet breathing in the supine position, the expiratory muscles are also silent but they may be recruited under various circumstances including a minute volume in excess of about 40 l/min (page 121).

Anatomical location of the medullary neurons

Respiratory neurons in the medulla are mainly concentrated in two groups, the ventral and dorsal respiratory groups, which have numerous interconnections (Mitchell and Berger, 1981; von Euler, 1991).

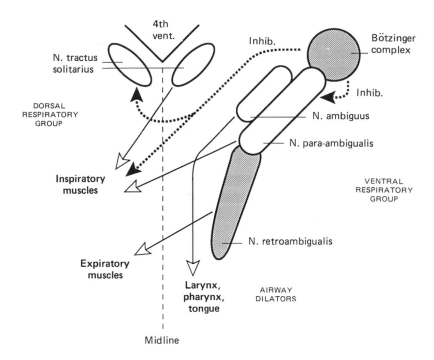

Figure 5.2 Dorsal view of the organization of the respiratory neurons in the medulla. The dorsal respiratory group (nucleus tractus solitarius) is shown on both sides. For clarity, the ventral respiratory group (Bötzinger complex, nucleus ambiguus, nucleus para-ambigualis and nucleus retroambigualis) is shown only on the right side. Areas with predominantly expiratory activity are shaded. Fibres which decussate are shown crossing the midline. Inspiration is jointly controlled by the nucleus tractus solitarius and the nucleus para-ambigualis. The broken lines are expiratory pathways which inhibit inspiratory neurons. Expiratory muscles (controlled by the nucleus retroambigualis) normally remain silent during quiet breathing. See text for details.

The dorsal respiratory group lies in close relation to the tractus solitarius, where visceral afferents from cranial nerves IX and X terminate (Figure 5.2). It is predominantly composed of inspiratory neurons with upper motor neurons passing to the inspiratory anterior horn cells of the opposite side. The dorsal group is primarily concerned with timing of the respiratory cycle.

The ventral respiratory group comprises four nuclei. The most caudal is the nucleus retroambigualis, which is predominantly expiratory with upper motor neurons passing to the expiratory muscles of the other side. The nucleus ambiguus controls the dilator functions of larynx, pharynx and tongue. The nucleus para-ambigualis (lying parallel to it) is mainly inspiratory and controls the force of contraction of the inspiratory muscles of the opposite side. The Bötzinger complex (within the nucleus retrofacialis) has widespread expiratory functions.

Role of the pons

There is no doubt of the existence of pontine neurons firing in synchrony with different phases of respiration, but this is not to say that they are essential for the generation of the respiratory rhythm. Bertrand, Hugelin and Vibert (1974) described discrete temporal and spatial distributions of three types of neurons in the pneumotaxic region. According to their firing patterns the three types were defined as inspiratory, expiratory and phase-spanning. Although the pontine pneumotaxic centre is no longer thought to be the dominant controller of the respiratory rhythm, the pattern of firing of these neurons suggests a role in modification and fine control of the respiratory rhythm as, for example, in setting the lung volume at which inspiration is terminated.

Influence of volition and wakefulness

Breathing can be voluntarily interrupted and the pattern of respiratory movements altered within limits determined mainly by changes in arterial blood gas tensions. This is essential for such acts as speech, singing, sniffing, coughing, expulsive efforts and the performance of tests of ventilatory function. There are numerous reports of alteration in the pattern of breathing when various cortical areas are stimulated (Berger and Hornbein, 1987). In addition to volitional changes in the pattern of breathing, there are numerous suprapontine reflex interferences with respiration such as sneezing, swallowing and reflex coughing. There are usually minor changes in the respiratory pattern when subjects focus their attendance on their breathing as when physiological mouthpieces or breathing masks are used (Western and Patrick, 1988).

Douglas and Haldane (1909) observed periods of apnoea following voluntary hyperventilation by subjects aware of the classic paper of Haldane and Priestley (1905) describing the major role of carbon dioxide in the regulation of breathing. The apnoea was ascribed to reduction of P_{CO_2} below the apnoeic threshold (see below). However, Fink (1961) found that 13 naive conscious subjects all continued to breathe rhythmically during recovery from reduction of end-expiratory P_{CO_2} to 3.3 kPa (25 mmHg) or less. Bainton and Mitchell (1965) and Moser, Rhodes and Kwaan (1965) observed apnoea after hyperventilation in some, but not all, of their conscious subjects. Conscious drive may well maintain breathing in those subjects not showing post-hyperventilation apnoea, since apnoea may be consistently produced by moderate hypocapnia in anaesthetized patients (Hanks, Ngai and Fink, 1961).

Ondine's curse and primary alveolar hypoventilation

Severinghaus and Mitchell (1962) described three patients who exhibited long periods of apnoea, even when awake, but who breathed on command. They termed the condition 'Ondine's curse' from its first description in German legend. The water nymph, Ondine, having been jilted by her mortal husband, took from him all automatic functions, requiring him to remember to breathe. When he finally fell asleep he died. The condition is seen in patients with primary alveolar hypoventilation occurring as a feature of many different diseases, including chronic poliomyelitis and the pickwickian syndrome, although upper airway obstruction is now recognized as a more important cause of apnoea in these patients (page 334). Characteristics include a raised P_{CO_2} in the absence of pulmonary pathology, a flat CO_2/ventilation response curve and periods of apnoea which may be central or obstructive. A similar condition is also produced by overdosage with opiates. The influence of sleep is discussed further in Chapter 14.

Motor pathways concerned in breathing

Three groups of upper motor neurons converge on the anterior horn cells from which arise the lower motor neurons supplying the respiratory muscles (see Figure 6.1). Integration of respiratory control takes place at the anterior horn cell (Mitchell and Berger, 1975, 1981) as well as at the pontomedullary level (Berger and Hornbein, 1987).

The first group of upper motor neurons is from the dorsal and ventral respiratory groups of the medulla (see Figure 5.1), and are mainly concerned with involuntary rhythmic breathing. This group descends in the ventrolateral quadrant of the cord. The second group is concerned with voluntary control of breathing (speech, respiratory gymnastics, etc.) and lies in the dorsolateral and ventrolateral quadrants of the cord. The third group is concerned with involuntary non-rhythmic respiratory control (swallowing, cough, hiccup, etc.). This group does not occupy a single compact location in the cord but appears to be separate from the tracts concerned with rhythmic input to the diaphragm (Newsom-Davis and Plum, 1972). Selective cordotomies can interfere with rhythmic but not voluntary respiration, particularly during sleep, while Newsom-Davis (1974) described a patient with partial transverse cervical myelitis who had normal rhythmic breathing but could not voluntarily alter his ventilation.

The respiratory muscles, in common with other skeletal muscles, have their tension controlled by a servo mechanism mediated by muscle spindles. They appear to play a more important role in the intercostal muscles than in the diaphragm (Corda, von Euler and Lennerstrand, 1965). There was, in fact, some doubt about the existence of spindles in the human diaphragm until a small number were demonstrated by Muller et al. (1979). Their function is largely inferred from knowledge of their well established role in other skeletal muscles not concerned with respiration (Granit, 1955).

Two types of cell can be distinguished in the motor neuron pool of the anterior horn cell. The alpha motor neuron has a thick efferent fibre (12–20 μm diameter) and passes in the ventral root directly to the neuromuscular junction of the muscle fibre (Figure 5.3). The gamma motor neuron has a thin efferent fibre (2–8 μm) which also passes in the ventral root, but terminates in the intrafusal fibres of the muscle spindle. Contraction of the intrafusal fibres alone (without overall shortening of the muscle) increases the tension in the central part of the spindle (the nuclear bag), causing stimulation of the annulospiral endings. Impulses so generated are then transmitted via fibres which lie in the dorsal root to reach the anterior horn where they have an excitatory effect on the alpha motor neurons. It will be seen that an efferent impulse transmitted by the gamma system may cause reflex contraction of the main muscle mass by means of an arc through the annulospiral afferent and the alpha motor neuron. Thus contraction of the whole muscle may be controlled entirely by efferents travelling in the gamma fibres and this has been suggested in relation to breathing (Robson, 1967).

Alternatively, muscle contraction may in the first instance result from discharge of the alpha and gamma motor neurons. If the shortening of the muscle is unopposed, main (extrafusal) and intrafusal fibres will contract together and the tension in the nuclear bag of the spindle will be unchanged. If, however, the shortening of the muscle is opposed, the intrafusal fibres will shorten more than the extrafusal fibres, causing the nuclear bag to be stretched (Figure 5.3b). The consequent stimulation of the annulospiral endings results in afferents which raise

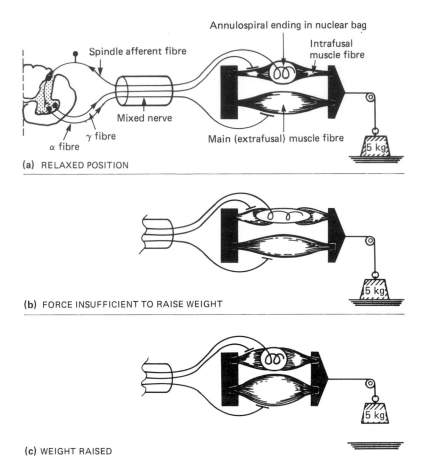

(a) RELAXED POSITION

(b) FORCE INSUFFICIENT TO RAISE WEIGHT

(c) WEIGHT RAISED

Figure 5.3 Diagrammatic representation of the servo mechanism mediated by the muscle spindles. (a) The resting state with muscle and intrafusal fibres of spindle relaxed. (b) The muscle is attempting to lift the weight following discharge of both alpha and gamma systems. The force developed by the muscle is insufficient: the weight is not lifted and the muscle cannot shorten. However, the intrafusal fibres are able to shorten and stretch the annulospiral endings in the nuclear bag of the spingle. Afferent discharge causes increased excitation of the motor neuron pool in the anterior horn. (c) Alpha discharge is augmented and the weight is finally lifted by the more powerful contraction of the muscle. When the weight is lifted, the tension on the nuclear bag is relieved and the afferent discharge from the spingle ceases. This series of diagrams relates to the lifting of a weight but it is thought that similar action of spindles is brought into play when the inspiratory muscles contract against augmented airway resistance.

the excitatory state of the motor neurons, causing the main muscle fibres to increase their tension until the resistance is overcome, allowing the muscle to shorten and the tension in the nuclear bag of the spindle to be reduced (Figure 5.3c).

By this mechanism, fine control of muscle contraction is possible. The message from the upper motor neuron is in the form: 'muscles should contract with whatever force may be found necessary to effect such and such a shortening', and not simply: 'muscles should contract with such and such a force'. The former message is typical of input into a servo system and far more satisfactory when the load is not known in advance. Relay to cortical levels is probably the mechanism of detection of external changes in compliance (Campbell et al., 1961) or resistance (Bennett et al., 1962). Campbell and Howell (1962) presented evidence for believing that a spindle servo system governs the action of the respiratory muscles.

The use of the servo loop implies that the action of the respiratory muscles must be dependent upon the integrity of the dorsal roots which contain the efferents from the annulospiral endings. This appears to be the case, and dorsal root section at the appropriate level causes temporary paralysis of the respiratory muscles in man (Nathan and Sears, 1960).

The spindle servo mechanism provides an excellent mechanism for rapid response to sudden changes in airway resistance. The nature and magnitude of the response of the inspiratory muscles to added resistance to breathing is described in Chapter 4 (page 83), and the immediate response is easily explicable in terms of muscle spindles.

Chemical control of breathing

Pflüger in his classic paper of 1868 gave the first convincing evidence that breathing could be stimulated either by a reduction of oxygen content or by an increase of carbon dioxide content of the arterial blood. However, the importance of the role of carbon dioxide was not fully established until the work of Haldane and Priestley (1905). In one paper they presented their technique for sampling alveolar gas, showed the constancy of the alveolar PCO_2 under a wide range of circumstances, and also demonstrated the great sensitivity of ventilation to small changes in alveolar PCO_2.

Until 1926 it was thought that changes in the chemical composition of the blood influenced ventilation solely by direct action on the respiratory centre, which was presumed to be sensitive to these influences although direct experimental proof was lacking. However, between 1926 and 1930 there occurred a major revision following the histological studies of de Castro (1926) which led him to suggest a chemoreceptor function for the carotid bodies. These receptors were found to be sensitive to hypoxia and the role of the carotid bodies in the control of breathing was clearly established (Heymans and Heymans, 1927; Heymans, Bouckaert and Dautrebande, 1930). A similar function for the aortic bodies was reported in 1939 by Comroe, and C. Heymans received a Nobel prize for his work in 1938.

Division of the afferent nerves from the peripheral chemoreceptors does not greatly diminish the ventilatory response to elevation of the arterial PCO_2 and until recently it was generally believed that the respiratory centre itself was sensitive to carbon dioxide. However, it is now known that the central chemoreceptors, as they have come to be called, are actually separate from the respiratory neurons of the medulla although located only a short distance away.

An overall view of the chemical control of breathing is shown schematically in Figure 5.4. The plan of this section of the chapter is first to give a separate account of the peripheral and central chemoreceptors and then to consider the quantitative aspects of their function in combination.

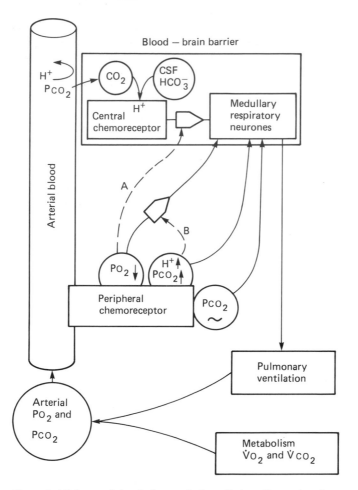

Figure 5.4 Scheme of chemical control of ventilation. For explanation, see text.

The peripheral chemoreceptors
(reviews by McDonald, 1981; McQueen and Pallot, 1983; Lahiri, 1991)

The peripheral chemoreceptors are fast-responding monitors of the arterial blood, responding to a fall in PO_2, a rise in PCO_2 or H^+ concentration, or a fall in their perfusion rate. The bilaterally paired carotid bodies, rather than the aortic bodies, are almost exclusively responsible for the respiratory response. Their structure/function relationships have been exhaustively reviewed by McDonald (1981). Each is only about 6 mm³ in volume and they are located close to the bifurcation of the common carotid artery. The carotid bodies undergo hypertrophy and hyperplasia under conditions of chronic hypoxia and are usually lost in the operation of carotid endarterectomy.

Histology. The carotid bodies contain large sinusoids with a very high rate of perfusion which is about ten times the level which would be proportional to their metabolic rate, which is itself very high (Fidone et al., 1991). Therefore the arterial/venous PO_2 difference is small. This accords with their role as a sensor of arterial blood gas tensions, and their rapid response which is within the range 1–3 seconds (Ponte and Purves, 1974).

At the cellular level, the main feature is the glomus or type 1 cell, which is in synaptic contact with nerve endings derived from an axon with its cell body in the petrosal ganglion of the glossopharyngeal nerve (Figure 5.5). These endings are mainly postsynaptic to the glomus cell. Type I cells are partly encircled by type II or sheath cells whose function is still obscure. Efferent nerves, which are known to modulate receptor afferent discharge, include preganglionic sympathetic fibres from the superior cervical ganglion, amounting to 5% of the nerve endings on the glomus cell. In addition, the glossopharyngeal terminations on the glomus cell are partly presynaptic. Glomus cells secrete dopamine, which is known to alter chemoreceptor sensitivity, and possibly also noradrenaline, serotonin, acetylcholine and polypeptides.

Types of stimulant

Discharge in the afferent nerves increases in response to the following forms of stimulation.

Decrease of arterial PO_2. Stimulation is by decreased PO_2 and not by reduced oxygen content (at least down to about half the normal value). Thus there is little stimulation in anaemia, carboxyhaemoglobinaemia or methaemoglobinaemia (Comroe and Schmidt, 1938). The response of ventilation to reduction of arterial PO_2, approximates to a rectangular hyperbola asymptotic to a PO_2 of about 4.3 kPa (32 mmHg) and to the level of ventilation at high PO_2 (Figure 5.6). Quantitative aspects of the response to PO_2 are considered in greater detail below.

A small number of otherwise normal subjects lack a measurable ventilatory response to hypoxia when studied at normal PCO_2 (see data of subjects 4 and 5 reported by Cormack, Cunningham and Gee, 1957). This is of little importance under normal circumstances, because the PCO_2 drive from the central chemoreceptors will normally ensure a safe level of PO_2. However, in certain therapeutic and abnormal environmental circumstances, it could be dangerous. Such people would certainly do badly at high altitude.

Decrease of arterial pH. Acidaemia of perfusing blood causes stimulation, the magnitude of which is the same whether it is due to carbonic or to 'non-respiratory' acids such as lactic (Hornbein and Roos, 1963). Quantitatively, the change produced by elevated PCO_2 on the peripheral chemoreceptors is only about one-sixth of that caused by the action on the central chemosensitive areas (see below).

Respiratory oscillations of PCO_2. A series of square waves of raised PCO_2 in the carotid artery of the dog results in a higher level of ventilation than is obtained when the PCO_2 is maintained steady at the same mean value (Dutton, Fitzgerald and Gross, 1968). Respiratory oscillations in PO_2 do not appear to have this effect.

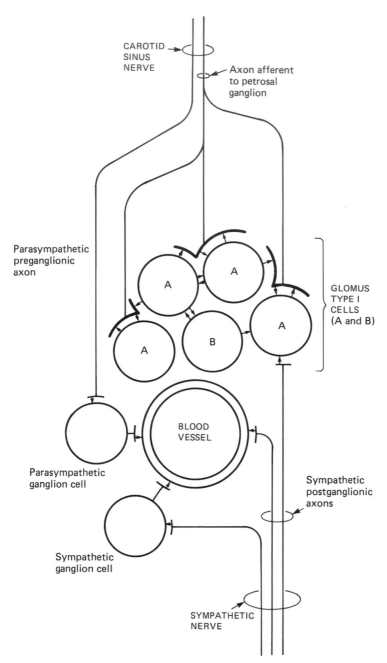

Figure 5.5 Grouping of glomus type I cells around a blood vessel in the carotid body, showing innervation. This grouping would be surrounded by a sheath cell which is not shown, and is sometimes termed a glomoid.

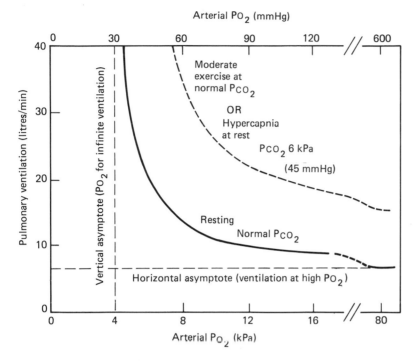

Figure 5.6 The heavy curve represents the normal P_{O_2}/ventilation response curve at constant (normal) P_{CO_2}. It has the form of a rectangular hyperbola asymptotic to the ventilation at high P_{O_2} and the P_{O_2} at which ventilation becomes infinite. The curve is displaced upwards by both hypercapnia and exercise at normal P_{CO_2}. The curve is depressed by anaesthetics. See text for references.

The mechanism of the stimulation of the central chemoreceptors is too slow to respond to these changes, but the output of the peripheral chemoreceptor in the sinus nerve has been found to vary during the respiratory cycle (Hornbein, Griffo and Roos, 1961). The timing of the nerve discharge suggests that the response is to the rate of rise of P_{CO_2} as well as to its magnitude.

The effect of oscillations of P_{CO_2} has been demonstrated in the dog, cat and rat, but in man direct investigation is not possible and recourse has to be made to elaborate experiments involving artificially imposed changes in the composition of the inspired gas (Cunningham and Ward, 1975a, b). In contrast to animal experiments, there is no evidence that the overall ventilation in man is higher than it would be with the same mean P_{CO_2} held at a steady level, and this applies even to hypoxic conditions. However, if the P_{CO_2} is made to rise sharply during inspiration then an augmentation of ventilation occurs (Cunningham, Howson and Pearson, 1973). This mechanism may have relevance to hyperventilation of exercise when the increased mixed venous/arterial P_{CO_2} difference causes a more abrupt rise in arterial P_{CO_2} during expiration.

Hypoperfusion of peripheral chemoreceptors causes stimulation, possibly by causing a 'stagnant hypoxia' of the chemoreceptor cells. Hypoperfusion may result from hypotension.

Blood temperature elevation causes stimulation of breathing via the peripheral chemoreceptors.

Chemical stimulation by a wide range of substances is known to cause increased ventilation through the mmmedium of the peripheral chemoreceptors. These substances fall into two groups. The first comprises agents such as nicotine and acetylcholine which stimulate sympathetic ganglia. Action of this group of drugs can be blocked with ganglion-blocking agents (e.g. hexamethonium). The second group of chemical stimulants comprises substances such as cyanide and carbon monoxide which block the cytochrome system and so prevent oxidative metabolism. Respiration is also stimulated through the carotid bodies by the drugs doxapram and almitrine.

The gain of the carotid bodies is under neural control. There is an efferent pathway in the sinus nerve which, on excitation, decreases chemoreceptor activity. Excitation of the sympathetic nerve supply to the carotid body causes an increase in activity (Biscoe and Willshaw, 1981). Hypotension does not stimulate the carotid body down to an arterial pressure of 60 mmHg.

Mechanism of action

In 1926, de Castro postulated that glomus cells excited the carotid sinus nerve endings by products of their own metabolism in response to hypoxia (the so-called 'metabolic hypothesis'). His view has stood the test of time. Arterial hypoxaemia causes a reduction in the intracellular level of adenosine triphosphate (ATP) in the carotid body at levels of PO_2 which have little effect elsewhere in the body, and this is accompanied by increased glucose uptake. In response to hypoxaemia (and also cyanide administration) there is release of a number of neurotransmitters from the type I cell including dopamine, noradrenaline, acetylcholine, substance P and enkephalins.

Increased PCO_2 causes a similar release of neurotransmitters. The action is dependent on carbonic anhydrase (present in the type I cell) and there is therefore the possibility of both raised PCO_2 and decreased arterial pH acting through an increase in intracellular hydrogen ion concentration. However, for hypoxia, raised PCO_2 and decreased pH, the full transductive cascade of events between the stimulus and the release of the neurotransmitters is not yet clear. Neither is it certain what is the role of the various transmitters (Fidone et al., 1991). Dopamine is abundant in type I cells, and both carotid sinus nerve endings and type I cells have dopamine (D-2) receptors. Nevertheless, exogenous dopamine *inhibits* carotid sinus nerve activity. It is impossible at this stage to define any one critical neurotransmitter between the type I cell and the carotid sinus nerve endings. No single receptor blocker prevents the hypoxic ventilatory response.

An entirely different mechanism was proposed by Mills and Jöbsis (1972), who reported the presence in the carotid of a special type of cytochrome with a particularly high P_{50} which would be sensitive to small changes in normal arterial PO_2. However, its presence has not been confirmed by other workers (Fidone et al., 1991).

Other effects of stimulation. Apart from the well known increase in depth and rate of breathing, peripheral chemoreceptor stimulation causes a number of other effects, including bradycardia, hypertension, increase in bronchiolar tone and adrenal secretion. Stimulation of the carotid bodies has predominantly respiratory effects, while the aortic bodies have a greater influence on circulation.

Iatrogenic loss of peripheral chemoreceptor sensitivity

Reference has been made above to the studies of bilateral vagal block in man (Guz et al., 1964, 1966a, b), which also blocked the glossopharyngeal nerve, so denervating the carotid bodies. This was confirmed by loss of ventilatory response to hypoxia produced by inhaling 8% oxygen in nitrogen. The carotid bodies are usually lost during bilateral carotid endarterectomy (Wade et al., 1970), which provides evidence that the carotid bodies are not essential for the maintenance of reasonably normal breathing under conditions of rest and mild exercise. Anaesthetics have a powerful depressant effect on peripheral chemoreceptor sensitivity (page 390), and all patients without peripheral chemoreceptor sensitivity are dangerously at risk if exposed to low partial pressures of oxygen or if they lose their central chemosensitivity (see below).

The central chemoreceptors
(reviews by Bledsoe and Hornbein, 1981; Loeschcke, 1983)

About 85 per cent of the total respiratory response to inhaled carbon dioxide originates in the central medullary chemoreceptors (Mitchell, 1966; Cunningham, 1974). The central response is thus the major factor in the regulation of breathing by carbon dioxide, and it had long been thought that the actual neurons of the 'respiratory centre' were themselves sensitive either to PCO_2 (Haldane and Priestley, 1905) or to pH (Winterstein, 1911; Gessell, 1923).

   More recently attention has been turned to the role of the cerebrospinal fluid (CSF) in the control of breathing. This followed the important studies of Leusen (1950, 1954) who showed that the ventilation of anaesthetized dogs was stimulated by perfusion of the ventriculocisternal system with mock CSF of elevated PCO_2 and reduced pH.

Localization of the central chemoreceptors

Leusen's work touched off a long series of studies aimed at localizing central chemoreceptors. They were thought to lie superficially and in contact with one or other of the reservoirs of CSF, since it seemed unlikely that changes in the composition of the CSF could influence the respiratory neurons within the substance of the medulla in the few minutes required for full development of the ventilatory response to inhaled carbon dioxide.

   It has now been shown that the central chemosensitive areas lie within 0.2 mm of the anterolateral surfaces of the medulla, close to the origins of the glossopharyngeal and vagus nerves, and crossed by the anterior inferior cerebellar arteries (Mitchell et al., 1963). In the cat, there are bilateral rostral (Mitchell) and caudal (Loeschcke) areas which are sensitive to pH (Figure 5.7). It seems likely that their connections pass through a third intermediate area and all chemosensitivity is lost if the intermediate areas are destroyed (Berger and Hornbein, 1987).

   Sato, Severinghaus and Basbaum (1991) used c-fos immunochemistry to identify the medullary neurons which responded to stimulation by carbon dioxide. Evi-

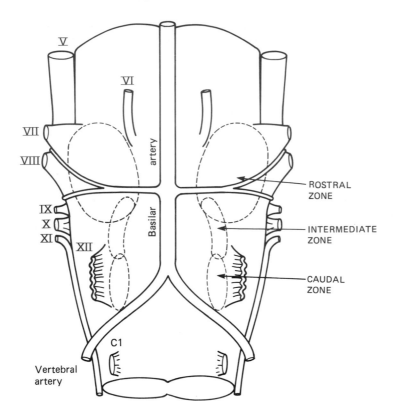

Figure 5.7 Location of the chemoreceptor zones on the anterolateral surface of the medulla of the cat. (Redrawn after Schläfke et al. (1975) with permission of the Editors of the Bulletin de Physio-Pathologie Respiratoire)

dence of stimulation was found in the rostral and caudal areas known to be chemosensitive and most stimulated cells lay within 0.2 mm of the surface. c-fos staining was also found in neurons of the dorsal respiratory group.

Mechanism of action

An elevation of arterial P_{CO_2} causes an approximately equal rise of CSF, cerebral tissue and jugular venous P_{CO_2}, which are all about 1.3 kPa (10 mmHg) more than the arterial P_{CO_2}. Over the short term, and without change in CSF bicarbonate, a rise in CSF P_{CO_2} causes a fall in CSF pH, and it was postulated by Mitchell et al. (1963) that the reduction in pH stimulated the respiratory neurons indirectly through receptors in the chemosensitive area. The theory was especially attractive because the time course of change in CSF pH accorded with the well known delay in the ventilatory response to a change in arterial P_{CO_2} (Lambertsen, 1963; Loeschcke, 1965). The blood/brain barrier (operative between blood and CSF) is permeable to carbon dioxide but not hydrogen ions, and in this respect resembles the membrane of a P_{CO_2}-sensitive electrode (page 244). In both cases, carbon dioxide crosses the barrier and hydrates to carbonic acid, which then ionizes to give a pH inversely proportional to the log of the P_{CO_2}. A hydrogen ion sensor is thus made to respond to P_{CO_2}. This accords with the old observation that the ventilatory response to respiratory acidosis is greater than to a metabolic acidosis with the same change in *blood* pH. Ventilation is, in fact, a single function of CSF pH in both conditions (Fencl, Miller and Pappenheimer, 1966).

The precise mechanism by which a change in pH causes stimulation of neurons is not firmly established, but it could clearly influence the action of an enzyme. Decreased pH inhibits the metabolism of acetylcholine by choline esterase and it has been observed that atropine blocks the CO_2 sensitivity of the central chemoreceptors (Dev and Loeschcke, 1979) and this effect has been shown to occur at M-2 receptors.

Compensatory bicarbonate shift in the CSF. If the P_{CO_2} is maintained at an abnormal level, the CSF pH gradually returns towards normal over the course of a few days as a result of changes in the CSF bicarbonate level. This is analogous to and proceeds in parallel with the partial restoration of blood pH in patients with chronic hyper- or hypocapnia. The mechanism of the shift in bicarbonate was originally thought to be due to active transport of bicarbonate ion (Severinghaus et al., 1963). It was later shown that CSF pH was not completely restored to normal (Dempsey, Forster and doPico, 1974; Forster, Dempsey and Chosy, 1975) and compensatory changes were found to be similar in CSF and blood, suggesting that changes were due to passive ion distribution. Further studies by Pavlin and Hornbein (1975a, b, c) and Hornbein and Pavlin (1975) also indicated that the bicarbonate shift could be explained by passive distribution although the possibility of active ion transfer could not be excluded.

A shift in CSF bicarbonate is a major factor in the early partial reversal of the hypocapnia which occurs in response to hypoxia at altitude (page 344). Similar changes in CSF bicarbonate occur during prolonged periods of hypocapnic artificial ventilation. Semple (1965) pointed out that CSF bicarbonate would be significantly reduced after 1 hour of hyperventilation, and Christensen (1974) reported that CSF pH had returned to normal 30 hours after commencing passive hyperventilation. Hornbein and Pavlin (1975) found substantial resetting of the CSF pH within $4\frac{1}{2}$ hours of a step increase in the ventilation of an anaesthetized paralysed dog. This offers one reason why patients subjected to this treatment may demand high minute volumes, and often continue to hyperventilate after resumption of spontaneous breathing.

Compensatory changes in CSF bicarbonate and the restoration of its pH are not confined to respiratory alkalosis, but are also found in chronic respiratory acidosis and metabolic acidosis and alkalosis (Mitchell et al., 1965). Mean values of CSF pH in Mitchell's study did not differ by more than 0.011 units from the normal value (7.326) in spite of mean arterial pH values ranging from 7.334 to 7.523.

If the bicarbonate of the CSF is altered by pathological factors, the pH is changed and ventilatory disturbances follow. Froman and Crampton-Smith (1966) described three patients who hyperventilated after intracranial haemorrhages. In each case the CSF pH and bicarbonate were persistently below the normal values and it was postulated that this was due to the metabolic breakdown products of blood which contaminated the CSF. In a later communication, Froman (1966) reported correction of hyperventilation by intrathecal administration of 3–5 mmol of bicarbonate.

Central hypoxic depression of breathing

Unlike the peripheral chemoreceptors, the central chemoreceptors are not stimulated by hypoxia. In fact, the central respiratory neurons are depressed by hypoxia, and apnoea follows severe medullary hypoxia whether due to ischaemia or to hypoxaemia.

With denervated peripheral chemoreceptors, phrenic motor activity becomes silent when the medullary PO_2 falls to about 1.7 kPa (13 mmHg) (see review by Edelman and Neubauer, 1991). More intense hypoxia causes a resumption of breathing with an abnormal pattern, possibly driven by a 'gasping' centre. This pattern of central hypoxic depression appears to be particularly marked in neonates and may be the relic of a mechanism to prevent the fetus from attempting to breathe *in utero* (see page 374).

Mechanisms of hypoxic depression of ventilation. Medullary PCO_2 may be reduced by increased cerebral blood flow induced by hypoxia, and severe hypoxia causes depletion of high energy phosphates. However, it has also been shown that neonatal hypoxia results in decreased levels of excitatory neurotransmitters (glutamate and aspartate) and increased levels of inhibitory substances, particularly gamma-amino butyric acid (GABA) and endogenous opioids, both powerful respiratory depressants. Naloxone may reverse apnoea following neonatal asphyxia.

Quantitative aspects of the chemical control of breathing

It was originally thought that the various factors interacted according to the algebraic sum of the individual effects caused by changes of PCO_2, PO_2, pH, etc. Hypoxia and hypercapia were, for example, thought to be simply additive in their effects. It is now realized that the interactions between PCO_2 and PO_2 are far more complex (Lloyd and Cunningham, 1963), especially during exercise (Chapter 13).

The PO_2/ventilation response curve

The approach developed by Lloyd, Jukes and Cunningham (1958) considers the response as a rectangular hyperbola (see Appendix F), asymptotic to the ventilation at high PO_2 (zero hypoxic drive) and to the PO_2 at which ventilation theoretically becomes infinite (known as 'C' and about 4.3 kPa (32 mmHg)). Figure 5.6 shows typical examples but there are very wide individual variations. Note that there is a small but measurable difference in ventilation between normal and very high PO_2.

The ventilatory response to PO_2 may be expressed as $W/(PO_2-C)$, where W is a multiplier (i.e. the gain of the system) and partly dependent upon the PCO_2. The ventilatory response is here the difference between the actual ventilation and the ventilation at high PO_2, PCO_2 being unchanged. Others have suggested that the PO_2/ventilation response curve be considered as an exponential function but curve-fitting to available data does not give a clear-cut answer as to which model is the better.

The inconvenience of the non-linear relationship between ventilation and PO_2 may be overcome by plotting ventilation against oxygen saturation. The relationship is linear with a negative slope, at least down to a saturation of 70% (Rebuck and Campbell, 1974). This approach is the basis of a simple non-invasive method of measurement of the hypoxic ventilatory response (see below).

The ventilatory response to hypoxia is enhanced at elevated P_{CO_2} (Cormack, Cunningham and Gee, 1957) as shown by the upper broken curve in Figure 5.6. This interaction contributes to the ventilatory response in asphyxia being greater than the sum of the response to be expected from the rise in P_{CO_2} and the fall in P_{O_2} considered separately. Simple elicitation of the ventilatory response to hypoxia will normally result in hypocapnia and the response is then a combination of the hypoxic drive and the resultant hypocapnic depression of breathing. Precise measurement of the hypoxic drive *per se* requires that the P_{CO_2} be maintained at a constant level.

The response to hypoxia is also enhanced by exercise even if the P_{CO_2} is not raised (Weil et al., 1972). This may be due to lactacidosis, oscillations of P_{CO_2} or perhaps to catecholamine secretion. The upper broken curve in Figure 5.6 would also correspond to the response during exercise at an oxygen consumption of about 800 ml/min. It is important to note that the slope of the curve at normal P_{O_2} is considerably increased under both these circumstances, so that there will then be an appreciable 'hypoxic' drive to ventilation at normal P_{O_2}. Enhanced response to P_{O_2} during exercise appears to be an important component in the overall ventilatory response to exercise (page 328). The P_{O_2}/ventilation response is virtually abolished during anaesthesia (page 390).

Time course of hypoxic ventilatory response. Sudden acute imposition of a constant degree of hypoxia causes complex changes in the level of ventilatory stimulation. Hypoxia results in initial stimulation of ventilation within the lung-to-carotid body circulation time (about 6 seconds). Within a minute, the response is decreased by hypocapnia resulting from the hyperventilation caused by the hypoxia (see above). In the course of the next few minutes there is a further decrease in ventilation (the 'roll-off') which is particularly evident in neonates. However, even if P_{CO_2} is maintained constant, there is still a very marked decrease over 30 minutes. Although this is thought to be mediated by central hypoxic depression, it is not reversed by naloxone (Kagawa et al., 1982). This contrasts with the comparable condition in neonates (see above). Over the first 6 days of hypoxia there is a steady increase in hypoxic ventilatory response (Severinghaus et al., 1991) which supplements the beneficial effect on ventilation of bicarbonate shifts in the CSF (see above). Finally, over many years, there is a loss of hypoxic drive which is grossly attenuated in residents at very high altitude (Weil et al., 1971).

The P_{CO_2}/ventilation response curve

The response is slower than that to hypoxia but a steady ventilation is usually achieved after a few minutes. The response is linear over the range which is usually studied and may therefore be defined in terms of two parameters, slope and intercept (see Appendix F and Lloyd, Jukes and Cunningham, 1958):

$$\text{ventilation} = S(P_{CO_2} - B)$$

where S is the slope (l min^{-1} kPa^{-1} or l/min/mmHg) and B is the intercept at zero ventilation (kPa or mmHg). The heavy continuous line in Figure 5.8 is a typical normal curve with an intercept (B) of about 4.8 kPa (36 mmHg) and a slope (S) of about 15 l min^{-1} kPa^{-1} (2 l/min/mmHg). There is in fact a very wide individual variation in P_{CO_2}/ventilation response curves and the response may be decreased by disease or drugs. Actual values of P_{CO_2} and ventilation depend on the inspired carbon dioxide concentration and the metabolic rate (page 233). The broken curve in Figure 5.8 shows the effect of changing ventilation on arterial P_{CO_2} when the inspired carbon dioxide concentration is negligible, and is a section of a rectangular hyperbola (page 129). The normal resting P_{CO_2} and ventilation are indicated by the intersection of this curve with the normal P_{CO_2}/ventilation response curve, which is usually obtained by varying the carbon dioxide concentration in the inspired gas.

The P_{CO_2}/ventilation response curve is the response of the entire respiratory system to the challenge of a raised P_{CO_2}. Apart from reduced sensitivity of the central chemoreceptors, the overall response may be blunted by neuromuscular blockade or by obstructive or restrictive lung disease (see Figure 21.2). These factors must be taken into account in drawing conclusions from a reduced response, and diffuse airway obstruction is a most important consideration (Clark, Clarke and Hughes, 1966). Nevertheless the slope of the P_{CO_2}/ventilation response curve remains one of the most valuable parameters in the assessment of the responsiveness of the respiratory system to carbon dioxide and its depression by drugs.

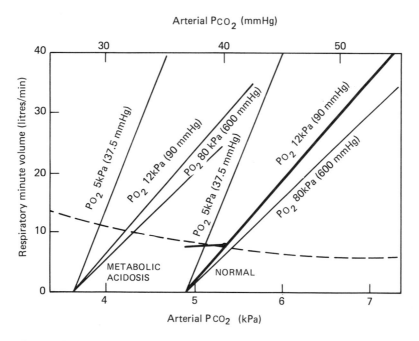

Figure 5.8 Two fans of P_{CO_2}/ventilation response curves at different values of P_{O_2}. The right-hand fan is at normal metabolic acid–base state (zero base excess). The left-hand fan represents metabolic acidosis. The broken line represents the P_{CO_2} produced by the indicated ventilation for zero inspired P_{CO_2}, at basal metabolic rate. The intersection of the broken curve and any response curve indicates the resting P_{CO_2} and ventilation for the relevant metabolic acid–base state and P_{O_2}. The heavy curve is the normal curve. For details, see text.

Slopes and intercepts of P_{CO_2}/ventilation response curves are subject to very wide individual variation. The curves in this diagram are intended to indicate only general principles, and considerable deviations may be found in healthy subjects

Figure 5.8 shows two possible extensions to the response curves below the dotted curve, which defines the effect of ventilation on PCO_2. These extensions are of two types. The first is an extrapolation of the curve to intersect the X axis (zero ventilation) at a PCO_2 known as the apnoeic threshold. If PCO_2 is depressed below this point, apnoea may result, and this represents Haldane's post-hyperventilation apnoea. The second type of extension is shown on the middle line of the right-hand fan. It is horizontal and to the left, like a hockey stick, representing the response of a subject who continues to breathe regardless of the fact that his PCO_2 has been reduced (see above). The resting arterial point at resting ventilation is in fact 0.3 kPa (2.3 mmHg) to the left of the extrapolated response curve (Lumb and Nunn, 1991b).

As PCO_2 is raised, a point of maximal ventilatory stimulation is reached, probably within the range 13.3–26.7 kPa (100–200 mmHg). Thereafter the ventilatory stimulation is reduced until, at very high PCO_2, the ventilation is actually depressed below control value and finally apnoea results, at least in the dog (Graham, Hill and Nunn, 1960) and almost certainly in man as well. It does not appear to be possible to arrest breathing in the cat by this means in spite of elevation of PCO_2 to more than 67 kPa or 500 mmHg (Hornbein, personal communication; Raymond and Standaert, 1967).

Interaction of PCO_2, PO_2 and metabolic acidosis

The broken line (A) in Figure 5.4 shows the influence of the chemoreceptor drive from PO_2 on the central ventilatory response to PCO_2. Typical quantitative relationships are shown in Figure 5.8, with hypoxia at the left of the fan and hyperoxia on the right. The curve marked PO_2 80 kPa represents total abolition of chemoreceptor drive obtained by the inhalation of 100% oxygen. A similar result follows carotid endarterectomy (see above).

Metabolic acidosis displaces the whole fan of curves to the left as shown in Figure 5.8. The intercept (B) is reduced but the slope of the curves at each value of PO_2 is virtually unaltered. Display of the fan of PCO_2/ventilation response curves at different PO_2 is a particularly comprehensive method of representing the state of respiratory control in a patient, but it is unfortunately laborious to determine.

The influence of increased PCO_2 on the hypoxic ventilatory response is illustrated in Figure 5.6.

Reflex control of breathing

We have already considered the reflex arcs with afferent limbs arising in the peripheral chemoreceptors in relation to chemical control. In addition, there are the ventilatory reflexes in response to pain, which are similar in many respects to the arousal state. There remain, however, a number of neural control mechanisms which are more appropriately considered specifically under the heading of reflexes.

Baroreceptor reflexes

The most important groups of arterial baroreceptors are in the carotid sinus and around the aortic arch. These receptors are primarily concerned with regulation of the circulation, but a decrease in pressure produces hyperventilation, while a rise in pressure causes respiratory depression and, ultimately, apnoea (Heymans and Neil, 1958). This is the likely cause of apnoea produced by a massive dose of catecholamines. Baroreceptors are sensitized by diethyl ether (Robertson, Swan and Whitteridge, 1956), cyclopropane (Price and Widdicombe, 1962) and halothane (Biscoe and Millar, 1964). This effect has been considered mainly in relation to circulatory control during anaesthesia, and the respiratory implications are not yet established.

Pulmonary stretch reflexes

There are a large number of different types of receptors in the lungs (see reviews by Widdicombe, 1981; Sant'Ambrogio and Sant'Ambrogio, 1991) sensitive to inflation, deflation, mechanical and chemical stimulation. Afferents from all are conducted by the vagus, although some fibres may be additionally carried in the sympathetic. The stretch receptors are predominantly in the airways rather than in the alveoli, and the slowly adapting receptors are in the tracheobronchial smooth muscle and the rapidly adapting receptors in the superficial mucosal layer. These receptors have attracted much attention since the associated inflation and deflation reflexes were described by Hering (1868) and Breuer (1868). Breuer was a clinical assistant to Professor Hering but apparently the work was at his own instigation. However, Hering, who was a corresponding member of the Vienna Academy of Science, published Breuer's work under his own name, in accord with the custom of the time. Breuer's role was clearly stated in Hering's paper but he was not a co-author. Later the same year, Breuer published a much fuller account of his work under his own name. The extent of the individual contributions of Hering and Breuer has been discussed by Ullmann (1970), who also appended an English translation of the original papers.

The inflation reflex consists of inhibition of inspiration in response to an increased pulmonary transmural pressure gradient (as in sustained inflation of the lung). An exactly similar effect may be obtained by obstructing expiration so that an inspiration is retained in the lungs.

Generations of medical students have been brought up with the unquestioned belief in the important role of the Hering–Breuer reflex in man. However, there appears to be a most important species difference between man and the laboratory animals in whom the reflex is so easy to demonstrate. Widdicombe (1961) compared the strength of the inflation reflex in eight species and found the reflex weakest in man, concluding that '...caution must be exercised before ascribing any important role to the Hering–Breuer reflexes in modifying the pattern of breathing in healthy man'. This is borne out in studies showing no effect of bilateral vagal block on breathing patterns in volunteers (see earlier). It is also well known that patients have normal ventilatory patterns after bilateral lung transplant. It has also been noted (page 85) that end-expiratory obstruction *augments* the force of the inspiratory muscles. Although the Hering–Breuer inflation reflex appears to have minimal functional significance in man, its actual existence has been demonstrated by both Widdicombe (1961) and Gautier, Bonora and Gaudy (1981).

The pulmonary stretch receptors are stimulated by a decrease of P_{CO_2}, but it is unlikely that this effect is of great practical importance (Widdicombe, 1981). The receptors are unaffected by changes in P_{O_2}. An increase in pulmonary venous pressure of 4 kPa (30 mmHg) causes an augmentation of stretch receptor activity by about 20% (Marshall and Widdicombe, 1958).

The deflation reflex consists of an augmentation of inspiration in response to deflation of the lung and can be demonstrated in man (Guz et al., 1971). Guz concluded that his results were consistent with the hypothesis that lung deflation has a reflex excitatory effect on breathing, but that the threshold is higher than for other mammalian species. The deflation reflex in the rabbit is blocked by breathing a local anaesthetic aerosol (Jain et al., 1973).

The inflation and deflation reflexes were the basis of the *Selbststeuerung* (self-steering) hypothesis of Hering and Breuer. This concept has played a major role in theories of the control of breathing and, even though its role in man may be questionable, it remains a classic example of a physiological autoregulating mechanism. The ventilatory response to loaded breathing is considered in Chapter 4 on pages 83 et seq.

Head's paradoxical reflex. Head, working in Professor Hering's laboratory, described a reversal of the inflation reflex, which could be elicited during partial block of the vagus nerves in the course of thawing after cold block. Under these conditions, inflation of the lung of the rabbit caused strong maintained contractions of an isolated diaphragmatic slip (curve VI, Plate I in Head, 1889). Many authors have reported that, with normal vagal conduction, sudden inflation of the lungs of many species may cause a transient inspiratory effort before the onset of apnoea due to the inflation reflex (Widdicombe, 1961). A similar response may also be elicited in newborn infants (Cross et al., 1960), but it has not been established whether this 'gasp reflex' is analogous to Head's paradoxical reflex. All anaesthetists are aware that, after administration of respiratory depressants, transient increases in airway pressure often cause an immediate deep gasping type of inspiration. There is a possible relationship between the reflex and the mechanism of sighing which may be considered a normal feature of breathing (Bendixen, Smith and Mead, 1964).

Other pulmonary afferents

Pulmonary embolization and pneumothorax may each cause rapid shallow breathing by a reflex arc with afferents carried in the vagi. Changes in blood gas tensions may also produce secondary changes in ventilation. The pattern of discharge of medullary neurons in these conditions was reported by Katz and Horres (1972). More recent work suggests the stretch receptors are sensitized after microembolism.

C-fibre endings (J receptors). These endings lie in close relationship to the capillaries. One group is in relation to the bronchial circulation and the other to the pulmonary microcirculation. The latter correspond to Paintal's juxtapulmonary capillary receptors (J receptors, for short) which were reviewed by him in 1983 and by Coleridge and Coleridge in 1984. Afferent unmyelinated fibres are in the vagus.

These receptors are relatively silent during normal breathing but appear to be stimulated under various pathological conditions. They appear to be nociceptive and activated by tissue damage, accumulation of interstitial fluid and release of various mediators (Widdicombe, 1981). In the laboratory they can be activated by intravascular injection of capsaicin to produce the so-called pulmonary chemoreflex which comprises bradycardia, hypotension, apnoea or shallow breathing, bronchoconstriction and increased mucus secretion. They may well be concerned in the dyspnoea of pulmonary vascular congestion and the ventilatory response to exercise and pulmonary embolization. C-fibre endings have been characterized in physiological studies but have never been identified histologically, although non-myelinated nerve fibres have been seen in the alveolar walls.

Lung chemoreceptors. Various phenomena such as the hyperventilation of exercise could be very conveniently explained by the existence of chemoreceptors on the arterial side of the pulmonary circulation, which would be sensitive to mixed venous blood gas tensions. Widdicombe (1981) has reviewed the evidence for believing their existence to be unlikely.

Reflexes arising from the upper respiratory tract
(see review by Sant'Ambrogio and Sant'Ambrogio, 1991)

The nose. Water and stimulants such as ammonia or cigarette smoke may cause apnoea as part of the diving reflex (page 361). Subatmospheric pressure can activate the pharyngeal dilator muscles (page 16). Irritants can initiate sneezing which, unlike coughing, cannot be undertaken voluntarily. There are also cold receptors which initiate bronchoconstriction in sensitive subjects.

The pharynx. Mechanoreceptors which respond to pressures play a major role in activation of the pharyngeal dilator muscles (page 16). There is ample evidence that local anaesthesia of the pharynx impairs their action. Irritants may cause bronchodilatation, hypertension, tachycardia, and secretion of mucus in the lower airway. Presence of solids or liquids may initiate the swallowing reflex, which involves powerful laryngeal closure (page 17).

The larynx. The larynx has a dense sensory innervation of which the superior laryngeal nerve is the most important. Subatmospheric pressure causes activation of the pharyngeal dilator muscles. Chemical and mechanical stimulation cause cough, laryngeal closure and bronchoconstriction. Distilled water is a powerful stimulant.

The cough reflex may be elicited by mechanical stimuli arising in the larynx, trachea, carina and main bronchi. Chemical stimuli are effective further down the respiratory tract (Widdicombe, 1964). Coughing can be undertaken voluntarily but the reflex is complex and comprises three main stages:

1. An inspiration, which takes into the lungs a volume of air sufficient for the expiratory activity.
2. Build-up of pressure in the lungs by contraction of expiratory muscles against a closed glottis.
3. Forceful expiration through narrowed airways with high linear velocity of gas flow which sweeps irritant material up towards the pharynx.

The mechanism of the narrowing of the airways is illustrated in Figure 4.8. Transient changes of pressure up to 40 kPa (300 mmHg) may occur in the thorax, arterial blood and the CSF during the act of coughing (Sharpey-Schafer, 1953). Tetraplegics augment their coughing with the clavicular fibres of pectoralis major.

Afferents from the musculoskeletal system

Kalia et al. (1972) showed that a variety of mechanical stimuli applied to the gastrocnemius muscle of the dog can produce a reflex increase in ventilation. This occurred when afferents from the pressure–pain receptors were blocked by antidromic stimulation. The afferents causing stimulation of ventilation were carried by non-medullated fibres. Afferents from the musculoskeletal system probably have an important role in the hyperventilation of exercise (Chapter 13).

Breath holding

Influence of P_{CO_2} and P_{O_2}

When the breath is held after air breathing, the arterial and alveolar P_{CO_2} are remarkably constant at the breaking point and values are normally close to 6.7 kPa (50 mmHg). This does not mean that P_{CO_2} is the sole or dominant factor and concomitant hypoxia is probably more important. Preliminary oxygen breathing delays the onset of hypoxia, and breath-holding times may be greatly prolonged with consequent elevation of P_{CO_2} at the breaking point. The relationship between P_{CO_2} and P_{O_2} at breaking point, after starting from different levels of oxygenation, is shown in Figure 5.9. The breaking point curve is displaced upwards and to the left by carotid body resection (Davidson et al., 1974). Guz et al. (1966b) observed marked prolongation of breath holding after vagal and glossopharyngeal block, but advanced cogent reasons for believing that this was not due primarily to block of the chemoreceptors. Oxygen breathing would also prevent the chemoreceptor drive but this did not prolong breath holding to the same extent as the nerve block.

Effect of lung volume

Breath-holding time is directly proportional to the lung volume at the onset of breath holding, partly because this has a major influence on oxygen stores (page 288). There are, however, other effects of lung volume and its change, which are mediated by afferents arising from both chest wall and the lung itself. Guz et al. (1966b) reported substantial prolongation of breath-holding times after bilateral vagal and glossopharyngeal block. As a sequel to these studies, Campbell et al. (1967, 1969) reported prolongation of breath-holding time following curarization of conscious subjects. Their explanation was that much of the distress leading to the termination of breath holding is caused by frustration of the involuntary contractions of the respiratory muscles, which increase progressively during breath holding (Agostoni, 1963). It appears that the inappropriateness arises in the diaphragm (Noble et al., 1971), rather than in the intercostals (Eisele et al., 1968), in spite of the paucity of afferents from the former (Corda, von Euler and Lennerstrand, 1965).

The importance of frustration of involuntary respiratory movements was strikingly demonstrated by Fowler's experiment (1954). After normal air breathing, the breath is held until breaking point. If the expirate is then taken in a bag and immediately reinhaled, there is a marked sense of relief although it may be shown that the rise of P_{CO_2} and fall of P_{O_2} are uninfluenced.

Extreme durations of breath holding may be attained after hyperventilation and preoxygenation. Times of 14 minutes have been reached and the limiting factor is

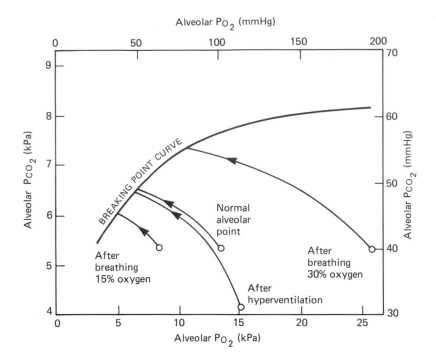

Figure 5.9 The 'breaking point' curve defines the coexisting values of alveolar P_{O_2} and P_{CO_2}, at the breaking point of breath holding, starting from various states. The normal alveolar point is shown (P_{O_2}, 13.3 kPa or 100 mmHg; P_{CO_2}, 5.3 kPa or 40 mmHg) and the curved arrow shows the changes in alveolar gas tensions which occur during breath holding. Starting points are displaced to the right by preliminary breathing of oxygen-enriched gas mixtures, and to the left by breathing mixtures containing less than 21% oxygen. Hyperventilation displaces the point representing the alveolar gas tensions to the right and downwards. The length of the arrows from starting point to the 'breaking point' curve gives an approximate indication of the possible duration of breath holding. This can clearly be prolonged by oxygen breathing or by hyperventilation, maximal prolongation occurring after hyperventilation with 100% oxygen. (Data for construction of the 'breaking point' curve have been taken from Ferris et al. (1946) and Otis, Rahn and Fenn (1948))

then reduction of lung volume to residual volume, as oxygen is removed from the alveolar gas by the circulating pulmonary blood (Klocke and Rahn, 1959).

Outline of methods of assessment of factors in control of breathing

Sensitivity to hypoxia

There is often some reluctance to test sensitivity to hypoxia because of the reduction in P_{O_2} to which the patient is exposed. Various approaches to the problem have been reviewed by Rebuck and Slutsky (1981).

The steady state method is the classic technique and is best undertaken by preparing P_{CO_2}/ventilation response curves at different levels of P_{O_2}, which are presented as a fan (see Figure 5.8). The spread of the fan is an indication of peripheral chemoreceptor sensitivity but it is also possible to present the data in the form of the rectangular hyperbola (see Figure 5.6) by plotting the ventilatory response for different values of PO_2 at the same PCO_2 (intercepts of components of the fan with a vertical line drawn through a particular value of PCO_2). The parameters of the hyperbola may then be derived as outlined above.

A minimum of 5 minutes is required to reach a steady state for PCO_2 although it is possible to speed up the process by varying PO_2 while keeping PCO_2 constant. Alternatively the ventilation may be kept approximately constant while PCO_2 and PO_2 are both raised by appropriate amounts so that the PCO_2 stimulus increases by the same amount as the hypoxic drive diminishes (Lloyd and Cunningham, 1963). Nevertheless, it is a laborious undertaking to determine the oxygen response by these methods and patients may be distressed, particularly by the run at low PO_2 and high PCO_2.

The rebreathing method has been adapted to measure the response to hypoxia (Rebuck and Campbell, 1974). The oxygen concentration of the rebreathed gas is reduced by the oxygen consumption of the subject, but active steps have to be taken to maintain the PCO_2 at a constant level. Calculation of the response is greatly simplified by measuring the oxygen saturation (usually non-invasively by means of an ear oximeter) and plotting the response as ventilation against saturation. This normally approximates to a straight line and the slope is a function of the chemoreceptor sensitivity. However, even if PCO_2 is held constant, the response is directly influenced by the patient's sensitivity to PCO_2.

Intermittent inhalation of high oxygen concentration. This method avoids exposing subjects to hypoxia. Temporary withdrawal of peripheral chemoreceptor drive by inhalation of oxygen should reduce ventilation by about 15%. This may be used as an indication of the existence of carotid body activity (Dejours, 1962) but clearly it is much less sensitive than the steady state method.

Sensitivity to carbon dioxide

It has been stressed above that the ventilatory response may be reduced as a result of impaired function anywhere between the medullary neurons and the mechanical properties of the lung (see Figure 21.2). Thus it cannot be assumed that a decreased ventilation/PCO_2 response is necessarily due to failure of the central chemoreceptor mechanism.

The steady state method requires the simultaneous measurement of minute volume and PCO_2 after PCO_2 has been raised by increasing the concentration of carbon dioxide in the inspired gas. The ventilation is usually reasonably stable after 5 minutes of inhaling a fixed concentration of carbon dioxide. Severinghaus' pseudo steady state method (1976) measures ventilation after 4 minutes and is a useful compromise giving highly repeatable results (Lumb and Nunn, 1991b). PCO_2 is best measured in arterial blood but end-expiratory gas is more usual. Several points are needed to define the PCO_2/ventilation response curve and it is a time-consuming process which may be distressing to some patients. Methods of measurement of ventilation are outlined on page 130 and PCO_2 on page 243.

The rebreathing method introduced by Read (1967) has greatly simplified determination of the slope of the P_{CO_2}/ventilation response curve. The subject rebreathes for up to 4 minutes from a 6-litre bag originally containing 7% carbon dioxide and about 50% oxygen, the remainder being nitrogen. The carbon dioxide concentration rises steadily during rebreathing while the oxygen concentration should remain above 30%. Thus there should be no appreciable hypoxic drive and ventilation is driven solely by the rising arterial P_{CO_2}, which should be very close to the P_{CO_2} of the gas in the bag. Ventilation is measured by any convenient means and plotted against the P_{CO_2} of the gas in the bag. Milledge, Minty and Duncalf (1974) described an automated technique by which the P_{CO_2}/ventilation response curve is automatically determined and presented on an X–Y plotter.

The P_{CO_2}/ventilation response curve measured by the rebreathing technique is displaced to the right by about 0.7 kPa (5 mmHg) compared with the steady state method, but the slope agrees closely with the steady state method (Read, 1967; Clark, 1968; Lumb and Nunn, 1991b).

The $P_{CO_2}/P_{0.1}$ response. It was suggested by Whitelaw, Derenne and Milic-Emili (1975) that a better indication of the output of the respiratory centre may be obtained by measuring the effect of P_{CO_2} on the subatmospheric pressure developed in the airways when obstructed for 0.1 second at the beginning of inspiration ($P_{0.1}$). This eliminates any effect due to increased airway resistance or reduced compliance. Nevertheless, it is still influenced by impaired performance in the lower motor neurons or respiratory muscles.

The ventilatory response to P_{CO_2} may be separated into rib cage and abdominal components most easily by using inductive respiratory plethysmography (page 132).

Chapter 6

Pulmonary ventilation: mechanisms and the work of breathing

Breathing consists of rhythmic changes in lung volume. During spontaneous breathing, the lungs passively follow the changes in the contours of the thorax produced by contraction of the respiratory muscles. During artificial ventilation by the application of intermittent positive pressure to the airways, the lungs and chest wall move passively in response to the changing transmural pressures. Adequate ventilation may be obtained by either means but there are subtle differences between the two types of ventilation. This chapter is concerned solely with pulmonary ventilation achieved by use of the respiratory muscles. Artificial ventilation is considered in Chapter 22. Muscles governing the patency of the pharynx are considered in Chapter 2.

The spirogram in Figure 3.9 shows the tidal volume in relation to the total lung capacity. Figure 6.1 shows the corresponding radiographic appearance of the

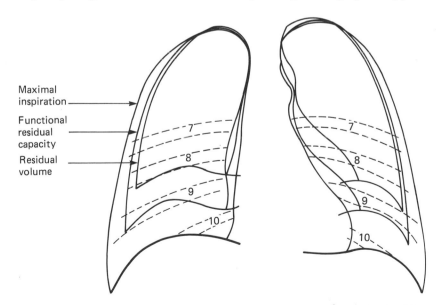

Maximal
inspiration

Functional
residual
capacity

Residual
volume

Figure 6.1 Outlines of chest radiographs of a normal subject at various levels of lung inflation. The numbers refer to ribs as seen in the position of maximal inspiration. (I am indebted to Dr R.L. Marks who was the subject)

117

thorax at residual volume, the normal expiratory level and at maximal inspiration. Expiration normally proceeds passively to the functional residual capacity (FRC), which may be considered as the equilibrium position governed by the balance of elastic forces, unless modified by residual end-expiratory tone in certain muscle groups. Inspiration is the active phase, entering the inspiratory capacity but normally leaving a substantial volume unused (the inspiratory reserve volume). Similarly, there is a substantial volume (the expiratory reserve volume) between FRC and the residual volume. By voluntary effort it is possible to effect a satisfactory tidal exchange anywhere within the vital capacity, but the work of breathing is minimal at FRC.

Geometrical confines of thorax and abdomen

It is necessary first to consider the very complex structures on which the respiratory muscles act to produce changes in lung volume. Nomenclature is not intuitively explicit, and sometimes the same words are used by different authors in different senses.

The trunk (referred to as chest wall by De Troyer) may be divided into rib cage and abdomen, separated by the diaphragm. The former may be regarded as a cylinder, with length governed primarily by the diaphragm and secondarily by flexion and extension of the spine. The cross-sectional area of the cylinder is governed by bucket-handle and pump-handle movement of the ribs which are manifest as changes in lateral and anteroposterior diameter of the rib cage. Upper ribs are inserted into the sternum and do not necessarily behave in the same way as the lower floating ribs. The abdomen is essentially an incompressible volume held between the diaphragm and the abdominal muscles. Contraction of either will cause a corresponding passive displacement of the other.

The respiratory muscles
(see review by De Troyer, 1991)

Under resting conditions in the supine position, only inspiratory muscles are active. Work overcoming elastic resistance during inspiration is stored as potential energy and used to provide the work of expiration. As ventilation or resistance to breathing is increased, additional inspiratory muscles are recruited and eventually expiratory muscles become active in a pull–push pattern of breathing.

Although we tend to think of the respiratory muscles individually, it is important to remember that they act together in an extraordinarily complex interaction which may differ between species and, within a species, is influenced by factors including posture, minute volume, respiratory load and anaesthesia. Figure 6.2 illustrates some features of the interaction and is developed from the model proposed by Hillman and Finucane (1987) and further developed by Drummond (1989b).

The inspiratory muscles

The inspiratory muscles are not easy of access for electromyographic or other methods of study and this has greatly hampered elucidation of their pattern of contraction. Measurement of pressures within the thorax and abdomen is particu-

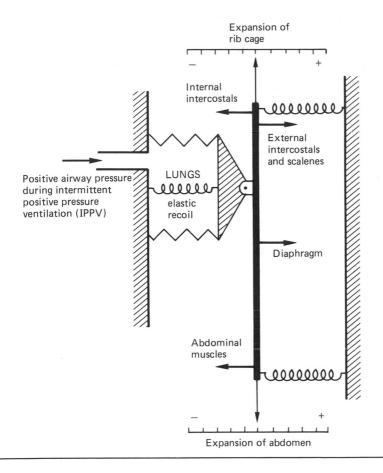

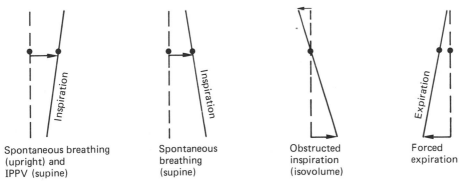

THE BROKEN LINE REPRESENTS FUNCTIONAL RESIDUAL CAPACITY

Figure 6.2 This is the model of the balance of static and dynamic forces seen earlier as Figure 3.10. Action of the various inspiratory or expiratory muscles causes changes, not only in the lung volume but also in the inclination of the bar which represents relative changes in cross-sectional area of rib cage and abdomen. See text for details.

larly useful to distinguish between active and passive movements of the diaphragm. Radiographic and a wide range of other imaging and stethographic methods will indicate the change in shape of the confines of thorax, abdomen and lungs, but do not necessarily indicate the muscle groups responsible for the observed changes (Figure 6.2). Inspiratory muscle activity does not terminate abruptly at the end of inspiration. There is a gradual let-down of their tone during early expiration, which does not therefore assume the pattern of exponential decay as seen in the paralysed patient.

The diaphragm. The diaphragm is the most important inspiratory muscle, with motor innervation solely from the phrenic nerves (C3, 4, 5). The origins of the *crural* part are the lumbar vertebrae and the arcuate ligaments, while the *costal* parts arise from the lower ribs and xiphisternum. Both parts are inserted into the central tendon. During inspiration, the origins and insertion are approximated, resulting both in descent of the domes of the diaphragm and in elevation and rotation of the lower ribs. The upper ribs, in contrast, are drawn inwards when the diaphragm contracts alone (De Troyer, 1991). The normal excursion of the domes is 1.5 cm, increasing to 6–7 cm during deep breathing (Wade and Gilson, 1951). The diaphragm has considerable reserve of function, and unilateral phrenic block causes little decrement of overall ventilatory capacity. Although the diaphragm is the most important inspiratory muscle, bilateral phrenic interruption is still compatible with good ventilatory function (Dowman, 1927; Eisele et al., 1972). There is general agreement that the diaphragm is only sparsely provided with spindles.

Electromyographic activity in the crura may be recorded with a bipolar oesophageal lead (Agostoni, Sant'Ambrogio and Carrasco, 1960; Agostoni, 1962). Muller et al. (1979) recorded from the costal part by silencing overlying intercostal muscle activity with a nerve block. They reported tonic expiratory electrical activity, which has not been reported from the crural part.

The intercostal muscles. These muscles are divided into the external group (deficient anteriorly), the less powerful internal group (deficient posteriorly) and the feeble strands of intercostalis intima. In 1749, mechanical consideration led Hamberger to suggest that the external intercostals were primarily inspiratory, and the internal intercostals primarily expiratory. This has generally been confirmed by electromyography, although the parasternals (part of the internal intercostals) are inspiratory, particularly in the dog. Levator costalis is also inspiratory. The intercostals are richly provided with spindles.

Scalenes are not accessory respiratory muscles as was originally thought, but are active in inspiration during quiet breathing of man, though not the dog (De Troyer, 1991). Their action is elevation of the rib cage and this counteracts the tendency of the diaphragm to cause inward displacement of the upper ribs (see above). Innervation is C1–5.

Sternocleidomastoids are silent in normal breathing in man but are potent accessory muscles in hyperventilation or when the respiratory load is increased. As innervation is mainly from the 11th cranial nerve they have a crucial role in high tetraplegia. Their action is similar to that of the scalenes.

The expiratory muscles

In the supine position, the expiratory muscles are normally silent during quiet breathing. They become active when the minute volume exceeds about 40 l/min, in the face of substantial expiratory resistance, during phonation and when making expulsive efforts. However, their use in breathing is complicated by their role in the maintenance of posture. Thus the abdominal muscles are normally active in the upright position but silent during quiet breathing in the supine position.

The most important expiratory muscles are rectus abdominis, external and internal obliques, and tranversalis. The muscles of the pelvic floor have a supportive role. Their obvious expiratory role is to force the diaphragm upwards and pull the rib cage downwards. However, the fixation of the central tendon of the diaphragm increases the efficiency with which the diaphragm can elevate the rib cage. External oblique is usually monitored as an indication of expiratory muscle activity but gastric pressure is a valuable index of their activity because they cannot contract without causing an increase in intra-abdominal pressure.

Active hyperventilation

As ventilation is increased, the inspiratory muscles contract more vigorously and accessory muscles are recruited. Considerable hyperventilation (about 50 l/min) is usually attained before the sternomastoids and extensors of the vertebral column are brought into play (Campbell, 1958). Maximal hyperventilation requires the use of many groups of muscles. The pectorals, for example, reverse their usual origin/insertion and help to expand the chest, provided the arms are fixed by grasping a suitable support. Expiratory muscle activity is evident when the minute volume exceeds about 40 l/min (Campbell, 1952). Thereafter it becomes progressively more important until ventilation assumes a quasi sine wave push–pull pattern in extreme hyperventilation (Cooper, 1961).

Effect of posture

The diaphragm tends to lie some 4 cm higher in the supine position (Wade and Gilson, 1951) and this accords with the reduction in FRC (see Figure 3.4). The dimensions of the rib cage are probably little altered. Although there is a greater tendency to airway closure at the reduced FRC, the diaphragm is able to contract more effectively the higher it rises into the chest. In the lateral position (Figure 6.3), the lower dome of the diaphragm is pushed higher into the chest by the weight of the abdominal contents while the upper dome is flattened. It follows that the lower dome can contract more effectively than the upper, and the ventilation of the lower lung is about twice that of the upper. This is fortunate because gravity causes a preferential perfusion of the lower lung (page 163).

Separation of volume contribution of rib cage and abdomen

Konno and Mead (1967) proposed that the separate volume contribution of changes in rib cage (RC) and abdomen (AB) could be measured (as anteroposterior diameter). Essentially similar results may be obtained by measuring circumference (strain gauge) or cross-sectional area (respiratory inductance plethy-

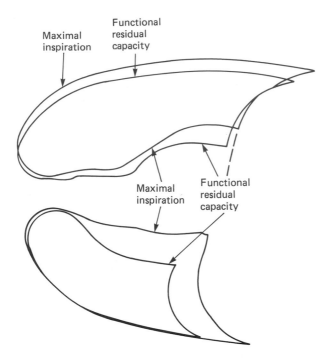

Figure 6.3 Radiographic outlines of the lungs at two levels of lung volume in a conscious subject during spontaneous breathing in the lateral position (right side down). This is the same subject as in Figure 6.1: comparison will show that, in the lateral position at FRC, the lower lung is close to residual volume while the upper lung is close to inspiratory capacity. The diaphragm therefore lies much higher in the lower half of the chest. Both these factors contribute to the greater volume changes which occur in the lower lung during inspiration. The mediastinum seems to rest on a pneumatic cushion at FRC and rises during inspiration.

smography − RIP). The sum of RC and AB correlates well with tidal volume and provides an excellent non-invasive measure of ventilation. RC/(RC + AB) indicates the proportion of total ventilation which can be attributed to expansion of the rib cage. However, such is the complexity of the muscular system described above that changes in RC/(RC + AB) cannot be attributed to changes in the force of contraction of any particular muscle.

Effects of posture and hypercapnia. There is widespread agreement that RC is about 33% of total in the supine position, but 67% in the upright subject. In the supine position, the diaphragm lies higher in the chest, its fibre length is greater and it can therefore contract more effectively. In the prone and lateral position, RC contribution does not differ significantly from that in the supine position (Lumb and Nunn, 1991a). Hyperventilation in response to hypercapnia in the supine position results in a small increase in RC contribution (0.13% per kPa P_{CO_2} or 1% per mmHg P_{CO_2}) (Lumb and Nunn, 1991b).

The work of breathing
(see review by Milic-Emili, 1991)

When expiration is passive during quiet breathing, the work of breathing is performed entirely by the inspiratory muscles. Approximately half of this work is dissipated during inspiration as heat in overcoming the frictional forces opposing inspiration. The other half is stored as potential energy in the deformed elastic tissues of lung and chest wall. This potential energy is thus available as the source of energy for expiration and is then dissipated as heat in overcoming the frictional forces resisting expiration. Energy stored in deformed elastic tissue thus permits the work of *expiration* to be transferred to the *inspiratory* muscles. This remains true with moderate increases of either inspiratory or expiratory resistance, lung volume and therefore elastic recoil being increased in the latter condition (page 85).

The actual work performed by the respiratory muscles is very small in the healthy resting subject. Under these circumstances the oxygen consumption of the respiratory muscles is only about 3 ml/min or less than 2% of the metabolic rate. Furthermore, the efficiency of the respiratory muscles is only about 10%. The efficiency is further reduced in many forms of respiratory disease, certain deformities, pregnancy and when the minute volume is increased (Figure 6.4).

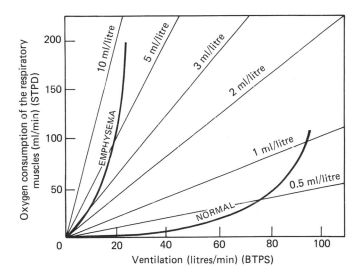

Figure 6.4 Oxygen consumption of the respiratory muscles plotted against minute volume of respiration. The isopleths indicate the oxygen cost of breathing in millilitres of oxygen consumed per litre of minute volume. The curve obtained from the normal subject shows the low oxygen cost of breathing up to a minute volume of 70 l/min. Thereafter the oxygen cost rises steeply. In the emphysematous patient, the oxygen cost of breathing is not only much higher at the resting minute volume but also rises steeply as ventilation is increased. At a minute volume of 20 l/min, the respiratory muscles are consuming 200 ml oxygen per minute, and a further increase of ventilation would consume more oxygen than it would make available to the rest of the body. (Reproduced after Campbell, Westlake and Cherniak (1957) by permission of the Editor of the Journal of Applied Physiology)

When maximal ventilation is approached, the efficiency falls to such a low level that additional oxygen made available by further increases in ventilation will be entirely consumed by the respiratory muscles (Otis, 1954).

Units of measurement of work

Work is performed when a force moves its point of application, and the work is equal to the product of force and distance moved. Similarly, work is performed when force is applied to the plunger of a syringe raising the pressure of gas contained therein. In this case the work is equal to the product of the mean pressure and the change in volume, or alternatively the product of the mean volume and the change in pressure. The units of work are identical whether the product is *force × distance* or *pressure × volume*. A multiplicity of units have been used for measuring work and are listed in Appendix A.

Power is a measure of the rate at which work is being (or can be) performed. The term 'work of breathing', as it is normally used and when expressed in watts, is thus a misnomer since we are referring to the rate at which work is being performed and *power* is the correct term. 'Work of breathing' would be appropriate for a single event such as one breath, and joules would then be the appropriate units.

Dissipation of the work of breathing

The work of breathing overcomes two main sources of impedance. The first is the elastic recoil of the lungs and chest wall (Chapter 3) and the second is the non-elastic (mainly frictional) resistance to gas flow (Chapter 4).

Work against elastic recoil. When an elastic body is deformed, no work is dissipated as heat and all work is stored as potential energy. Figure 6.5a shows a section of the alveolar pressure/volume plot for the total respiratory system (see Figure 3.8). As the lungs are inflated, the plot forms the hypotenuse of a triangle, whose area represents the work done against elastic resistance. The area of the triangle (half the base times the height) will thus equal either half the tidal volume times the pressure change or the mean pressure times the volume change. Either product has the units of work or energy (joules) and represents the potential energy available for expiration. In Figure 6.5b, the pressure/volume curve is flatter, indicating stiffer or less compliant lungs. For the same tidal volume, the area of the triangle is increased. This indicates the greater amount of work performed against elastic resistance and the greater potential energy available for expiration.

Work against resistance to gas flow. Frictional resistance was ignored in Figure 6.5. Additional pressure is required to overcome frictional resistance to gas flow which is reflected in the mouth pressure which, during inspiration, is above the alveolar pressure by the driving pressure required to overcome frictional resistance. When mouth pressure is plotted as in Figure 6.6, the inspiratory curve is bowed to the right and the area shaded with vertical lines to the right of the pressure volume curve indicates the additional work performed in overcoming inspiratory frictional resistance. Figure 6.6b represents a patient with increased airway resistance. The expiratory curve, not shown in Figure 6.6, would be bowed to the left as the mouth-to-alveolar pressure gradient is reversed during expiration.

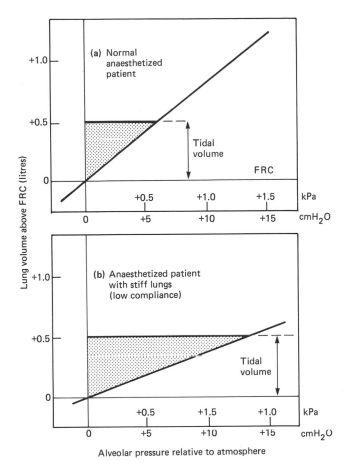

Figure 6.5 Work of breathing against elastic resistance during passive inflation. Pressure/volume plots of the lungs of anaesthetized patients (see Figure 3.8). The length of the pressure/volume curve covered during inspiration forms the hypotenuse of a right-angled triangle whose area equals the work performed against elastic resistance. Note that the area is greater when the pressure/volume curve is flatter (indicating stiffer or less compliant lungs).

The minimal work of breathing

For a constant minute volume, the work performed against elastic resistance is increased when breathing is slow and deep. Conversely, the work performed against air flow resistance is increased when breathing is rapid and shallow. If the two components are summated and the total work is plotted against respiratory frequency, it will be found that there is an optimal frequency at which the total work of breathing is minimal (Figure 6.7). If there is increased elastic resistance (as in patients with pulmonary fibrosis), the optimal frequency is increased, while in the presence of increased air flow resistance the optimal frequency is decreased. Man and animals tend to select a respiratory frequency which is close to that which minimizes respiratory work (McIlroy et al., 1956). This applies to different species, different age groups and also to pathological conditions.

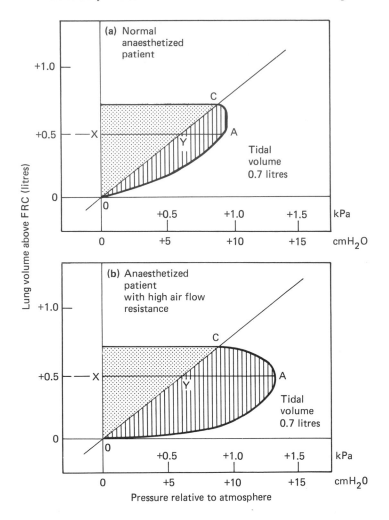

Figure 6.6 Work of breathing against air flow resistance during passive inflation. The sloping line (OYC) is the alveolar pressure/volume curve. The curve (OAC) is the mouth pressure/volume curve during inflation of the lungs. The area shaded with vertical stripes indicates the work of inspiration performed against air flow resistance. This work is increased in the patient with high resistance (b). At the point when 500 ml gas has entered the patient, XY represents the pressure distending the lungs, while YA represents the pressure overcoming air flow resistance. XA is the inflation pressure at that moment. The stippled areas represent work done against elastic resistance (see Figure 6.5).

Respiratory muscle fatigue
(see reviews by Moxham, 1990, and McKenzie and Gandevia, 1991)

In 1977, Roussos and Macklem showed that the diaphragm, like other striated muscles, was subject to fatigue. While resistive loads less than 40% of maximum could be sustained indefinitely, loads greater than 40% of maximum could only be

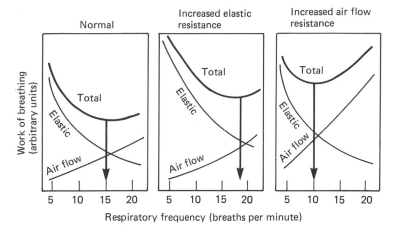

Figure 6.7 The diagrams show the work done against elastic and air flow resistance separately and summated to indicate the total work of breathing at different respiratory frequencies. The total work of breathing has a minimum value at about 15 breaths per minute under normal circumstances. For the same minute volume, minimum work is performed at higher frequencies with stiff (less compliant) lungs and at lower frequencies when the air flow resistance is increased.

sustained for short times. Central drive may be greatly increased in patients with chronic obstructive airway disease and the respiratory muscles may be hypertrophied. Conversely, there may be muscle wasting in malnutrition, or disuse atrophy following a period of artificial ventilation. An increased FRC results in a flattened diaphragm with shortened fibre length which contracts less efficiently.

When working against an unsustainable load, striated muscle shows a progressive loss of the high frequency component of the electromyogram (EMG) relative to lower frequencies. A reduction in the high/low frequency ratio of the EMG is an indication of impending fatigue.

It seems probable that respiratory muscle fatigue may be an important factor in ventilatory failure and failure to wean from artificial ventilation. Although many aspects of the clinical significance are still unclear, steps can be taken to minimize the oxygen demand of patients, to minimize respiratory impedance, to optimize the efficiency of the ventilatory pump and to rest the respiratory muscles by the use of assisted ventilation.

Dyscoordinated breathing

Under a wide range of pathological circumstances, there may occur a type of breathing in which there is lack of co-ordination between thoracic and diaphragmatic components. In its extreme form there is failure to synchronize, and the chest wall moves inwards during inspiration. Pontoppidan, Geffin and Lowenstein (1972) discussed this problem in their review of acute respiratory failure, and pointed out that it is relatively common and may exist between the two sides of the diaphragm which is difficult to diagnose without recourse to imaging techniques. Respiratory muscle dyscoordination increases the work of breathing and reduces the effective tidal volume.

Effect of disuse

The diaphragm may be rested by artificial ventilation with or without neuromuscular blockade, and the effect on diaphragmatic performance is clearly important. In adult hamsters, 2 weeks of unilateral phrenic nerve block or section resulted in a decrease in maximal contractile strength but increased resistance to fatigue (Zhan and Sieck, 1992). These changes were consistent with the observation that type I fibres were hypertrophied whilst type II fibres were atrophied.

The minute volume of pulmonary ventilation

The primary function of the respiratory system is to ensure the normality of oxygen and carbon dioxide partial pressures in the arterial blood. The adequacy of minute volume depends upon the corresponding alveolar ventilation, which equals the product of respiratory frequency and (tidal volume less dead space). Dead space is considered in detail on pages 169 et seq. As alveolar ventilation increases, the composition of the alveolar gas tends to approach that of the inspired gas. The difference between inspired and alveolar gas concentrations is equal to the ratio of the output (or uptake) of the gas to the alveolar ventilation according to the universal alveolar air equation:

$$\begin{matrix} \text{alveolar} \\ \text{concentration} \\ \text{of gas X} \end{matrix} = \begin{matrix} \text{inspired} \\ \text{concentration} \\ \text{of gas X} \end{matrix} + (\text{or} -) \frac{\text{output (or uptake) of gas X}}{\text{alveolar ventilation}}$$

Note:

1. Concentrations are here expressed as fractions and must be multiplied by 100 to give the more familiar percentages.
2. The equation is only approximate and does not correct for any difference between inspired and expired minute volumes. Corrections for this factor are considered on page 196.
3. The sign on the right-hand side is + for output of a gas (e.g. carbon dioxide) and − for uptake (e.g. oxygen).
4. The tension or partial pressure of gas X may be obtained by multiplying the fractional concentration by the dry barometric pressure (page 256).

Alveolar P_{CO_2} and P_{O_2} (the latter for different values of inspired oxygen concentration) are plotted against alveolar ventilation in Figure 6.8 and receive individual consideration for carbon dioxide on page 232 and for oxygen on page 257. The curves are rectangular hyperbolas (explained in Appendix F, page 580) and have great practical and clinical relevance, making clear many aspects of the effect of changes in ventilation.

Rectangular hyperbolas relating alveolar gas concentrations to alveolar ventilation all obey the following general rules:

1. The vertical asymptote is zero alveolar ventilation.
2. The horizontal asymptote is the ambient concentration of the gas under consideration (i.e. effectively zero for carbon dioxide and approximately 21 kPa or % for oxygen while breathing air).

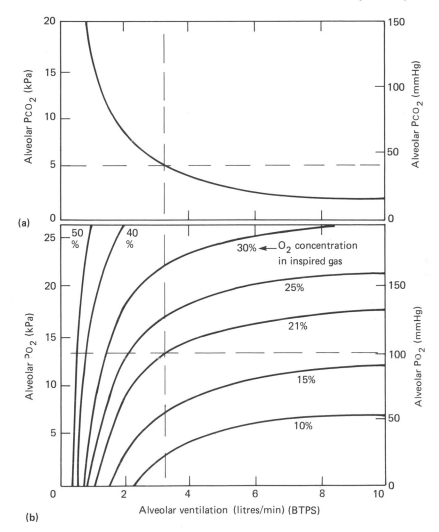

Figure 6.8 Alveolar gas tensions produced by different levels of alveolar ventilation. (a) The hyperbolic relationship between alveolar P_{CO_2} and alveolar ventilation. (b) The relationship between alveolar P_{O_2} and alveolar ventilation for different levels of oxygen concentration in the inspired gas. The broken vertical line indicates an alveolar ventilation of 3.2 l/min. Dry barometric pressure, 95 kPa = 713 mmHg; carbon dioxide output, 150 ml/min (STPD) = 180 ml/min (BTPS); oxygen uptake, 190 ml/min (STPD) = 225 ml/min (BTPS). No allowance has been made for the difference between inspired and expired minute volumes.

3. The curve is concave upwards for gases being eliminated from the body and concave downwards for gas being taken up into the body.
4. The curves move away from the intersection of the asymptotes as the volume of the gas being exchanged increases.

Failure of ventilation is considered in Chapter 21.

Measurement of ventilation

Volume is the integral of gas flow rate and may be measured either directly or, alternatively, by the integration of instantaneous gas flow rate (Figure 6.9). It is important to distinguish between the instantaneous flow rate of gases during breathing and the minute volume of the subject which is of the order of one-quarter of the maximal flow rate (see Figure 4.13). Both differ from the peak flow rate which the patient is able to achieve (see below).

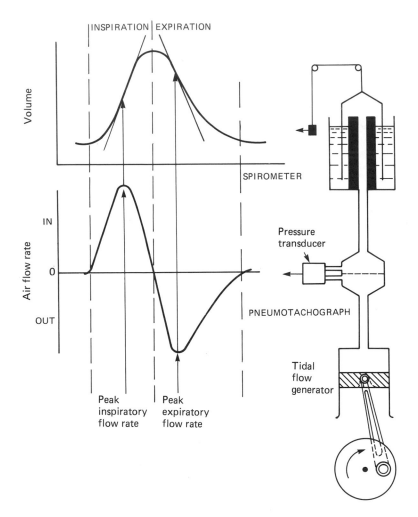

Figure 6.9 Relationship between volume and flow rate. The upper graph shows volume plotted against time; this type of tracing may be obtained with a spirometer. The lower graph shows instantaneous air flow rate plotted against time; this type of tracing may be obtained with a pneumotachograph. At any instant, the flow-rate trace indicates the slope of the volume trace, while the volume trace indicates the cumulative area under the flow-rate trace. Flow is the differential of volume; volume is the integral of flow rate. Differentiation of the spirometer trace gives a 'pneumotachogram'. Integration of the pneumotachogram gives a 'spirometer trace'.

Direct measurement of respired volumes

Inspiratory and expiratory tidal volumes and minute volumes may be markedly different and the difference is important in calculations of gas exchange. The normal respiratory exchange ratio of about 0.8 means that inspiratory minute volume is about 50 ml larger than the expiratory minute volume in the resting subject. Much larger differences can arise during exercise and during uptake or wash-out of an inert gas such as nitrogen or, to a greater extent, nitrous oxide.

Water-sealed spirometers provide the reference method for the measurement of ventilation (Figure 6.9), and may be precisely calibrated by water displacement. They provide negligible resistance to breathing and, by suitable design, may have a satisfactory frequency response up to very high respiratory frequencies (Bernstein and Mendel, 1951; Bernstein, D'Silva and Mendel, 1952). Tissot spirometers have a capacity of about 200 litres and are used either as inspiratory gas reservoirs or for the collection of expired gas.

The box–bag spirometer (Figure 6.10) permits accurate measurement of both inspiratory and expiratory tidal volumes without rebreathing (Donald and Christie, 1949). It provides a useful solution to a number of difficult problems of spirometry but suffers from the disadvantage of being very temperature sensitive and having a capacity which is sufficient for only a few breaths. It may be adapted to continuous flow (Nunn, 1956).

Dry spirometers are hinged bellows, usually with electrical read-out of both volume and instantaneous flow rate. Their accuracy approaches that of a water-filled spirometer and they are far more convenient in use.

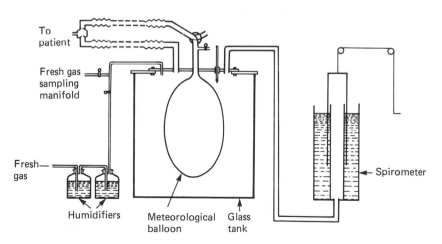

Figure 6.10 In the box–bag spirometer system, the patient inhales from the box and exhales into the bag. The tidal volume and the difference between the inspiratory and expiratory volumes are read directly from the spirometer. Inspiratory and expiratory gas may be sampled and analysis permits measurement of exchange of all gaseous components. The system may be reversed (i.e. inspiration from the bag) for studying the response to different inhaled gas mixtures. (Reproduced from Nunn and Pouliot (1962) by permission of the Editor of the British Journal of Anaesthesia)

The wet gas meter consists of a type of paddle wheel which is sealed with water. These instruments are rather cumbersome but are highly accurate for the measurement of a volume which is passed steadily through the meter. It is particularly suitable for the measurement of the expired volume collected in a Douglas bag.

Dry gas meters are based on two bellows which alternately drive a spindle by means of cranks. The principle is similar to the long-established design of meters used for measuring domestic gas consumption. They are not accurate for small volumes such as a single tidal volume but are very reliable for the measurement of larger volumes such as the volume exhaled over a few minutes. Errors in the use of dry gas meters were exhaustively discussed by Cooper (1959).

Impellers and turbines. The best known of these instruments is the respirometer developed by Wright (1955). Alternating gas flow is mechanically rectified and the dead space (22 ml) is sufficiently small for the patient to breathe to and fro through it. The essential mechanism is entirely mechanical with indication of volume on a dial but the output may be converted to an electrical signal to indicate either tidal volume or minute volume. The accuracy of the instrument was assessed by Nunn and Ezi-Ashi (1962). In general the respirometer tends to read low at low minute volumes and high at high minute volumes. Departure from normality is thus exaggerated and the instrument is essentially safe.

There are, in addition, a wide range of dry rotary meters, all somewhat larger than the Wright respirometer. Each has its own characteristics and with a generic tendency to under-reading at low minute volumes.

Respiratory inductance plethysmography. Reference has been made above (page 121) to this method of measurement of cross-sectional area of rib cage (RC) and abdomen (AB) (Milledge and Stott, 1977). RC and AB can be made to provide proportional signals by means of an 'iso-volume' manoeuvre in which the subject changes the relative volumes of his rib cage and abdomen against a closed glottis. The sum of RC and AB signals correlates well with lung volume and changes in the summated signals provide a very useful non-invasive method of measurement or monitoring of ventilation, uninfluenced by the presence of a mouthpiece or mask.

Measurement of ventilatory volumes by integration of instantaneous gas flow rate

Technical advances in electronic circuitry have increased the attractions of measuring ventilatory volumes by integration of instantaneous flow rate. There are many methods of measurement of rapidly changing gas flow rates of which the original was pneumotachography. This employs measurement of the pressure gradient across a laminar resistance, which ensures that the pressure drop is directly proportional to flow rate (page 62). This is illustrated in Figure 6.9 where the resistor is a wire mesh screen. It is necessary to take precautions to prevent errors due to different gas composition and temperature, and to prevent condensation of moisture on the screen. The pressure drop need not exceed a few millimetres of water and the volume can be very small. The pneumotachograph should not therefore interfere with respiration. Sources of error were considered in detail by Smith (1964).

Alternative flow detectors include Venturi tubes which give a pressure signal proportional to the square of flow, Pitot tubes and the hot wire anemometer. The last device depends on the cooling of a very thin platinum wire heated to about 400°C. The hot wire anemometer is capable of considerable accuracy when run at high temperature and is little influenced by the temperature of the gas.

Measurement of ventilatory capacity

Measurement of ventilatory capacity is the most commonly performed test of respiratory function. The ratio of ventilatory capacity to actual ventilation is a measure of ventilatory reserve and of the comfort of breathing. In the normal subject the maximal breathing capacity is about 15–20 times the resting minute volume.

Maximal breathing capacity (MBC)

MBC is defined as the maximal minute volume of ventilation which the subject can maintain for 15 seconds. The subject simple breathes in and out of a spirometer without the need for removal of carbon dioxide. The test, although simple, is exhausting to perform and is now seldom used. MBC cannot be sustained indefinitely but 75% of MBC can be sustained with difficulty by young fit subjects for 15 minutes (Shephard, 1967). Dyspnoea ensues when ventilation reaches about a third of MBC. The average fit young male adult should have an MBC of about 170 l/min but normal values depend upon body size, age and sex, the range being 47–253 min for men and 55–139 l/min for women (Cotes, 1975).

Forced expiration

A more practical test of ventilatory capacity is the forced expiratory volume (1 second) or $FEV_{1.0}$, which is the maximal volume exhaled in the first second starting from a maximal inspiration. A simple spirometer is all that is required. It is far more convenient to perform than the MBC and less exhausting for the patient. It correlates well with the MBC, which is about 35 times the $FEV_{1.0}$.

Peak expiratory flow rate

Most convenient of all the indirect tests of ventilatory capacity is the peak expiratory flow rate. This can be measured with simple and inexpensive hand-held devices. This is most commonly done with the Wright peak flow meter, described in its original form by Wright and McKerrow (1959). Alternatively, the peak flow may be derived from a pneumotachogram but this is sensitive to very short transients and may give a spuriously high value. The Wright peak flow meter tends to give values about 5.7 times the MBC.

Interpretation of measurements of maximal expirations may be misleading. It should be remembered that these tests measure active expiration which plays no part in normal breathing. They are most commonly performed as a measure of airway obstruction and are extensively used in asthma and chronic obstructive airway disease. However, the results also depend on many other factors, including chest restriction, motivation and muscular power. The measurements may also be inhibited by pain. A more specific indication of airway resistance is the ratio of $FEV_{1.0}$ to vital capacity. This should exceed 75% in the normal subject.

Use of bronchodilators

When there is a reduction in the ventilatory capacity measured by the techniques outlined above, it is helpful to administer a bronchodilator such as a beta-sympathomimetic agent. Any improvement in ventilatory capacity will then indicate the extent to which bronchoconstriction had been responsible. No change indicates that the reduction in ventilatory capacity was mainly caused by structural factors such as trapping or pulmonary fibrosis. No improvement is to be expected when reduced ventilatory capacity is due to non-pulmonary factors such as pain or muscle weakness.

Chapter 7

The pulmonary circulation

*Fit autem comunicatio haec non per parierem cordis medium, ut vulgo creditur sed magno artificio a dextro cordis ventriculo, longo per pulmones ductu agitatur sanguis subtilis: a pulmonibus praeparatur, flavus efficitur...*etc. (Michael Servetus, 1553). In a few words, interspersed in a theological writing, Michael Servetus was the first to suggest that venous blood did not pass through the middle wall of the heart, as was generally believed, but pursued a long course through the lungs starting from the right side of the heart.

The entire blood volume passes through the lungs during each circulation. This is an appropriate arrangement for gas exchange but is equally suitable for the filtering and metabolic functions of the lungs, which are considered in Chapter 12.

Although blood flow is continuous while gas flow is tidal, it is sometimes helpful to represent both flows as continuous and to consider the lung as a exchanger with a gas inflow and outflow, and a blood inflow and outflow (Figure 7.1). There is near-equilibrium of oxygen and carbon dioxide tensions between the two outflow streams from the exchanger itself. However, each side has a bypass causing contamination of both outflows with part of the corresponding inflow. This model has been deliberately drawn without countercurrent flow, which would be far more efficient. Such a system operates in the gills of fishes, and brings the PO_2 of arterial blood close to the PO_2 of the environment.

Pulmonary blood volume

Table 2.3 shows the anatomical distribution of the pulmonary blood volume within the pulmonary arterial tree which has a volume of the order of 150 ml. Pulmonary capillary volume may be calculated from measurements of diffusing capacity (Chapter 9), and this technique yields values of the order of 80 ml. The pulmonary veins have less vasomotor tone than the arterial tree and consequently have a larger volume. Methods of measurement are outlined at the end of this chapter and, for practical purposes, the pulmonary (or central) blood volume is defined as the volume which lies between the two anatomical sites chosen for injection and sampling of dye. Typical values are of the order of 0.5–1.0 litre or 10–20% of total blood volume.

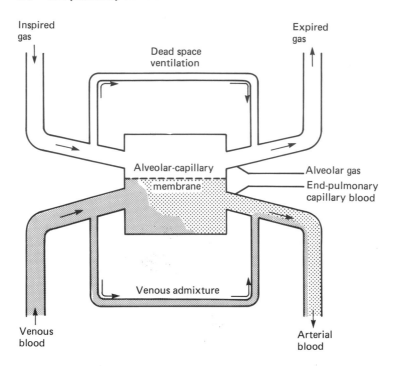

Figure 7.1 In this functional representation of gas exchange in the lungs, the flow of gas and blood is considered as a continuous process with movement from left to right. Under most circumstances, equilibrium is obtained between alveolar gas and end-pulmonary capillary blood, the gas tensions in the two phases being almost identical. However, alveolar gas is mixed with dead space gas to give expired gas. Meanwhile, end-pulmonary capillary blood is mixed with shunted venous blood to give arterial blood. Thus both expired gas and arterial blood have gas tensions which differ from those in alveolar gas and end-pulmonary capillary blood.

Haemodynamic and anatomical considerations

As a first approximation the right heart pumps blood into the pulmonary circulation, while the left heart pumps away the blood which returns from the lungs. Therefore, provided that the output of the two sides is the same, the pulmonary blood volume will remain constant. However, very small differences in the outputs of the two sides must result in large changes in pulmonary blood volume if they are maintained for more than a few beats.

In fact, the relationship between the inflow and outflow of the pulmonary circulation is much more complicated (Figure 7.2). The lungs receive a significant quantity of blood from the bronchial arteries which usually arise from the arch of the aorta. Blood from the bronchial circulation returns to the heart in two ways. From a plexus around the hilum, blood from the pleurohilar part of the bronchial circulation returns to the systemic veins via the azygos veins, and this fraction may thus be regarded as normal systemic flow, neither arising from nor returning to the pulmonary circulation. However, another fraction of the bronchial circulation, distributed more peripherally in the lung, passes through postcapillary anastomoses to join the pulmonary veins, constituting an admixture of venous blood with the

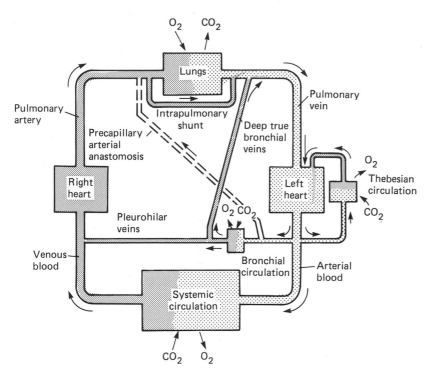

Figure 7.2 Schema of bronchopulmonary anastomoses and other forms of venous admixture in the normal subject. Part of the bronchial circulation returns venous blood to the systemic venous system (pleurohilar veins) while another part returns venous blood to the pulmonary veins and so constitutes venous admixture. Other forms of venous admixture are the thebesian circulation of the left heart and flow through atelectatic parts of the lungs. The existence of precapillary bronchopulmonary anastomoses in the normal subject is controversial. It will be clear from this diagram why the output of the left heart must be slightly greater than that of the right heart.

arterialized blood from the alveolar capillary networks (Marchand, Gilroy and Wilson, 1950).

The situation may be further complicated by blood flow through precapillary anastomoses from the bronchial arteries to the pulmonary arteries. The communications (so-called 'sperr arteries') have muscular walls and are thought to act as sluice gates (Verloop, 1948; von Hayek, 1960). They may have special functional importance in cases of pulmonary oligaemia. Flow has been demonstrated after experimental ligation of a branch of the pulmonary artery in dogs (Cockett and Vass, 1951), but congenital pulmonary atresia is the most important natural cause. It should be noted that a Blalock–Taussig bronchopulmonary anastomosis achieved the same purpose.

There are many possible abnormal communications between the pulmonary and systemic circulations. It is not unusual for aberrant pulmonary veins to drain into the right atrium. Furthermore, flow may be reversed through normally occurring channels. Thus, in pulmonary venous hypertension due to mitral stenosis, pulmonary venous blood may traverse the bronchial venous system to gain access to the azygos system.

Factors influencing pulmonary blood volume

The pulmonary volume fluctuates during the cardiac cycle since inflow exceeds outflow during systole. It is also likely that the cyclical pressure changes caused by respiration will influence pulmonary blood volume which decreases initially during a Valsalva manoeuvre (page 457), and during positive pressure breathing (Fenn et al., 1947). Conversely, pulmonary blood volume is increased during negative pressure breathing (Slome, 1965).

Posture. Pulmonary blood volume is directly influenced by posture (Harris and Heath, 1962). Change from the supine to the erect position decreases the pulmonary blood volume by 27%, which is about the same as the corresponding change in cardiac output. Both changes are probably due to pooling of blood in dependent parts of the systemic circulation.

Drugs. Since the systemic circulation has much greater vasomotor activity than the pulmonary circulation, an overall increase in vascular tone will tend to squeeze blood from the systemic into the pulmonary circulation. This may result from the administration of vasoconstrictor drugs or from release of endogenous catechol-amines. Similar changes result from passive compression of the body in a G-suit. Conversely, it seems likely that pulmonary blood volume would be diminished when systemic tone is diminished, as for example by sympathetic ganglion blockade. Large decreases in pulmonary blood volume have been reported during spinal anaesthesia, but increases sometimes occurred when the patient was in the Trendelenburg position (Johnson, 1951).

Left heart failure. Pulmonary venous hypertension (due, for example, to mitral stenosis) would be expected to result in an increased pulmonary blood volume. There has, however, been difficulty in the experimental demonstration of any significant change.

Pulmonary blood flow

The flow of blood through the pulmonary circulation is approximately equal to the flow through the whole of the systemic circulation. It therefore varies from about 6 l/min under resting conditions to as much as 25 l/min in severe exercise. It is remarkable that such an increase can normally be achieved with minimal increase in pressure. Pulmonary vascular pressures and vascular resistance are much less than those of the systemic circulation. Consequently the pulmonary circulation has only limited ability to control the distribution of blood flow within the lung fields and is markedly affected by gravity, which results in overperfusion of the dependent parts of the lung fields. Maldistribution of the pulmonary blood flow has important consequences for gaseous exchange, and these are considered in Chapter 8.

Methods for the measurement of pulmonary blood flow are outlined at the end of this chapter, but at this stage it should be pointed out that most methods of measurement of cardiac output (Fick, dye and thermal dilution) measure the total pulmonary blood flow, together with the venous admixture (see Figure 7.1). On the other hand, the body plethysmograph measures only the pulmonary capillary blood flow. In this method, the alveoli are filled with nitrous oxide at a concentration of about 15%, and the amount of nitrous oxide taken up by the blood is measured by whole body plethysmography. The method clearly shows that capillary blood flow is pulsatile.

Pulmonary vascular pressures

Pulmonary arterial pressure is only about one-sixth of systemic arterial pressure, although the capillary and venous pressures are not greatly different for the two circulations (Figure 7.3). There is thus only a small pressure drop along the pulmonary arterioles and therefore little possibility for active regulation of the distribution of the pulmonary circulation. This also explains why there is little damping of the arterial pressure wave, and the pulmonary capillary blood flow is markedly pulsatile.

Consideration of pulmonary vascular pressures carries a special difficulty in the selection of the reference pressure. Systemic pressures are customarily measured with reference to ambient atmospheric pressure, but this is not always appropriate when considering the pulmonary arterial pressure, which is relatively small in comparison with the intrathoracic and pulmonary venous pressures. This may be important under two circumstances. Firstly, the extravascular (intrathoracic) pressure may have a major influence on the intravascular pressure and should be taken into account. Secondly, the driving pressure through the pulmonary circulation may be markedly influenced by the pulmonary venous pressure which must be taken into account in measurement of pulmonary vascular resistance. We therefore require to distinguish between pressures within the pulmonary circulation expressed in the three different forms listed below. Measurement techniques may be adapted to indicate these pressures directly (Figure 7.4).

Intravascular pressure is the pressure at any point in the circulation relative to atmosphere. This is the customary way of expressing pressures in the systemic

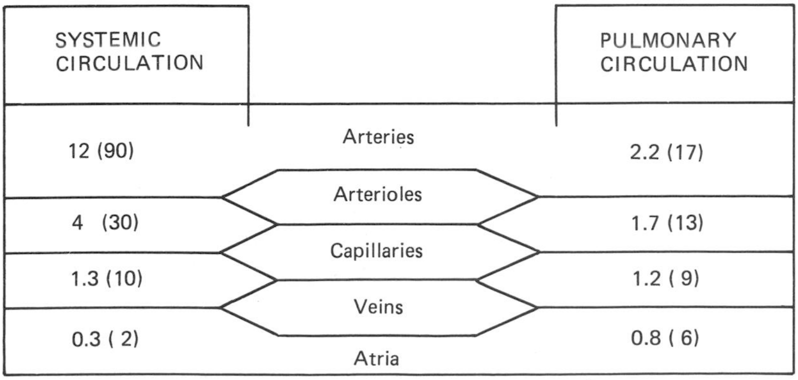

SYSTEMIC CIRCULATION		PULMONARY CIRCULATION
12 (90)	Arteries	2.2 (17)
	Arterioles	
4 (30)		1.7 (13)
	Capillaries	
1.3 (10)		1.2 (9)
	Veins	
0.3 (2)		0.8 (6)
	Atria	

Figure 7.3 Comparison of typical mean pressure gradients along the systemic and pulmonary circulations. (Mean pressures relative to atmosphere in kPa, with mmHg in parentheses)

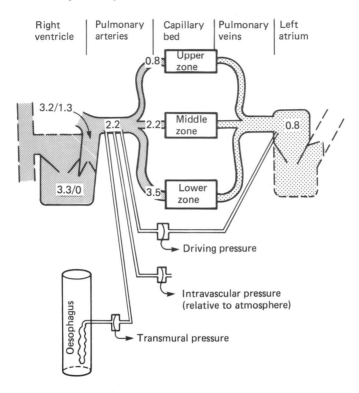

Figure 7.4 Normal values for pressures in the pulmonary circulation relative to atmosphere (kPa). Systolic and diastolic pressures are shown for the right ventricle and pulmonary trunk. Note the effect of gravity on pressures at different levels in the lung fields. Three differential manometers are shown connected to indicate driving pressure, intravascular pressure and transmural pressure.

circulation, and is also the commonest method of indicating the pulmonary vascular pressures.

Transmural pressure is the difference in pressure between the inside of a vessel and the tissue surrounding the vessel. In the case of the larger pulmonary vessels, the outside pressure is the intrathoracic pressure (commonly measured as the oesophageal pressure as in Figure 7.4). This method should be used to exclude the physical effect of major changes in intrathoracic pressure.

Driving pressure is the difference in pressure between one point in the circulation and another point downstream. The driving pressure of the pulmonary circulation as a whole is the pressure difference between pulmonary artery and left atrium. This is the pressure which overcomes the flow resistance and should be used for determination of vascular resistance.

   These differences are far from being solely academic. Changes in intrathoracic pressure transmit a direct physical effect to pulmonary intravascular pressures, and it is necessary to exclude this factor before it is possible to determine the physiological effect of the change in intrathoracic pressure. The difference between pulmonary arterial intravascular pressure (relative to atmosphere) and the pulmonary driving pressure is of importance in distinguishing between different causes of pulmonary hypertension. If the primary lesion is a raised left atrial pressure, the pulmonary arterial intravascular pressure will be raised but the driving pressure will not be increased unless there is a secondary rise in pulmonary vascular resistance.

Left atrial pressure represents pulmonary venous pressure and is measured by one of four possible techniques.

1. Wedge pressures are obtained by advancing the Swan–Ganz catheter into a branch of the pulmonary artery and inflating the balloon to the point at which the arterial pulsation disappears. There should then be no flow in the column of blood between the tip of the catheter and the left atrium, and the manometer will indicate left atrial pressure.
2. The left atrium may be punctured by a needle at bronchoscopy.
3. The atrial septum may be pierced from a catheter in the right atrium.
4. A catheter may be passed retrogradely from a peripheral systemic artery.

Typical normal values within the pulmonary circulation are shown in Figure 7.4. The effect of gravity on the pulmonary vascular pressure may be seen, and it will be clear why pulmonary oedema is most likely to occur in the lower zones of the lungs where the intravascular pressures and the transmural pressure gradients are highest.

Factors influencing pulmonary vascular pressures

Many very important factors which influence pulmonary vascular resistance have a direct effect on pulmonary vascular pressures. These are discussed below under the heading 'Pulmonary vascular resistance' and will not be considered here. However, it is convenient at this point to mention cardiac output, changes in alveolar pressure, posture and disease.

Cardiac output. The pulmonary circulation can adapt to large changes in cardiac output with only small increases in pulmonary arterial pressure. Thus, after pneumonectomy, the remaining lung will normally take the entire resting pulmonary blood flow without rise in pulmonary arterial pressure. The pulmonary circulation adapts to increased flow partly by recruitment of vessels and partly by passive dilatation, the latter now being considered the most important factor (Marshall and Marshall, 1992). Thus pulmonary vascular resistance decreases as flow increases.

There is, however, a limit to the flow which can be accommodated without an increase in pressure, and this will be less if the pulmonary vascular bed is diminished by disease or surgery. Furthermore the pulmonary blood flow may be abnormally increased. The most important pathological cause of increased flow is left-to-right shunting through a patent ductus arteriosus or through atrial or ventricular septal defects. Under these circumstances the pulmonary circulation is greater than the systemic circulation and may be sufficient to result in pulmonary hypertension, even with normal vascular resistance. However, secondary changes commonly result in an increase in vascular resistance, causing a further rise in pulmonary arterial pressure.

Changes of intra-alveolar pressure cause changes in intrathoracic pressure according to the following relationship:

Intrathoracic pressure = Alveolar pressure − Alveolar transmural pressure

Alveolar transmural pressure is a function of lung volume (Figures 3.7 and 3.8) and, when the lungs are passively inflated, the intrathoracic pressure will normally increase by rather less than half the inflation pressure. The increase will be even less if the lungs are stiff, and thus a low compliance protects the circulation from inflation pressure. Intravascular pressures are normally increased directly and instantaneously by changes in intrathoracic pressure, and this explains the initial rise in systemic arterial pressure during a Valsalva manoeuvre (page 458). It also explains the cyclical changes in pulmonary arterial pressure during spontaneous respiration, with pressures greater during expiration than during inspiration. Such changes would not be seen if transmural pressure was measured (see Figure 7.4).

In addition to the immediate physical effect of an increase in intrathoracic pressure on intravascular pressures, there is a secondary physiological effect due to interference with venous filling. This accounts for the secondary decline in systemic pressure seen in the Valsalva manoeuvre.

Posture. It is difficult to study the effect of change of posture on pulmonary blood pressure, since the actual levels of pressure are so low that they are markedly influenced by movement of the reference level. However, it seems likely that the upright position is associated with a lower pulmonary arterial pressure in patients with pulmonary hypertension (Donald et al., 1953). Wedge pressures are also reduced. Intrathoracic pressure is also lower in the upright position, so it is unlikely that capillary transmural pressure is greatly affected.

Disease. There are many causes of pulmonary hypertension. Pulmonary vascular resistance is increased in many forms of pulmonary disease which result in chronic hypoxia (see below), and similar changes occur with intermittent hypoxia caused by sleep apnoea (Chapter 14). The change is initially temporary and reversible but progresses to become permanent. Pulmonary vascular resistance is also increased in many forms of chronic interstitial lung disease, and in pulmonary thrombo-embolism. Severe pulmonary hypertension results from pulmonary atresia and this induces an increased flow through precapillary anastomoses from the bronchial circulation (Figure 7.2), collateral flow sometimes being as great as 1 l/min.

Mitral stenosis and incompetence cause an elevation of pressure in the left atrium. The maintenance of the pulmonary driving pressure requires a corresponding increase of the pulmonary arterial pressure. This may progress to a secondary increase in pulmonary vascular resistance resulting in further elevation of the pulmonary arterial pressure. The work of the right ventricle is increased and, in severe cases, increased vascular resistance limits the benefit of mitral valvotomy, since the mitral valve is no longer the only site of increased resistance to the circulation. Furthermore, a low cardiac output results in reduction of mixed venous PO_2, which also causes increased pulmonary vascular resistance (see below). In a small number of patients pulmonary hypertension appears to be primary and analogous to systemic hypertension.

Whatever the cause, pulmonary hypertension will ultimately lead to dyspnoea and right ventricular hypertrophy, which may progress to failure (cor pulmonale) and an increase in systemic venous pressure. Treatment should first be directed towards relief of chronic or intermittent hypoxia, and the role of long-term oxygen therapy is considered below. Vasodilator therapy is complicated by the lack of drugs with specific action on the pulmonary circulation. The only truly specific drugs are acetylcholine (infused into the pulmonary artery) and nitric oxide (by inhalation), but both require continuous administration. Since nitric oxide by inhalation preferentially dilates the circulation to ventilated alveoli, it not only relieves pulmonary hypertension but also improves gas exchange (page 311). Diuretics may relieve some of the effects of venous congestion. In severe intractable cases lung transplant should be considered.

Pulmonary vascular resistance

Vascular resistance is an expression of the relationship between driving pressure and flow, as in the case of resistance to gas flow (see Figure 4.1). It may be expressed in similar terms as follows:

$$\text{pulmonary vascular resistance} = \frac{\text{pulmonary driving pressure}}{\text{cardiac output}}$$

There are, however, important caveats and the concept of pulmonary vascular resistance is not a simple parallel to Ohm's law, appropriate to laminar flow (page 63). When gases flow through rigid tubes the flow is laminar or turbulent, or a mixture of the two. In the first case pressure increases in direct proportion to flow rate and the resistance remains constant (Poiseuille's law). In the second case pressure increases according to the square of the flow rate, and the resistance increases with flow. When the type of flow is mixed, the pressure rises in proportion to the flow rate raised to a power between one and two.

The circumstances are two stages more complicated in the case of blood. Firstly, the tubes through which the blood flows are not rigid but tend to expand as flow is increased, particularly in the pulmonary circulation with its low vasomotor tone. Consequently the resistance tends to fall as flow increases and the plot of pressure against flow rate is neither linear (see Figure 4.2) nor curved with the concavity upwards (see Figure 4.3) but curved with the concavity downwards. The second complication is that blood is a non-newtonian fluid (due to the presence of the corpuscles) and its viscosity varies with the shear rate, which is a function of its linear velocity.

Although the relationship between flow and pressure is very far removed from simple linearity, there is a widespread convention that pulmonary vascular resistance should be expressed in a form of the equation above. This is directly analogous to electrical resistance, as though there were laminar flow of a newtonian fluid through rigid pipes (see Figure 4.2). It would, of course, be quite impractical in the clinical situation to measure pulmonary driving pressure at different values of cardiac output to determine the true nature of their relationship. Driving pressure is the difference in mean pressures between pulmonary artery and left atrium, the latter usually measured as the 'wedge pressure'. Flow rate is usually taken as cardiac output.

Vascular resistance is expressed in units derived from those which are used for expression of pressure and flow rate. Using conventional units, vascular resistance is usually expressed in units of mmHg litre^{-1} minute. In absolute CGS units, vascular resistance is usually expressed in units of dynes/square centimetre per cubic centimetre/second (i.e. dyn sec cm^{-5}). The appropriate SI units will probably be kilopascal litre^{-1} minute. Normal values for the pulmonary circulation in the various units are as follows:

	Driving pressure	Pulmonary blood flow	Pulmonary vascular resistance
SI units	1.2 kPa	5 l/min	0.24 kPa l^{-1} min
Conventional units	9 mmHg	5 l/min	1.8 mmHg l^{-1} min
Absolute CGS units	12 000 dyn/cm^2	83 cm^3/sec	144 dyn sec cm^{-5}

The measurement of pulmonary vascular resistance is important, not only in the diagnosis of the primary cause of pulmonary hypertension, but also for the detection of increased pulmonary vascular resistance, which often develops in patients in whom the primary cause of pulmonary hypertension is raised left atrial pressure.

Localization of the pulmonary vascular resistance

By far the greatest part of the systemic resistance is within the arterioles, along which the pressure falls from a mean value of about 12 kPa (90 mmHg) down to about 4 kPa (30 mmHg) (see Figure 7.3). This pressure drop largely obliterates the pulse pressure wave, and the systemic capillary flow is not pulsatile to any great extent. In the pulmonary circulation, the pressure drop along the arterioles is very much smaller than in the systemic circulation and, as an approximation, the pulmonary vascular resistance is equally divided between arteries, capillaries and veins. If the whole of the pulmonary microcirculation (i.e. vessels without muscular walls – page 33) is considered, then well over half of the total resistance lies in these vessels. Thus in the pulmonary circulation, vessels without the power of active vasoconstriction play a major role in governing total vascular resistance and the distribution of the pulmonary blood flow.

Autonomic control

The pulmonary circulation has both sympathetic and, to a less extent, parasympathetic control. There are both alpha- and beta-adrenergic endings, the former vasoconstrictor and the latter vasodilator, both acting on the smooth muscle of arteries and arterioles of diameter greater than 30 μm (Fishman, 1985). Noradrenaline is vasoconstrictor and isoprenaline vasodilator. The influence of the sympathetic system is not as strong as in the systemic circulation and appears to have little influence under resting conditions. There is no obvious disadvantage in this respect in patients with lung transplant (Chapter 24). The sympathetic system does, however, have an appreciable effect when there is general activation, as for example under conditions of flight, fright or fight. Pulmonary vasoconstriction may be demonstrated when the stellate ganglion is stimulated, and also when the peripheral chemoreceptors are stimulated by hypoxia (see below).

The parasympathetic system causes pulmonary vasodilatation by release of acetylcholine which is well established as a pulmonary vasodilator when injected into the pulmonary artery. It is now known to act by release of nitric oxide from the endothelium (page 312).

Effect of changes in oxygen and carbon dioxide tensions

Hypoxia has a vasoconstrictor effect on the pulmonary circulation, which is the reverse of its effect on the systemic circulation. The effect is mediated both by the alveolar P_{O_2} and the mixed venous (pulmonary arterial) P_{O_2} (Figure 7.5). The response to P_{O_2} is non-linear. This may be deduced from Figure 7.5 by noting the pressure response for different values of the isobaric P_{O_2} (the broken line), and it will be seen that the general shape of the response curve resembles an oxyhae-moglobin dissociation curve with a P_{50} of about 4 kPa (30 mmHg). The combined effect of hypoxia in alveolar gas and mixed venous blood may be considered as acting at a single point (Marshall, Marshall and Frasch, 1992), which exerts a 'stimulus' P_{O_2} as follows:

$$P(stimulus)O_2 = P\bar{v}_{O_2}^{0.375} \times P_{A_{O_2}}^{0.626}$$

In addition to the effect of mixed venous and alveolar P_{O_2}, the bronchial arterial P_{O_2} influences tone in the larger pulmonary arteries via the vasa vasorum (Marshall et al., 1991).

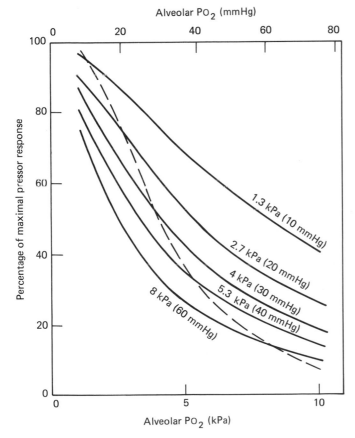

Figure 7.5 Pulmonary vasoconstriction (ordinate) as a function of alveolar P_{O_2} (abscissa) for different values of mixed venous P_{O_2} (indicated for each curve). The broken line shows the response when the alveolar and mixed venous P_{O_2} are identical. (Drawn from the data of Marshall and Marshall (1983))

Regional hypoxic pulmonary vasoconstriction is beneficial as a means of diverting the pulmonary blood flow away from regions in which the oxygen tension is low (Marshall et al., 1981). This is an important factor in the optimization of ventilation/perfusion relationships (Marshall, 1990). It is also important in the fetus to minimize perfusion of the unventilated lung. However, overall chronic or intermittent hypoxic pulmonary vasoconstriction results in pulmonary hypertension, and this response is disadvantageous in a range of clinical conditions (see above). The long-term administration of oxygen to such patients, during the day and during sleep, retards the development of pulmonary hypertension, partially reverses established hypertension and improves survival (Abraham, Cole and Bishop, 1968; Abraham et al., 1969; Flenley, 1985a; Timms, Khaja and Williams, 1985).

The pressor response to hypoxia appears to result from constriction of vessels of less than 1 mm diameter on the arterial side of the pulmonary capillaries. No hypoxic receptors have been identified and neither is there any evidence for release of a vasoconstrictor substance in response to hypoxia although histamine has been investigated for this possibility (Fishman, 1985). Some pulmonary vasoconstriction may result from hypoxic stimulation of the peripheral chemoreceptors by way of sympathetic efferent pathways (Daly and Daly, 1959) but this is manifestly less important than the local effect which is well known to operate in the isolated lung.

There is now substantial evidence that endothelium-derived relaxing factor (EDRF), which is probably nitric oxide (see below and page 311), has an important role in the mechanism of hypoxic pulmonary vasocontriction. Production of EDRF was reduced when PO_2 was reduced in cultured pulmonary arterial endothelial cells from calves (Warren et al., 1989) and rats (Rodman et al., 1990). Inhibition of the action of endothelium-derived relaxing factors augmented hypoxic pulmonary vasoconstriction (Brashers, Peach and Rose, 1988), and inhalation of low concentrations of nitric oxide (5–80 p.p.m.) prevented hypoxic pulmonary vasconstriction (Frostell et al., 1991). Johns, Linden and Peach (1989) showed that the hypoxic vasoconstriction was greater in vessels with intact endothelium. However, hypoxic contraction was still observed in endothelium-denuded bovine pulmonary arteries (Burke-Wolin and Wolin, 1990) and isolated pulmonary artery smooth muscle cells (Murray et al., 1990). The exact role of EDRF in hypoxic pulmonary vasoconstriction is still not clear and it may well be a modulator rather than the primary mechanism. Positive end-expiratory pressure has been observed to inhibit hypoxic pulmonary vasoconstriction (Lejeune et al., 1991).

Hyperoxia has little effect upon pulmonary arterial pressure in the normal subject.

Hypercapnia has a slight pressor effect and reinforces hypoxic vasoconstriction, probably by causing acidosis. Hypoventilation of one lobe of a dog's lung reduces perfusion of that lobe, although its ventilation/perfusion ratio is still reduced (Suggett et al., 1982).

Chemical mediators

Acetylcholine has been used extensively in studies of the pulmonary circulation. When introduced into the pulmonary artery, the rate of hydrolysis is so rapid that the drug is destroyed before it can act upon the systemic circulation. Acetylcholine results in a relaxation of vasomotor tone, causing the pulmonary vascular resistance and arterial pressure to fall by an amount which depends on the tone present before the administration of the drug. The response to acetylcholine may thus be used as an indicator of the degree of vasomotor tone which exists in the pulmonary circulation. Small falls of pressure occur in the normal subject but much greater falls occur in hypoxic subjects and those with pulmonary hypertension resulting from congenital heart disease, emphysema or mitral stenosis (Harris and Heath, 1962). A number of references cited by those authors concur in the view that atropine does not affect pulmonary arterial pressure and is without vasomotor action on the pulmonary circulation. However, Daly, Ross and Behnke (1963) reported a fall in pressure following 2 mg of atropine (intravenously), and Nunn and Bergman (1964) suggested that this might be a cause of the increase in alveolar dead space which they found to follow the administration of atropine.

Furchgott and Zawadzki (1980) showed that the vasodilatory action of acetylcholine is dependent on an intact endothelium. This observation led directly to the discovery of EDRF (Cherry et al., 1982), which is almost certainly nitric oxide (Palmer, Ferrige and Moncada, 1987) (see above and pages 311 and 312). The continuous inhalation of nitric oxide has been shown to be a powerful vasodilator of *ventilated* alveoli but without effect on the systemic circulation (Rossaint et al., 1993).

Catecholamines. Adrenaline and dopamine, which act primarily upon the alpha receptors, result in an increase in pulmonary vascular resistance and arterial pressure. Isoprenaline and drugs which act primarily upon the beta receptors cause a fall of pressure, particularly when this is elevated. Ganglion-blocking agents generally cause a fall in pressure, and this has also been noted in the case of aminophylline.

Other pulmonary vasoconstrictors include 5-hydroxytryptamine (serotonin), thromboxane A_2 and the prostaglandins $PGF_{2\alpha}$ and PGE_2. Histamine causes vasoconstriction by action at the H_1 receptors.

Other pulmonary vasodilators include bradykinin and the prostaglandins PGE_1 and PGE_2 (prostacyclin), the latter being released from capillary endothelium in response to sheer stress (Fishman, 1985). Histamine causes vasodilatation when acting at the H_2 receptors.

Almitrine is a drug which acts primarily to increase the drive of the peripheral chemoreceptors (page 102). However, it may improve arterial PO_2 without necessarily increasing pulmonary ventilation. Romaldini et al. (1983) have observed that it enhances hypoxic pulmonary vasoconstriction, and there is therefore the possibility that it improves the relative distribution of ventilation and perfusion, particularly in patients with diseased lungs.

Physical factors

Recruitment and distension in the pulmonary capillary bed. Reference has been made above (page 138) to the ability of the pulmonary circulation to adapt to large increases in flow with minimal increase in pressure. Therefore, the pulmonary vascular resistance is reduced at the higher flow rate, implying an increase in the total cross-sectional area of the pulmonary vascular bed and particularly the capillaries. This is achieved partly by recruitment of new capillaries, with opening of new passages in the network lying in the alveolar septa (see Plate 5). Sections cut in lungs rapidly frozen while perfused with blood have shown that the number of open capillaries increase with rising pulmonary arterial pressure, particularly in the mid-zone of the lung (Glazier et al., 1969; Warrell et al., 1972).

In addition to recruitment, there is distension of the entire pulmonary vasculature in response to increased transmural pressure gradient. This is particularly true of the capillary bed which is devoid of any vasomotor control. Sobin et al. (1972) showed the diameter increasing from 5 to 10 μm as the transmural pressure increased from 0.5 to 2.5 kPa (5 to 25 cmH$_2$O). Distension plays the major role in zone 3 (page 150) where most of the capillaries are already open (Glazier et al., 1969). Marshall and Marshall (1992) have recently reviewed the evidence for believing that distension plays a more important role than recruitment.

Effects of inflation of the lung. Reference has been made above (page 139) to the effect of alveolar pressure on pulmonary vascular pressures. The effect on pulmonary vascular resistance is complex. Confusion has arisen in the past because of failure to appreciate that pulmonary vascular resistance must be derived from driving pressure and not from pulmonary arterial or transmural pressure (Figure 7.4). This is important because inflation of the lungs normally influences the pressure in the oesophagus, pulmonary artery and left atrium and so can easily conceal the true effect on vascular resistance.

When pulmonary vascular resistance is correctly calculated from the driving pressure, there is reasonable agreement that, in the open-chested or isolated preparation, the pulmonary vascular resistance is minimal at an inflation pressure of the order of 0.5−1 kPa (5−10 cmH$_2$O). Change in inflation pressure in either direction usually causes a small increase in resistance. It seems likely that inflation of the lungs increases the calibre and the volume of the larger blood vessels due to traction from the surrounding lung tissue (Howell et al., 1961). However, the smaller vessels are collapsed as the lung is expanded by inflation.

The effect of lung collapse. The effect of lung collapse on pulmonary blood flow is clinically important because of the physiological advantage in minimizing the perfusion of parts of the lung without ventilation. Barer and her colleagues (1969) clearly showed that it was the PO_2 within the collapsed lung which was important and not the volume or the inflation pressure. With total collapse, the 'alveolar' PO_2 is controlled by the pulmonary arterial PO_2 which thus becomes the main factor governing vascular resistance. Reduction in 'stimulus' PO_2 (see above) increased vascular resistance and decreased flow. These changes could be reversed by vasodilator drugs, and the authors concluded that there was no evidence for any mechanical cause of increased vascular resistance in the collapsed lobe, as had been suggested in the past. Nevertheless, in long-standing collapse, the circulation is further reduced by structural changes in the vessels.

The vascular weir. The interplay of alveolar pressure, flow rate and vascular resistance is best considered by dividing the lung field into three zones (West, Dollery and Naimark, 1964; West and Dollery, 1965). Figure 7.6 shows behaviour as a Starling resistor (see Figure 4.5) and also the analogy of a weir. This is more helpful than the familiar vascular waterfall (Permutt and Riley, 1963), as we can extend the analogy to the situation when the weir is totally submerged (representing zone 3 conditions). In zone 1 of Figure 7.6, the pressure within the arterial end

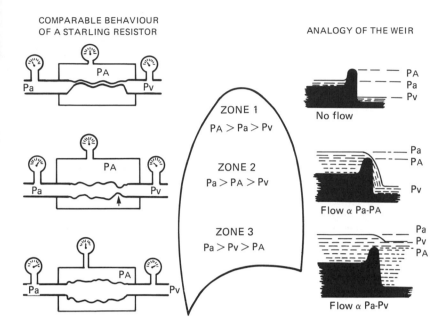

Figure 7.6 The effect of gravity upon pulmonary vascular resistance is shown by comparison with a Starling resistor (left) and with a weir (right). Pa, pressure in pulmonary artery; PA, pressure in alveoli; Pv, pressure in pulmonary vein (all pressures relative to atmosphere). This analogy does not illustrate zone 4 in which perfusion is reduced, apparently due to interstitial pressure acting on the larger vessels (Hughes et al., 1968). See text for full discussion.

of the collapsible vessels is less than the alveolar pressure, and therefore insufficient to open the vessels which remain collapsed as in a Starling resistor. The upstream water is below the top of the weir and so there can be no flow. The downstream (venous) pressure is irrelevant. Zone 1 corresponds to conditions which may apply in the uppermost parts of the lungs.

In the mid-zone of the lungs (zone 2 of Figure 7.6), the pressure at the arterial end of the collapsible vessels exceeds the alveolar pressure and, under these conditions, a collapsible vessel, behaving like a Starling resistor, permits flow in such a way that the flow rate depends upon the arterial/alveolar pressure difference. Resistance in the Starling resistor is concentrated at the point marked with the arrows in Figures 4.5 and 7.6. The greater the difference between arterial and alveolar pressure, the more widely the collapsible vessels will open and the greater will be the flow. Note that the venous pressure is still not a factor which affects flow or vascular resistance. This condition is still analogous to a weir with the upstream depth (head of pressure) corresponding to the arterial pressure, and the height of the weir corresponding to alveolar pressure. Flow depends solely on the difference in height between the upstream water level and the top of the weir. The depth of water below the weir (analogous to venous pressure) cannot influence the flow of water over the weir unless it rises above the height of the weir.

In the lower zone of the lungs (zone 3 of Figure 7.6), the pressure in the venous end of the capillaries is above the alveolar pressure, and under these conditions a collapsible vessel behaving like a Starling resistor will be held wide open and the flow rate will, as a first approximation, be governed by the arterial/venous pressure difference (the driving pressure) in the normal manner for the systemic circulation. However, as the intravascular pressure increases in relation to the alveolar pressure, the collapsible vessels will be further distended and their resistance will be correspondingly reduced. Returning to the analogy of the weir, the situation is now one in which the downstream water level has risen until the weir is completely submerged and offers little resistance to the flow of water, which is largely governed by the difference in the water level above and below the weir. However, as the levels rise further, the weir is progressively more and more submerged and what little resistance it offers to water flow is diminished still further.

To the three-zone model shown in Figure 7.6, Hughes et al. (1968) added a fourth zone of reduced blood flow in the most dependent parts of the lung. This reduction in blood flow appears to be due to compression of the larger blood vessels by increased interstitial pressure. This effect is more pronounced at reduced lung volumes. It is not shown in the weir analogy.

So far we have not mentioned the critical opening pressure of the pulmonary vessels (Burton, 1951). Current views suggest that the vessels of the lungs open or close at a pressure which is very near to the alveolar pressure; that is to say, their critical opening pressure, if it exists at all, is extremely low (West and Dollery, 1965). Marshall and Marshall (1992) stress that there is no obvious physical reason why there should be a critical opening pressure at all.

If the lungs are passively inflated by positive pressure, the pulmonary capillaries would clearly collapse if the pulmonary vascular pressures were to remain unchanged. In fact, the pulmonary vascular pressures normally rise by an amount almost exactly equal to the change in alveolar pressure up to inflation pressures of about 1.1 kPa (8 mmHg) (Lenfant and Howell, 1960). Beyond this the rise in intravascular pressure is less than the rise in alveolar pressure and flow is reduced by the mechanism of the Starling resistor. This has been demonstrated as an increase in physiological dead space during positive pressure breathing (Folkow and Pappenheimer, 1955; Bitter and Rahn, 1965) and by the application of positive end-expiratory pressure during artificial ventilation (Bindslev et al., 1981).

Structural factors which influence pulmonary vascular resistance

Organic obstruction of pulmonary blood vessels is important in a wide variety of conditions. Obstruction from within the lumen may be caused by emboli (thrombus, fat or gas) or by thrombosis. Obstruction arising within the vessel wall is probably the cause of eventual reduction of flow through collapsed areas, and medial hypertrophy is a major cause of pulmonary hypertension. Kinking of vessels may cause partial obstruction during surgery although probably not in atelectasis. Obstruction arising from outside the vessel wall may be due to a variety of pathological conditions (tumour, abscess, etc.) or to surgical manipulations during thoracotomy. Finally, vessels may be destroyed in emphysema and certain inflammatory conditions, which cause a reduction in the total pulmonary vascular bed and therefore an increase in vascular resistance.

Principles of measurement of the pulmonary circulation

Detailed consideration of haemodynamic measurement techniques must lie outside the scope of this book. The following section presents only the broad principles of measurement such as may be required in relation to respiratory physiology.

Pulmonary blood volume

Available methods are based on the technique used for measurement of cardiac output by dye dilution (see below). Dye is injected into a central vein and its concentration is recorded in samples aspirated from some point in the systemic arterial tree. Cardiac output is determined by the method described below, and multiplied by the interval between the time of the injection of the dye and the mean arrival time of the dye at the sampling point. This product indicates the amount of blood lying between injection and sampling sites. Assumed values for the extrapulmonary blood are then subtracted to indicate the intrapulmonary blood volume. It is not at all easy to obtain satisfactory results with this method. The mean arrival time of the dye is difficult to determine, and the correction for the extrapulmonary blood volume can be little more than an inspired guess.

Pulmonary capillary blood volume may be measured as a byproduct of the measurement of pulmonary diffusing capacity (page 210).

Pulmonary vascular pressures

Pressure measurements within the pulmonary circulation are almost always made with electronic differential pressure transducers. These have a diaphragm which is deformed by a pressure difference across it. The movement of the diaphragm may influence a variable resistor (strain gauge), act as a variable capacitance, or move the core of a coil thereby altering its inductance. Any of these electrical quantities can be detected, amplified and displayed as indicative of the pressures across the diaphragm of the transducer.

The space on the reference side of the diaphragm is normally in communication with atmosphere, but may be connected to an oesophageal balloon or left atrial blood, as required to yield differential pressures (see Figure 7.4). The other side of the diaphragm is filled with a liquid (usually heparinized saline) which is in direct communication with the blood of which the pressure is being measured.

If the system is to have the ability to respond to rapid changes of pressure, damping must be reduced to a minimum. This requires the total exclusion of bubbles of air from the manometer and connecting tubing, and the intravascular cannula must be unobstructed. Electrical manometry then yields a plot of instantaneous pressure against time (Figure 7.7a). Mean pressure (integrated with respect to time) is the height of a rectangle (ABCD in Figure 7.7a) with length equal to one cardiac cycle and area equal to that under the pressure curve over the same interval. In practice, mean pressure is more commonly derived by use of a smoothing circuit in the amplifier (Figure 7.7b), but hydraulic damping in the manometer tubing can achieve the same result. As a rough approximation, mean arterial pressure is often taken to be diastolic plus one-third of pulse pressure.

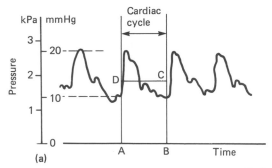

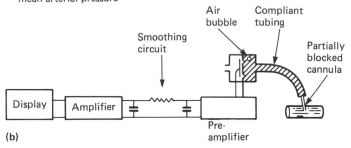

(b)

Figure 7.7 Determination of mean pulmonary arterial pressure. (a) An actual trace of instantaneous intravascular pulmonary arterial pressure during four cardiac cycles. For the second cycle, a rectangle has been constructed (ABCD) which has an area equal to that under the curve over the same time interval. The height of the rectangle (AD) indicates the effective integrated mean pressure. It will be seen to be approximately equal to diastolic pressure plus one-third of the pulse pressure. (b) Factors which tend to damp the recording of instantaneous pressure (i.e. lower the indicated systolic pressure and raise the indicated diastolic pressure) tending towards an indication of the integrated mean pressure. Some of these factors are accidental (e.g. air bubble or blocked cannula) but others (e.g. smoothing circuit) may be employed deliberately to avoid the tedious method of calculation of mean pressure shown in (a).

Pulmonary blood flow

The total flow of blood through the pulmonary circulation may be measured by four groups of methods, each of which contains many variants.

The Fick principle states that the amount of oxygen extracted from the respired gases equals the amount added to the blood which flows through the lungs. Thus the oxygen uptake of the subject must equal the product of pulmonary blood flow and arteriovenous oxygen content difference:

$$\dot{V}O_2 = \dot{Q} \, (Ca_{O_2} - C\bar{v}_{O_2})$$

therefore:

$$\dot{Q} = \frac{\dot{V}O_2}{Ca_{O_2} - C\bar{v}_{O_2}}$$

All the quantities on the right-hand side can be measured, although determination of the oxygen content of the mixed venous blood requires catheterization of the right ventricle or, preferably, the pulmonary artery. Measurement of oxygen consumption is discussed at the end of Chapter 11.

Interpretation of the result is less easy. The calculated value includes the intrapulmonary arteriovenous shunt, but the situation is complicated beyond the possibility of easy solution if there is appreciable extrapulmonary admixture of venous blood (see Figure 7.2). The second major problem is that spirometry measures the total oxygen consumption, including that of the lung. The Fick equation excludes the lung (see Figure 11.22) but the difference is negligible with healthy lungs. There is now strong evidence that the oxygen consumption of infected lungs may be very large (page 510) and therefore the Fick method of measurement of cardiac output would appear to be invalid under such circumstances.

Methods based on uptake of inert tracer gases. A modified Fick method of measurement of cardiac output may be employed with fairly soluble inert gases such as acetylene (Grollman, 1929). A single breath of a dilute acetylene mixture is taken and held. It is then exhaled and the alveolar (or, more correctly, end-expiratory) concentration of acetylene determined. Analysis of volume and composition of expired gas permits measurement of acetylene uptake. Since the duration of the procedure does not permit recirculation, it may be assumed that the mixed venous concentration of acetylene is zero. The Fick equation then simplifies to the following:

cardiac output — acetylene uptake/arterial acetylene concentration

The arterial acetylene concentration equals the product of the arterial acetylene tension (assumed equal to the alveolar acetylene tension) and the solubility coefficient of acetylene in blood. This method is thus relatively non-invasive.

This technique fell into disuse for a variety of technical reasons, but the concept came back into use following the introduction of the body plethysmograph, which can be used for the measurement of the uptake of an inert tracer gas (usually nitrous oxide at the present time). The subject inhales a mixture of about 15% nitrous oxide, and holds his breath with his mouth open inside the body plethysmograph. Nitrous oxide uptake is measured directly from the fall of the pressure within the box, and the arterial nitrous oxide content is derived as the product of the alveolar nitrous oxide tension and its solubility coefficient in blood (Lee and DuBois, 1955). It is assumed that the mixed venous nitrous oxide concentration is zero and the calculation is as described above for acetylene.

All the methods based on the uptake of inert tracer gases have the following characteristics:

1. They measure pulmonary capillary blood flow, excluding any flow through shunts. This is in contrast to the Fick and dye methods.
2. The assumption that the tension of the tracer gas is the same in end-expiratory gas and arterial blood is invalid in the presence of either alveolar dead space or shunt (see Chapter 8).
3. Some of the tracer gas dissolves in the tissues lining the respiratory tract and is carried away by blood perfusing these tissues. The indicated blood flow is therefore greater than the actual pulmonary capillary blood flow.

When the body plethysmograph is used to measure tracer gas uptake, it is possible to detect phasic changes in uptake, in time with the cardiac cycle and maximal during systole. This is taken as evidence that pulmonary capillary blood flow is pulsatile.

Dye or thermal dilution. Currently the most popular technique for measurement of cardiac output is by dye dilution. Measurement can be repeated at least 20 times at 3-minute intervals with dye and indefinitely with a thermal indicator.

An indicator substance is introduced as a bolus into a large vein and its concentration is measured continuously at a sampling site in the systemic arterial tree. Figure 7.8a shows the method as it is applied to continuous non-circulating flow as, for example, of fluids through a pipeline. The downstream concentration of dye is displayed on the Y axis of the graph against time on the X axis. The dye is injected at time t_1 and is first detected at the sampling point at time t_2. The uppermost curve shows the form of a typical curve. There is a rapid rise to maximum concentration followed by a decay which is an exponential wash-out in form (see Appendix F), reaching insignificant levels at time t_3. The second graph shows the concentration (Y axis) on a logarithmic scale when the exponential part of the decay curve becomes a straight line (see Figure F.5). Between times t_2 and t_3, the mean concentration of dye equals the amount of dye injected, divided by the volume of fluid flowing past the sampling point during the interval t_2–t_3, which is the product of the fluid flow rate and the time interval t_2–t_3. The equation may now be rearranged to indicate the flow rate of the fluid as the following expression:

$$\frac{\text{amount of dye injected}}{\text{mean concentration of dye} \times \text{time interval } t_2 - t_3}$$

The amount of dye injected is known and the denominator is the area under the curve.

Figure 7.8b shows the more complicated situation when fluid is flowing round a circuit. Under these conditions, the front of the dye-laden fluid may lap its own tail so that a recirculation peak appears on the graph before the primary peak has decayed to insignificant levels. This commonly occurs when cardiac output is determined in man, and steps must be taken to reconstruct the tail of the primary curve as it would have been had recirculation not taken place. This is done by extrapolating the exponential wash-out which is usually established before the recirculation peak appears. This is shown as the broken lines in the graphs of Figure 7.8b. The calculation of cardiac output then proceeds as described above for non-recirculating flow. This laborious procedure used to be undertaken manually. Nowadays it is almost invariably undertaken by a dedicated computer which is an integral part of the apparatus for measuring cardiac output.

Many different indicators have been used for the dye dilution technique, but currently the most satisfactory appears to be 'coolth'. A bolus of cold saline is injected and the dip in temperature is recorded downstream with the temperature record corresponding to the dye curve. No blood sampling is required and temperature is measured directly with a thermometer mounted on the catheter. The 'coolth' is dispersed in the systemic circulation and therefore there is no recirculation peak to complicate the calculation. The thermal method is particularly suitable for repeated measurements.

Direct measurements of intravascular flow rate. The instantaneous flow through a blood vessel may be measured with an electromagnetic flow meter probe in the

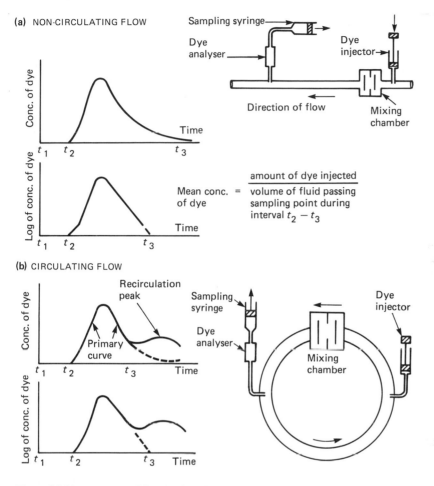

Figure 7.8 Measurement of flow by dye dilution. (a) The measurement of continuous non-circulating flow rate of fluid in a pipeline. The bolus of dye is injected upstream and its concentration is continuously monitored downstream. The relationship of the relevant quantities is shown in the equation. Mean concentration of dye is determined from the area under the curve as shown in Figure 7.7. (b) The more complicated situation when recirculation occurs and the front of the circulating dye laps its own tail, giving a recirculation peak. Reconstruction of the primary curve is based on extrapolation of the primary curve before recirculation occurs. This is facilitated by the fact that the down curve is exponential and therefore a straight line on a logarithmic plot.

form of a cuff attached directly to the blood vessel. The method is clearly of limited application to man but has been extremely useful in animal studies.

The velocity of blood flow in a vessel may be measured by the Doppler shift using ultrasound. This can be translated into flow rate only if the diameter of the vessel is known. Practical difficulties arise in being sure that the signal arises solely from the vessel under consideration. Furthermore, it is erroneous to assume that the velocity profile is constant across the diameter of the vessel. Methods of measurement of distribution of pulmonary blood flow are considered in Chapter 8.

Chapter 8

Distribution of pulmonary ventilation and perfusion

Gas exchange will clearly be optimal if ventilation and perfusion are distributed in the same proportion to one another throughout the lung. Conversely, to take an extreme example, if ventilation were distributed entirely to one lung and perfusion to the other, there could be no gas exchange, although total ventilation and perfusion might each be normal. This chapter begins with consideration of the spatial and temporal distribution of ventilation, followed by similar treatment for the pulmonary circulation. Distribution of ventilation and perfusion are then considered in relation to one another. Finally the concepts of dead space and shunt are presented.

Distribution of ventilation

Spatial and anatomical distribution of inspired gas

Distribution between the two lungs may be grossly affected by disease or trauma, affecting the patency of the bronchi or the integrity of the chest wall. However, in the normal subject it is influenced by posture and by the manner of ventilation. The right lung normally enjoys a ventilation slightly greater than the left lung in both the upright and the supine position (Table 8.1). The studies of Svanberg (1957) showed that, in the lateral position, the lower lung is always better ventilated regardless of the side on which the subject is lying although there still remains a bias in favour of the right side. The preferential ventilation of the dependent lung is due to the lower diaphragm lying higher in the chest and so being more sharply curved and with increased length of muscle fibres. It will therefore contract more effectively during inspiration (see Figure 6.3). Fortunately, the preferential ventilation of the lower lung accords with increased perfusion of the same lung, so the ventilation/perfusion ratios of the two lungs are not greatly altered on assuming the lateral position. However, the upper lung tends to be better ventilated in the anaesthetized patient in the lateral position, particularly with an open chest (Table 8.1).

Spatial distribution in relation to the external anatomy of the trunk may be determined by a variety of techniques (considered at the end of this chapter) which yield many different types of information. Distinction between tidal expansion of

Table 8.1 Distribution of resting lung volume (FRC) and ventilation between the two lungs in man
(The first figure is the unilateral FRC (litres) and the second the percentage partition of ventilation)

	Supine		Right lateral (left side up)		Left lateral (right side up)	
	Right lung	*Left lung*	*Right lung*	*Left lung*	*Right lung*	*Left lung*
Conscious man	1.69	1.39	1.68	2.07	2.19	1.38
(Svanberg, 1957)	53%	47%	61%	39%	47%	53%
Anaesthetized man –	1.18	0.91	1.03	1.32	1.71	0.79
spontaneous breathing	52%	48%	45%	55%	56%	44%
(Rehder and Sessler, 1973)						
Anaesthetized man –	1.36	1.16	1.33	2.21	2.29	1.12
artificial ventilation	52%	48%	44%	56%	60%	40%
(Rehder et al., 1972)						
Anaesthetized man – thoracotomy	—	—	—	—	—	—
(Nunn, 1961a)	—	—	—	—	83%	17%

Each study refers to separate subjects or patients.

rib cage and abdomen is now usually made by respiratory inductive plethysmography. There is predominantly rib cage expansion in the upright position but mainly abdominal expansion in the supine, prone or lateral positions (see Table 3.1). This probably relates to the position of the diaphragm as considered on pages 42 and 120. The change in rib cage dimensions is predominantly in the anteroposterior diameter, and a mean inspiratory cephalad displacement of the sternum of 5.7 mm has been observed in supine anaesthetized patients (Logan and Drummond, 1991).

Distribution to horizontal slices of lung was first studied by West (1962) using a radioactive isotope of oxygen. He found the ventilation of the uppermost slices to be one-third those at the bases of the lungs in the upright position (Figure 8.1). However, these studies were carried out with slow vital capacity inspirations starting from residual volume, and circumstances are very different during normal tidal ventilation. A slow inspiration from functional residual capacity (FRC) showed a mean ratio of only 1.5:1 for basal ventilation compared with apical (Hughes et al., 1972). Fast inspirations from FRC reversed the distribution of ventilation, with preferential ventilation of the upper parts of the lungs (Figure 8.1). It will be seen below that this is contrary to the distribution of pulmonary blood flow. Bake et al. (1974) reported that the preferential ventilation of the dependent parts of the lung was present only at flow rates below 1.5 l/s, starting from FRC. At higher flow rates, distribution was approximately uniform. However, normal inspiratory flow rate is much less than 1.5 l/s (see Figure 4.13).

Posture affects distribution since *inter alia* the vertical height of the lung is reduced by about 30% in the supine position. Therefore the gravitational force generating maldistribution is much less. Hulands et al. (1970) investigated normal tidal breathing in the supine position and found slight preferential ventilation of the posterior slices of the lungs compared with the anterior slices

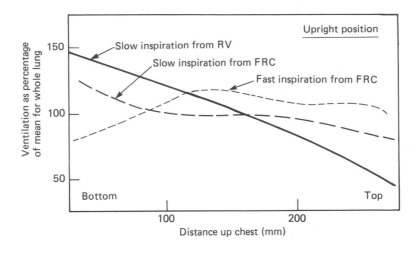

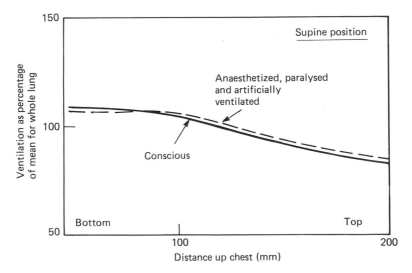

Figure 8.1 Relative distribution of ventilation in horizontal strata of the lungs. Data for the upright position from West (1962) and Hughes et al. (1972). Data for the supine position from Hulands et al. (1970), comprising inspirations of 1 litre from FRC with normal inspiratory flow rate.

(Figure 8.1). Over all, the effect of gravity on ventilation seems to be of minor importance in comparison to its effect on perfusion, which will be considered below.

Distribution of inspired gas in relation to the rate of alveolar filling

The rate of inflation of the lung as a whole is a function of inflation pressure, compliance and airway resistance (page 435). It is convenient to think in terms of the time constant (explained in Appendix F) which is the product of the compliance and resistance and is:

1. The time required for inflation to 63% of the final volume attained if inflation is prolonged indefinitely.

or

2. The time which would be required for inflation of the lungs if the initial gas flow rate were maintained throughout inflation (see Appendix F, Figure F.6).

These considerations apply equally to large and small areas of the lungs; Figure 3.6 shows fast and slow alveoli, the former with a short time constant and the latter with a long time constant. Figure 8.2 shows some of the consequences of different *functional units* of the lung having different time constants. The considerations are fundamentally similar for spontaneous respiration and for artificial ventilation with a constant or sine-wave flow generator (see Figures 22.4 and 22.5). However, consideration of the special case of passive inflation of the lungs by development of a constant mouth pressure (see Figures 22.1 and 22.2) simplifies the presentation.

Figure 8.2a shows two functional units of identical compliance and resistance. If the mouth pressure is increased to a constant level, there will be an increase in volume of each unit equal to the mouth pressure multiplied by the compliance of the unit. The time course of inflation will follow the wash-in type of exponential function (Appendix F), and the time constants will be equal to the product of compliance and resistance of each unit and therefore identical. If the inspiratory phase is terminated at any instant, the pressure and volume of each unit will be identical and no redistribution of gas will occur between the two units.

Figure 8.2b shows two functional units, one of which has half the compliance but twice the resistance of the other. The time constants of the two will thus be equal. If a constant inflation pressure is maintained, the one with the lower compliance will increase in volume by half the volume change of the other. Nevertheless, the pressure build-up within each unit will be identical. Thus, as in the previous example, the relative distribution of gas between the two functional units will be independent of the rate or duration of inflation. If the inspiratory phase is terminated at any point, the pressure in each unit will be identical and no redistribution will occur between the different units.

In Figure 8.2c, the compliances of the two units are identical but the resistance of one is twice that of the other. Therefore, its time constant is double that of its fellow and it will fill more slowly, although the volume increase in both units will be the same if inflation is prolonged indefinitely. Relative distribution between the units is thus dependent upon the rate and duration of inflation. If inspiration is checked by closure of the upper airway after 2 seconds (for example), the pressure will be higher in the unit with the lower resistance. Gas will then be redistributed from one unit to the other as shown by the arrow in the diagram.

Figure 8.2d shows a pair of units with identical resistances but the compliance of one being half that of the other. Its time constant is thus half that of its fellow and it has a faster time course of inflation. However, since its compliance is half that of the other, the ultimate volume increase will only be half that of the other unit when the inflation is prolonged indefinitely. The relative distribution of gas between the two units is dependent upon the rate and duration of inflation. Pressure rises more rapidly in the unit with the lower compliance, and if inspiration is checked by closure of the upper airway at 2 seconds (for example), gas will be redistributed from one unit to the other as shown by the arrow.

An interesting and complex situation occurs when one unit has an increased resistance and the other a reduced compliance (Figure 8.2e). This combination also

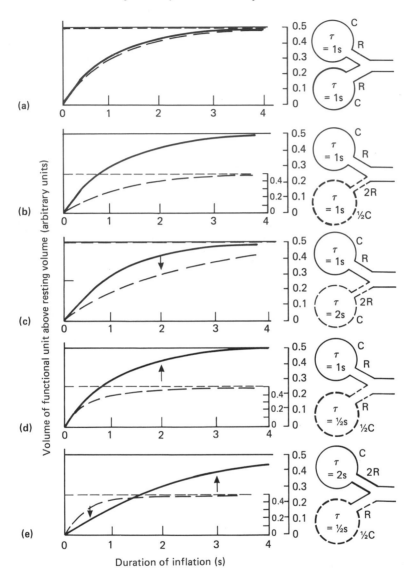

Figure 8.2 The effect of mechanical characteristics on the time course of inflation of different functional units of the lung when exposed to a sustained constant inflation pressure. The Y co-ordinate is volume change, but a scale showing intra-alveolar pressure is shown on the right. The continuous curve relates to the upper unit and the broken curve to the lower unit, in each case. Separate pressure scales are necessary when the compliances are different. Arrows show the direction of gas redistribution if inflow is checked by closure of the upper airway at the times indicated. See text for explanation of the changes.

features in the presentation of the concept of fast and slow alveoli in Figure 3.6. In the present example the time constant of one unit is four times that of the other, while the ultimate volume changes are determined by the compliance as in Figure 8.2d. When the inflation pressure is sustained, the unit with the lower resistance (the 'fast alveolus') shows the greater volume change at first, but rapidly approaches its equilibrium volume. Thereafter the other unit (the 'slow alveolus') undergoes the major volume changes, the inflation of the two units being out of phase with one another. Throughout inspiration, the pressure build-up in the unit with the shorter time constant is always greater and, if inspiration is checked by closure of the upper airway, gas will be redistributed from one unit to the other as shown by the arrows in Figure 8.2e.

These complex relationships may be summarized as follows. If the inflation pressure is sustained indefinitely, the volume change in different units of the lungs will depend solely upon their regional compliances. *If their time constants are equal*, the build-up of pressure in the different units will be identical at all times during inflation and therefore:

1. Distribution of inspired gas will be independent of the rate, duration or frequency of inspiration.
2. Dynamic compliance (so far as it is influenced by considerations discussed in relation to Figure 3.6) will not be affected by changes in frequency and should not differ greatly from static compliance.
3. If inspiration is checked by closure of the upper airway, there will be no redistribution of gas within the lungs.

If, however, *the time constants of different* units are different, for whatever cause, it follows that:

1. Distribution of inspired gas will be dependent on the rate, duration and frequency of inspiration.
2. Dynamic compliance will be decreased as respiratory frequency is increased and should differ significantly from static compliance.
3. If inspiration is checked by closure of the upper airway, gas will be redistributed within the lungs.

Spontaneous versus artificial ventilation

Intermittent positive pressure ventilation (IPPV) results in a spatial pattern of distribution which is determined by inflation pressure, regional compliance and time constants (Figure 8.2). It is still not clear how far similar considerations apply to spontaneous breathing. On the one hand there is the view that, during spontaneous breathing, the lungs simply expand passively in response to the reduction in intrapleural pressure created by the inspiratory muscles. On the other hand, it seems possible that the anatomical pattern of contraction of the inspiratory muscles may directly influence spatial distribution.

During anaesthesia, spontaneous respiration is predominantly abdominal, while there is a slight excess of rib cage movement during IPPV (page 387). However, in spite of the major differences in the spatial distribution of inspired gas, various indices of the efficiency of gas exchange (such as dead space and shunt) are not significantly different for the two modes of breathing (pages 405 et seq.). It thus seems that, although the spatial distribution of gas appears to be altered by IPPV, the functional effect is minimal.

Effect of maldistribution of inspired air on gas mixing

Various therapeutic manoeuvres require the replacement of the nitrogen in the alveolar gas with a different gas. Examples are the administration of 100% oxygen, the replacement of nitrogen with helium to diminish the resistance to breathing, and the administration of an inhalational anaesthetic. Replacement takes place, not only in the alveolar gas but also in all the tissues of the body and this is relatively more important in the case of the more soluble gases. Oxygen is a special case since it is consumed within the body and so can never come into equilibrium between the different tissues.

If we ignore the exchange of gases within the tissue compartments, the wash-in and wash-out of gases in the lungs may be considered as an exponential function (Appendix F). Thus if a patient inhales 100% oxygen, the alveolar nitrogen concentration falls according to a wash-out exponential function (Figure F.5). If, on the other hand, he inhales a helium mixture, the alveolar helium concentration rises according to a wash-in exponential function (Figure F.6) towards a plateau concentration equal to that in the inspired gas. In each case the time constant of change in the composition of the alveolar gas is the same and equals the functional volume of the lungs (usually the FRC) divided by the alveolar ventilation. If, for example, the lung volume is 3 litres and the alveolar ventilation is 6 l/min, the time constant will be 30 seconds. (This time constant should not be confused with the time constant of lung inflation and deflation which equals the product of compliance and resistance.)

This makes the important assumption that every alveolus is ventilated in proportion to its volume. If this is not the case, there will be a whole family of time constants for different functional units of the lungs. Some units will exchange rapidly and some more slowly. The overall picture is that of delayed equilibrium, and after a finite interval (say 7 minutes) it will be found that the mixed alveolar gas concentration has not changed as rapidly as would otherwise be expected. It may, furthermore, be shown that the wash-out curve is not that of a simple exponential, but shows two or more components, the areas with short time constants being dominant early and the areas with long time constants being dominant later.

If a patient breathes 100% oxygen, the alveolar nitrogen will normally be reduced to less than 2.5% after 7 minutes. Clearly this must be influenced to a certain extent by FRC and alveolar ventilation but, if these are reasonably normal, the disappearance of the nitrogen may be delayed by maldistribution. The rate of decrease of the nitrogen concentration is the basis of the 'nitrogen wash-out test'.

Helium wash-in has already been considered as a method of measurement of FRC (page 60). The rate at which equilibrium of helium is attained between spirometer and lungs is also a measure of the equality of distribution. Thus the measurement of FRC may be conveniently combined with a test of distribution.

Effect of maldistribution on the alveolar 'plateau'

If different functional units of the lung empty synchronously during expiration, the composition of the expired air will be approximately constant after the anatomical dead space has been flushed. However, this will not occur when there is maldistribution with fast and slow units as shown in Figure 3.6. The slow units are slow both to fill and to empty, and thus are hypoventilated for their volume; therefore they tend to have a high PCO_2 and low PO_2 and are slow to respond to a change in the inspired gas composition. This forms the basis of the single-breath test of maldistribution (page 188) in which a single breath of oxygen is used to increase alveolar PO_2 and decrease alveolar PN_2. The greatest increase will clearly occur of PO_2 in the functional units with the best ventilation per unit volume which will usually have the shortest time constants. The *slow* units will make the predominant contribution to the *latter* part of exhalation when the mixed exhaled P_{O_2} will decline and the P_{N_2} will increase (see Figure 8.14 below). Thus the expired alveolar plateau of nitrogen will be sloping upwards in patients with maldistribution. It should, however, be stressed that this test will be positive only if maldistribution is accompanied by sequential emptying of units due to differing time constants. For example, Figure 8.2b shows definite maldistribution, due to the different regional compliances which directly influence the regional ventilation. However, since time constants are equal, there will be a constant mix of gas from both units during the course of expiration (i.e. no sequential emptying) and therefore the alveolar plateau would remain flat in spite of P_{O_2} and P_{N_2} being different for the two units. However, maldistribution due to the more common forms of lung disease is usually associated with different time constants and sequential emptying. Therefore, under these circumstances the single-breath nitrogen test has proved to be a useful test of maldistribution.

Distribution of perfusion

Since the pulmonary circulation operates at low pressure, it is never distributed evenly to all parts of the lung, except at zero gravity (Michels and West, 1978), and the degree of non-uniformity is usually much greater than for gas. Maldistribution of pulmonary blood flow is the commonest cause of impaired oxygenation of the arterial blood. Uneven distribution may be present between the two lungs and between different lobes but always between successive horizontal slices of the lungs, except under conditions of zero gravity.

Distribution between the two lungs

There are considerable difficulties in measuring unilateral pulmonary blood flow in man. However, Defares et al. (1960) studied supine subjects using an indirect method based on the Fick principle for CO_2, and obtained values for unilateral flow which agree closely with the distribution of ventilation observed in the supine position by Svanberg (1957) (see Table 8.1).

The lateral position. In man the lateral diameter of the thorax is of the order of 30 cm and so, in the lateral position, the column of blood in the pulmonary circulation exerts a hydrostatic pressure which is high in relation to the mean pulmonary arterial pressure. A fairly gross maldistribution is therefore to be expected with much of the upper lung comprising zone 2 and much of the lower lung comprising zone 3 (see Figure 7.6). Using the ^{133}Xe technique, Kaneko et al. (1966) showed uniform high perfusion of the dependent lung (apparently in zone 3) but with reduced perfusion of the upper lung which appeared to be mainly in zone 2. There was no evidence of the existence of a zone 1 (absent perfusion). In the dog, with its narrow chest, the effect is not large, and Rehder, Theye and Fowler (1961) reported only small increases in perfusion of the dependent lung when dogs were turned from the supine to the lateral position. Surprisingly, the effect was reversed when the thorax was opened.

The increased perfusion of the lower lung is advantageous because of the proportionately greater ventilation of the lower lung in conscious man (see Table

8.1). During anaesthesia in the lateral position, preferential ventilation of the upper lung, particularly during thoracotomy, negates this advantage. Conversely, one-lung anaesthesia *in the lateral position* diverts ventilation to the better perfused lung. Nevertheless, the high perfusion of the dependent lung, combined with its low relative lung volume (see Figure 6.3), causes the dependent lung to be at increased risk of absorption collapse (Potgieter, 1959).

Distribution in horizontal slices of the lung

In the previous chapter, it was shown how the pulmonary vascular resistance is mainly in the capillary bed and is governed by the relationship between alveolar, pulmonary arterial and pulmonary venous pressures. Figure 7.6 presented the concept of the vascular weir with pulmonary vascular resistance decreasing and pulmonary blood flow increasing with distance down the lung. The first studies with radioactive gases took place at total lung capacity and showed flow increasing progressively down the lung in the upright position (West, 1963). However, it was later found that there was a significant reduction of flow in the most dependent parts of the lung (zone 4) which became progressively more important as lung volume was reduced from total lung capacity towards the residual volume (Hughes et al., 1968). Figure 8.3 is redrawn from the work of Hughes' group, and shows that pulmonary perfusion (per alveolus) is, in fact, reasonably uniform at the lung volumes relevant to normal tidal exchange. However, the dependent parts of the lung contain more but smaller alveoli than the apices at FRC, and the perfusion *per unit lung volume* is increased at the bases (Kaneko et al., 1966).

In the *supine* position the differences in blood flow between apices and bases are replaced by differences between anterior and posterior aspects. Over the 20 cm height of the lung field in the average supine adult, the perfusion *per unit lung*

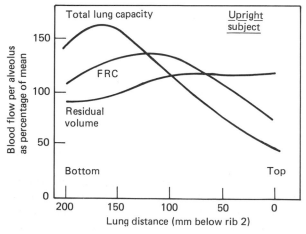

Figure 8.3 Pulmonary perfusion per alveolus as a percentage of that expected if all alveoli were equally perfused. At total lung capacity, perfusion increases down to 150 mm, below which perfusion is slightly decreased (zone 4). At FRC, zone 4 conditions apply below 100 mm, and at residual volume the perfusion gradient is actually reversed. It should be noted that perfusion has been calculated per alveolus. If shown as perfusion per unit lung volume, the non-uniformity at total lung capacity would be the same because alveoli are all the same size at total lung capacity. At FRC there are more but smaller alveoli at the bases and the non-uniformity would be greater. (Data are redrawn from Hughes et al. (1968))

volume increases progressively, with the most dependent parts receiving approximately double the perfusion of the uppermost parts at FRC (Kaneko et al., 1966; Hulands et al., 1970).

Ventilation in relation to perfusion

Inspired gas distributed to regions which have no pulmonary capillary blood flow cannot take part in gas exchange and, conversely, pulmonary blood flow distributed to regions without ventilation cannot become oxygenated. This principle was appreciated by John Hunter who, in the eighteenth century, wrote:

> In animals where there is no circulation, there can be no lungs: for lungs are an apparatus for the air and blood to meet, and can only accord with motion of blood in vessels...As the lungs are to expose the blood to the air, they are so constructed as to answer this purpose exactly with the blood brought to them, and so disposed in them as to go hand in hand.

It is convenient to consider the relationship between ventilation and perfusion in terms of the ventilation/perfusion ratio (abbreviated to $\dot{V}/\dot{Q}$). Each quantity is measured in litres per minute although ventilation is tidal and perfusion is continuous flow. Taking the lungs as a whole, typical resting values might be 4 l/min for alveolar ventilation and 5 l/min for pulmonary blood flow. Thus the overall ventilation/perfusion ratio would be 0.8 (which happens to be close to the respiratory exchange ratio but this is coincidental). If ventilation and perfusion of all alveoli were uniform then each alveolus would have an individual $\dot{V}/\dot{Q}$ ratio of 0.8.

In fact, ventilation and perfusion are not uniformly distributed but may range all the way from unventilated alveoli to unperfused alveoli with every gradation in between. Unventilated alveoli will have a $\dot{V}/\dot{Q}$ ratio of zero and the unperfused alveoli a $\dot{V}/\dot{Q}$ ratio of infinity. $\dot{V}/\dot{Q}$ ratios of other alveoli are ranged between these two extremes.

Alveoli with no ventilation ($\dot{V}/\dot{Q}$ ratio of zero) will have PO_2 and PCO_2 values which are the same as those of mixed venous blood since the trapped air in the unventilated alveoli will equilibrate with mixed venous blood. Alveoli with no perfusion ($\dot{V}/\dot{Q}$ ratio of infinity) will have PO_2 and PCO_2 values which are the same as those of the inspired gas since there is no gas exchange to alter the composition of the inspired gas which is drawn into these alveoli. Alveoli with intermediate values of $\dot{V}/\dot{Q}$ ratio will thus have PO_2 and PCO_2 values which are intermediate between those of mixed venous blood and inspired gas. Figure 8.4 is a PO_2/PCO_2 plot with the thick line joining the mixed venous point to the inspired gas point. This line covers all possible combinations of alveolar PO_2 and PCO_2, with an indication of the $\dot{V}/\dot{Q}$ ratios which determine them.

The inhalation of higher than normal partial pressures of oxygen moves the inspired point of the curve to the right. The mixed venous point also moves to the right but only by a small amount for reasons which are explained on page 538. A new curve must be prepared for each combination of values for mixed venous blood and inspired gas (see appendix 2 of West, 1990). The curve can then be used to demonstrate the gas tensions in the horizontal strata of the lung according to their different $\dot{V}/\dot{Q}$ ratios (Figure 8.4).

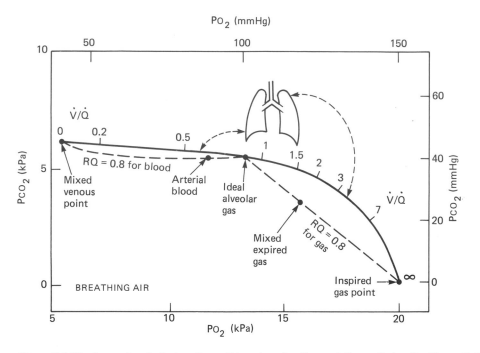

Figure 8.4 The heavy line indicates all possible values for Po$_2$ and Pco$_2$ of alveoli with ventilation/ perfusion (V̇/Q̇) ratios ranging from zero to infinity (subject breathing air). Values for normal alveoli are distributed as shown in accord with their vertical distance up the lung field. Mixed expired gas may be considered as a mixture of 'ideal' alveolar and inspired gas (dead space). Arterial blood may be considered as a mixture of blood with the same gas tensions as 'ideal' alveolar gas and mixed venous blood (the shunt).

The use of collimated counters with ^{133}Xe to measure ventilation and perfusion in horizontal strata of the lung can discriminate only rather thick slices of the lung and is unable to detect changes in small areas of lung within the slices. This limitation has been overcome by the multiple inert gas technique developed by West's group in San Diego. The methodology, which is outlined on page 194, permits the plotting of the distribution of pulmonary ventilation and perfusion, not in relation to anatomical location, but in large numbers of compartments defined by their V̇/Q̇ ratios, expressed on a logarithmic scale.

Figure 8.5 shows typical plots for healthy subjects (Wagner et al., 1974). For the young adult, both ventilation and perfusion are mainly confined to alveoli with V̇/Q̇ ratios in the range 0.5–2.0. There is no measurable distribution to areas of infinite V̇/Q̇ (i.e. alveolar dead space) or zero V̇/Q̇ ratio (i.e. shunt), but the method does not detect extrapulmonary shunt which must be present to a small extent (page 178). For the older subject (Figure 8.5b) there is a widening of the distribution of V/Q ratios, with the main part of the curve now in the range of V/Q ratios 0.3–5.0. In addition, there is the appearance of a 'shelf' of distribution of blood flow to areas of low V̇/Q̇ ratio in the range 0.01–0.3. This probably represents gross underventi- lation of dependent areas of the lung due to airway closure when the closing capacity exceeds the functional residual capacity (see Figure 3.13). The effects of increased spread of V̇/Q̇ ratios on gas exchange is considered below (page 185).

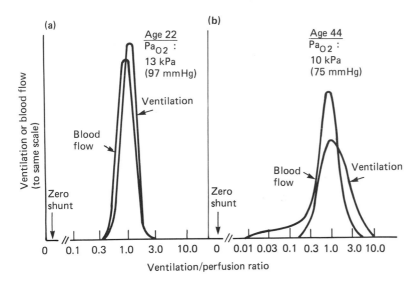

Figure 8.5 The distribution of ventilation and blood flow in relation to ventilation/perfusion ratios in two normal subjects. (a) A male aged 22 years with typical narrow spread and no measureable intrapulmonary shunt or alveolar dead space. This accords with high arterial Po₂, while breathing air. (b) The wider spread in a male aged 44 years. Note in particular the 'shelf' of blood flow distributed to alveoli with V̇/Q̇ ratios in the range 0.01 0.1. There is still no measurable intrapulmonary shunt or alveolar dead space. However, the appreciable distribution of blood flow to underperfused alveoli is sufficient to reduce the arterial Po₂ to 10 kPa (75 mmHg) while breathing air. (Redrawn from Wagner et al. (1974) by permission of the authors and copyright permission of the American Society for Clinical Investigation)

The pattern of distribution of V̇/Q̇ ratios shows characteristic changes in a number of pathological conditions such as pulmonary oedema and pulmonary embolus (Wagner et al., 1975; West, 1990). Some examples are shown in Figure 8.6. Changes occurring during anaesthesia are described in Chapter 20, and the effects of breathing different concentrations of oxygen in Chapter 27.

Quantification of spread of V̇/Q̇ ratios as if it were due to dead space and shunt

The types of analysis illustrated in Figures 8.4, 8.5 and 8.6 are technically complex and unfortunately beyond the scope of all but a few centres in the world. A less precise but highly practical approach derived from the studies of Riley and his colleagues in Baltimore in the years 1945−1951. The essence of the 'Riley' approach is to consider the lung *as if* it were a three-compartment model (Figure 8.7) comprising:

1. Ventilated but unperfused alveoli.
2. Perfused but unventilated alveoli.
3. Ideally perfused and ventilated alveoli.

The ventilated but unperfused alveoli comprise alveolar dead space (described below). The perfused but unventilated alveoli are here represented as a shunt. Gas exchange can occur only in the 'ideal' alveolus. There is no suggestion that this is an accurate description of the actual state of affairs, which is more accurately depicted

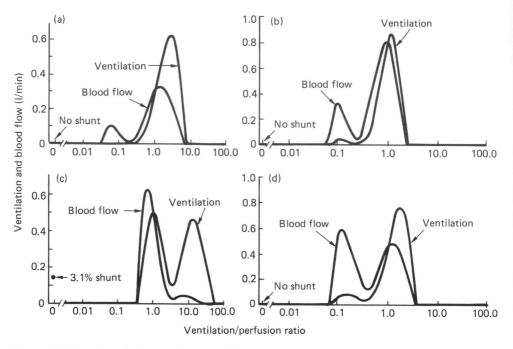

Figure 8.6 Examples of abnormal patterns of maldistribution of ventilation and blood flow, to be compared with normal curves in Figure 8.5. (a) Chronic obstructive lung disease, predominantly chronic bronchitis. The blood flow to units of very low ventilation/perfusion ratio would cause arterial hypoxaemia and simulate a shunt. (b) Asthma with a more pronounced bimodal distribution of blood flow than the patient shown in (a). (c) Bimodal distribution of ventilation in a 60-year-old patient with chronic obstructive lung disease, predominantly emphysema. A similar pattern is seen after pulmonary embolization. (d) Pronounced bimodal distribution of perfusion after a bronchodilator was administered to the patient shown in (b). (Redrawn from West (1990) by permission of the author and publishers)

by the type of plot shown in Figure 8.5, where the analysis would comprise some 50 compartments in contrast to the three compartments of the Riley model. However, the parameters of the three-compartment model may be easily determined with equipment to be found in any department which is concerned with respiratory problems. Furthermore, the values obtained are of direct relevance to therapy. Thus an increased dead space can usually be offset by an increased minute volume, and arterial PO_2 can be restored to normal with shunts up to about 30% by an appropriate increase in the inspired oxygen concentration (see Figure 8.10 below).

    Methods of calculation of dead space and shunt for the three-compartment model are described at the end of the chapter, but no analytical techniques are required beyond measurement of blood and gas PCO_2 and PO_2. It is then possible to determine what fraction of the inspired tidal volume does not participate in gas exchange and what fraction of the cardiac output constitutes a shunt or venous admixture. However, it is most important to remember that the measured value for 'dead space' will include a fraction representing ventilation of *relatively* underperfused alveoli, and the measured value for 'shunt' will include a fraction representing perfusion of *relatively* underventilated alveoli. Furthermore, although perfusion of relatively underventilated alveoli will reduce arterial PO_2, the pattern of change,

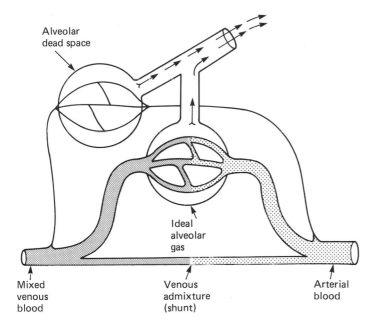

Figure 8.7 The assessment of the efficiency of gas exchange in the lungs considered as a three-compartment model. The lung is imagined to consist of three functional units comprising alveolar dead space, 'ideal' alveoli and venous admixture or shunt. Gas exchange occurs only in the 'ideal' alveoli. The measured alveolar dead space consists of true alveolar dead space together with a component caused by $\dot{V}/\dot{Q}$ scatter. The measured venous admixture consists of true venous admixture (shunt) together with a component caused by $\dot{V}/\dot{Q}$ scatter. Note that 'ideal' alveolar gas is exhaled contaminated with alveolar dead space gas (if present). Under such circumstances it is not possible to sample 'ideal' alveolar gas, the P_{CO_2} and P_{O_2} of which must therefore be derived indirectly.

in relation to the inspired oxygen concentration, is quite different from that of a true shunt (see Figure 8.11 below).

The concept of ideal alveolar gas is considered below (page 195), but it will be clear from Figure 8.7 that ideal alveolar gas cannot be sampled for analysis. There is a convention that ideal alveolar P_{CO_2} is assumed to be equal to the arterial P_{CO_2} and that the respiratory exchange ratio of ideal alveolar gas is the same as that of expired air.

Dead space

It was realized in the last century that an appreciable part of each inspiration did not penetrate to those regions of the lungs in which gas exchange occurred and was therefore exhaled unchanged. This fraction of the tidal volume has long been known as the dead space, while the effective part of the minute volume of respiration is known as the alveolar ventilation. The relationship is as follows:

alveolar ventilation = respiratory frequency (tidal volume − dead space)

$$\dot{V}_A = f\,(V_T - V_D)$$

It is often useful to think of two ratios. The first is the dead space/tidal volume ratio (often abbreviated to VD/VT and expressed as a percentage). The second useful ratio is the alveolar ventilation/minute volume ratio. The first ratio indicates the wasted part of the breath, while the second gives the utilized portion of the minute volume. The sum of the two ratios is unity and so one may easily be calculated from the other.

Components of the dead space

The preceding section considers dead space as though it were a single homogeneous component of expired air. The situation is actually more complicated and Figure 8.8 shows in diagrammatic form the various components of a single expirate.

The first part to be exhaled will be from the *apparatus dead space* if the subject is employing any form of external breathing apparatus. The next component will be from the *anatomical dead space*, which is related to the volume of the conducting air passages. Thereafter gas is exhaled from the alveolar level and the diagram shows two representative alveoli, corresponding to the two ventilated compartments of the three-compartment lung model shown in Figure 8.7. One alveolus is perfused and, from this, *'ideal' alveolar gas* is exhaled. The other alveolus is

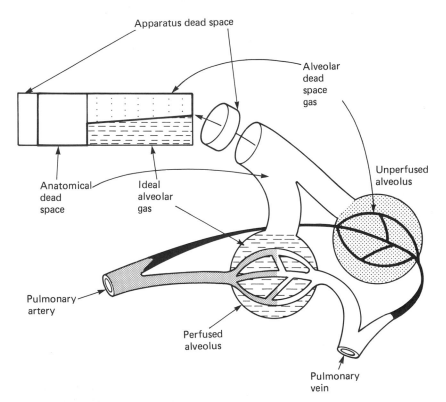

Figure 8.8 Components of expired gas. The rectangle is an idealized representation of a single expirate. The physiological dead space equals the sum of the anatomical and alveolar dead spaces and is outlined in the heavy black line. The alveolar dead space does not equal the volume of the unperfused spaces at alveolar level but only the part of their contents which is exhaled. This varies with the tidal volume.

unperfused and so without gas exchange. From this alveolus is exhaled gas approximating in composition to inspired gas. This component of the expirate is known as *alveolar dead space gas* which is important in many pathological conditions. *The physiological dead space* is the sum of the anatomical and alveolar dead spaces. It is defined as the sum of all parts of the tidal volume which do not participate in gas exchange, as defined by the appropriate Bohr equation (see below).

In Figure 8.8, the final part of the expirate consists of a mixture of 'ideal' alveolar gas and alveolar dead space gas. A sample of this gas is called an *end-tidal* or, preferably, an *end-expiratory* sample and corresponds to the alveolar sample defined by Haldane and Priestley (1905) as gas sampled at the end of a forced expiration. The composition of such a sample approximates to that of 'ideal' alveolar gas in a healthy resting subject. However, in many pathological states (and during anaesthesia), an end-expiratory sample is contaminated by alveolar dead space gas and it is then necessary to distinguish between end-tidal gas and 'ideal' alveolar gas, as shown in Figure 8.7, and defined by Riley et al. (1946) (see page 195). For symbols, the small capital A relates to 'ideal' alveolar gas as in PA_{CO_2}, while end-expiratory gas is distinguished by a small capital E, suffixed with a prime (e.g. PE'_{CO_2}). The term 'alveolar/arterial PO_2 difference' always refers to 'ideal' alveolar gas. Unqualified, the term 'alveolar' may mean either end-tidal or 'ideal' alveolar, depending on the context. This is a perennial source of confusion and it is better to specify either 'ideal' alveolar gas or end-expiratory gas.

It must again be stressed that Figure 8.8 is only a model to simplify quantification and there may be an infinite gradation between $\dot{V}/\dot{Q}$ ratios of zero and infinity. However, it is often helpful from the quantitative standpoint, particularly in the clinical field, to consider alveoli *as if* they fell into the three categories shown in Figure 8.7.

The Bohr equation

Bohr introduced his equation in 1891 when the dead space was considered simply as gas exhaled from the conducting airways (i.e. anatomical dead space only). It may be simply derived as follows. During expiration all the CO_2 eliminated is contained in the alveolar gas. Therefore:

> The quantity of CO_2 eliminated in the alveolar gas
> = quantity of CO_2 eliminated in the mixed expired gas

that is to say:

> Alveolar CO_2 concentration × alveolar ventilation
> = mixed-expired CO_2 concentration × minute volume

or, for a single breath:

> alv. CO_2 conc. × (tidal volume − dead space)
> = mixed-expired CO_2 conc. × tidal volume

There are four terms in this equation. There is no serious difficulty in measuring two of them, the tidal volume and the mixed-expired CO_2 concentration. This leaves the alveolar CO_2 concentration and the dead space. Therefore the alveolar CO_2 concentration may be derived if the dead space be known or, alternatively, the dead space may be derived if the alveolar CO_2 concentration be known. In the nineteenth century, it was not realized that alveolar gas could be sampled and the Bohr equation was used to calculate the alveolar CO_2 concentration, substituting an assumed value for the dead space. After the historic discovery of the constancy of the alveolar gas (Haldane and Priestley, 1905), the position was reversed and the alveolar CO_2 concentration was measured directly and the Bohr equation used to calculate the dead space.

More recently the use of this equation has been expanded to measure various components of the dead space by varying the interpretation of the term 'alveolar'. In the paragraph above, the word 'alveolar' means end-expiratory gas, and therefore this use of the Bohr equation indicates the anatomical dead space. If the 'ideal' alveolar CO_2 concentration were used, then the equation would indicate the physiological dead space comprising the sum of the anatomical and alveolar dead spaces (Figure 8.8). 'Ideal' alveolar gas cannot be sampled but Enghoff (1938) suggested that arterial P_{CO_2} should be substituted for alveolar P_{CO_2} in the Bohr equation. The value so derived is now widely accepted as the definition of the physiological dead space:

$$V_D/V_T = (Pa_{CO_2} - P\bar{E}_{CO_2})/Pa_{CO_2}$$

In the healthy conscious resting subject, there is no significant difference between P_{CO_2} of end-expiratory gas and arterial blood. The former may therefore be used as a substitute for the latter, since the anatomical and physiological dead spaces should be the same (the normal alveolar dead space being too small to measure). However, the use of the end-expiratory P_{CO_2} in the Bohr equation may cause difficulties in certain situations. In exercise, in acute hyperventilation or if there is maldistribution of inspired gas with sequential emptying, the alveolar P_{CO_2} rises, often steeply, during expiration of the alveolar gas, and the end-tidal P_{CO_2} will depend on the duration of expiration. The dead space so derived will not necessarily correspond to any of the compartments of the dead space shown in Figure 8.8. Fletcher (1984) has suggested that it be simply termed the Bohr dead space, which commits us to nothing beyond a tribute to Bohr's historic contribution. The distinction between different meanings of the term 'alveolar gas' is fundamental for understanding dead space and is the clue to the controversy which existed for many years between Haldane and Krogh (reviewed by Bannister, Cunningham and Douglas, 1954).

Anatomical dead space

The gills of fishes are perfused by a stream of water which enters by the mouth and leaves by the gill slits. All of the water is available for gaseous exchange. Mammals, however, employ tidal ventilation which suffers from the disadvantage that a considerable part of the inspired gas comes to rest in the conducting air passages and is thus not available for gaseous exchange. The anatomical dead space is, in effect, the volume of the conducting air passages with the qualifications considered below.

This imperfection was understood in the nineteenth century when the volume of the anatomical dead space was calculated from *post mortem* casts of the respiratory tract (Zuntz, 1882; Loewy, 1894). The value so obtained was used in the calculation of the composition of the alveolar gas according to the Bohr equation (1891) as described above. The anatomical dead space is now generally defined as the volume of gas exhaled before the CO_2 concentration rises to its alveolar plateau, according to the technique of Fowler (1948) and outlined at the end of this chapter (see Figure 8.15). Fowler originally termed it the *physiological* dead space and Folkow and Pappenheimer (1955) suggested the term *series* dead space using an electrical analogy to distinguish it from alveolar dead space (*parallel* dead space).

The volume of the anatomical dead space, in spite of its name, is not constant and is influenced by many factors, some of which are of considerable clinical importance. Since many of these factors are not primarily anatomical, Fletcher (1984) has introduced the term 'airway dead space', but still with the Fowler definition.

The following factors influence the true or the functional volume of the anatomical dead space.

Size of the subject must clearly influence the dimensions of the conducting air passages, and Radford (1955) drew attention to the fact that the volume of the air passages (in millilitres) approximates to the weight of the subject in pounds (1 pound = 0.45 kg).

Posture influences many lung volumes, including the anatomical dead space; Fowler (1950a) quoted the following mean values:

sitting	147 ml
semi-reclining	124 ml
supine	101 ml

Position of the neck and jaw has a pronounced effect on the anatomical dead space; studies by Nunn, Campbell and Peckett (1959) indicated the following mean values in three conscious subjects (not intubated):

neck extended, jaw protruded	143 ml
normal position	119 ml
neck flexed, chin depressed	73 ml

It is noteworthy that the first position is that which is used by resuscitators and anaesthetists to procure the least possible airway resistance. Unfortunately, it also results in the maximum dead space.

Age is usually accompanied by an increase in anatomical dead space but this may be associated with an increased incidence of chronic bronchitis which usually results in an enlarged calibre of the major air passages (Fowler, 1950b).

Lung volume at the end of inspiration affects the anatomical dead space, since the volume of the air passages changes in proportion to the lung volume. The increase is of the order of 20 ml additional anatomical dead space for each litre increase in lung volume (Shepard et al., 1957).

Tracheal intubation or tracheostomy will bypass the extrathoracic anatomical dead space. This was found to be 72 ml in six cadavers, while the intrathoracic anatomical dead space was found to be 66 ml in three intubated patients (Nunn, Campbell and Peckett, 1959). Intrathoracic anatomical dead space of 12 intubated anaesthetized patients had a mean value of 63 ml (Nunn and Hill, 1960). Thus tracheal intubation or tracheostomy will bypass approximately half of the total anatomical dead space, although this advantage will clearly be lost if a corresponding volume of apparatus dead space is added to the circuit.

Pneumonectomy will result in a reduction of anatomical dead space if the excised lung was functional (Fowler and Blakemore, 1951).

Hypoventilation results in a marked reduction of the anatomical dead space as measured by Fowler's method, and this limits the fall of alveolar ventilation resulting from small tidal volumes. This is important in the case of comatose or anaesthetized patients who are left to breathe for themselves, with tidal volumes as small as 140 ml (Nunn, 1958a). Tidal volumes of less than the supposed anatomical dead space are commonly used during high frequency ventilation, and this problem is discussed on page 446.

There are probably two factors which reduce the anatomical dead space during hypoventilation. Firstly, there is a tendency towards streamline or laminar flow of gas through the air passages. Inspired gas advances with a cone front and the tip of the cone penetrates the alveoli before all the gas in the conducting passages has been washed out (see Figure 4.2). This, in effect, reduces what we may call the 'functional anatomical dead space' below its value morphologically defined. The reduction of functional anatomical dead space at low tidal volumes was predicted by Rohrer in 1915 and, in the same year, Henderson, Chillingworth and Whitney demonstrated the axial flow of tobacco smoke through glass tubing. The second factor reducing dead space during hypoventilation is the mixing effect of the heartbeat which tends to mix all gas lying below the carina. This effect is negligible at normal rates of ventilation, but becomes more marked during hypoventilation and during breath holding. Thus in one hypoventilating patient, Nunn and Hill (1960) found alveolar gas at the carina at the beginning of expiration. A similar effect occurs during breath holding when alveolar gas mixes with dead space gas as far up as the glottis.

In conscious subjects some inspired gas may be detected in the alveoli with tidal volumes as small as 60 ml (Briscoe, Forster and Comroe, 1954). In anaesthetized patients with tidal volumes less than 350 ml, Nunn and Hill (1960) found the 'functional' anatomical dead space (below the carina) to be about one-fifth of the tidal volume, a number of patients having values less than 25 ml at tidal volumes below 250 ml (see Figure 20.13). Above a tidal volume of about 300 ml the anatomical dead space was constant and accorded roughly with the volume of the airways.

Drugs acting on the bronchiolar musculature will affect the anatomical dead space, and an increase was noted after atropine by Higgins and Means (1915), Severinghaus and Stupfel (1955) and Nunn and Bergman (1964). Nunn and Bergman found a mean increase of 18 ml in six normal subjects, while Severinghaus and Stupfel reported an increase of 45 ml. The latter also reported significant increases with the ganglion-blocking agents hexamethonium and trimetaphan. Histamine caused a small decrease in anatomical dead space.

Hypothermia was reported to increase anatomical dead space in dogs (Severinghaus and Stupfel, 1955) but there seems to be little change in man (Nunn, 1961a).

Alveolar dead space

Alveolar dead space may be defined as that part of the inspired gas which passes through the anatomical dead space to mix with gas at the alveolar level, but which does not take part in gas exchange. The cause of the failure of gas exchange is lack of effective perfusion of the spaces to which the gas is distributed at the alveolar level. Parallel dead space (Folkow and Pappenheimer, 1955) is synonymous with alveolar dead space. Measured alveolar dead space must sometimes contain a component due to the ventilation of *relatively* underperfused alveoli which have a very high (but not infinite) $\dot{V}/\dot{Q}$ ratio (Figure 8.6). The alveolar dead space is too small to be measured with confidence in healthy supine man, but becomes appreciable in many conditions considered below.

Pulmonary hypotension may result in failure of perfusion of the uppermost parts of the lungs (zone 1 in Figure 7.6). This cannot be detected in the normal subject but may occur with pulmonary hypotension, which accompanies many forms of low-output circulatory failure. This is the probable cause of the large increase in physiological dead space after haemorrhage (Gerst, Rattenborg and Holaday, 1959; Freeman and Nunn, 1963), and during anaesthesia with deliberate hypotension, when some patients were found to have a physiological dead space in excess of 75% of the tidal volume (Eckenhoff et al., 1963).

Posture. In the supine position, the vertical height of the lungs, and therefore the hydrostatic head of pressure in the pulmonary arteries, is reduced to about 20 cm and this would tend to improve the unformity of distribution of pulmonary blood flow. However, in the lateral position, the vertical height is about 30 cm, and approximately two-thirds of the pulmonary blood flow is distributed to the dependent side. During spontaneous respiration the greater part of the ventilation is also distributed to the lower lung and it is unlikely that there is any significant alveolar dead space. If, however, a patient is ventilated artificially in the lateral position, ventilation is distributed in favour of the upper lung (see Table 8.1), particularly in the presence of an open pneumothorax (Nunn, 1961a). Under these conditions, part of the ventilation of the upper lung will constitute alveolar dead space. This problem is discussed further on page 415.

Embolism. Pulmonary embolism is considered separately in Chapter 28. Partial embolization of the pulmonary circulation results in the development of an alveolar dead space which may reach massive proportions.

Ventilation of non-vascular air space. This occurs in obstructive lung disease following widespread destruction of alveolar septa and the contained vessels. This is the principal cause of the very marked increase in physiological dead space reported in patients with chronic lung disease (Donald et al., 1952). Preferential ventilation of a lung cyst in communication with a bronchus may cause a massive increase in alveolar dead space.

Constriction of precapillary pulmonary vessels. It is conjectural whether alveolar dead space may be increased by precapillary constriction of the pulmonary blood vessels.

Obstruction of the pulmonary circulation by external forces. There may be kinking, clamping or blocking of a pulmonary artery during thoracic surgery. This may be expected to result in an increase in dead space depending on the ventilation of the section of lung supplied by the obstructed vessel.

Physiological dead space

The physiological dead space is the sum of all parts of the tidal volume which do not participate in gaseous exchange. Nowadays it is universally defined by the Bohr mixing equation with substitution of arterial P_{CO_2} for alveolar P_{CO_2} as described above.

Enghoff (1931) was the first to demonstrate that the physiological dead space remained a fairly constant fraction of the tidal volume over a wide range of tidal volumes. It is, therefore, generally more useful to use the V_D/V_T ratio: the alveolar ventilation will then be $(1 - V_D/V_T) \times$ the respiratory minute volume. Thus if the physiological dead space is 30% of the tidal volume (i.e. $V_D/V_T = 0.3$), the alveolar ventilation will be 70% of the minute volume. This approach is radically different from the assumption of a constant 'dead space' which is subtracted from the tidal volume, the difference then being multiplied by the respiratory frequency to indicate the alveolar ventilation.

Factors influencing the physiological dead space

This section summarizes information on the value of the total physiological dead space, but reasons for the changes have been considered above in the sections on the anatomical and alveolar dead space.

Age and sex. There is a tendency for V_D and also the V_D/V_T ratio to increase with age, with V_D increasing by slightly less than 1 ml per year (Harris et al., 1973). These authors found values for V_D in men of the order of 50 ml greater than in women but the former group had larger tidal volumes and there was a smaller sex difference in the V_D/V_T ratios (33.2–15.1% for men; 29.4–9.4% for women). All subjects were seated. The authors reviewed other studies of normal values for V_D/V_T ratios which tended to be slightly less than their own values, although there was general agreement that V_D/V_T increased with age.

Body size. It is evident that V_D, in common with other pulmonary volumes, will be larger in larger people. Harris' group recommended correlation with height, and reported that V_D increased by 17 ml for every 10 cm increase in height.

Posture. Craig et al. (1971) showed that the V_D/V_T ratio decreased from a mean value of 34% in the upright position to 30% in the supine position. This is largely explained by the change in anatomical dead space (see above).

Duration of inspiration and breath holding. It is well known that prolongation of inspiration reduces dead space by allowing gas mixing to take place between dead space and alveolar gas.

Smoking. Craig et al. (1971) showed a highly significant increase in the V_D/V_T ratio of smokers in whom the values were 37% (upright) and 32% (supine), compared with 29% (upright) and 26% (supine) for non-smokers. Smokers were evenly distributed among their age groups.

Pulmonary disease. The previous part of this chapter has considered the enlargement of the alveolar dead space which occurs when parts of the lung are deprived of circulation. Very large increases in VD/VT occur in pulmonary embolus and, to a lesser extent, in pulmonary hypoperfusion and emphysema. Patients with emphysema suffer a further increase in the VD/VT ratio following induction of anaesthesia (Pietak et al., 1975).

Anaesthesia. Many studies have now shown that the VD/VT ratio of a healthy, anaesthetized intubated patient is of the order of 30–35% *below the carina*, whether breathing spontaneously or ventilated artifically (see Chapter 20).

Artificial ventilation. Artificial ventilation itself seems to have little effect upon the VD/VT ratio compared with the value obtained during anaesthesia with spontaneous breathing. However, it seems likely that prolonged use of positive end-expiratory pressure causes an increase in the dead space (page 456).

Apparatus dead space and rebreathing

When a subject or patient is connected to breathing apparatus, there will usually be apparatus dead space, which is in series with the anatomical dead space and is included in the value given by solution of Bohr's equation. Consideration of apparatus dead space as though it were always a simple extension of the patient's anatomical dead space is perfectly valid for simple breathing equipment but, with more complex devices, the whole of the gas space may not be washed out by the tidal volume. The functional volume may then be less than the geometric volume as determined by filling it with water. However, with certain breathing apparatus, the conceptual problems become really daunting (Nunn and Newman, 1964). The gas rebreathed may be end-expiratory gas (as with a simple facemask), mixed expired gas (as in circuit C, described by Mapleson, 1954), or even expired dead space gas (as in circuit A, described by Mapleson, 1954). In the last case, this will not influence gas exchange although, considered in terms of gas volumes, rebreathing has occurred. If expired alveolar gas is rebreathed from the apparatus dead space gas late in inspiration, it may penetrate no further than the patient's anatomical dead space and therefore have no effect on gas exchange.

The composition of gas rebreathed from apparatus dead space can be very difficult to define. It is commonly analysed in relation to time, whereas a true effective mean concentration must be volume biased. Thus inspired gas of changing composition should be sampled for analysis at a flow rate proportional to the instantaneous inspiratory flow rate (Bookallil and Smith, 1964). Even then, the effective 'mean inspired gas composition' has two alternative meanings. The first refers to the mean composition of the gas which enters the patient's respiratory tract. The second is restricted to the gas which enters functioning alveoli and is the only part which can influence gas exchange.

Effects of an increased physiological dead space

Regardless of whether an increase in physiological dead space is in the anatomical or the alveolar component, alveolar ventilation must be reduced, unless there is a compensatory increase in minute volume. Reduction of alveolar ventilation due to an increase in physiological dead space produces changes in the 'ideal' alveolar gas tensions which are identical to those produced when alveolar ventilation is decreased by reduction in respiratory minute volume (see Figure 6.8). It is usually possible to counteract the effects of an increase in physiological dead space by a corresponding increase in the respiratory minute volume. If, for example, the minute volume is 10 l/min and the V_D/V_T ratio 30%, the alveolar ventilation will be 7 l/min. If the patient were then subjected to pulmonary embolism resulting in an increase of the V_D/V_T ratio to 50%, the minute volume would need to be increased to 14 l/min to maintain an alveolar ventilation of 7 l/min. However, should the V_D/V_T increase to 80%, the minute volume would need to be increased to 35 l/min. Ventilatory capacity may be a limiting factor with massive increases in dead space, and this is a rare cause of ventilatory failure (page 423).

Venous admixture or shunt

Admixture of arterial blood with suboxygenated or mixed venous blood is a most important cause of arterial hypoxaemia. It is an ever-present clinical problem in intensive care.

Nomenclature of venous admixture

Venous admixture refers to the degree of admixture of mixed venous blood with pulmonary end-capillary blood which would be required to produce the observed difference between the arterial and the pulmonary end-capillary P_{O_2} (usually taken to equal ideal alveolar P_{O_2}), the principles of the calculation being shown in Figure 8.9. Note that the venous admixture is not the *actual* amount of venous blood which mingles with the arterial blood, but the *calculated* amount which would be required to produce the observed value for the arterial P_{O_2}. The difference is due to two factors. The first is that the thebesian and bronchial venous drainage does not necessarily have the same P_{O_2} as mixed venous blood. The second is the contribution to the arterial blood from alveoli having a ventilation/perfusion ratio of more than zero but less than the normal value (see Figure 8.5), this problem being discussed in greater detail below. *Venous admixture* is thus a convenient index but defines neither the precise volume nor the anatomical pathway of the shunt. Nevertheless, it is often loosely termed 'shunt'.

Anatomical shunt refers to the amount of venous blood which mingles with the pulmonary end-capillary blood on the arterial side of the circulation. The term embraces bronchial and thebesian venous blood flow and also admixture of mixed venous blood caused by atelectasis, bronchial obstruction, congenital heart disease with right-to-left shunting, etc. Clearly different components may have different oxygen contents which will not necessarily equal the mixed venous oxygen content. Anatomical shunt excludes blood draining any alveoli with a $\dot{V}/\dot{Q}$ ratio of more than zero.

Pathological shunt is sometimes used to describe the forms of anatomical shunt which do not occur in the normal subject.

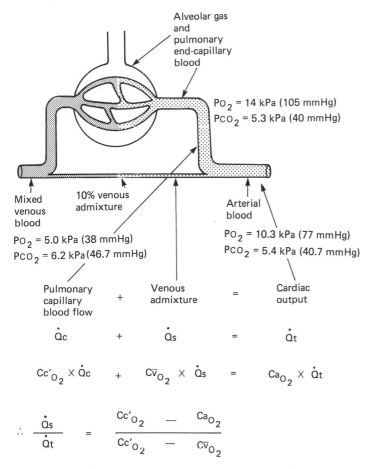

Figure 8.9 A schematic representation of venous admixture. It makes the simplifying assumption that all the arterial blood has come either from alveoli with normal $\dot{V}/\dot{Q}$ ratio or from a shunt. This is never true but it forms a convenient method of quantifying venous admixture and can be used as a basis for oxygen therapy. The shunt equation is similar to the Bohr equation and is based on the axiomatic relationship that the total amount of oxygen in 1 minute's flow of arterial blood equals the sum of the amount of oxygen in 1 minute's flow through the pulmonary capillaries and the amount of oxygen in 1 minutes's flow through the shunt. Amount of oxygen in 1 minute's flow of blood equals the product of the blood flow rate and the concentration of oxygen in the blood. $\dot{Q}t$, total cardiac output; $\dot{Q}c$, pulmonary capillary blood flow; $\dot{Q}s$, flow of blood through shunt; Ca_{O_2}, concentration of oxygen in arterial blood; Cc'_{O_2}, concentration of oxygen in pulmonary end-capillary blood; $C\bar{v}_{O_2}$, concentration of oxygen in mixed venous blood.

Physiological shunt. This term is, unfortunately, used in two senses. In the first sense it is used to describe the degree of venous admixture which occurs in a normal healthy subject. Differences between the actual measured venous admixture and the normal value for the 'physiological shunt' thus indicate the amount of venous admixture which results from the disease process. In its alternative sense, physiological shunt is synonymous with venous admixture as derived from the mixing equation (Figure 8.9). The term is probably best avoided.

Forms of venous admixture

Venae cordis minimae (thebesian veins). Some small veins of the left heart drain directly into the chambers of the left heart and so mingle with the arterial blood. The oxygen content of this blood is probably very low, and therefore the flow (believed to be about 0.3% of cardiac output; Ravin, Epstein and Malm, 1965) causes an appreciable fall in the mixed arterial oxygen tension. It was thought by Cole and Bishop (1963) that the venae cordis minimae constitute the major part of the observed venous admixture in healthy man.

Bronchial veins. Figure 7.2 shows that a part of the venous drainage of the bronchial circulation passes by way of the deep true bronchial veins to reach the pulmonary veins. It is uncertain how large this component is in the healthy subject but is probably less than 1% of cardiac output. In bronchial disease and coarctation of the aorta, the flow through this channel may be greatly increased, and in bronchiectasis and emphysema may be as large as 10% of cardiac output. Under these circumstances it becomes a major cause of arterial desaturation.

Congenital heart disease. Right-to-left shunting in congenital heart disease is the cause of the worst examples of venous admixture. When there are abnormal communications between right and left hearts, shunting will usually be from left to right unless the pressures in the right heart are raised above those of the left heart, as occurs, for example, with pulmonary atresia. Left-to-right shunts may be temporarily reversed by transient increases in right heart pressure, as may be caused by increasing alveolar pressure and therefore pulmonary vascular resistance (page 148).

Pulmonary infection. In the days when lobar pneumonia was common, it was a familiar sight to see a patient hyperventilating but deeply cyanosed. The hypoxaemia was due to a large shunt through the lobe which was affected by the pneumonic process. It seems likely that the infection increased the blood flow through the affected lobe above its normal value.

Although lobar pneumonia is now rare, bronchopneumonia is still relatively common, and is an important cause of venous admixture. The alveolar/arterial PO_2 difference is a useful aid to diagnosis and assessment of progress.

Pulmonary oedema. Pulmonary oedema is considered in detail in Chapter 26. Once alveolar flooding has occurred, perfusion through the affected alveoli constitutes venous admixture and the alveolar/arterial PO_2 difference increases. When froth enters the bronchial tree there is failure of ventilation of whole regions of the lungs and venous admixture reaches high levels, resulting in gross hypoxaemia.

Pulmonary collapse is considered separately in Chapter 27.

Pulmonary neoplasm. Any pulmonary neoplasm is likely to cause a shunt as its venous drainage mingles with the pulmonary venous blood. With bronchial or secondary carcinoma, the flow through the neoplasm may be high, resulting in appreciable arterial hypoxaemia. Pulmonary haemangioma is rare but may first present as an unexplained venous admixture.

Pulmonary arteriovenous shunts. Chapter 2 referred to the possibility of shunting through 'sperr' arteries and other forms of precapillary anastomoses (Krahl, 1964) but the functional significance of these potential shunts remains in doubt. Flow through them must be negligible in the healthy conscious subject.

Finger clubbing

It is believed that finger clubbing (hypertrophic pulmonary osteoarthropathy in its most advanced stage) is due to shunting rather than hypoxaemia since it is absent in certain forms of hypoxaemia without shunting such as residence at high altitude. The association with shunting is strong (Pain, 1964) and it has also been suggested that bronchopulmonary anastomoses may be responsible for the transfer of a substance to the systemic circulation which is normally detoxified in the lung (Weatherall, Ledingham and Warrell, 1983). These authors have suggested a role for reduced ferritin but the mechanism is not immediately obvious.

Effect of cardiac output on shunt

Cardiac output has an important bearing on shunt and this must be considered from three entirely separate standpoints. Firstly, a reduction of cardiac output causes a decrease in mixed venous oxygen content with the result that a given shunt causes a greater reduction in arterial PO_2 *provided the shunt fraction is unaltered*, a relationship which is illustrated in Figure 11.9. Secondly, it has been observed that, in a very wide range of pathological and physiological circumstances, a reduction in cardiac output causes an approximately proportional reduction in the shunt fraction (Lynch, Mhyre and Dantzker, 1979; Dantzker, Lynch and Weg, 1980), the only apparent exception being a shunt through regional pulmonary atelectasis (Cheney and Colley, 1980). It is remarkable that these two effects tend to have approximately equal and opposite effects on arterial PO_2. Thus with a decreased cardiac output there is usually a reduced shunt of a more desaturated mixed venous blood with the result that the arterial PO_2 is scarcely changed. Marshall and Marshall (1985) have advanced convincing reasons for believing that the reduction in shunt is due to pulmonary vasoconstriction in consequence of the reduction in PO_2 of the mixed venous blood flowing through the shunt. The magnitude of the flow diversion is inversely related to the size of the hypoxic segment (Marshall et al., 1981). The third consideration concerns the oxygen flux. Even though a reduced cardiac output may have little effect on arterial oxygen content, it must have a direct effect on the oxygen flux which is the product of cardiac output and arterial oxygen content (page 283).

Effect of venous admixture on arterial PCO_2 and PO_2

Qualitatively, it will be clear that venous admixture reduces the overall efficiency of gas exchange and results in arterial blood gas tensions which are closer to those of mixed venous blood than would otherwise be the case. Quantitatively, the effect is simple provided that we consider the *contents* of gases in blood. In the case of the anatomical shunt in Figure 8.9, conservation of mass (oxygen) is the basis of the equations, which simply state that the amount of oxygen flowing in the arterial system equals the sum of the amount of oxygen leaving the pulmonary capillaries and the amount of oxygen flowing through the shunt. For each term in this equation the amount of oxygen flowing may be expressed as the product of the blood flow rate and the oxygen content of blood flowing in the vessel (the symbols are explained in Figure 8.10 and Appendix D). Figure 8.9 shows how the equation may be cleared and solved for the ratio of the venous admixture to the cardiac output. The final equation has a form which is rather similar to that of the Bohr equation for the physiological dead space (page 172).

In terms of *content*, the shunt equation is very simple to solve for the effect of venous admixture on arterial oxygen content. If, for example:

Pulmonary end-capillary oxygen content is   20 ml/100 ml
and mixed venous blood oxygen content is   10 ml/100 ml

then a 50% venous admixture will result in an arterial oxygen content of 15 ml/100 ml, a 25% venous admixture will result in an arterial oxygen content of 17.5 ml/100 ml, and so on. It is then necessary to convert arterial oxygen content to PO_2 by reference to the haemoglobin dissociation curve (see page 272). Since arterial PO_2 is usually on the flat part of the dissociation curve, small changes in content tend to have a very large effect on PO_2.

The effect of venous admixture on arterial CO_2 *content* is roughly similar in magnitude to that of oxygen content. However, due to the steepness of the CO_2 dissociation curve near the arterial point (see Figure 10.2), the effect on arterial PCO_2 is very small and far less than the change in arterial PO_2 (Table 8.2). Two conclusions may be drawn:

1. Arterial PO_2 is the most useful blood gas measurement for the detection of venous admixture.
2. Venous admixture reduces the arterial PO_2 markedly, but has relatively little effect on arterial PCO_2 or on the content of either CO_2 or O_2 unless the venous admixture is large.

Elevations of PCO_2 are seldom caused by venous admixture and it is customary to ignore the effect of moderate shunts on arterial PCO_2. It is, in fact, more usual for venous admixture to lower the PCO_2 indirectly, since the decreased PO_2 commonly

Table 8.2 Effect of 5% venous admixture on the difference between arterial and pulmonary end-capillary blood levels of carbon dioxide and oxygen

	Pulmonary end-capillary blood	Arterial blood
CO_2 content (ml/100 ml)	49.7	50.0
PCO_2 (kPa)	5.29	5.33
(mmHg)	39.7	40.0
O_2 content (ml/100 ml)	19.9	19.6
O_2 saturation (%)	97.8	96.8
PO_2 (kPa)	14.0	12.0
(mmHg)	105	90

It has been assumed that the arterial/venous oxygen content difference is 4.5 ml/100 ml and that the haemoglobin concentration is 14.9 g/dl. Typical changes in PO_2 and PCO_2 have been shown for a 10% venous admixture in Figure 8.9.

causes hyperventilation, which more than compensates for the very slight elevation of P_{CO_2} which would otherwise result from the venous admixture (see Figure 21.1).

Since the effect of venous admixture on arterial P_{O_2} is so markedly influenced by the slope of the dissociation curve, it will clearly depend upon the section of the dissociation curve which is concerned in a particular situation. Thus if the pulmonary end-capillary P_{O_2} is high (above 40 kPa or 300 mmHg where the curve is flat), venous admixture causes a very marked fall in arterial P_{O_2} (approximately 2.3 kPa or 17 mmHg) for 1% venous admixture). If, however, the pulmonary end-capillary P_{O_2} is low (below 9.3 kPa or 70 mmHg), where the curve is steep, venous admixture has relatively little effect on arterial P_{O_2} (see Figure 11.8). It would probably be wrong to consider this from the teleological standpoint, but it is nevertheless convenient to remember that a given degree of venous admixture causes a greater fall of P_{O_2} in the better oxygenated patients and a smaller fall in the less well oxygenated patients.

The iso-shunt diagram

If we assume normal values for arterial P_{CO_2}, haemoglobin and arterial/mixed venous oxygen content difference, the arterial P_{O_2} is determined mainly by the inspired oxygen concentration and venous admixture considered in the context of the three-compartment model (Figure 8.7). The relationship between inspired oxygen concentration and arterial P_{O_2} is a matter for constant attention in such situations as intensive therapy, and it has been found a matter of practical convenience to prepare a graph of the relationship at different levels of venous admixture (Figure 8.10). The arterial/mixed venous oxygen content difference is often unknown in the clinical situation and therefore the diagram has been prepared for an assumed content difference of 5 ml oxygen per 100 ml of blood. Iso-shunt bands have then been drawn on a plot of arterial P_{O_2} against inspired oxygen concentration. The bands are sufficiently wide to encompass all values of P_{CO_2} between 3.3 and 5.3 kPa (25–40 mmHg) and haemoglobin levels between 10 and 14 g/dl. Normal barometric pressure is assumed. Since calculation of the venous admixture requires knowledge of the actual arterial/mixed venous oxygen content difference, the iso-shunt lines in Figure 8.10 refer to the 'virtual shunt', which is defined as the calculated shunt on the basis of an assumed value of the arterial/mixed venous oxygen content difference of 5 ml/100 ml. The calculations for preparation of an iso-shunt diagram are conceptually simple, but laborious in execution, requiring solution of complex equations and repeated conversions of blood P_{O_2} to oxygen content and vice versa, the last requiring an iterative approach. There is really no alternative to the use of a computer.

In practice, the iso-shunt diagram is useful for adjusting the inspired oxygen concentration to obtain a required level of arterial P_{O_2} to prevent hypoxaemia while avoiding the administration of an unnecessarily high concentration of oxygen. For example, if a patient is found to have an arterial P_{O_2} of 30 kPa (225 mmHg) while breathing 90% oxygen, he has a virtual shunt of 20% and, if it is required to attain an arterial P_{O_2} of 10 kPa (75 mmHg), this should be achieved by reducing the inspired oxygen concentration to 45%. The new value for arterial P_{O_2} should then be checked by direct measurement. After measuring arterial P_{O_2} while the patient breathes 100% oxygen, the virtual shunt may be read off the iso-shunt graph. Resolution of conditions such as pulmonary oedema, infection or collapse is

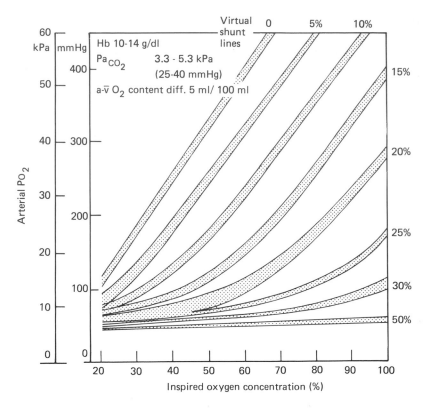

Figure 8.10 Iso-shunt diagram. On co-ordinates of inspired oxygen concentration (abscissa) and arterial P_{O_2} (ordinate), iso-shunt bands have been drawn to include all values of Hb, Pa_{CO_2} and a-v̄ oxygen content difference shown above. (Redrawn from Benatar, Hewlett and Nunn (1973) by permisson of the Editor of the British Journal of Anaesthesia)

shown by a reduction of the virtual shunt which may therefore be used as an indication of progress.

Under static pathological conditions, the author has found that changing the inspired oxygen concentration results in changes in arterial P_{O_2} which are reasonably well predicted by the iso-shunt diagram (Lawler and Nunn, 1984). Others have reported an increased shunt at high concentrations of inspired oxygen, the so-called hyperoxic shunt.

With inspired oxygen concentrations in excess of 35%, perfusion of alveoli with low (but not zero) V̇/Q̇ ratios has relatively little effect on arterial P_{O_2}. However, with inspired oxygen concentrations in the range 21–35%, increased scatter of V̇/Q̇ ratios has an appreciable effect on arterial P_{O_2} for reasons which are explained below. Therefore in these circumstances, the standard iso-shunt diagram is not applicable, since arterial P_{O_2} is less than predicted as the inspired oxygen concentration is reduced towards 21%. A new diagram, which provides a reasonable simulation of scatter of V̇/Q̇ ratios *plus* a shunt, is explained below, and this diagram (see Figure E.6) appears to be a satisfactory model for a wide range of patients requiring the administration of oxygen within this range (Petros, Doré and Nunn, 1993).

The effect of scatter of V̇/Q̇ ratios on arterial P_{O_2}

It is usually extremely difficult to say whether reduction of arterial P_{O_2} is due to true shunt (areas of zero V̇/Q̇) ratio, or increased scatter of V̇/Q̇ ratios with an appreciable contribution to arterial blood from alveoli with very low (but not zero) V̇/Q̇ ratio. In the clinical field, it is quite usual to ignore scatter of V̇/Q̇ ratios (which cannot usually be quantified) and treat blood gas results *as if* the alveolar/arterial P_{O_2} difference (page 261) was caused entirely by true shunt. In the example shown in Figure 8.11, it is quite impossible to distinguish between scatter of V̇/Q̇ ratios and

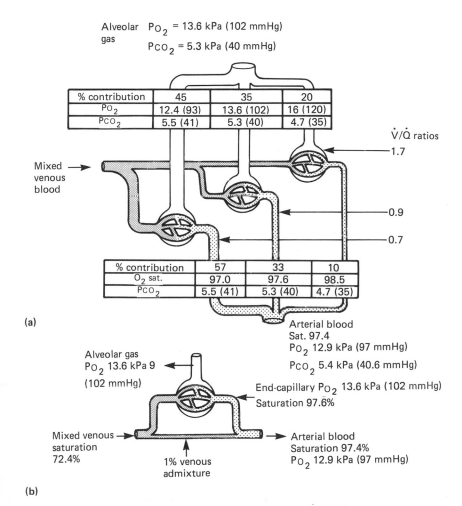

Figure 8.11 Alveolar/arterial P_{O_2} difference caused by scatter of V̇/Q̇ ratios and its representation by an equivalent degree of venous admixture. (a) Scatter of V̇/Q̇ ratios corresponding roughly to the three zones of the lung in the normal upright subject. Mixed alveolar gas P_{O_2} is calculated with allowance for the volume contribution of gas from the three zones. Arterial saturation is similarly determined and the P_{O_2} derived. There is an alveolar/arterial P_{O_2} difference of 0.7 kPa (5 mmHg). (b) An entirely imaginary situation which would account for the difference. This is a useful method of quantifying the functional effect of scatter of V̇/Q̇ ratios but should be carefully distinguished from the actual situation.

a shunt on the basis of a single measurement of arterial PO_2. However, the two conditions are quite different in the effect of different inspired oxygen concentrations on the alveolar/arterial PO_2 difference and therefore the apparent shunt.

Figure 8.10 shows that, for a true shunt, with increasing inspired oxygen concentration, the effect on arterial PO_2 increases to reach a plateau value of 2–3 kPa (15–22 mmHg) for each 1% of shunt. This is more precisely shown in terms of alveolar/arterial PO_2 difference, plotted as a function of alveolar PO_2 in Figure 11.8.

It is not intuitively obvious why an increased spread of $\dot{V}/\dot{Q}$ ratios should increase the alveolar/arterial PO_2 difference. There are essentially two reasons. Firstly, there tends to be more blood from the alveoli with low $\dot{V}/\dot{Q}$ ratio. For example, in Figure 8.11, 57% of the arterial blood comes from the alveoli with low $\dot{V}/\dot{Q}$ ratio and low PO_2, while only 10% is contributed by the alveoli with high $\dot{V}/\dot{Q}$ ratio and high PO_2. Therefore the latter cannot compensate for the former, when arterial oxygen levels are determined with due allowance for volume contribution. The second reason is illustrated in Figure 8.12. Alveoli with high $\dot{V}/\dot{Q}$ ratios are on a

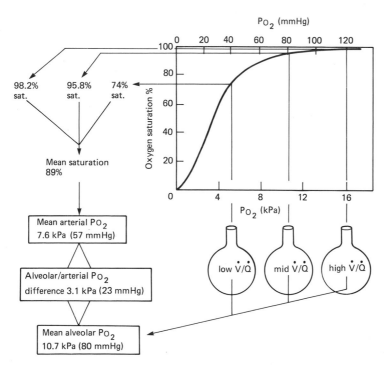

Figure 8.12 Alveolar/arterial PO_2 difference caused by scatter of $\dot{V}/\dot{Q}$ ratios resulting in oxygen tensions along the upper inflexion of the oxygen dissociation curve. The diagram shows the effect of three groups of alveoli with PO_2 values of 5.3, 10.7 and 16.0 kPa (40, 80 and 120 mmHg). Ignoring the effect of the different volumes of gas and blood contributed by the three groups, the mean alveolar PO_2 is 10.7 kPa. However, due to the bend of the dissociation curve, the saturations of the blood leaving the three groups are not proportional to their PO_2. The mean arterial saturation is, in fact, 89% and the PO_2 therefore is 7.6 kPa. The alveolar/arterial PO_2 difference is thus 3.1 kPa. The actual difference would be somewhat greater since gas with a high PO_2 would make a relatively greater contribution to the alveolar gas, and blood with a low PO_2 would make a relatively greater contribution to the arterial blood. In this example a calculated venous admixture of 27% would be required to account for the scatter of $\dot{V}/\dot{Q}$ ratios in terms of the measured alveolar/arterial PO_2 difference, at an alveolar PO_2 of 10.7 kPa.

flatter part of the haemoglobin dissociation curve than are alveoli with low $\dot{V}/\dot{Q}$ ratios. Therefore, the adverse effect on oxygen *content* is greater for alveoli with a low $\dot{V}/\dot{Q}$ (and therefore low PO_2) than is the beneficial effect of alveoli with a high $\dot{V}/\dot{Q}$ (and therefore high PO_2). Thus, the greater the spread of $\dot{V}/\dot{Q}$ ratios, the larger the alveolar/arterial PO_2 difference.

Modification of the iso-shunt diagram to include $\dot{V}/\dot{Q}$ scatter. Petros, Doré and Nunn (1993) described a series of calculations which indicated arterial PO_2 values at various inspired oxygen concentrations for a two-compartment model of $\dot{V}/\dot{Q}$ scatter, with increasing divergence of the $\dot{V}/\dot{Q}$ ratios for the two compartments (Table 8.3 and Figure 8.13). This model is clearly an oversimplification of such situations as those shown in Figure 8.6. Nevertheless, a combination of shunt and a grade of $\dot{V}/\dot{Q}$ mismatch, which increased progressively with the shunt (determined at high inspired oxygen concentration), was found to provide a close simulation of the relationship between arterial PO_2 and inspired oxygen concentration for a wide variety of patients with moderate respiratory dysfunction requiring oxygen therapy in the range 25–35% inspired oxygen concentration. The model accurately predicted the reduction of arterial PO_2 below the value derived from the standard iso-shunt diagram as the inspired oxygen was reduced below 35%. The patients, who were all breathing spontaneously, included 20 patients recovering in an intensive care unit (Petros, Doré and Nunn, 1993) and 10 patients recovering from abdominal surgery (Drummond and Wright, 1977). The modified iso-shunt diagram (see Figure E.6) is not appreciably different from the standard iso-shunt diagram at higher concentrations of inspired oxygen, but is more likely to be helpful at lower oxygen concentrations.

Principles of assessment of distribution of ventilation and pulmonary blood flow

Distribution of inspired gas

Much of the methodology has been outlined in the text above in the course of explaining basic principles and will not be repeated here.

Table 8.3 Ventilation/perfusion ratios for the bimodal two-compartment model of maldistribution of ventilation/perfusion ratios used in the construction of Figure 8.13 (Petros, Doré and Nunn, 1993)

	Compartment with high $\dot{V}/\dot{Q}$ ratio	*Compartment with low $\dot{V}/\dot{Q}$ ratio*
Perfect match (grade 0)	0.86	0.86
Mismatch grade 1	1.18	0.55
Mismatch grade 2	1.56	0.38
Mismatch grade 3	2.15	0.30
Mismatch grade 4	3.34	0.16

It is assumed that the ratio of actual perfusions is inversely related to the square root of the $\dot{V}/\dot{Q}$ ratios.

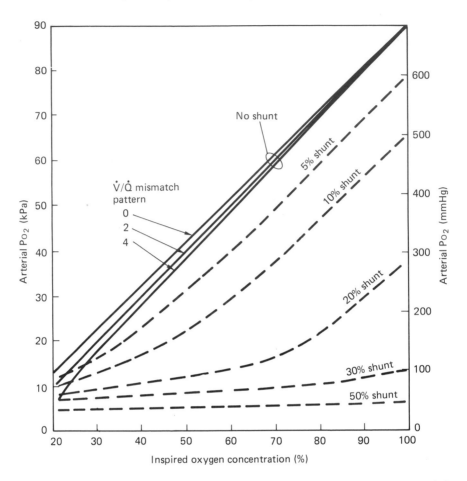

Figure 8.13 The continuous curves show the effect on arterial Po₂ of increasing degrees of V̇/Q̇ mismatch (using the bimodal two-compartment model of maldistribution specified in Table 8.3) for different values of inspired oxygen concentration in the absence of a true shunt. At lower inspired oxygen the arterial Po₂ is progressively decreased below normal for the reasons shown in Figures 8.11 and 8.12. These concave-downward curves may be compared with the concave-upward iso-shunt curves shown as broken lines. V̇/Q̇ mismatch patterns 1–4 are combined with iso-shunt curves in Appendix Figure E.6. This extends the clinical applicability of the iso-shunt curves.

Distribution to zones of the lung can be conveniently studied with the gamma camera following inhalation of a suitable radioactive gas which is not too soluble in blood. ^{133}Xe is suitable for this purpose and the technique has become a routine clinical investigation. The technique defines zones of the lung which can be related to anatomical subdivisions by comparing anteroposterior and lateral scans. The technique is useful for defining pathological causes of failure of regional ventilation and can be related to scans which indicate perfusion.

Single-breath maldistribution test

This test is shown diagrammatically in Figure 8.14. The subject, who has been breathing air, takes a single deep breath of 100% oxygen sufficient to raise the alveolar oxygen concentration to about 50%. The patient then exhales deeply and the nitrogen concentration is measured at the patient's lips. (It would be just as satisfactory to monitor the oxygen concentration, but in the past it has been more convenient to measure nitrogen concentration.) We may now consider what is found under four different circumstances (Figure 8.14a–d):

1. Figure 8.14a shows two identical functional units. Following the inspiration of a single breath of oxygen, the nitrogen concentration in each unit is reduced to the same value and the exhaled nitrogen concentration must therefore remain constant throughout the latter part of expiration.
2. Figure 8.14b shows functional units of identical mechanical properties but which are subjected to unequal forces during inspiration. As a result, the nitrogen concentration is reduced by a greater amount in the better ventilated unit. If expiration is passive, the expirate will consist of the same proportion from each unit throughout expiration. Therefore the exhaled nitrogen concentration will be constant throughout the latter part of expiration, at a value intermediate between that of the two units.
3. Figure 8.14c shows two units of different mechanical properties but which nevertheless have the same time constant. (The unit on the right may be considered as having double the resistance and half the compliance of the unit on the left.) In these circumstances, ventilation will be preferentially distributed to the unit with the higher compliance and lower resistance. However, since the time constants are the same, a passive expiration will again consist of the same proportion from each unit throughout expiration. Therefore the exhaled nitrogen concentration will remain constant throughout the latter part of expiration as in the previous example.
4. Figure 8.14d has two units with different time constants resulting from different mechanical properties, similar to the fast and slow alveoli in Figure 3.6. During inspiration of finite length, the faster unit will be preferentially ventilated, and its nitrogen concentration will therefore be lower. During expiration, the faster unit empties more rapidly at first while gas from the slower unit forms a proportionately greater part of the end-expiratory gas. Thus the proportion of gas from the two units changes during expiration and the nitrogen concentration rises progressively.

Even with perfect distribution the exhaled nitrogen concentration rises slightly during the latter part of the exhalation. This is because oxygen is being consumed in greater volume than carbon dioxide is being produced. Therefore, the alveolar nitrogen concentration always rises slightly as expiration proceeds. The upper limit of normal is a rise of 1.5% (more in older subjects) between the exhalation of 750 ml and 1250 ml after the inhalation of a large breath of oxygen.

Measurement of anatomical dead space

The anatomical dead space is most conveniently measured by the technique illustrated in Figure 8.15, originally developed for use with a nitrogen anlyser by Fowler (1948). The CO_2 concentration at the lips is measured continuously with a rapid gas analyser, and then displayed against the volume actually expired. The 'alveolar plateau' of CO_2 concentration is not flat but slopes gently. Anatomical dead space is easily derived by the graphical solution shown in the Figure.

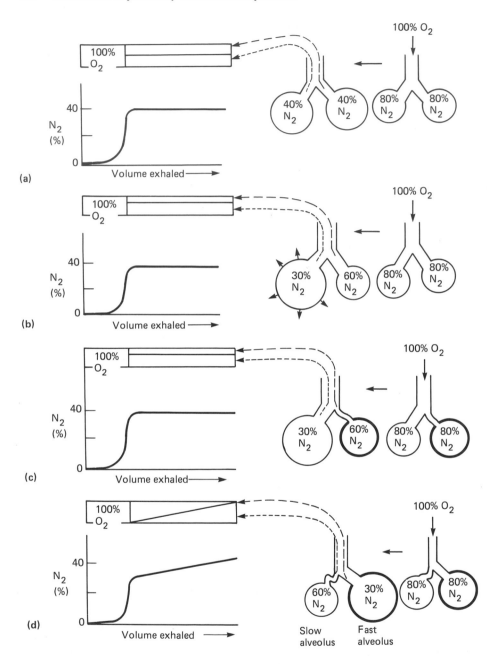

Figure 8.14 The single-breath nitrogen wash-out test in different types of maldistribution. Reading the diagram from right to left, the subject inhales a deep breath of 100% oxygen oxygen and then exhales into a nitrogen meter. (a) Normal subject with uniform distribution. (b) Maldistribution due to non-uniform pull of inspiratory muscles. (c) Maldistribution due to non-uniform mechanical factors in lung units but all having the same time constants. (d) Maldistribution due to non-uniform mechanical factors in lung units resulting in different time constants. Only this type of maldistribution alters the slope of the curve of the expired nitrogen.

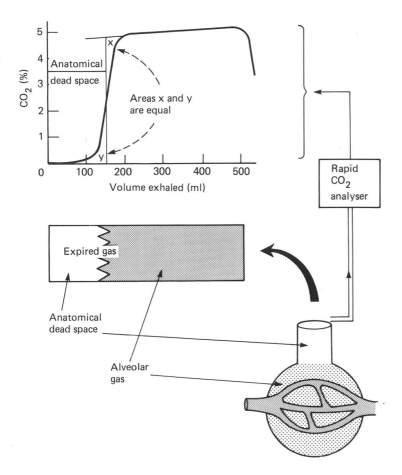

Figure 8.15 Measurement of the anatomical dead space using CO_2 as the tracer gas. If the gas passing the patient's lips is continuously analysed for CO_2 concentration, there is a sudden rise to the alveolar plateau level, after the expiration of gas from the anatomical dead space (conducting air passages). If the instantaneous CO_2 concentration is plotted against the volume exhaled (allowing for delay in the CO_2 analyser), a graph similar to that shown is obtained. A vertical line is constructed so that the two areas x and y are equal. This line will indicate the volume of the anatomical dead space.

Measurement of physiological dead space

Arterial blood and expired air are collected simultaneously over a period of 2–3 minutes (Figure 8.16). PCO_2 of blood and gas are then determined, the CO_2-sensitive electrode being suitable for both samples. Provided that the inspired gas is free from carbon dioxide, physiological dead space is indicated by the following form of the Bohr equation:

physiological dead space

$$= \text{tidal volume} \left(\frac{\text{arterial } PCO_2 - \text{mixed-expired gas } PCO_2}{\text{arterial } PCO_2} \right) - \text{apparatus dead space}$$

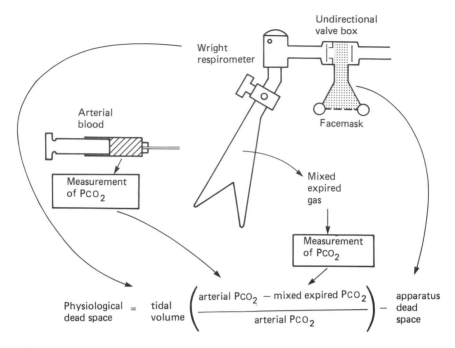

Figure 8.16 Clinical measurement of physiological dead space. Arterial blood and mixed expired gas are collected simultaneously over a period of 2–3 minutes. Values for P_{CO_2} are then substituted in the Bohr equation. Tidal volume is conveniently determined with a Wright respirometer and the apparatus dead space by water displacement.

Apparatus dead space includes such items as the facemask and unidirectional valve box and is usually measured by water displacement. Tidal volume may be determined by a variety of techniques; the Wright respirometer is the most convenient and may easily be incorporated in the gas-collection apparatus. The result is often most conveniently expressed as the ratio of the physiological dead space to the tidal volume.

Measurement of alveolar dead space

The alveolar dead space is measured as the difference between the physiological and anatomical dead space, determined separately but at the same time. When only the physiological dead space is measured, it is often possible to attribute a large increase in physiological dead space to an increase in the alveolar component, since there are few circumstances in which the anatomical dead space is greatly enlarged.

The arterial/end-expiratory P_{CO_2} difference is a convenient and relatively simple method of assessing the magnitude of the alveolar dead space. In Figure 8.8, end-expiratory gas is shown to consist of a mixture of 'ideal' alveolar gas and alveolar dead space gas. If the patient has an appreciable alveolar dead space, the end-expiratory P_{CO_2} will be less than the arterial P_{CO_2} which is assumed equal to the 'ideal' alveolar P_{CO_2}.

If, for example, 'ideal' alveolar gas has a P_{CO_2} of 5.3 kPa (40 mmHg) and the end-expiratory P_{CO_2} is found to be 2.65 kPa (20 mmHg), it follows that the end-expiratory gas consists of equal parts of 'ideal' alveolar gas and alveolar dead space gas. Thus if the tidal volume is 500 ml and the anatomical dead space 100 ml, the components of the tidal volume would be as follows:

anatomical dead space	100 ml
alveolar dead space	200 ml
'ideal' alveolar gas	200 ml

The physiological dead space would be $100 + 200 = 300$ ml and the V_D/V_T ratio 60%.

Sudden changes in the end-expiratory P_{CO_2} provide a very useful qualitative indication of such conditions as pulmonary air embolus which result in an abrupt increase in alveolar dead space. However, a sudden decrease in cardiac output will have the same effect.

Measurement of distribution of pulmonary blood flow

Unilateral pulmonary blood flow. Flow sensors, such as electromagnetic flow meters, may be applied to the pulmonary arteries but such methods are essentially very invasive. There is no simple method to estimate the partitioning of the pulmonary blood flow in man. The unilateral oxygen consumption can be measured with a divided airway and this gives an approximate indication of the relative perfusion of the two lungs. However, the Fick equation cannot be solved separately for the two lungs, because the anatomical arrangement of the pulmonary veins makes it impossible to sample representative pulmonary venous blood from the two lungs. It is, however, possible to make a very approximate estimate of the pulmonary venous oxygen content from the unilateral end-expiratory P_{O_2}.

The dummy pneumonectomy. Carlens, Hanson and Nordenström (1951) introduced the technique of occluding one pulmonary artery with a balloon, and so deflecting the entire pulmonary blood flow through one lung. This may be combined with occlusion of the bronchus (on the same side!) to reproduce the cardiorespiratory effects of pneumonectomy (Nemir et al., 1953).

Measurement of pulmonary lobar blood flow. By intubation, the right upper lobe bronchus may be isolated in man (Mattson and Carlens, 1955), and the oxygen consumption of this lobe may therefore be estimated. End-expiratory gases sampled from different lobes at bronchoscopy will give some qualitative indication of blood flow, although precise calculation of flow is not possible. A simple estimate of ventilation/perfusion ratio may be obtained from the respiratory exchange ratio (Armitage and Taylor, 1956). A more complete assessment has been made by the simultaneous analysis of a number of gases exhaled from various bronchi, using a mass spectrometer at bronchoscopy (Hugh-Jones and West, 1960).

Distribution to zones of the lung. The techniques most widely used in the clinical field are analogous to the methods for studying the zonal distribution of ventilation outlined above (page 188). A relatively insoluble gas such as ^{133}Xe may be dissolved in saline and injected into a systemic vein. The xenon is evolved in the lungs and may be counted in the alveolar gas with a gamma camera as explained above for ventilation scans. Xenon is rapidly cleared by pulmonary ventilation and the method is therefore suitable only if counting can be completed during a breath hold. The second method is to inject labelled particles which have a diameter greater than about 50 μm and so lodge in the pulmonary circulation. They can then be counted at leisure without the limitation of breath-holding time. Different isotopes with different energy levels of radiation can be used at different times to study changes in the pulmonary circulation. Counts may be obtained by stationary or moving scintillation counters and graphical representation of the circulation may be presented as a lung scan by means of a gamma camera. The use of ^{133}Xe to study blood flow to horizontal slices of the lung was introduced by West (1962). Ventilation and perfusion scans can be combined to give $\dot{V}/\dot{Q}$ scans.

Measurement of ventilation and perfusion as a function of $\dot{V}/\dot{Q}$ ratio

The information of the type displayed in Figure 8.5 is obtained by a technique developed by Wagner, Saltzman and West (1974) and reviewed by West (1990). It employs a range of tracer gases ranging from very soluble (e.g. acetone) to very insoluble (e.g. sulphur hexafluoride). Saline is equilibrated with these gases and infused intravenously at a constant rate. After about 20 minutes a steady state is achieved and samples of arterial blood and mixed expired gas are collected. Levels of the tracer gases in the arterial blood are then measured by gas chromatography (Wagner, Naumann and Laravuso, 1974), and levels in the mixed venous blood are derived by use of the Fick principle. It is then possible to calculate the retention of each tracer in the blood passing through the lung and the elimination of each in the expired gas. Retention and elimination are related to the solubility coefficient of each tracer in blood and then, by numerical analysis, it is possible to compute a distribution curve for pulmonary blood flow and alveolar ventilation respectively in relation to the spectrum of $\dot{V}/\dot{Q}$ ratios. In practice, a number of finite values of $\dot{V}/\dot{Q}$ are employed. The range of $\dot{V}/\dot{Q}$ ratios between 0.005 and 100 is divided equally on a logarithmic scale into 48 compartments which, together with zero (shunt) and infinity (alveolar dead space), make 50 in all.

The technique is technically demanding and laborious. It has not become widely used, but results from a small number of laboratories have made major contributions to our understanding of gas exchange in a wide variety of circumstances.

Measurement of venous admixture or shunt

Venous admixture, according to the Riley three-compartment model (see Figure 8.7) is calculated by solution of the equation shown in Figure 8.9. When the alveolar P_{O_2} is less than about 30 kPa (225 mmHg), scatter of $\dot{V}/\dot{Q}$ ratios contributes appreciably to the total calculated venous admixture (see Figure 8.13). When the subject breathes 100% oxygen, the component due to scatter of $\dot{V}/\dot{Q}$ ratios is minimal. Nevertheless, the calculated quantity still does not indicate the precise value of shunted blood since some of the shunt consists of blood of which the oxygen content is unknown (i.e. from bronchial veins and venae cordis minimae). The calculated venous admixture is thus at best an index rather than a precise measurement of contamination of arterial blood with venous blood.

In the equation shown in Figure 8.9, some of the quantities on the right-hand side are amenable to direct measurement. Arterial blood may be drawn from any convenient systemic artery, but the mixed venous blood must be sampled from the right ventricle or pulmonary artery. Blood from inferior and superior venae cavae and coronary sinus remains separate in the right atrium. An assumed value for arterial/mixed venous blood oxygen content difference is often made if it is not feasible to sample mixed venous blood, and this is inherent in the iso-shunt diagram (see Figure 8.10). For the measurement of shunt, there is no satisfactory substitute for a sample of arterial blood.

The major problem is measurement of the pulmonary end-capillary PO_2. This cannot be measured directly, and is assumed equal to the alveolar PO_2 (page 206). If Figure 8.7 is studied in conjunction with Figure 8.9, it will be seen that the 'alveolar' PO_2 required is the 'ideal' alveolar PO_2 and not the end-expiratory PO_2 which may be contaminated with alveolar dead space gas. The 'ideal' alveolar PO_2 is derived by solution of one of the alveolar air equations (see below).

Solution of the shunt equation requires blood oxygen *content* which must be calculated from PO_2 which is measured in the case of blood samples or derived in the case of the 'ideal' alveolar gas. The relevant calculations are described in Chapter 11 (page 262). This requires knowledge of haemoglobin concentration, shift of dissociation curve and haemoglobin saturation. The last two may be determined from the nomogram shown in Figure 11.13: if a computer is used, the following equation (Severinghaus, Stafford and Thunston, 1978) is highly convenient, but is valid only for PO_2 values above 4 kPa (30 mmHg).

$$SO_2 = \frac{100\ (PO_2{}^3 + 2.667 \times PO_2)}{PO_2{}^3 + 2.667 \times PO_2 + 55.47}$$

(PO_2 is in kPa; sat. in %)

Calculation of arterial PO_2 from a known degree of venous admixture. This involves clearing and solving the shunt equation (see Figure 8.9) for arterial PO_2. It is a notoriously difficult and tedious calculation requiring *inter alia* derivation of PO_2 from blood oxygen content. A computer is almost essential and the necessary steps in the calculation have been detailed by Petros, Doré and Nunn (1993).

The alveolar air equation

'Ideal' alveolar gas (see Figure 8.7) cannot be sampled and its PO_2 must be derived by indirect means. Derivation of the 'ideal' alveolar PO_2 was first suggested by Benzinger (1937) and later by Rossier and Méan (1943). It was formulated with greater precision by Riley et al. (1946). The alveolar air equation exists in several forms which appear to be very different but give the same result.

Derivation of the 'ideal' alveolar PO_2 is based on the following assumptions.

1. Quite large degrees of venous admixture or $\dot{V}/\dot{Q}$ scatter cause relatively little difference between PCO_2 of 'ideal' alveolar gas (or pulmonary end-capillary blood) and arterial blood (see Table 8.2). Therefore, 'ideal' alveolar PCO_2 is approximately equal to arterial PCO_2.
2. The respiratory exchange ratio of ideal alveolar gas (in relation to inspired gas) equals the respiratory exchange ratio of mixed expired gas (again in relation to inspired gas).

From these assumptions it is possible to derive an equation which indicates the 'ideal' alveolar PO_2 in terms of arterial PCO_2, inspired gas PO_2, respiratory exchange ratio or related quantities. As a very rough approximation, the oxygen and carbon dioxide in the alveolar gas replace the oxygen in the inspired gas. Therefore, very approximately:

$$\text{alveolar } PO_2 \doteqdot \text{inspired } PO_2 - \text{arterial } PCO_2$$

This equation is not sufficiently accurate for use except in the special case when 100% oxygen is breathed. In other situations, three corrections are required to overcome errors due to the following factors:

1. Usually, less carbon dioxide is produced than oxygen is consumed (effect of the respiratory exchange ratio).
2. The respiratory exchange ratio produces a secondary effect due to the fact that the expired volume does not equal the inspired volume.
3. The inspired and expired gas volumes may also differ because of inert gas exchange.

The simplest practicable form of the equation is that suggested by Benzinger (1937) and Rossier and Méan (1943). It makes correction for the principal effect of the respiratory exchange ratio (1), but not the small supplementary error due to the difference between the inspired and expired gas volumes (2):

$$\text{alveolar } PO_2 \doteqdot \text{inspired } PO_2 - \text{arterial } PCO_2/RQ$$

This form is suitable for rapid bedside calculations of alveolar PO_2, when great accuracy is not required.

One stage more complicated is an equation which allows for differences in the volume of inspired and expired gas due to the respiratory exchange ratio, but still does not allow for differences due to the exchange of inert gases. This equation exists in various forms, all algebraically identical:

$$\text{alveolar } PO_2 = PI_{O_2} - \frac{Pa_{CO_2}}{R}\left(1 - FI_{O_2}\left(1 - R\right)\right)$$

(derived from Riley et al., 1946)

This equation is suitable for use whenever the subject has been breathing the inspired gas mixture long enough for the inert gas to be in equilibrium. It is unsuitable for use when the inspired oxygen concentration has recently been changed, when the ambient pressure has recently been changed (e.g. during hyperbaric oxygen therapy) or when the inert gas concentration has recently been changed (e.g. soon after the start or finish of a period of inhaling nitrous oxide).

Perhaps the most satisfactory form of the alveolar air equation is that which was advanced by Filley, MacIntosh and Wright (1954). This equation makes no assumption that inert gases are in equilibrium and allows for the difference between inspired and expired gas from whatever cause. It also proves to be very simple in use and does not require the calculation of the respiratory exchange ratio:

$$\text{alveolar } PO_2 = PI_{O_2} - Pa_{CO_2}\left(\frac{PI_{O_2} - P\bar{E}_{O_2}}{P\bar{E}_{CO_2}}\right)$$

If the alveolar P_{O_2} is calculated separately according to the last two equations, the difference (if any) will be that due to inert gas exchange. This affords a method of study of such phenomena as the 'concentration' effect (page 260).

Distinction between shunt and the effect of $\dot{V}/\dot{Q}$ scatter

Shunt and scatter of $\dot{V}/\dot{Q}$ ratios will each produce an alveolar/arterial P_{O_2} difference from which a value for venous admixture may be calculated. It is usually impossible to say to what extent the calculated venous admixture is due to a true shunt or to perfusion of alveoli with low $\dot{V}/\dot{Q}$ ratio. Three methods are available for distinction between the two conditions.

If the inspired oxygen concentration is altered, the effect on the arterial P_{O_2} will depend upon the nature of the disorder. If oxygenation is impaired by a shunt, the arterial P_{O_2} will increase as shown in the iso-shunt diagram (see Figure 8.10). If, however, the disorder is due to scatter of $\dot{V}/\dot{Q}$ ratios, the arterial P_{O_2} will approach the normal value for the inspired oxygen concentration as the inspired oxygen concentration is increased (see Figure 8.13). $\dot{V}/\dot{Q}$ scatter has virtually no effect when the subject breathes 100% oxygen.

Measurement of the alveolar/arterial P_{N_2} difference is a specific method for quantification of $\dot{V}/\dot{Q}$ scatter, since the P_{N_2} difference is entirely uninfluenced by true shunt. The method has not come into general use. Subjects must be in a state of complete nitrogen equilibrium which may be difficult to achieve in the clinical environment. Furthermore, the method is technically difficult, requiring the measurement of P_{N_2} to an accuracy which is not easily obtainable. The method was described by Rahn and Farhi (1964).

The multiple inert gas wash-out technique for analysis of distribution of blood flow in relation to $\dot{V}/\dot{Q}$ ratio is the best method of distinction between shunt and areas of low $\dot{V}/\dot{Q}$ ratio (see above).

Chapter 9

Diffusion and alveolar/capillary permeability

Fundamentals of the diffusion process

Diffusion of a gas is a process by which a net transfer of molecules takes place from a zone in which the gas exerts a high partial pressure to a zone in which it exerts a lower partial pressure. The mechanism of transfer is the random movement of molecules and the term excludes both active biological transport and transfer by mass movement of gas in response to a total pressure difference (as occurs during expiration). The partial pressure (or tension) of a gas in a gas mixture is the pressure which it would exert if it occupied the space alone (equal to total pressure multiplied by fractional concentration). The tension of a gas in solution in a liquid is defined as being equal to the tension of the same gas in a gas mixture which is in equilibrium with the liquid. Gas molecules pass in each direction but at a rate proportional to the tension of the gas in the zone which they are leaving. The net transfer of the gas is the difference in the number of molecules passing in each direction, and is thus proportional to the difference in tension between the two zones. Typical examples of diffusion are shown in Figure 9.1.

In the living body oxygen is constantly being consumed, while carbon dioxide is being produced. Therefore, equilibrium cannot be attained as in the case of the open bottle of oxygen in Figure 9.1a. Instead, a dynamic equilibrium is attained with a cascade of oxygen tensions from 21 kPa (approx. 160 mmHg) in dry air, down to 1–3 kPa (7.5–22.5 mmHg) at the site of consumption in the mitochondria (see Figure 11.5). The maintenance of these tension gradients is, in fact, a characteristic of life.

In the case of gases which are not metabolized to any great extent, such as nitrogen and most inhalational anaesthetic agents, there is always a tendency towards a static equilibrium at which all tissue tensions become equal to the tension of the particular gas in the inspired air. This occurs with nitrogen (apart from the small effect of the respiratory exchange ratio), and would also be attained with an inhalational anaesthetic agent if it were administered for a very long time.

In each of the examples shown in Figure 9.1, there is a finite resistance to the transfer of the gas molecules. In Figure 9.1a, the resistance is concentrated at the restriction in the neck of the bottle. Clearly, the narrower the neck, the slower will be the process of equilibration with the outside air. In Figure 9.1b, the site of the resistance to diffusion is less circumscribed but includes gas diffusion within the alveolus, the alveolar/capillary membrane, the diffusion path through the plasma,

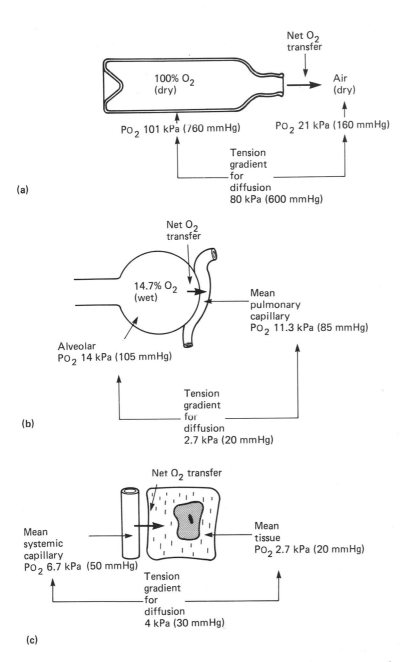

Figure 9.1 Three examples of diffusion of oxygen. In each case there is a net transfer of oxygen from left to right in accord with the tension gradient. (a) Oxygen passes from one gaseous phase to another. (b) Oxygen passes from a gaseous phase to a liquid phase. (c) Oxygen passes from one liquid phase to another.

and the delay in combination of oxygen with the reduced haemoglobin in the erythrocyte. In Figure 9.1c, the resistance commences with the delay in the release of oxygen by haemoglobin, and includes all the interfaces between the erythrocyte cell membrane and the site of oxygen consumption in the mitochondria. There may then be an additional component in the rate at which oxygen enters into chemical combination.

Quantification of resistance to diffusion

There is a clear analogy between the diffusion of gases in response to a partial pressure gradient and the passage of an electrical current in response to a potential difference in an electrical circuit. Diffusing capacity is analogous to conductance which is the reciprocal of resistance:

$$\text{diffusing capacity} = \frac{\text{net rate of gas transfer}}{\text{partial pressure gradient}}$$

$$\text{conductance} = \frac{\text{current flow (amps)}}{\text{potential difference (volts)}}$$

The unit of electrical conductance is the mho (reciprocal of the ohm). The usual biological unit of diffusing capacity is ml/min/mmHg, or, in SI units, ml min^{-1} kPa^{-1}.

Small molecules diffuse more easily than large molecules. Graham's law states that the rate of diffusion of a gas is inversely proportional to the square root of its density. Thus, nitrous oxide has a density of 1.4 times that of oxygen, but the rate of gaseous diffusion of oxygen is only 1.2 times that of nitrous oxide. Gases also diffuse more readily at higher temperatures.

When a gas is diffusing into or through an aqueous phase, the solubility of the gas in water becomes an important factor, and the diffusing capacity under these circumstances is considered to be directly proportional to the solubility. Nitrous oxide would thus be expected to have about 20 times the diffusing capacity of oxygen in crossing a gas/water interface. High solubility does not confer an increased 'agility' of the gas in its negotiation of an aqueous barrier, but simply means that, for a given tension, more molecules of the gas are present in the liquid.

Apart from these factors, inherent in the gas, the resistance to diffusion is related directly to the length of the diffusion path and inversely to the area of interface which is available for diffusion. In the case of the lungs, for example, the diffusion path extends from the gas side of the alveolar membrane to some unspecified reference point within the erythrocyte. The area of interface probably corresponds to the total area of pulmonary capillary endothelium in contact with alveolar epithelium. It is important to remember that the pulmonary diffusing capacity is as much a measure of the area of the interface as it is of the thickness of the tissues which comprise the diffusion path.

The diffusing capacity of oxygen in the lung is markedly influenced by the rate of combination of oxygen with reduced haemoglobin. Clearly, if this is slow, it will retard the whole process of oxygen transfer; similar considerations apply to release of carbon dioxide from chemical combination.

Tension versus concentration gradients

Non-volatile substances in solution diffuse in response to concentration gradients. This is also true for gas mixtures at the same total pressure, when the partial pressure of any component gas is directly proportional to its concentration. This is not the case when a gas in solution in one liquid diffuses into a different liquid in which it has a different solubility coefficient. When gases are in solution, the tension they exert is directly proportional to their concentration in the solvent but inversely to the solubility of the gas in the solvent. Thus, if water and oil have the same concentration of nitrous oxide dissolved in each, the tension of nitrous oxide in the oil will be only one-third of the tension in the water since the oil/water solubility ratio is about 3:1. If the two liquids are shaken up together, there will be a net transfer of nitrous oxide from the water to the oil until the tension in each phase is the same. At that time the concentration of nitrous oxide in the oil will be about three times the concentration in the water. There is thus a net transfer of nitrous oxide against the concentration gradient, but always with the tension gradient. Thus, it is useful to consider tensions rather than concentrations in relation to movement of gases and vapours from one compartment of the body to another. The same units of pressure may be used in gas, aqueous and lipid phases.

Diffusion of oxygen within the lungs

It is now widely accepted that oxygen passes from the alveoli into the pulmonary capillary blood by a passive process of diffusion according to physical laws. For a long time this view was contested by a school of thought which believed that oxygen was actively secreted into the blood (see review by Milledge, 1985b). A similar process was known to occur in the swim-bladders of certain fish, so the postulated mechanism was certainly feasible, but proof of secretion depended on the demonstration of an arterial PO_2 which was higher than the alveolar PO_2. In the earlier years of this century, a great controversy raged, with active secretion being upheld by Bohr and Haldane while the Kroghs and Barcroft took the opposite view.

There is now strong evidence for believing that diffusion equilibrium is very nearly achieved for oxygen during the normal pulmonary capillary transit time in the resting subject. Therefore, under these circumstances, the uptake of oxygen is limited by pulmonary blood flow and not by diffusing capacity. However, under conditions of exercise while breathing gas mixtures deficient in oxygen or at reduced barometric pressure, the diffusing capacity becomes important and may actually limit the oxygen uptake (page 349).

Components of the alveolar/capillary diffusion pathway

The gas space within the alveolus. At functional residual capacity, the diameter of the average human alveolus is of the order of 200 μm (Weibel and Gomez, 1962), and it is likely that mixing of normal alveolar gas is almost instantaneous over the very small distance from the centre to the periphery. Precise calculations are impossible on account of the complex geometry of the alveolus, but the overall efficiency of gas exchange within the lungs suggests that mixing must be complete within less than 10 ms (Forster, 1964b). Therefore, in practice it is usual to consider alveolar gas of normal composition as uniformly mixed.

This generalization does not seem to hold when subjects inhale gases of widely different molecular weights. Georg et al. (1965) studied intra-alveolar diffusion in normal subjects after inhaling mixtures of sulphur hexafluoride and helium. They showed that, as expiration of the alveolar fraction progressed, the relative concentration of sulphur hexafluoride was greater at first but then decreased at the expense of helium. Sulphur hexafluoride (molecular weight 146 daltons), would diffuse six times less readily than helium (molecular weight 4 daltons) according to Dalton's law, and would therefore tend to remain concentrated at the core of the alveolus. This would explain the higher concentration in the first part of the alveolar gas to be exhaled. This difference disappeared when the breath was held. Landon et al. (1993) found that a large proportion of the end-expiratory/arterial partial pressure gradient for the anaesthetic isoflurane (molecular weight 184.5 daltons) could not be explained by alveolar dead space or shunt and appeared to be due to failure to achieve uniformity within the alveolus. Nevertheless, it seems unlikely that non-uniformity within a single alveolus is an important factor limiting diffusing capacity under normal conditions with gases such as oxygen, nitrogen and carbon dioxide, which have molecular weights that are not greatly different.

The alveolar/capillary membrane. Electron microscopy has revealed details of the actual path between alveolar gas and pulmonary capillary blood, shown in Figures 2.6 and 2.8. Each alveolus is completely lined with epithelium which, with its basement membrane, is about 0.2 μm thick except where its nuclei bulge into the alveolar lumen. Beyond the basement membrane is a tissue space which is very thin where it overlies the capillaries, particularly on the active side; elsewhere it is thicker and contains collagen and elastic fibres. The pulmonary capillaries are lined with endothelium, also with its own basement membrane, which is approximately the same thickness as the alveolar epithelium, except where it is expanded to enclose the endothelial nuclei. The total thickness of the active part of the alveolar/capillary membrane is thus about 0.5 μm, containing four separate lipid bilayers. This arrangement is shown in Figure 2.8.

Pulmonary capillaries. Weibel (1962) suggested a mean diameter of 7 μm for the human pulmonary capillary. This is similar to the diameter of the erythrocyte, which is therefore forced into contact with the alveolar/capillary membrane. The space between the capillaries is normally less than the diameter of the capillaries themselves (see Plate 5, Figures 2.6 and 2.7).

Diffusion within the blood. Since the diameter of the erythrocytes is so close to that of the capillaries, the diffusion path through plasma may be very short indeed. Furthermore, since the diameter of the erythrocyte is about 14 times the thickness of the alveolar/capillary membranes, it is clear that the diffusion path within the erythrocyte is likely to be much longer than the path through the alveolar/capillary membrane. Once within the cell, diffusion of oxygen is aided by mass movement of the haemoglobin molecules caused by the deformation of the erythrocyte as it passes through the capillary bed. Other factors may be involved since oxygen diffuses through a layer of haemoglobin solution more rapidly than through a layer of water, which might have been expected to offer less resistance (Hemmingsen and Scholander, 1960).

Uptake of oxygen by haemoglobin. The greater part of the oxygen which is taken up in the lungs enters into chemical combination with haemoglobin. This chemical reaction takes a finite time and forms an appreciable part of the total resistance to the transfer of oxygen. Indeed, it now appears that the reaction of oxygen with haemoglobin is sufficiently slow to be the main limiting factor in the rate of transfer of oxygen from the alveolar gas into chemical combination within the erythrocyte. This important discovery by Staub, Bishop and Forster (1961) resulted in an extensive reappraisal of the whole concept of diffusing capacity. In particular, it became clear that measurements of 'diffusing capacity' did not necessarily give an indication of the degree of permeability of the alveolar/capillary membrane. This called into question the validity of the term 'diffusing capacity', and Forster (1987) clearly prefers the alternative 'transfer factor', adopted in Europe but not in the USA. It will be seen below that methods exist for analysing the diffusing capacity of carbon monoxide into two components, one through the alveolar/capillary membrane and the other within the pulmonary blood. The latter component is determined by the pulmonary capillary volume and the rate of chemical combination of carbon monoxide with haemoglobin.

Quantification of the diffusing capacity or transfer factor for oxygen
(see review by Forster, 1987)

The diffusing capacity of oxygen is simply the oxygen uptake (easily measured) divided by the tension gradient from alveolar gas to pulmonary capillary blood where the relevant tension is the mean pulmonary capillary PO_2:

$$\text{oxygen diffusing capacity} = \frac{\text{oxygen uptake}}{\text{alveolar } PO_2 - \text{mean pulmonary capillary } PO_2}$$

The alveolar PO_2, can be derived with some degree of accuracy (page 195) but there are very serious problems in estimating the mean capillary PO_2.

The mean pulmonary capillary PO_2. It is clearly impossible to make a direct measurement of the mean PO_2 of the pulmonary capillary blood, and therefore attempts have been made to derive this quantity indirectly from the presumed changes of PO_2 which occur as blood passes through the pulmonary capillaries.

The earliest analysis of the problem was made by Bohr (1909). He made the assumption that, at any point along the pulmonary capillary, the rate of diffusion of oxygen was proportional to the PO_2 difference between the alveolar gas and the pulmonary capillary blood at that point. Using this approach, and *assuming a value for the alveolar/pulmonary end-capillary PO_2 gradient*, it seemed possible to construct a graph of capillary PO_2, plotted against the time the blood had been in the pulmonary capillary. A typical curve drawn on this basis is shown as the broken line in Figure 9.2a. Once the curve has been drawn, it is relatively easy to derive the effective or integrated mean pulmonary capillary PO_2, which then permits calculation of the oxygen diffusing capacity. The validity of the assumption of the alveolar/pulmonary end-capillary PO_2 gradient is considered below.

Unfortunately this approach, known as the Bohr integration procedure, was shown to be invalid when it was found that the fundaamental assumption was untrue. The rate of transfer of oxygen is not proportional to the alveolar/capillary PO_2 gradient at any point along the capillary. It would no doubt be true if the

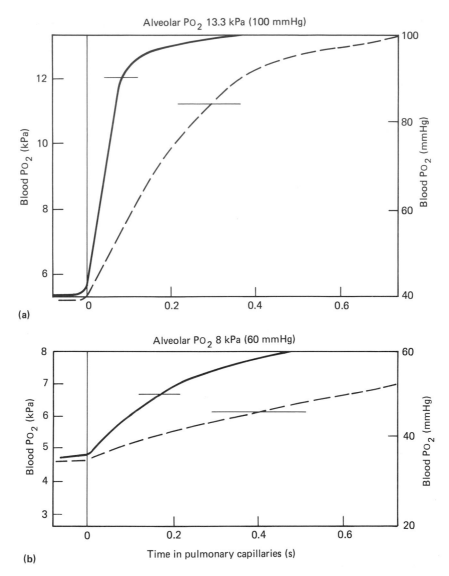

Figure 9.2 *Each graph shows the rise in blood PO₂ as blood passes through the pulmonary capillaries. The horizontal line at the top of the graph indicates the alveolar PO₂ which the blood PO₂ is approaching. In (a) the patient is breathing air, while in (b) the patient is breathing about 14% oxygen. The broken curve shows the rise in PO₂ calculated according to the Bohr procedure on an assumed value for the alveolar/end-capillary PO₂ gradient. The continuous curve shows the values obtained by forward integration (Staub, 1963a). Horizontal bars indicate mean pulmonary capillary PO₂ calculated from each curve.*

transfer of oxygen were a purely physical process (as in the case of nitrous oxide, for example) but the rate of transfer is actually limited by the chemical combination of oxygen with haemoglobin, which is sufficiently slow to comprise the greater part of the total resistance to transfer of oxygen.

In vitro studies of the rate of combination of oxygen with haemoglobin have shown that this is not directly proportional to the P_{O_2} gradient, for two distinct reasons:

1. The combination of the fourth molecule of oxygen with the haemoglobin molecule ($Hb_4(O_2)_3 + O_2 \rightleftharpoons Hb_4(O_2)_4$) has a much higher velocity constant than that of the combination of the other three molecules (Staub, Bishop and Forster, 1961). This is discussed further on page 272.
2. As the capillary oxygen saturation rises, the number of molecules of reduced haemoglobin diminishes and the velocity of the forward reaction must therefore diminish by the law of mass action. This depends upon the haemoglobin dissociation curve and is therefore not a simple exponential function of the actual P_{O_2} of the blood.

When these two factors are combined it is found that the resistance to 'diffusion' due to chemical combination of oxygen within the erythrocyte is fairly constant up to a saturation of about 80% ($P_{O_2} = 6$ kPa or 45 mmHg). Thereafter, it falls very rapidly to become zero at full saturation (Staub, Bishop and Forster, 1962). These authors proceeded to elaborate the Bohr integration procedure to allow for changes in the rate of combinations of haemoglobin with oxygen. Assuming traditional values for the alveolar/end-capillary P_{O_2} difference, they obtained a curve lying well to the left of the original Bohr curve as shown by the continuous curve in Figure 9.2a. This indicated a mean pulmonary capillary P_{O_2} greater than had previously been believed, and therefore an oxygen diffusing capacity which was substantially greater than the accepted value. The situation is actually more complicated still, since quick-frozen sections prepared by Staub showed that the colour of haemoglobin begins to alter to the red colour of oxyhaemoglobin within the pulmonary arterioles before the blood has entered the pulmonary capillaries. Furthermore, pulmonary capillaries do not cross a single alveolus but may pass over three or more (see Figures 2.6 and 2.7).

Uncertainties about the pulmonary end-capillary P_{O_2}. Both the classic and the modified Bohr integration procedures for calculation of mean capillary P_{O_2} depended critically on the precise value of the pulmonary end-capillary P_{O_2}. The constructed curve (Figure 9.2a) and therefore the derived mean capillary P_{O_2} were considerably influenced by very small variations in the value which was assumed. The 'ideal' alveolar/arterial P_{O_2} difference could be measured (page 195), but the problem was to separate this into its two components, the 'ideal' alveolar/pulmonary end-capillary P_{O_2} difference (due to diffusion block) and the pulmonary end-capillary/arterial P_{O_2} difference (due to venous admixture). Figure 8.7 will make this clear.

In 1946, Riley et al. proposed the ingenious two-level method of resolution of the alveolar/arterial P_{O_2} gradient into its two components. This was undertaken with the subject breathing air and then 11% oxygen, the former to minimize the effect of the diffusion component, and the latter to minimize the effect of venous admixture. Typical normal values obtained by this approach were as follows.

	Breathing air	*Breathing 11% oxygen*
Venous admixture component	1.2 kPa (9 mmHg)	0.1 kPa (1 mmHg)
'Diffusion' component	0.1 kPa (1 mmHg)	1.2 kPa (9 mmHg)
Total alveolar/arterial P_{O_2} difference	1.3 kPa (10 mmHg)	1.3 kPa (10 mmHg)

Unfortunately, the two-level oxygen study made two assumptions now known to be incorrect. Firstly, the component of the alveolar/arterial P_{O_2} difference due to venous admixture does not fall to small values when the alveolar P_{O_2} is reduced, because a considerable part of it is now known to be due to scatter of ventilation/perfusion ratios. This component actually increases as the alveolar P_{O_2} falls (Figure 8.13). The second fallacy is that the resistance to diffusion should be uninfluenced by the actual level of arterial P_{O_2}. It has been explained above that a major part of the resistance to 'diffusion' is due to the rate of chemical combination of oxygen with haemoglobin, which is very markedly influenced by the actual level of P_{O_2}. Thus, the two-level method of measuring the diffusing capacity of oxygen was based on false assumptions, and the results obtained by it cannot therefore be regarded as valid.

Forward integration. A new and entirely opposite approach was made by Staub in a most important paper in 1963 (Staub, 1963a). His approach was based on the new understanding of the kinetics of the combination of oxygen with haemoglobin (see above) and the pattern of blood flow through the pulmonary capillaries. Starting at the arterial end of the pulmonary capillaries, he calculated the P_{O_2} of the capillary blood progressively along the capillary until he was able to give an estimate of the remaining alveolar/capillary P_{O_2} gradient at the end of the capillary. This procedure of forward integration was thus the reverse of the classic approach which, starting from the alveolar/end-capillary P_{O_2} gradient, worked backwards to see what was happening along the capillary.

Staub's forward integrations gave important results (Table 9.1). They suggested that alveolar/end-capillary P_{O_2} gradients were very much smaller than had previously been thought, although papers by Asmussen and Nielsen (1960) and Thews (1961) had anticipated much of Staub's conclusion.

Table 9.1 Values for the alveolar/end-capillary P_{O_2} gradient suggested by the forward integration procedure of Staub (1963a)

Conditions	Capillary transit time(s)	Alveolar/end-capillary P_{O_2} gradient	
		kPa	*mmHg*
Resting subject ($\dot{V}_{O_2}$ = 270 ml/min)			
Breathing air	0.760	0.000 000 001	0.000 000 01
($P_{A_{O_2}}$ = 13.3 kPa = 100 mmHg)			
Breathing low oxygen	0.636	0.03	0.2
($P_{A_{O_2}}$ = 6.3 kPa = 47 mmHg)			
Moderate exercise ($\dot{V}_{O_2}$ = 1500 ml/min)			
Breathing low oxygen	0.476	0.5	4.0
($P_{A_{O_2}}$ = 7.3 kPa = 55 mmHg)			
Heavy exercise ($\dot{V}_{O_2}$ = 3000 ml/min)			
Breathing air	0.496	<0.000 1	<0.001
($P_{A_{O_2}}$ = 16 kPa = 120 mmHg)			
Breathing low oxygen	0.304	2.1	16.0
($P_{A_{O_2}}$ = 7.9 kPa = 59 mmHg)			

Abbreviations: $\dot{V}_{O_2}$, oxygen consumption; $P_{A_{O_2}}$, alveolar P_{O_2}.

Importance of the capillary transit time. Capillary transit time is a most important factor determining both the pulmonary end-capillary PO_2 and the diffusing capacity. It will be seen from Figure 9.2a that, if the capillary transit time is reduced below 0.2 second, there will be an appreciable gradient between the alveolar and end-capillary PO_2. Since the diffusion gradient from alveolar gas to mean pulmonary capillary blood will be increased, the oxygen diffusing capacity must be decreased.

The mean pulmonary capillary transit time equals the pulmonary capillary blood volume divided by the pulmonary blood flow (approximately equal to cardiac output). This gives a normal time of the order of 0.8 second with a subject at rest. However, there appears to be a wide range of values on either side of the mean, and times as short as 0.1 second have been suggested (McHardy, 1972). Blood from capillaries with the shortest time will yield desaturated blood and this will not be compensated by blood from capillaries with longer than average transit times, for the reason shown in Figure 8.12. Variation in capillary transit time is one cause of spread of diffusing capacity/perfusion (D/Q̇) ratios, which is a potential cause of hypoxaemia (Piiper, 1961; Piiper, Haab and Rahn, 1961.

Possible causes of a reduction in oxygen 'diffusing capacity'

At this stage it is helpful to consider the possible causes of a reduction in the value of the oxygen diffusing capacity as defined by the equation on page 203.

Decreased capillary transit time. In the section above, it has been explained how a reduction in capillary transit time may reduce the diffusing capacity. The mean transit time is reduced when the cardiac output is raised (as in anaemia or exercise), and the scatter of transit times may be increased in a number of diseases of the lungs.

The total area of the alveolar/capillary membrane may be reduced by any disease process or surgery which removes a substantial number of alveoli. In fact, occlusion of blood flow through one lung has little effect on the alveolar/arterial PO_2 difference in patients, even with pulmonary fibrosis (Staněk et al., 1967), but emphysema is thought to reduce the diffusing capacity mainly by destruction of alveolar septa.

A reduction in pulmonary capillary blood volume, sufficient to leave a substantial part of the lung unperfused, must reduce the diffusing capacity since the functioning interface is reduced in area.

Pulmonary congestion may reduce diffusing capacity by increasing the length of the diffusion pathway for oxygen within the pulmonary capillaries.

Severe maldistribution of ventilation relative to perfusion results in a physiological dysfunction which presents many of the features of a reduction in diffusing capacity. If, for example, most of the ventilation is distributed to the left lung and most of the pulmonary blood flow to the right lung, then the effective interface must be reduced. Minor degrees of maldistribution greatly complicate the interpretation of a reduced diffusing capacity. Both maldistribution and impaired diffusing capacity have a similar effect on the alveolar/arterial PO_2 gradient in relation to inspired oxygen concentration (see Figure 8.13), and a distinction cannot be made by simple means.

Alveolar/capillary block. At first sight, the most obvious cause of reduced diffusing capacity would seem to be an impediment at the alveolar/capillary membrane itself, which might either be thickened or else have its permeability to gas transfer reduced by some chemical abnormality. The term 'alveolar/capillary block' was introduced by Austrian et al. (1951) to describe a syndrome characterized by reduced lung volume, reasonably normal ventilatory capacity, hyperventilation and normal arterial PO_2 at rest, but with desaturation on exercise. A reduction in the measured 'diffusing capacity' suggested an impermeability of the alveolar/capillary membrane, which was supported by the light microscopy appearance in such conditions as scleroderma, sarcoidosis, asbestosis, pulmonary fibrosis and pulmonary oedema. Evidence for such a condition at the magnification offered by electron microscopy has proved elusive. Interstitial pulmonary oedema, for example, tends to accumulate on the inactive side of the pulmonary capillary, leaving the active side relatively normal in appearance and thickness (see Figure 2.8). This suggests that diffusion across the membrane should remain normal in spite of the presence of considerable pulmonary oedema. Similar sparing of the active side of the pulmonary capillary has been described for idiopathic interstitial pulmonary fibrosis (Hamman–Rich syndrome or fibrosing alveolitis) (Gracey, Divertie and Brown, 1968).

It will be clear that the oxygen diffusing capacity may be influenced by many factors which are really nothing at all to do with diffusion *per se*. In fact, there is considerable doubt as to whether a true defect of diffusion (e.g. by a thickened alveolar/capillary membrane) is ever the limiting factor in transfer of oxygen from the inspired gas to the arterial blood. In view of these considerations, Cotes (1975) suggested that the term 'diffusing capacity' be abandoned and replaced by the term 'transfer factor' which implies that factors other than just diffusion may be involved. The symbol T may be used instead of D but the definition and methods of measurement remain the same. It is unfortunate that the term 'transfer factor' has an entirely different meaning in immunology.

The cause of hypoxaemia, previously thought to be due to alveolar/capillary block. The previous section suggests that a true impairment of diffusion is seldom or never the limiting factor in the transfer of oxygen to the arterial blood. Nevertheless, alveolar/capillary block was formerly a well-recognized clinical entity, characterized by dyspnoea, hyperventilation (usually with reduced PO_2), cyanosis on exercise (if not at rest), and with radiological evidence of widespread involvement of the lungs by any one of a wide variety of pathological processes. The syndrome was clearly distinguished from obstructive airway disease with FEV/VC ratio normal or only slightly reduced, but the vital capacity substantially reduced.

When doubts were cast on the validity of the concept of impaired diffusing capacity, Finley, Swenson and Comroe (1962) studied a group of patients previously diagnosed as having alveolar/capillary block and found that, in each case, the arterial hypoxaemia could be explained by disturbances of distribution of ventilation and/or perfusion, without the need to invoke an alveolar/end-capillary PO_2 gradient. Arndt, King and Briscoe (1970) investigated a further 10 patients with the clinical syndrome of alveolar/capillary block. In 2 patients (alveolar cell carcinoma and idiopathic interstitial pulmonary fibrosis) hypoxaemia could be explained by the existence of large shunts. In 4 patients (sarcoidosis, sarcoidosis with pulmonary fibrosis, desquamative interstitial pneumonia and eosinophilic granuloma), hypoxaemia could be explained in terms of a 'slow compartment' having a low $\dot{V}/\dot{Q}$ ratio, corresponding to the 'shelf' in Figure 8.5b. In the remaining 4 patients (interstitial pulmonary oedema, sarcoidosis with pulmonary fibrosis and systemic sclerosis with pulmonary fibrosis), there was no appreciable shunt and identical $\dot{V}/\dot{Q}$ ratios in fast and slow alveolar compartments. However, this group had a normal saturation when breathing air at rest, although this presumably fell during exercise.

Diffusion of carbon monoxide within the lungs

Diffusing capacity is usually measured for carbon monoxide, for the very practical reason that affinity of carbon monoxide for haemoglobin is so high that the tension of the gas in the pulmonary capillary blood remains effectively zero. The formula for calculation of this quantity then simplifies to the following:

$$\text{diffusing capacity for carbon monoxide} = \frac{\text{carbon monoxide uptake}}{\text{alveolar } P\text{CO}}$$

(compare with corresponding equation for oxygen, page 203).

There are no insuperable difficulties in the measurement of either of the remaining quantities on the right-hand side of the equation, and the methods are outlined at the end of the chapter.

Measurement of the carbon monoxide diffusing capacity is firmly established as a valuable routine pulmonary function test, which may show changes in a range of conditions in which other tests yield normal values. It does in fact provide an index which shows that something is wrong, and changes in the index provide a useful indication of progress of the disease. However, it is much more difficult to explain a reduced diffusing capacity for carbon monoxide in terms of the underlying pathophysiology (see below).

The diffusion path for carbon monoxide

Diffusion of carbon monoxide within the alveolus, through the alveolar/capillary membrane and through the plasma is governed by the same factors which apply to oxygen and have been outlined above. The quantitative difference is due to the different vapour density and water solubility of the two gases. These factors indicate that the rate of diffusion of oxygen up to the point of entry into the erythrocyte is 1.23 times the corresponding rate for carbon monoxide.

Uptake of carbon monoxide by haemoglobin

The affinity of haemoglobin for carbon monoxide is about 250 times as great as for oxygen. Nevertheless, it does not follow that the *rate* of combination of carbon monoxide with haemoglobin is faster than the *rate* of combination of oxygen with haemoglobin: it is, in fact, rather slower (Forster, 1964a). The reaction is slower still when oxygen is displaced from oxyhaemoglobin according to the equation:

$$CO + HbO_2 \rightarrow O_2 + HbCO$$

Therefore the reaction rate of carbon monoxide with haemoglobin is reduced when the oxygen saturation of the haemoglobin is high. The inhalation of different concentrations of oxygen thus causes changes in the reaction rate of carbon monoxide with the haemoglobin of a patient. This has been used to study different components of the resistance to diffusion of carbon monoxide in man (Forster, 1987).

Quantification of the components of the resistance to diffusion of carbon monoxide

When two resistances are arranged in series, the total resistance of the pair is equal to the sum of the two individual resistances. Diffusing capacity is analogous to conductance, which is the reciprocal of resistance. Therefore, the reciprocal of the diffusing capacity of the total system equals the sum of the reciprocals of the diffusing capacities of the two components.

$$\frac{1}{\text{total diffusing capacity for CO}} = \frac{1}{\substack{\text{diffusing capacity} \\ \text{of CO through the} \\ \text{alveolar/capillary} \\ \text{membrane}}} + \frac{1}{\substack{\text{'diffusing capacity'} \\ \text{of CO within the} \\ \text{erythrocyte}}}$$

The second component on the right-hand side is not really a matter of diffusion, since the limiting factor to the passage of carbon monoxide within the erythrocyte is the rate of chemical combination with haemoglobin (exactly as in the case of oxygen). This 'diffusing capacity' within the erythrocyte is equal to the product of the pulmonary capillary blood volume (Vc) and the rate of reaction of carbon monoxide with haemoglobin (θCO), a parameter which varies with the oxygen saturation of the haemoglobin. The equation may now be rewritten:

$$\frac{1}{\text{total diffusing capacity for CO}} = \frac{1}{\substack{\text{diffusing capacity} \\ \text{of CO through the} \\ \text{alveolar/capillary} \\ \text{membrane}}} + \frac{1}{\substack{\text{pulmonary} \\ \text{capillary} \\ \text{blood} \\ \text{volume}} \times \substack{\text{reaction rate} \\ \text{of CO with} \\ \text{haemoglobin}}}$$

The usual symbols for representation of this equation are as follows:

$$\frac{1}{DL_{CO}} = \frac{1}{DM_{CO}} + \frac{1}{Vc \times \theta CO}$$

The term DM_{CO} equals $0.8\ DM_{O_2}$ under similar conditions (Table 9.2).

The total diffusing capacity for carbon monoxide is a routine clinical measurement (see the methods section at the end of this chapter): θCO may be determined, at different values of oxygen saturation, by *in vitro* studies. This leaves two unknowns – the diffusing capacity through the alveolar/capillary membrane and the pulmonary capillary blood volume. By repeating the measurement of total diffusing capacity at different values of θCO (obtained by inhaling different concentrations of oxygen and so varying the oxygen saturation of the haemoglobin), it is possible to obtain

Table 9.2 The influence of physical properties on the diffusion of gases through a gas/liquid interface

Gas	Density relative to oxygen	Water solubility relative to oxygen	Diffusing capacity relative to oxygen
Oxygen	1.00	1.00	1.00
Carbon monoxide	0.88	0.75	0.80
Nitrogen	0.88	0.515	0.55
Carbon dioxide	1.37	24.0	20.5
Nitrous oxide	1.37	16.3	14.0
Helium	0.125	0.37	1.05
Ether	2.30	580	380
Halothane	5.07	27.3	12.1

two simultaneous equations with two unknowns. It is then possible to solve and derive values for the following:

1. Total diffusing capacity of carbon monoxide at different levels of oxygenation of the blood.
2. Diffusing capacity of the alveolar/capillary membrane (presumably independent of oxygenation)
3. Pulmonary capillary blood volume.
4. The 'diffusing capacity' of carbon monoxide within the erythrocyte at different values of oxygen saturation.

This elegant approach was introduced by Roughton and Forster (1957). Although the original data appeared to undergo an unreasonable amount of manipulation, confidence in the whole operation is engendered by the observed fact that the total diffusing capacity of carbon monoxide is undoubtedly reduced by the inhalation of high concentrations of oxygen (Figure 9.3). The change occurs too quickly to be caused by changes in the alveolar/capillary membrane. The technique yields normal values for pulmonary capillary blood volume within the range 60–110 ml, which agrees well with a morphometric estimate of about 100 ml at a lung volume of 2.5 litres (Weibel, 1962). Normal values are shown in Table 9.3.

Interpretation of the carbon monoxide diffusing capacity

Factors which may affect the oxygen diffusing capacity have been described above. Similar considerations apply to the carbon monoxide diffusing capacity and it will be clear that a low value does not necessarily imply a thickened impermeable alveolar/capillary membrane. It does, in fact, indicate that there is an impediment to gas transfer from alveolar gas to arterial blood. This excludes hypoventilation as a cause, but the result may be influenced by shunt or by well-perfused areas of low $\dot{V}/\dot{Q}$ ratio (see above). However, there remain some patients in whom the defect of gas transfer cannot be entirely explained by maldistribution. Even this does not mean that the patient has a thickened impermeable membrane. For reasons given above, the defect may be due to short capillary transit time or to excessive destruction of the alveolar/capillary membrane. The effective area of the membrane may also be reduced by pulmonary hypoperfusion. In spite of these uncertainties, the carbon monoxide diffusing capacity, or more correctly its transfer factor, remains a valuable diagnostic aid. It has the advantage of being sensitive and it may show changes long before these are reflected in altered blood gas values or other simple tests of pulmonary function.

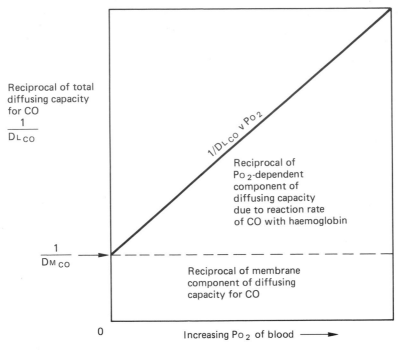

Figure 9.3 The reciprocal of the total diffusing capacity for carbon monoxide (i.e. resistance to diffusion) decreases with decreasing P_{O_2} of the blood in the pulmonary capillaries. The reciprocal of the component due to the reaction rate of carbon monoxide with haemoglobin depends on displacing oxygen from haemoglobin, and so decreases with decreasing P_{O_2}. Extrapolation to zero P_{O_2} removes this component entirely, and so indicates the reciprocal of the true membrane component which is independent of P_{O_2} (see Forster, 1987).

Table 9.3 Values obtained by various methods of measurement of diffusing capacity (transfer factor) of carbon monoxide

Technique of measurement	Total diffusing capacity for CO		Membrane component of diffusing capacity		Pulmonary capillary blood volume
	ml min^{-1} kPa^{-1}	*ml/min/ mmHg*	*ml min^{-1} kPa^{-1}*	*ml/min/ mmHg*	*(ml)*
Steady state	113	15	195	26	73
Single breath	225	30	428	57	79
Rebreathing	203	27	300	40	110

(Data from Forster, 1964b)

Non-pathological factors which influence diffusing capacity

Body size influences diffusing capacity directly. This is inevitable since alveolar/capillary gas tension gradients are not greatly different in different species or in different-sized individuals, while gas exchange volumes are related to body size.

Lung volume. Diffusing capacity is markedly increased when the lung volume is increased (Gurtner and Fowler, 1971).

Exercise results in an increase in diffusing capacity (Chapter 13) and it has been suggested that the increase proceeds to a plateau value which is known as the maximal diffusing capacity (Riley et al., 1954).

Age results in a diminution of both the diffusing capacity and the maximal diffusing capacity.

Posture. Diffusing capacity is substantially increased when the subject is supine rather than standing or sitting (Ogilvie et al., 1957), in spite of the fact that lung volume is reduced. This change is probably explained by the increase in pulmonary blood volume, and the more uniform distribution of perfusion of the lungs in the supine position.

Diffusion of carbon dioxide within the lungs

Carbon dioxide has a much higher water solubility than oxygen and, although its vapour density is greater, it may be calculated to penetrate an aqueous membrane about 20 times as rapidly as oxygen (see Table 9.2). Therefore it was formerly believed that diffusion problems could not exist for carbon dioxide because the patient would have succumbed from hypoxia before hypercapnia could attain measurable proportions. All of this ignored the fact that chemical reactions of the respiratory gases were sufficiently slow to affect the measured 'diffusing capacity', and in fact were generally the limiting factor in gas transfer. The carriage of carbon dioxide in the blood is discussed in Chapter 10, but for the moment it is sufficient to note the essential reactions in the release of chemically combined dioxide:

1. Release of some carbon dioxide from carbamino carriage.
2. Conversion of bicarbonate ions to carbonic acid followed by dehydration to release molecular carbon dioxide.

The latter reaction involves the movement of bicarbonate ions across the erythrocyte membrane (Hamburger effect), but its rate is probably limited by the dehydration of carbonic acid. This reaction would be very slow indeed if it were not catalysed by carbonic anhydrase which is present in abundance in the erythrocyte and also on the endothelium. The important limiting role of the rate of this reaction was elegantly shown in a study by Cain and Otis (1961) of the effect of inhibition of carbonic anhydrase on carbon dioxide transport. This resulted in a large increase in the arterial/alveolar P_{CO_2} gradient, corresponding to a gross decrease in the apparent 'diffusing capacity' of carbon dioxide.

Equilibrium of carbon dioxide is probably very nearly complete within the normal pulmonary capillary transit time. However, even if it were not so, it would be of little significance since the mixed venous/alveolar P_{CO_2} difference is itself quite small (about 0.8 kPa or 6 mmHg). Therefore an end-gradient as large as 20 per cent of the initial difference would still be too small to be of any importance and, indeed, could hardly be measured by modern analytical methods.

Hypercapnia is, in fact, never caused by decreased 'diffusing capacity' except when carbonic anhydrase is inhibited by drugs such as acetazolamide (Diamox).

Pathological hypercapnia may always be explained by other causes, usually an alveolar ventilation which is inadequate for the metabolic rate of the patient.

The assumption that there is no measurable difference between the P_{CO_2} of the alveolar gas and the pulmonary end-capillary blood is used when the alveolar P_{CO_2} is assumed to be equal to the arterial P_{CO_2} for the purpose of derivation of the 'ideal' alveolar P_{O_2} (page 195). The assumption is also made that there is no measurable difference between end-capillary and arterial P_{CO_2}. We have seen in the previous chapter (Table 8.2) that this is not strictly true and a large shunt of 50% will cause an arterial/end-capillary P_{CO_2} gradient of about 0.4 kPa.

Diffusion of 'inert' gases within the lungs

In the biological sense, inert gases are those which do not undergo chemical changes within the body. This definition includes nitrogen, helium, sulphur hexafluoride and, for practical purposes, most of the anaesthetic gases and vapours. Diffusion of inert gases is important to the diver, and is an essential consideration in the pharmacokinetics of the inhalational anaesthetic agents.

Since inert gases are carried in the blood by purely physical means, their diffusing capacity consists only of the membrane component, and there is no limitation due to chemical reaction as in the case of oxygen, carbon monoxide and carbon dioxide. Their diffusing capacities are therefore governed primarily by their water solubilities (Table 9.2), and the diffusing capacities of the anaesthetic agents should therefore be very much higher than for oxygen. Gases and vapours with high molecular weight may fail to achieve uniform gas mixing within the alveolus (see above), but it is unclear whether high molecular weight has any appreciable effect on transit through the alveolar/capillary membrane.

Diffusion of gases in the tissues

Oxygen

Oxygen leaves the systemic capillaries by the reverse of the process by which it entered the pulmonary capillaries. Chemical release from haemoglobin is followed by diffusion through the endothelium and thence through the tissues to its site of utilization in the mitochondria. Diffusion may possibly be aided by protoplasmic streaming. Diffusion paths are much longer in tissues than in the lung. In well-vascularized tissue, such as brain, each capillary serves a zone of radius about 20 μm, but the corresponding distance is about 200 μm in skeletal muscle and greater still in fat and cartilage.

It is impracticable to talk about mean tissue P_{O_2} since this varies from one organ to another and must also depend on perfusion in relation to metabolic activity. Furthermore, within an organ there must be some cells occupying more favourable sites towards the arterial ends of capillaries, while others must accept oxygen from the venous ends of the capillaries, where the P_{O_2} is lower. This is well demonstrated in the liver where the centrilobular cells must exist at a lower P_{O_2} than those at the periphery of the lobule. Even within a single cell, there can be no uniformity of P_{O_2}. Not only are there 'low spots' around the mitochondria, but those mitochondria nearest to the capillaries presumably enjoy a higher P_{O_2} than those lying further away.

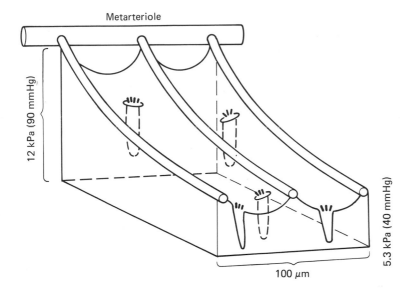

Figure 9.4 Diagrammatic representation of P_{O_2} within the tissues. The vertical axis represents the actual P_{O_2}; in the horizontal plane is represented the course of three parallel capillaries from the metarteriole to the point of entry into the venule (not shown). The P_{O_2} falls exponentially along the course of each capillary with a trough of P_{O_2} between the capillaries. The pits represent the low spots of P_{O_2} from about 12 kPa (90 mmHg) in the tissue close to the arterial end of the capillaries down to less than 1 kPa at the mitochondria near the venous end of the capillaries. This is the simplest of many possible models of tissue perfusion.

Figure 9.4 shows a model in which an area of tissue is perfused by three parallel capillaries. Vertical height indicates P_{O_2} which falls exponentially along the line of the capillaries, with troughs lying in between the capillaries. Five 'low spots' corresponding to mitochondria are shown. This diagram makes no pretence to histological accuracy but merely illustrates the difficulty of talking about the 'mean tissue P_{O_2}', which is not an entity like the arterial or mixed venous P_{O_2}.

There is uncertainty about the actual P_{O_2} within a mitochondrion. It is known that oxidative phosphorylation will continue down to a P_{O_2} of about 0.13 kPa (1 mmHg) (page 253), and some mitochondria may habitually operate at this level. Others, particularly those close to the arterial end of the capillaries, may have a much higher P_{O_2}.

Carbon dioxide

Little is known about the magnitude of carbon dioxide gradients between the mitochondria and the tissue capillaries. It is, however, thought that the tissue/venous P_{CO_2} gradient can be increased by two methods. The first is by inhibition of carbonic anhydrase which blocks the uptake of carbon dioxide by the blood. The second is by hyperoxygenation of the arterial blood caused by breathing 100% oxygen at high pressures. If the P_{O_2} of the arterial blood exceeds about 300 kPa (2250 mmHg), the dissolved oxygen will be sufficient for the usual tissue requirements. Therefore there will be no significant amount of reduced haemoglobin, which is more effective than oxyhaemoglobin for carbamino carriage of carbon dioxide. This results in partial blocking of the uptake of carbon dioxide by the blood, and was advanced by Gessell (1923) as the cause of oxygen convulsions. In fact the effect on tissue P_{CO_2} is likely to be too small to be clinically significant, and the alternative method of carbon dioxide carriage as bicarbonate seems to be adequate. There are alternative explanations of oxygen convulsions (page 552).

Inert gases and anaesthetic agents

Inert gases will ultimately attain equilibrium in the tissues because, unlike oxygen, they are not constantly being consumed which must result in permanent tension gradients. The rate of attaining equilibrium with inert gases depends upon the perfusion of the tissue relative to its bulk and the solubility of the agent in the tissue. Relatively rapid equilibration occurs in well-perfused tissues such as brain, heart and liver. In poorly perfused tissues, inert gases tend to diffuse slowly, forming tension gradients in the form of the cylinders and cones. Such tissues include fat, cartilage and, to a certain extent, resting muscle. Before equilibrium is attained, the tension of the gas in the venous blood draining the tissue does not give a representative value for the mean tissue tension, being higher during loading and lower during unloading of the agent. This greatly complicates measurement of exchange and also theoretical consideration of long-term changes in tissue levels. Appreciation of this problem has been important in improving techniques for prevention of the 'bends' after prolonged dives.

Alveolar/capillary permeability to non-volatile substances

The alveolar epithelium and the capillary endothelium have a very high permeability to water, most gases, alcohol and lipophilic substances such as the tracer antipyrene. However, for many hydrophilic substances of larger molecular diameter and for molecules carrying a charge, there is an effective barrier. Passage of these substances is mainly through the gaps between the cells and must be considered separately for epithelium and endothelium. It was explained in Chapter 2 that the alveolar epithelial type I cells have very tight junctions, effectively limiting the molecular radius to about 0.6 nm. Endothelial junctions are much larger, with gaps of the order of 4–6 nm

Passage of solutes across the alveolar/capillary membrane is usually quantified as the half-time of clearance or, alternatively, as the fractional clearance per minute, the one parameter being related to the reciprocal of the other. Clearance from the alveoli (i.e. across the epithelium) bears an approximate inverse relationship to the molecular weight (Effros and Mason, 1983). Urea (60 daltons) had a clearance of the order of 0.07/min, while for sucrose (342 daltons) the corresponding figure is 0.003/min and for albumin (64 000 daltons) is of the order of 0.0001/min. All of these clearances may be greatly increased if the alveolar epithelium is damaged as in the permeability type of pulmonary oedema (page 489).

A useful tracer molecule is ^{99m}Tc-DTPA (diethylene triamine penta-acetate) with a molecular weight of 492 daltons (Jones, Royston and Minty, 1983). After being aerosolized into the lungs, its concentration can be continuously measured over the lung fields *in vivo* by detection of its gamma emission. In the healthy non-smoker, the clearance is very slow, about 0.01/min (half-time about 1 hour).The clearance is dramatically increased in many different types of pulmonary damage – including, for example, smoking, in which there is a threefold increase. It is, in fact, the very sensitivity of this test which limits its value.

Electrolytes such as sodium ions can cross the epithelial barrier fairly freely, but the rate of passage is governed by concentration gradients. Thus, isotonic sodium solutions are cleared from the alveoli more quickly than hypertonic solutions (Efros and Mason, 1983). The normal alveolar epithelium is almost totally impermeable to protein, the half-time for turnover of albumin between plasma and the alveolar compartment being of the order of 36 hours (Staub, 1983).

The microvascular endothelium, with its larger intercellular gaps, is far more permeable for all molecular sizes and there is normally an appreciable leak of protein. Thus the concentration of albumin in pulmonary lymph is about half the concentration in plasma and may increase to approximate the plasma concentration in conditions of enhanced alveolar/capillary permeability (Staub, 1984). This problem is discussed further in relation to pulmonary oedema in Chapter 26 (pages 486 et seq.)

It should be noted that many lung diseases tend to decrease the carbon monoxide diffusing capacity, while the commonest pathological change in alveolar/capillary permeability is an increase.

Principles of methods of measurement of carbon monoxide diffusing capacity

All the methods are based on the general equation:

$$D_{CO} = \frac{\dot{V}_{CO}}{P_{A_{CO}} - P\bar{c}_{CO}}$$

In each case it is usual to assume that the mean tension of carbon monoxide in the pulmonary capillary blood ($P\bar{c}_{CO}$) is effectively zero. It is, therefore, only necessary to measure the carbon monoxide uptake ($\dot{V}_{CO}$), and the alveolar carbon monoxide tension ($P_{A_{CO}}$). The diffusing capacity (D_{CO}) is the total diffusing capacity including that of the alveolar/capillary membrane and the component due to the reaction of carbon monoxide with haemoglobin.

The steady state method

The subject breathes a gas mixture containing about 0.3% carbon monoxide for about a minute. After this time, expired gas is collected when the alveolar P_{CO} is steady but the mixed venous P_{CO} has not yet reached a level high enough to require consideration in the calculation.

The carbon monoxide uptake ($\dot{V}_{CO}$) is measured in exactly the same way as oxygen consumption by the open method (page 301): the amount of carbon monoxide expired ($V_E \times F_{E_{CO}}$) is subtracted from the amount of carbon monoxide inspired ($\dot{V}_I \times F_{I_{CO}}$). The alveolar P_{CO} is calculated from the form of the alveolar air equation derived by Filley, MacIntosh and Wright (1954):

$$P_{A_{CO}} = P_{I_{CO}} - P_{A_{CO_2}} \left(\frac{F_{I_{CO}} - F\bar{E}_{CO}}{F\bar{E}_{CO_2}} \right)$$

Measurement of inspiratory and expiratory carbon monoxide and expiratory carbon dioxide concentrations presents no serious difficulty, and infrared analysis has proved satisfactory. Alveolar P_{CO_2} may be determined by sampling arterial blood and assuming that the alveolar P_{CO_2} is equal to the arterial P_{CO_2}. This is not strictly true in the presence of maldistribution. As an alternative, some workers measure the end-expiratory P_{CO_2} but neither does this equal the arterial P_{CO_2} in the presence of alveolar dead space (see Figure 8.8).

The single-breath method

This method has a long history of progressive refinement. The patient is first required to exhale maximally. He then draws in a vital-capacity breath of a gas mixture containing about 0.3% carbon monoxide and about 10% helium. The breath is held for 10 seconds and a gas sample is then taken after the exhalation of the first 0.75 litre, which is sufficient to wash out the patient's dead space. The breath-holding time is sufficient to overcome maldistribution of the inspired gas.

It is assumed that no significant amount of helium has passed into the blood and, therefore, the ratio of the concentration of helium in the inspired gas to the concentration in the end-expiratory gas, multiplied by the volume of gas drawn into the alveoli during the maximal inspiration, will indicate the total alveolar volume during the period of breath holding. The alveolar P_{CO} at the commencement of breath holding is equal to the same ratio multiplied by the P_{CO} of the inspired gas mixture. The end-expiratory P_{CO} is measured directly.

From these data, together with the time of breath holding, it is possible to calculate the carbon monoxide uptake and the mean alveolar P_{CO}. A neat mathematical solution is available, and the interested reader is referred to Cotes (1979). Methodology was presented in detail by Bates, Macklem and Christie (1971) and reviewed by Forster (1987).

The rebreathing method

Somewhat similar to the single-breath method is the rebreathing method by which a gas mixture containing about 0.3% carbon monoxide and 10% helium is rebreathed rapidly from a rubber bag. The bag and the patient's lungs are considered as a single system, with gas exchange occurring in very much the same way as during breath holding. The calculation proceeds in a similar way to that for the single breath method.

Measurement of oxygen diffusing capacity

For reasons which were developed in this chapter, it now appears that the measurement of oxygen diffusing capacity is based on assumptions which can no longer be considered valid. Therefore, the method is not described here but, for historical purposes, reference may be made to Comroe et al. (1962).

Measurement of alveolar/capillary permeability

Reference has been made above to the use of [99m]TC-DPTA described by Jones, Royston and Minty (1983)

Chapter 10
Carbon dioxide

Carbon dioxide is the end-product of aerobic metabolism. It is produced almost entirely in the mitochondria where the P_{CO_2} is highest. From its point of origin, there are a series of tension gradients as carbon dioxide passes through the cytoplasm and the extracellular fluid into the blood. In the lungs, the P_{CO_2} of the blood entering the pulmonary capillaries is normally higher than the alveolar P_{CO_2}, and therefore carbon dioxide diffuses from the blood into the alveolar gas, where a dynamic equilibrium is established. The equilibrium concentration equals the ratio between carbon dioxide output and alveolar ventilation (page 128). Blood leaving the alveoli has, for practical purposes, the same P_{CO_2} as alveolar gas, and arterial blood P_{CO_2} is usually very close to 'ideal' alveolar P_{CO_2}.

Abnormal levels for arterial P_{CO_2} occur in a number of pathological states and have many important physiological effects throughout the body, some as a result of changes in pH. There are many clinical situations in which the P_{CO_2} must be maintained at an optimal level. Fundamental to the problem is the mechanism by which carbon dioxide is carried in the blood.

Carriage of carbon dioxide in blood

In physical solution

Carbon dioxide belongs to the group of gases with moderate solubility in water, which includes many of the anaesthetic gases. According to Henry's law of solubility:

$$P_{CO_2} \times \text{solubility coefficient} = CO_2 \text{ concentration in solution} \qquad \ldots(1)$$

The solubility coefficient of carbon dioxide (α) is expressed in units of mmol l^{-1} kPa^{-1} (or mmol/l/mmHg). The value depends on temperature, and values are listed in Table 10.1. The contribution of dissolved carbon dioxide to the total carriage of the gas in blood is shown in Table 10.2.

As carbonic acid

In solution, carbon dioxide hydrates to form carbonic acid:

$$CO_2 + H_2O \rightleftharpoons H_2CO_3 \qquad \ldots(2)$$

Table 10.1 Values for solubility of carbon dioxide in plasma and pK' at different temperatures

Temperature (°C)	Solubility of CO_2 in plasma		pK'		
	$mmol\ l^{-1}\ kPa^{-1}$	$mmol/l/mmHg$	at pH 7.6	at pH 7.4	at pH 7.2
40	0.216	0.0288	6.07	6.08	6.09
39	0.221	0.0294	6.07	6.08	6.09
38	0.226	0.0301	6.08	6.09	6.10
37	0.231	0.0308	6.08	6.09	6.10
36	0.236	0.0315	6.09	6.10	6.11
35	0.242	0.0322	6.10	6.11	6.12
33	0.253	0.0337	6.10	6.11	6.12
30	0.272	0.0362	6.12	6.13	6.14
25	0.310	0.0413	6.15	6.16	6.17
20	0.359	0.0478	6.17	6.19	6.20
15	0.416	0.0554	6.20	6.21	6.23

(Values from Severinghaus, Stupfel and Bradley, 1956a, b)

Table 10.2 Normal values for carbon dioxide carriage in blood P_{CO_2}

	Arterial blood (Hb 95% sat.)	Mixed venous blood (Hb 70% sat.)	Arterial/venous difference
Whole blood			
pH	7.40	7.367	−0.033
P_{CO_2} (kPa)	5.3	6.1	+0.8
(mmHg)	40.0	46.0	+6.0
Total CO_2 (mmol/l)	21.5	23.3	+1.8
(ml/dl)	48.0	52.0	+4.0
Plasma (mmol/l)			
Dissolved CO_2	1.2	1.4	+0.2
Carbonic acid	0.0017	0.0020	+0.0003
Bicarbonate ion	24.4	26.2	+1.8
Carbamino CO_2	Negligible	Negligible	Negligible
Total	25.6	27.6	+2.0
Erythrocyte fraction of 1 litre of blood			
Dissolved CO_2	0.44	0.51	+0.07
Bicarbonate ion	5.88	5.92	+0.04
Carbamino CO_2	1.10	1.70	+0.60
Plasma fraction of 1 litre of blood			
Dissolved CO_2	0.66	0.76	+0.10
Bicarbonate ion	13.42	14.41	+0.99
Total in 1 litre of blood (mmol/l)	21.50	23.30	+1.80

These values have not been drawn from a single publication but represent the mean of values reported in a large number of studies.

The equilibrium of this reaction is far to the left under physiological conditions. Published work shows some disagreement on the value of the equilibrium constant, but it seems likely that less than 1 per cent of the molecules of carbon dioxide are in the hydrated form. There is a very misleading medical convention by which both forms of carbon dioxide in equation (2) are sometimes shown as carbonic acid. Thus the term H_2CO_3 may, in some situations, mean the total concentrations of dissolved CO_2 and H_2CO_3 and, to avoid confusion, it is preferable to use $\alpha P CO_2$ as in equation (7) below. This does not apply to equations (4) and (5) below, where H_2CO_3 has its correct meaning.

It would be theoretically more correct to indicate the thermodynamic activities rather than concentrations, the two quantities being related as follows:

$$\frac{\text{activity}}{\text{concentration}} = \text{activity coefficient}$$

At infinite dilution the activity coefficient is unity, but in physiological concentrations it is significantly less than unity. Activity is therefore less than the concentration. However, in practice it is usual to work in concentrations, and values for the various equilibrium constants are adjusted accordingly, as indicated by a prime after the symbol K thus – K'. This is one of the reasons why these 'constants' are not in fact constant but should be considered as parameters which vary slightly under physiological conditions.

Carbonic anhydrase (see review by Maren, 1967). The reaction of carbon dioxide with water (equation 2) is non-ionic and slow, requiring a period of minutes for equilibrium to be attained. This would be far too slow for the time available for gas exchange in pulmonary and systemic capillaries if the reaction were not speeded up enormously in both directions by the enzyme carbonic anhydrase which is present in endothelium (Effros, Mason and Silverman, 1981) and erythrocytes, but not in plasma. In addition to its role in the respiratory transport of carbon dioxide, this enzyme is concerned with the transfer and accumulation of hydrogen and bicarbonate ions in secretory organs, including the kidney.

Carbonic anhydrase is a zinc-containing enzyme of low molecular weight, discovered by Meldrum and Roughton (1933). It is inhibited by a large number of unsubstituted sulphonamides (general formula $R—SO_2NH_2$). Sulphonilamide is an active inhibitor but the later antibacterial sulphonilamides are substituted ($R—SO_2NHR'$), and therefore inactive. Other active sulphonamides include the thiazide diuretics and various heterocyclic sulphonamides, of which acetazolamide is the most important. This drug produces complete inhibition at 5–20 mg/kg in all organs and has no other pharmacological effects of importance. Acetazolamide has been much used in the study of carbonic anhydrase and has revealed the surprising fact that it is not essential to life. With total inhibition, $P CO_2$ gradients between tissues and alveolar gas are increased, pulmonary ventilation is increased and alveolar $P CO_2$ is decreased.

As bicarbonate ion

The largest fraction of carbon dioxide in the blood is in the form of bicarbonate ion which is formed by ionization of carbonic acid thus:

$$H_2CO_3 \rightleftharpoons H^+ + HCO_3^- \rightleftharpoons 2H^+ + CO_3^{2-} \qquad \ldots(3)$$

$$\underset{\text{first}}{\underset{\text{dissociation}}{}} \qquad \underset{\text{second}}{\underset{\text{dissociation}}{}}$$

The second dissociation occurs only at high pH (above 9) and is not a factor in the carriage of carbon dioxide by the blood. The first dissociation is, however, of the greatest importance within the physiological range. The pK_1' is about 6.1 and carbonic acid is about 96% dissociated under physiological conditions (Morris, 1968).

According to the law of mass action:

$$\frac{[H^+] \times [HCO_3^-]}{[H_2CO_3]} = K_1' \qquad \ldots(4)$$

where K_1' is the equilibrium constant of the first dissociation. The subscript 1 indicates that it is the first dissociation, and the prime indicates that we are dealing with concentrations rather than the more correct activities.

Rearrangement of equation (4) gives the following:

$$[H^+] = K_1' \frac{[H_2CO_3]}{[HCO_3^-]} \qquad \ldots(5)$$

The left-hand side is the hydrogen ion concentration, and this equation is the non-logarithmic form of the Henderson–Hasselbalch equation (Henderson, 1909). The concentration of carbonic acid cannot be measured and the equation may be modified by replacing this term with the total concentration of dissolved CO_2 and H_2CO_3, most conveniently quantified as $\alpha P CO_2$ as described above. The equation now takes the form:

$$[H^+] = K' \frac{\alpha P CO_2}{[HCO_3^-]} \qquad \ldots(6)$$

The new constant K' is the *apparent* first dissociation constant of carbonic acid, and includes a factor which allows for the substitution of total dissolved carbon dioxide concentration for carbonic acid.

The equation is now in a useful form and permits the direct relation of plasma hydrogen ion concentration, $P CO_2$ and bicarbonate concentration, all quantities which can be measured. The value of K' cannot be derived theoretically and is determined experimentally by simultaneous measurements of the three variables. Under normal physiological conditions, if $[H^+]$ is in nmol/l, $P CO_2$ in kPa, and HCO_3 in mmol/l, the value of the combined parameter $(\alpha K')$ is about 180. If $P CO_2$ is in mmHg, the value of the parameter is 24. This equation is very simple to use and was strongly recommended by Campbell (1962).

Most people prefer to use the pH scale, following the approach of Hasselbalch (1916) and take logarithms of the reciprocal of each term in equation (6) with the following familiar result:

$$pH = pK' + \log \frac{[HCO_3^-]}{\alpha P CO_2} = pK' + \log \frac{[CO_2] - \alpha P CO_2}{\alpha P CO_2} \qquad \ldots(7)$$

where pK' has an experimentally derived value of the order of 6.1, but variable with temperature and pH (see Table 10.1). '$[CO_2]$' refers to the total concentration of carbon dioxide in all forms (dissolved CO_2, H_2CO_3 and bicarbonate) as indicated by Van Slyke analysis.

It is sometimes useful to clear equation (7) for P_{CO_2}:

$$P_{CO_2} = \frac{[CO_2]}{\alpha\{\text{antilog (pH} - pK') + 1\}} \qquad \ldots(8)$$

It is important to remember that $[CO_2]$ refers to the carbon dioxide concentration in plasma and not in whole blood.

Carbamino carriage

Amino groups in the uncharged $R\text{—}NH_2$ form have the ability to combine directly with carbon dioxide to form a carbamic acid (Klocke, 1991). The carbamic acid then dissociates almost completely to carbamate at body pH:

$$R\text{—}\overset{\overset{\displaystyle H}{|}}{N}\text{—}H + CO_2 \rightleftharpoons R\text{—}\overset{\overset{\displaystyle H}{|}}{N}\text{—}\overset{\underset{\displaystyle \|}{\underset{\displaystyle O}{}}}{C}\text{—}OH \rightleftharpoons R\text{—}\overset{\overset{\displaystyle H}{|}}{N}\text{—}\overset{\underset{\displaystyle \|}{\underset{\displaystyle O}{}}}{C}\text{—}O^- + H^+$$

In a protein, the amino groups involved in the peptide linkages between amino acid residues cannot combine with carbon dioxide. The potential for carbamino carriage is therefore restricted to the one terminal amino group in each protein and to the side chain amino groups in lysine and arginine. Since both hydrogen ions and carbon dioxide compete to react with uncharged amino groups, the ability to combine with carbon dioxide is markedly pH dependent. The terminal α-amino groups are the most effective at physiological pH, and one binding site per protein monomer is more than sufficient to account for the quantity of carbon dioxide carried as a carbamino compound.

Only very small quantities of carbon dioxide are carried in carbamino compounds with plasma protein. Almost all is carried by haemoglobin, and reduced haemoglobin is about 3.5 times as effective as oxyhaemoglobin (Figure 10.1). The actual P_{CO_2} has very little effect upon the quantity of carbon dioxide carried in this manner, throughout the physiological range of P_{CO_2} (Ferguson, 1936).

The Haldane effect. Although the amount of carbon dioxide carried in the blood in carbamino carriage is small, the *difference* between the amount carried in venous and arterial blood is about a third of the total arterial venous difference (see Table 10.2). This accounts for the major part of the Haldane effect, which is the difference in the quantity of carbon dioxide carried, at constant P_{CO_2}, in oxygenated and reduced blood (Figure 10.2). The remainder of the effect is due to the increased buffering capacity of reduced haemoglobin, which is discussed below. When the Haldane effect was described by Christiansen, Douglas and Haldane (1914) they believed that the whole effect was due to altered buffering capacity; carbamino carriage was not demonstrated until much later (Ferguson and Roughton, 1934).

Formation of carbamino compounds does not require the dissolved carbon dioxide to be hydrated and so is independent of carbonic anhydrase. The reaction is very rapid and would be of particular importance in a patient who had received a carbonic anhydrase inhibitor.

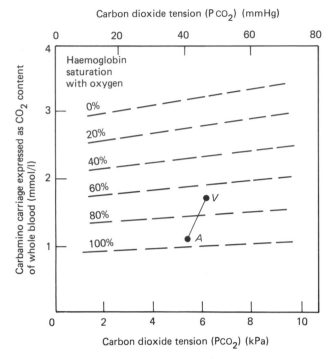

Figure 10.1 The broken lines on the graph indicate the carbamino carriage of carbon dioxide at different levels of saturation of haemoglobin with oxygen (15 g Hb/dl blood). It will be seen that this has a far greater influence on carbamino carriage than the actual P_{CO_2} (abscissa). A represents arterial blood (95% saturation and P_{CO_2} 5.3 kPa or 40 mmHg); V represents mixed venous blood (70% saturation and P_{CO_2} 6.1 kPa or 46 mmHg). Note that the arterial/venous difference in carbamino carriage is large in relation to the actual level of carbamino carriage, and accounts for about a third of the total arterial/venous blood CO_2 content difference (see Table 10.2). (These values have not been drawn from a single publication but present the mean of values reported from a number of studies.)

The arterial/venous difference in carbamino carriage is lost in certain regions of the body when a patient inhales 100% oxygen at a pressure of about 3 atmospheres absolute (ATA), since the oxygen dissolved in the arterial blood is then sufficient for metabolic requirements and very little reduced haemoglobin appears in the venous blood. Gessell (1923) suggested that the loss of the arterial/venous difference in carbamino carriage of carbon dioxide under these conditions resulted in tissue retention of carbon dioxide, and was a major factor in the cerebral toxic effects produced by high tensions of oxygen (page 552). It is, however, unlikely that this would cause a rise of tissue P_{CO_2} greater than 1 kPa (7.5 mmHg), and it is known that such a rise can be tolerated without any of the symptoms characteristic of oxygen toxicity. Furthermore, administration of carbonic anhydrase inhibitors does not produce a condition resembling oxygen toxicity.

Effect of buffering power of proteins on carbon dioxide carriage

Amino and carboxyl groups concerned in peptide linkages have no buffering power. Neither have most side chain groups (e.g. in lysine and glutamic acid) since

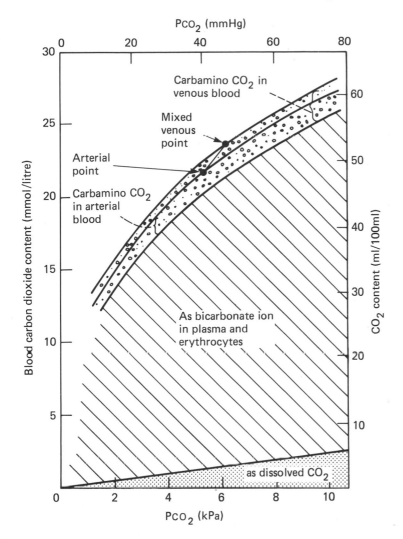

Figure 10.2 Components of the CO_2 dissociation curve for whole blood. Dissolved CO_2 and bicarbonate ion vary with P_{CO_2} but are little affected by the state of oxygenation of the haemoglobin. (Increased basic properties of reduced haemoglobin causes slight increase in formation of bicarbonate ion.) Carbamino carriage of CO_2 is strongly influenced by the state of oxygenation of haemoglobin but hardly at all by P_{CO_2}. (These values have not been drawn from a single publication but represent the mean of values reported in a large number of studies.)

their pK values are far removed from the physiological range of pH. In contrast is the imidazole group of the amino acid histidine, which is almost the only amino acid to be an effective buffer in the normal range of pH. Imidazole groups constitute the major part of the considerable buffering power of haemoglobin, each tetramer containing 38 histidine residues. The buffering power of plasma proteins is less and is proportional to their histidine content.

$$\text{Basic form} + H^+ \rightleftharpoons \text{Acidic form}$$

Basic form of histidine   *Acidic form of histidine*

The four haem groups of a molecule of haemoglobin are attached to the corresponding four amino acid chains at one of the histidine residues on each chain (page 270). The following is a section of a beta chain of human haemoglobin:

haem O_2
 \   /
  Fe
  |
—leucine—histidine—cysteine—aspartic — lysine —leucine—histidine—valine—
  91   92   93   acid   95   96   97   98
                                94

The figures indicate the position of the amino acid residue in the chain. The histidine in position 92 is one to which a haem group is attached. The histidine in position 97 is not. Both have buffering properties but the dissociation constant of the imidazole groups of the four histidine residues to which the haem groups are attached is strongly influenced by the state of oxygenation of the haem. Reduction causes the corresponding imidazole group to become more basic. The converse is also true: in the acidic form of the imidazole group of the histidine, the strength of the oxygen bond is weakened. Each reaction is of great physiological interest and both effects were noticed many decades before their mechanisms were elucidated.

1. *The reduction of haemoglobin causes it to become more basic.* This results in increased carriage of carbon dioxide as bicarbonate, since hydrogen ions are removed, permitting increased dissociation of carbonic acid (first dissociation of equation 3). This accounts for part of the Haldane effect, the other and greater part being due to increased carbamino carriage (see above).
2. *Conversion to the basic form of histidine causes increased affinity of the corresponding haem group for oxygen.* This is, in part, the cause of the Bohr effect (page 274).

Total reduction of the haemoglobin in blood would raise the pH by about 0.03 pH units if the P_{CO_2} were held constant at 5.3 kPa (40 mmHg), and this would correspond roughly to the addition of 3 mmol of base to 1 litre of blood. The normal degree of desaturation in the course of the change from arterial to mixed venous blood is about 25%, corresponding to a pH increase of about 0.007 if

P_{CO_2} remains constant. In fact, P_{CO_2} rises by about 0.8 kPa (6 mmHg), which would cause a decrease of pH of 0.040 units if the oxygen saturation were to remain the same. The combination of a increase of P_{CO_2} of 0.8 kPa and a decrease of saturation of 25 per cent thus results in a fall of pH of 0.033 units (see Table 10.2).

Distribution of carbon dioxide within the blood

Table 10.2 shows the forms in which carbon dioxide is carried in normal arterial and mixed venous blood. Although the amount carried in solution is small, most of the carbon dioxide enters and leaves the blood as CO_2 itself (Figure 10.3). Within the plasma there is little chemical combination of carbon dioxide, for three reasons. Firstly, there is no carbonic anhydrase in plasma and therefore carbonic acid is formed only very slowly. Secondly, there is little buffering power in plasma to promote the dissociation of carbonic acid. Thirdly, the formation of carbamino compounds by plasma proteins is not great, and must be almost identical for arterial and venous blood.

Carbon dioxide can, however, diffuse freely into the erythrocyte, where two courses are open. Firstly, carbamino carriage by haemoglobin is increased, not so much because the P_{CO_2} is increased, but rather because the oxygen saturation is likely to be reduced at the same time as the P_{CO_2} is increased. Reduced saturation favours carbamino carriage (see Figure 10.1). The second course is hydration and dissociation. Hydration is greatly facilitated by the presence of carbonic anhydrase in the erythrocyte, and dissociation is facilitated by the buffering power of the imidazole groups on the histidine residues of the haemoglobin, particularly reduced haemoglobin. In this way considerable quantities of bicarbonate ion are formed and these are able to diffuse into the plasma in exchange for chloride ions which diffuse in the opposite direction (Hamburger, 1918).

Dissociation curves of carbon dioxide

Figure 10.2 shows the classic form of the dissociation curve of carbon dioxide relating blood content to tension. Recently, there has been much greater interest in curves which relate any pair of the following: (1) plasma bicarbonate concentration; (2) P_{CO_2}; (3) pH. These three quantities are related by the Henderson–Hasselbalch equation and therefore the third variable can always be derived from the other two. For this reason the three possible plots may be used interchangeably and choice is largely a matter of custom or convenience.

A slight modification of the conventional CO_2 dissociation curve relates plasma bicarbonate to P_{CO_2} (Figure 10.2). The Davenport plot (Figure 10.4) relates plasma bicarbonate to pH. The Siggaard-Andersen plot (1964) relates log P_{CO_2} to pH (Figure 10.5). Any one of the graphs can be used to explore the effects of changes in respiratory and metabolic acid–base balance. However, if the P_{CO_2} of an entire patient is altered, the pH changes are not the same as those of a blood sample of which the P_{CO_2} is altered *in vitro*. This is because the blood of a patient is in continuity with the extracellular fluid (of very low buffering capacity) and also with intracellular fluid (of high buffering capacity). Bicarbonate ions pass rapidly and freely across the various interfaces, and experimental studies have shown the following changes to occur in the arterial blood of an intact subject when the P_{CO_2} is acutely changed.

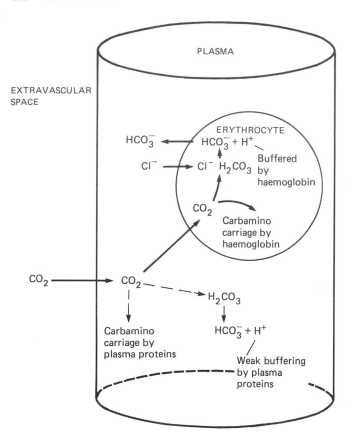

Figure 10.3 How carbon dioxide enters the blood in molecular form. Within the plasma, there is only negligible carbamino carriage due to the structure of the plasma proteins, and a slow rate of hydration to carbonic acid due to the absence of carbonic anhydrase. The greater part of the carbon dioxide diffuses into the erythrocytes where conditions for carbamino carriage are much more favourable. In addition, hydration to carbonic acid occurs rapidly in the presence of carbonic anhydrase and subsequent ionization is promoted by the buffering capacity of haemoglobin for the hydrogen ions.

1. The arterial pH reaches a steady state within minutes of establishment of the new level of $P\text{CO}_2$.
2. The change in arterial pH is intermediate between the pH changes obtained *in vitro* with plasma and whole blood after the same change in $P\text{CO}_2$. That is to say, the *in vivo* change in pH is greater than the *in vitro* change in the patient's blood when subjected to the same change in $P\text{CO}_2$.

   Numerous studies have been carried out in animals, and there is indication of some species differences (Shaw and Messer, 1932). Studies in conscious man show *in vivo* changes close to the *in vitro* changes obtained in plasma (Cohen, Brackett and Schwartz, 1964). Prys-Roberts, Kelman and Nunn (1966) studied step changes of $P\text{CO}_2$ in anaesthetized patients and obtained *in vivo* dissociation curves of similar slope to those which would be obtained with the patient's blood *in vitro* if the haemoglobin concentration were reduced by a third (shown by the broken lines in Figures 10.4 and 10.5).

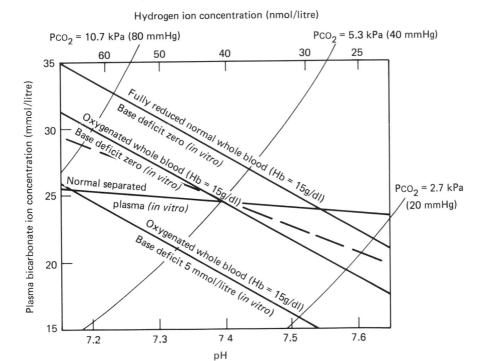

Figure 10.4 A number of CO_2 equilibration curves plotted on the co-ordinates $pH/[HCO_3^-]$. (Isobars are shown for P_{CO_2} 10.7, 5.3, 2.7 kPa = 80, 40 and 20 mmHg.) For most biological fluids, the plot is linear over the physiological range. pH = 7.40, P_{CO_2} = 5.3 kPa (40 mmHg) and HCO_3^- = 24.4 mmol/l is the accepted normal point through which all curves for normal oxygenated blood or plasma pass. The steepest curve passing through that point is the curve of normal oxygenated whole blood; the flattest is that of plasma, both curves being obtained in vitro. The broken curve describes blood of haemoglobin 10 g/dl equilibrated in vitro, or alternatively the arterial blood (Hb = 15 g/dl) equilibrated in vivo of a normal anaesthetized patient whose P_{CO_2} is acutely changed (Prys-Roberts, Kelman and Nunn, 1966). The uppermost curve is that of reduced but otherwise normal blood equilibrated in vitro. The lowermost curve is that of oxygenated blood with a metabolic acidosis (base deficit) of 5 mmol/l equilibrated in vitro.

This effect introduces a small potential error into the calculation of base excess in a patient whose P_{CO_2} is well outside the normal range. The error may be determined from Figures 10.4 and 10.5. The measured base excess will be about 2 mmol/l low (apparent metabolic acidosis) if blood is sampled when the P_{CO_2} is 10.7 kPa (80 mmHg), and the measured base excess will be about 2 mmol/l high (apparent metabolic alkalosis) if blood is sampled when the P_{CO_2} is 2.7 kPa (20 mmHg).

Transfer of carbon dioxide across cell membranes

Membranes made of most plastic materials (e.g. polytetrafluorethylene or Teflon) permit the free diffusion of carbon dioxide but will not permit the passage of hydrogen ions. This is the principle of the CO_2-sensitive electrode (page 244). Somewhat similar selectivity exists across cell membranes in the living body and

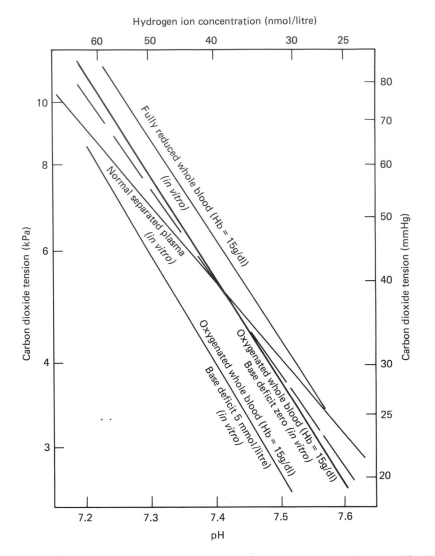

Figure 10.5 A number of CO$_2$ equilibration curves plotted on the co-ordinates pH/log PCO_2. For most biological fluids the plot is linear over the physiological range. pH = 7.40 and PCO_2 = 5.3 kPa (40 mmHg) is the accepted normal value through which all curves for normal oxygenated blood or plasma pass. The steepest curve passing through this point is that of normal oxygenated blood; the flattest is that of plasma, both curves being obtained in vitro. *The broken curve describes blood of haemoglobin 10 g/dl, equilibrium* in vitro, *or alternatively the arterial blood, equilibrated* in vivo, *(Hb = 15 g/dl), of a normal anaesthetized patient whose PCO_2 is acutely changed (Prys-Roberts, Kelman and Nunn, 1966). The uppermost curve is that of reduced but otherwise normal blood equilibrated* in vitro. *The lowermost curve is that of oxygenated blood with a metabolic acidosis (base deficit) of 5 mmol/l, equilibrated* in vitro.

particularly in the case of the blood/brain barrier, which is impervious to hydrogen ions but permits the rapid diffusion of carbon dioxide. Therefore, the intracellular hydrogen ion concentration is relatively uninfluenced by changes in extracellular pH, but does repond to changes in PCO_2. Carbon dioxide passes through the membrane and, once inside the cell, is able to hydrate and ionize, thus producing hydrogen ions. This property is unique to carbon dioxide, which is the only substance normally present in the body, which is able to diffuse through cell membranes and alter the intracellular pH in this manner.

The passage of carbon dioxide through the cell membrane to release hydrogen ions within the cell is reminiscent of the siege of Troy (Virgil, 19 BC). The city of Troy is analogous to the cell and its walls were impervious to Greek soldiers (hydrogen ions). However, the wooden horse (carbon dioxide) passed through the walls without difficulty and, once within the city (cell), was able to release the Greek soldiers (hydrogen ions).

This effect of carbon dioxide is of great physiological importance, and accounts for many of the effects of carbon dioxide, including its effect on the central chemoreceptors (page 104), which function in a manner very similar to the PCO_2-sensitive electrode.

Factors influencing the carbon dioxide tension in the steady state

In common with other catabolites, the level of carbon dioxide in the body fluids depends upon the balance between production and elimination. There is a continuous gradient of PCO_2 from the mitochondria to the expired air and thence to ambient air. The PCO_2 in all cells is not identical, but is lowest in tissues with the lowest metabolic activity and the highest perfusion (e.g. skin) and highest in tissues with the highest metabolic activity for their perfusion (e.g. the myocardium). Therefore the PCO_2 of venous blood differs from one tissue to another, and the mixed venous PCO_2 is the mean for the whole body, integrated with respect to organ perfusion.

In the pulmonary capillaries, carbon dioxide passes into the alveolar gas and this causes the alveolar PCO_2 to rise steadily during expiration. During inspiration, the inspired gas dilutes the alveolar gas and the PCO_2 falls by about 0.4 kPa, imparting a sawtooth curve to the alveolar PCO_2 when it is plotted against time (Figure 10.6). The amplitude of the oscillations of alveolar PCO_2 is increased during exercise and this has implications in the control of breathing (page 328).

Blood leaving the pulmonary capillaries has a PCO_2 which is very close to that of the alveolar gas and, therefore, varies with time in the same manner as the alveolar PCO_2. There is also a regional variation with PCO_2 inversely related to the ventilation/perfusion ratio of different parts of the lung (see Figure 8.11). The mixed arterial PCO_2 is the integrated mean of blood from different parts of the lung, and a sample drawn over several seconds will average out the cyclical variations.

It is more convenient to consider tension than content, because carbon dioxide always moves in accord with tension gradients even if they are in the opposite direction to concentration gradients. Also, the concept of tension may be applied with equal significance to gas and liquid phases, content having a rather different connotation in the two phases. Furthermore, the effects of carbon dioxide (e.g. upon respiration) are a function of tension rather than content. Finally, it is easier to measure blood PCO_2 than CO_2 content. Normal values for tension and content are shown in Figure 10.7.

Each factor which influences the PCO_2 has already been mentioned in this book and in this chapter they will be drawn together, illustrating their relationship to one

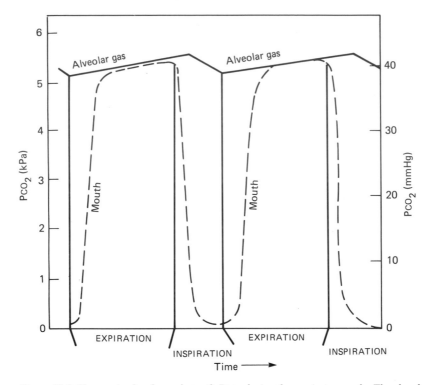

Figure 10.6 Changes in alveolar and mouth P_{CO_2} during the respiratory cycle. The alveolar P_{CO_2} is shown by a continuous curve, and the mouth P_{CO_2} (as determined by a rapid analyser) by the broken curve. The mouth P_{CO_2} falls at the commencement of inspiration but does not rise during expiration until the anatomical dead space gas is washed out. The alveolar P_{CO_2} rises during expiration and also during the early part of inspiration until fresh gas penetrates the alveoli after the anatomical dead space is washed out. The alveolar P_{CO_2} then falls until expiration commences. This imparts a sawtooth curve to the alveolar P_{O_2}.

another. It is convenient first to summarize the factors influencing the alveolar P_{CO_2}, and then to consider the factors which influence the relationship between the alveolar and the arterial P_{CO_2} (Figure 10.8).

The alveolar P_{CO_2} ($P_{A_{CO_2}}$)

Carbon dioxide is constantly being added to the alveolar gas from the pulmonary blood and removed from it by the alveolar ventilation. The concentration of carbon dioxide is equal to the ratio of the two, provided that carbon dioxide is not inhaled:

$$\text{alveolar } CO_2 \text{ concentration} = \frac{\text{carbon dioxide output}}{\text{alveolar ventilation}}$$

This axiomatic relationship is the basis of all the methods of predicting alveolar concentrations of all gases which enter or leave the body. In Chapter 6 it was used as the basis of the universal alveolar air equation and the following is the version for carbon dioxide, arranged to indicate partial pressure:

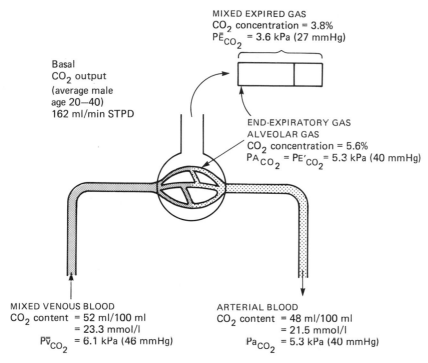

Figure 10.7 Normal values of CO₂ levels. These normal values are rounded off and ignore the small difference in PCO₂ between end-expiratory gas, alveolar gas and arterial blood. Actual values of PCO₂ depend mainly on alveolar ventilation but the differences depend upon maldistribution; the alveolar/end-expiratory PCO₂ difference depends on alveolar dead space and the very small arterial/alveolar PCO₂ difference on shunts. Scatter of V̇/Q̇ ratios makes a small contribution to both alveolar/end-expiratory and arterial/alveolar PCO₂ gradients. The arterial/mixed venous CO₂ content difference is directly proportional to CO₂ output and inversely proportional to cardiac output. Secondary symbols Ē, mixed expired; E′, end-expiratory′; A, alveolar; a, arterial; v̄, mixed venous.

$$\begin{array}{c} \text{alveolar} \\ \text{PCO}_2 \end{array} = \begin{array}{c} \text{dry} \\ \text{barometric} \\ \text{pressure} \end{array} \left(\begin{array}{c} \text{mean} \\ \text{inspired CO}_2 \\ \text{concentration} \end{array} + \dfrac{\text{CO}_2 \text{ output}}{\text{alveolar ventilation}} \right)$$

This equation includes all the more important factors influencing the alveolar PCO_2 (Figure 10.8), and examples of the relationship between PCO_2 and alveolar ventilation are shown in Figure 10.9. The hyperbolic nature of this relationship was discussed on page 128. Individual factors will now be considered.

The dry barometric pressure is not a factor of much importance in the determination of alveolar PCO_2, and normal variations of barometric pressure at sea level are unlikely to influence the PCO_2 by more than 0.3 kPa (2 mmHg). At high altitude, the hypoxic drive to ventilation lowers the PCO_2 (page 344). At very high pressures, alveolar PCO_2 tends to remain fairly constant, while the fractional concentration is reduced inversely to the barometric pressure (see Table 16.2).

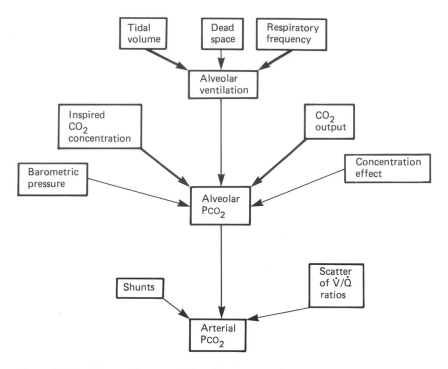

Figure 10.8 Summary of factors which influence P_{CO_2}; the more important ones are indicated with the thicker arrows. In the steady state, the CO_2 output of a resting subject usually lies within the range 150–200 ml/min and the alveolar P_{CO_2} is largely governed by the alveolar ventilation, provided that the inspired CO_2 concentration is zero. The barometric pressure is the only limit to the elevation of P_{CO_2} which may be brought about by the inhalation of gas mixtures containing CO_2. See text for explanation of the concentration effect.

The mean inspired CO_2 concentration is a more difficult concept than it appears at first sight (Nunn and Newman, 1964), and has been considered in relation to apparatus dead space on page 177. Essentially the effect of inspired carbon dioxide on the alveolar P_{CO_2} is additive. If, for example, a patient breathes gas containing 4.2% carbon dioxide (P_{CO_2} = 4.0 kPa or 30 mmHg), the alveolar P_{CO_2} will be raised 4.0 kPa above the level that it would be if there were no carbon dioxide in the inspired gas, *and other factors, including ventilation, remained the same.* The barometric pressure is the only limit to the elevation of P_{CO_2} which may be obtained by the inhalation of carbon dioxide mixtures. Arterial tensions of over 27 kPa (200 mmHg) have been obtained by inhaling a few breaths of 30% carbon dioxide.

Carbon dioxide output. It is carbon dioxide output and not production which directly influences the alveolar P_{CO_2}. Output equals production in a steady state, but they may be quite different during unsteady states (Nunn and Matthews, 1959). During acute hypoventilation, much of the carbon dioxide production is diverted into the body stores, so that the output may temporarily fall to very low figures until the alveolar carbon dioxide concentration has risen to its new level.

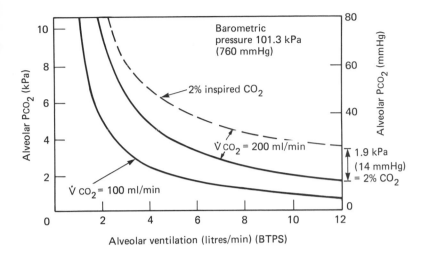

Figure 10.9 The effect of CO_2 output, alveolar ventilation and inspired CO_2 concentration on alveolar PCO_2. The lowest continuous curve shows the relationship between ventilation and alveolar PCO_2 for a carbon dioxide output of 100 ml/min (STPD). The upper continuous curve shows the relationship when the carbon dioxide output is 200 ml/min (STPD). The broken curve represents the relationship when the carbon dioxide output is 200 ml/min and there is an inspired CO_2 concentration of 2%. Two per cent CO_2 is equivalent to about 1.9 kPa (14 mmHg) and each point on the broken curve is 1.9 kPa above the upper of the two continuous curves. The continuous curves are rectangular hyperbolas with identical asymptotes (zero alveolar PCO_2 and zero alveolar ventilation). The broken curve is also a rectangular hyperbola but the horizontal asymptote is PCO_2 1.9 kPa (14 mmHg) which is the tension in the inspired gas.

Conversely, acute hyperventilation results in a transient increase in carbon dioxide output. A sudden fall in cardiac output decreases the carbon dioxide output until the carbon dioxide concentration in the mixed venous blood rises. The unsteady state is considered in more detail later (page 238).

Alveolar ventilation for present purposes means the product of the respiratory frequency and the difference between the tidal volume and the physiological dead space (page 128). It can change over very wide limits and is the most important factor influencing alveolar PCO_2. Factors governing ventilation are considered in Chapter 5, and dead space in Chapter 8.

  With gas circuits which result in rebreathing, it is possible for the fresh gas inflow rate to replace the alveolar ventilation in the relationship defined in the equation above. When the alveolar ventilation is considerably in excess of the fresh gas inflow rate, the latter may then be used to control the level of the PCO_2 (Schofield and Williams, 1974).

The concentration effect. Apart from the factors shown in the equation above and in Figure 10.9, the alveolar PCO_2 may be temporarily influenced by net transfer of soluble inert gases across the alveolar/capillary membrane. Uptake of an inert gas increases the concentration (and tension) of carbon dioxide (and oxygen) in the alveolar gas. This occurs, for example, at the beginning of an anaesthetic when large quantities of nitrous oxide are passing from the alveolar gas into the body stores, and a much smaller quantity of nitrogen is passing from the body into the alveolar gas. The converse occurs during elimination of the inert gas and results in transient reduction of alveolar P_{CO_2} and P_{O_2}. Implications for oxygenation are discussed on page 260.

The end-expiratory P_{CO_2} (PE'_{CO_2})

In the normal, healthy, conscious subject, the end-expiratory gas consists almost entirely of alveolar gas. If, however, appreciable parts of the lung are ventilated but not perfused, they will contribute a significant quantity of CO_2-free gas from the alveolar dead space to the end-expiratory gas (see Figure 8.8). As a result, the end-expiratory P_{CO_2} (end-tidal or Haldane–Priestley sample) will have a lower P_{CO_2} than that of the alveoli which are perfused. Gas cannot be sampled selectively from the perfused alveoli but Chapter 8 explains why the arterial P_{CO_2} usually approximates closely to the mean value of the perfused alveoli in spite of scatter of ventilation/perfusion ratios. It is therefore possible to compare the arterial P_{CO_2} with the end-expiratory P_{CO_2} to demonstrate the existence of an appreciable proportion of unperfused alveoli. Studies during anaesthesia have, for example, shown an arterial/end-tidal P_{CO_2} gradient of about 0.7 kPa (5 mmHg) in patients without lung disease (Ramwell, 1958; Nunn and Hill, 1960).

The alveolar/arterial P_{CO_2} gradient

For reasons which have been discussed in Chapter 9, we may discount the possibility of any significant gradient between the P_{CO_2} of alveolar gas and that of pulmonary end-capillary blood. Arterial P_{CO_2} may, however, be slightly greater than the mean alveolar P_{CO_2} because of shunting or scatter of ventilation/perfusion ratios. Factors governing the magnitude of the gradient were considered in Chapter 8 (page 181), where it was shown that a shunt of 10% will cause an alveolar/arterial P_{CO_2} gradient of only about 0.1 kPa (0.7 mmHg) (Figure 8.9). Since the normal degree of ventilation/perfusion ratio scatter causes a gradient of the same order, neither has much significance for carbon dioxide (in contrast to oxygen), and there is an established convention by which the arterial and 'ideal' alveolar P_{CO_2} values are taken to be identical. It is only in exceptional patients with, for example, a shunt in excess of 30% that the gradient is likely to exceed 0.3 kPa (2 mmHg).

The arterial P_{CO_2}

Pooled results for the normal arterial P_{CO_2} reported by various authors show a mean of 5.1 kPa (38.3 mmHg) with 95% limits (2 s.d.) of 1.0 kPa (7.5 mmHg). Five per cent of normal patients will lie outside these limits and it is therefore preferable to call it the reference range rather than the normal range. There is no evidence that P_{CO_2} is influenced by age in the healthy subject.

Causes of hypocapnia (respiratory alkalosis)

Hypocapnia can result only from an alveolar ventilation which is excessive in relation to carbon dioxide production. Low values of arterial P_{CO_2} are very commonly found, due to artificial ventilation with a generous minute volume, or to voluntary hyperventilation, often resulting from drawing an arterial sample. Persistently low values may be due to an excessive respiratory drive resulting from one or more of the following causes.

Hypoxaemia is a common cause of hypocapnia, occurring in congenital heart disease with right-to-left shunting, residence at high altitude, pulmonary collapse or consolidation and any other condition which reduces the arterial P_{O_2} below about 8 kPa (60 mmHg). Hypocapnia, secondary to hypoxaemia, opposes the ventilatory response to the hypoxaemia (page 237).

Metabolic acidosis produces a compensatory hyperventilation (air hunger) which minimizes the fall in pH which would otherwise occur. This is a pronounced feature of diabetic ketosis and severe haemorrhagic shock. Arterial P_{CO_2} values below 3 kPa (22.5 mmHg) are not uncommon in severe metabolic acidosis.

Mechanical abnormalities of the lung may drive respiration through the vagus, resulting in moderate reduction of the P_{CO_2}. Thus conditions such as pulmonary fibrosis and asthma are usually associated with a low to normal P_{CO_2} until the patient passes into respiratory failure.

Hypotension may drive respiration directly but, in cases of haemorrhage, metabolic acidosis is usually a more important factor.

Hysteria, head injuries and various neurological disorders may result in hyperventilation.

The effects of hypocapnia are considered in Chapter 30.

Causes of hypercapnia (respiratory acidosis)

It is uncommon to encounter an arterial P_{CO_2} above the normal range in a healthy subject. Any value of more than 6.1 kPa (46 mmHg) should be considered abnormal, but values up to 6.7 kPa (50 mmHg) may be attained by breath holding. It is difficult for the healthy subject to exceed this level by any respiratory manoeuvre other than by breathing mixtures of carbon dioxide in oxygen.

When a patient is found to be hypercapnic, there are only four possible causes. These should be considered systematically as follows.

Increased concentration of carbon dioxide in the inspired gas

This iatrogenic cause of hypercapnia is very uncommon but it is dangerous and differs fundamentally from the other causes listed below. It should therefore be excluded at the outset in any patient unexpectedly found to be hypercapnic when breathing from or being ventilated by external equipment. The carbon dioxide may be endogenous or exogenous, the former resulting from rebreathing while the latter is usually therapeutic or accidental. The only essential difference between the two is the rate at which the P_{CO_2} can increase. If all the carbon dioxide produced by metabolism is retained and distributed in the body stores, arterial P_{CO_2} can increase no faster than about 0.4–0.8 kPa/min (3–6 mmHg/min. This limits the rate of increase of P_{CO_2} during rebreathing. In contrast, the P_{CO_2} may rise extremely rapidly when exogenous carbon dioxide is inhaled (see page 240).

Increased carbon dioxide production

If the pulmonary minute volume is fixed by artificial ventilation and carbon dioxide production is increased by, for example, malignant hyperpyrexia, then hypercapnia is inevitable. Like the previous category, this is a rare but dangerous cause of hypercapnia, which should be excluded when there is no other obvious explanation for hypercapnia.

Hypoventilation

An inadequate pulmonary minute volume is by far the commonest cause of hypocapnia. Pathological causes of hypoventilation leading to hypercapnia are considered in Chapter 21. In respiratory medicine, the commonest cause of long-standing hypercapnia is chronic bronchitis. The type of patient known as the 'blue bloater' has reduced ventilatory capacity combined with reduced ventilatory response to carbon dioxide. There are many other possible causes (see Figure 21.2), including medullary depression by drugs, neuromuscular blockade, respiratory obstruction and restriction of lungs or chest wall.

While breathing air, it is not possible for a hypoventilating patient to have a P_{CO_2} in excess of about 13 kPa (100 mmHg) because, at that level of ventilation, the accompanying hypoxaemia will become critical (see Figure 21.1). P_{CO_2} values in excess of 13 kPa can occur only in patients breathing either oxygen-enriched gas mixtures or gas containing carbon dioxide: the condition can therefore be regarded as iatrogenic.

In many conditions with reduced ventilatory capacity, including asthma, pulmonary fibrosis, poliomyelitis and emphysema ('pink puffers'), the ventilatory response to carbon dioxide is better preserved and the arterial P_{CO_2} is usually subnormal even in the presence of dyspnoea. A rise in P_{CO_2} occurs late and is a serious development.

Increased dead space

This very rare cause of hypercapnia is usually diagnosed by a process of exclusion when a patient has a high P_{CO_2}, with a normal minute volume and no evidence of a hypermetabolic state or inhaled carbon dioxide. The cause may be incorrectly connected breathing apparatus, or an excessively large alveolar dead space (page 175). This might be due to pulmonary embolism or a cyst communicating with the tracheobronchial tree and receiving preferential ventilation.

The effects of hypercapnia are considered in Chapter 30.

Carbon dioxide stores and the unsteady state

The quantity of carbon dioxide and bicarbonate ion in the body is very large – about 120 litres, which is almost 100 times greater than the volume of oxygen (page 288). Therefore, when ventilation is altered out of accord with metabolic

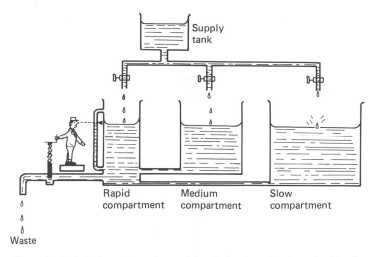

Rapid compartment   Medium compartment   Slow compartment

Waste

Figure 10.10 A hydrostatic analogy of the elimination of carbon dioxide. See text for full discussion.

activity, carbon dioxide levels change only slowly and new equilibrium levels are attained only after about 20–30 minutes. In contrast, corresponding changes in oxygen levels are very rapid.

Figure 10.10 shows a three-compartment hydraulic model in which depth of water represents $P\text{co}_2$ and the volume in the various compartments corresponds to volume of carbon dioxide. The metabolic production of carbon dioxide is represented by the variable flow of water from the supply tank. The outflow corresponds to alveolar ventilation and the controller watching the $P\text{co}_2$ represents the central chemoreceptors. The rapid compartment represents circulating blood, brain, kidneys and other well perfused tissues. The medium compartment represents skeletal muscle (resting) and other tissues with a moderate blood flow. The slow compartment includes bone, fat and other tissues with a large capacity for carbon dioxide. Each compartment has its own time constant (see Appendix F), and the long time constants of the medium and slow compartments buffer changes in the rapid compartment.

Hyperventilation is represented by a wide opening of the outflow valve with subsequent exponential decline in the levels in all three compartments, the rapid compartment falling most quickly. The rate of decrease of $P\text{co}_2$ is governed primarily by ventilation and the capacity of the stores. Hypoventilation is fundamentally different. The rate of increase of $P\text{co}_2$ is now limited by the metabolic production of carbon dioxide which is the *only* factor directly increasing the quantity of carbon dioxide in the body compartments. Therefore, the time course of the increase of $P\text{co}_2$ following step decrease of ventilation is not the mirror image of the time course of decrease of $P\text{co}_2$ when ventilation is increased. The rate of rise is much slower than the rate of fall, which is fortunate for patients in asphyxial situations.

When *all* metabolically produced carbon dioxide is retained, the rate of rise of arterial $P\text{co}_2$ is of the order of 0.4–0.8 kPa/min (3–6 mmHg/min). This is the resultant of the rate of production of carbon dioxide and the capacity of the body stores for carbon dioxide. During actual hypoventilation, the rate of increase in

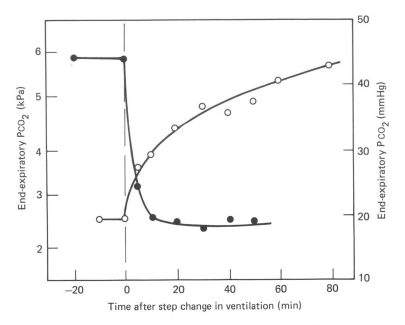

Figure 10.11 Time course of changes in end-expiratory P_{CO_2} following step changes in ventilation. The solid circles indicate the changes in end-expiratory P_{CO_2} which followed a step change in ventilation from 3.3 to 14 l/min. The open circles show the change following a step change in ventilation from 14 to 3.3 l/min in the same patient. During the fall of P_{CO_2}, half the total change is completed in about 3 minutes. During the rise of P_{CO_2}, half-change takes approximately 16 minutes.

P_{CO_2} will be less than this and Figure 10.11 shows typical curves for P_{CO_2} increase and decrease following step changes in ventilation of anaesthetized patients. The time course of rise of P_{CO_2} after step reduction of ventilation is faster when the previous level of ventilation has been of short duration (Ivanov and Nunn, 1968).

In a later study, Ivanov and Nunn (1969) compared the rapidity with which P_{CO_2} could be elevated by three different techniques in a previously hyperventilated patient. Reduction of minute volume was the slowest method. Rebreathing with oxygen replenishment was the fastest practicable method without using exogenous carbon dioxide, which was much the quickest technique. The use of an inspired gas mixture containing 5% carbon dioxide elevated the P_{CO_2} by 2.3 kPa (17.3 mmHg) in 2 minutes, most of the change occurring in the first minute.

Laparoscopy with carbon dioxide as the inflating gas seems at first sight to carry a hazard of exogenous carbon dioxide intoxication. However, a number of studies have shown that the elevation of P_{CO_2} is minimal provided that pulmonary ventilation is properly maintained (Kelman et al., 1972). Surprisingly, the elevation of P_{CO_2} appears to be greater if nitrous oxide is used as the inflating gas.

The difference in the rate of change of P_{CO_2} and P_{O_2} after a step change in ventilation (see Figure 11.20) has two important implications for monitoring and measurement. Firstly, changes in P_{O_2} (or the output of a pulse oximeter) will often provide an earlier warning of acute hypoventilation than will the capnogram, provided that the alveolar P_{O_2} is not much above the normal range. However, *in the steady state* P_{CO_2} gives the best indication of the adequacy of ventilation, because oxygenation is so heavily influenced by intrapulmonary shunting (see Figure 8.10) and the inspired oxygen concentration (see Figure 6.8). Secondly, step changes in ventilation are followed by temporary changes in the respiratory exchange ratio because, in the unsteady state, carbon dioxide output changes more than oxygen uptake. However, if the ventilation is held constant at its new level, the respiratory exchange ratio must eventually return to the value determined by the metabolic process of the body. Carbon dioxide stores were reviewed by Farhi (1964).

Apnoeic mass-movement oxygenation
(formerly known as **diffusion respiration**)

When a patient becomes apnoeic while breathing air, alveolar gas reaches equilibrium with mixed venous blood, within a few minutes. Assuming normal starting conditions and ignoring changes in the composition of the recirculated mixed venous blood, this would entail a rise of alveolar PCO_2 from 5.3 to 6.1 kPa (40 to 46 mmHg) and a fall of PO_2 from 14 to 5.3 kPa (105 to 40 mmHg). These changes correspond to the uptake of 230 ml of oxygen but the output of only 21 ml of carbon dioxide. Carbon dioxide appears to reach equilibrium within about 10 seconds (Stock et al., 1988), while oxygen would take about a minute, being limited by the ability of the cardiac output and the arterial/mixed venous oxygen content difference to remove some two-thirds of the oxygen in the alveolar gas (normally about 450 ml).

These calculations assume that alveolar gas is not replenished from outside the patient. What actually happens to the arterial blood gases in apnoea depends upon the patency of the airway and the composition of the ambient gas if the airway is patent.

With airway occlusion. As described above, there is rapid attainment of equilibrium between alveolar and mixed venous PCO_2. Thereafter, arterial, alveolar and mixed venous PCO_2 values remain close, and, with recirculation of the blood, increase together at the rate of about 0.4–0.8 kPa/min (3–6 mmHg/min), with more than 90% of the metabolically produced carbon dioxide passing into the body stores. Alveolar PO_2 decreases close to the mixed venous PO_2 within about a minute, and then decreases further as recirculation continues. The lung volume falls by the difference between the oxygen uptake and the carbon dioxide output. Initially the rate would be $230 - 21 = 209$ ml/min. The change in alveolar PO_2 may be calculated, and gross hypoxia supervenes after about 90 seconds if apnoea with airway occlusion follows air breathing at the functional residual capacity.

With patent airway and air as ambient gas. The initial changes are as described above. However, instead of the lung volume falling by the net gas exchange rate (initially 209 ml/min), this volume of ambient gas is drawn in by mass movement down the trachea. If the ambient gas is air, the oxygen in it will be removed but the nitrogen will accumulate and rise above its normal concentration until gross hypoxia supervenes after about 2 minutes. This is likely to occur when the accumulated nitrogen has reached 90% since the alveolar carbon dioxide concentration will then have reached about 8%. Carbon dioxide elimination cannot occur as there is mass-movement of air down the trachea, preventing loss of carbon dioxide by either convection or diffusion. Measured at the mouth, there is oxygen uptake but no carbon dioxide output: the respiratory exchange ratio is thus zero.

With patent airway and oxygen as the ambient gas. Oxygen is continuously removed from the alveolar gas as described above, but is replaced by oxygen drawn in by mass-movement. No nitrogen is added to the alveolar gas, and the alveolar P_{O_2} only falls as fast as the P_{CO_2} rises (about 0.4–0.8 kPa/min or 3–6 mmHg/min). Therefore the patient will not become seriously hypoxic for several minutes. If the patient has been breathing oxygen prior to the respiratory arrest, the starting alveolar P_{O_2} would be of the order of 88 kPa (660 mmHg) and therefore the patient could theoretically survive about 100 minutes of apnoea *provided that his airway remained clear and he remained connected to a supply of 100% oxygen.* This does, in fact, happen and has been demonstrated in both animals and man (Draper and Whitehead, 1944; Enghoff, Holmdahl and Risholm, 1951; Holmdahl, 1956; Frumin, Epstein and Cohen, 1959).

The phenomenon enjoyed a brief vogue in anaesthetic practice as a means of maintaining oxygenation during apnoea, particularly for bronchoscopy (Holmdahl, 1953; Barth, 1954; Payne, 1962). However, hypercapnia is an inevitable feature of the technique, and arterial P_{CO_2} values as high as 18.7 kPa (140 mmHg) were reported by Payne (1962).

Therapeutic uses of carbon dioxide

The varied and powerful effects of increased P_{CO_2} (see Chapter 30) suggest that the inhalation of carbon dioxide gas mixtures would have a clear place in therapy. In fact, this is not so and its therapeutic role is very limited.

The main indication for the administration of carbon dioxide is to stimulate respiration. It has been used to expedite the uptake and elimination of inhalational anaesthetic agents, and also to raise the arterial P_{CO_2} above the apnoeic threshold in order to encourage the resumption of spontaneous breathing after passive hyperventilation. It is, of course, useless for the stimulation of breathing in any patient whose hypoventilation is due to diminished or absent chemoreceptor sensitivity to carbon dioxide. Carbon dioxide is also likely to be ineffective or harmful if ventilation is limited by malfunction of the efferent motor pathway, the respiratory muscles or by raised airway resistance. Such patients will already have a raised P_{CO_2} and a flattened P_{CO_2}/ventilation response curve.

Carbon monoxide poisoning remains one of the clearest indications for the administration of carbon dioxide gas mixtures. Not only will stimulation of respiration hasten the elimination of carbon monoxide, but also the venous (and therefore the tissue) P_{O_2} will be substantially increased by the rightward shift of the dissociation curve of the remaining normal haemoglobin (see Figure 11.14). Increasing P_{CO_2} will usually improve both cardiac output and regional perfusion of certain organs, particularly the brain, but raised intracranial pressure is a hazard. If carbon dioxide is used clinically, careful attention must be paid to dosimetry. It would be unwise to exceed 5% carbon dioxide, which is available in oxygen as carbogen.

Accidental administration of carbon dioxide is considered in Chapter 30.

Outline of methods of measurement of carbon dioxide

Fractional concentration in gas mixtures

Chemical absorption. This remains the reference method of analysis. In medical circles the most accurate method usually employed is Lloyd's modification of the Haldane apparatus (Cormack, 1972). A simpler version of Haldane's apparatus, which is sufficiently accurate for clinical work, was described by Campbell (1960a). The popularity of the Scholander apparatus has declined in Great Britain in recent years, but it may still be useful for the analysis of samples of less than 1 ml (Scholander, 1947). All these methods are markedly influenced by the presence of nitrous oxide in gas samples, and modifications of technique are required (Nunn, 1958a; Glossop, 1963; Meade and Owen-Thomas, 1975).

Infrared analysis. This is the most widely used method for rapid breath-to-breath analysis. It is also very convenient for analysis of discrete gas samples. Most diatomic gases absorb infrared radiation, and errors may arise due to overlap of absorption bands and collision broadening (Cooper, 1957). These effects are best overcome by filtering and calibrating with a known concentration of carbon dioxide in a diluent gas mixture which is similar to the gas sample for analysis. Infrared analysers are available with a response time of less than 300 μs and will follow the respiratory cycle provided the respiratory frequency is not too high. Breathe-through cells have a better frequency response. Cormack and Powell (1972) described refinements of technique which permit greater accuracy. The broken line in Figure 10.6 shows a typical capnogram from which much information, including the following, may be derived:

1. The end-expiratory carbon dioxide concentration (FE'_{CO_2}).
2. The inspiratory carbon dioxide concentration.
3. The anatomical dead space may be derived from a plot of the expired carbon dioxide concentration against the expired volume (see Figure 8.15).
4. The slope of the plateau and its relationship to the arterial P_{CO_2} give useful information on other components of the dead space (page 192).
5. The demonstration of the capnogram is a reliable indication of the correct placement of a tracheal tube.
6. Sudden decrease in FE'_{CO_2} at a fixed level of ventilation is a valuable indication of pulmonary embolism.
7. Cardiac arrest during artificial ventilation will cause FE'_{CO_2} to fall to zero.

Mass spectrometry. This powerful technique has at last become established as an alternative method for the rapid analysis of carbon dioxide. The cost is much greater than for infrared analysis, but response times tend to be shorter and there is usually provision for analysis of up to four gases at the same time. Time sharing permits the monitoring of several patients with a single analyser.

Blood carbon dioxide concentration

For more than half a century the concentration of carbon dioxide in blood or plasma was measured by vacuum extraction followed by chemical absorption in the manometric apparatus of Van Slyke and Neill (1924). The microapparatus of

Natelson (1951) was considerably easier to handle. An even simpler technique is dissociation of bicarbonate by adding a large volume of acid to blood followed by measurement of PCO_2 of the blood-plus-acid (Linden, Ledsome and Norman, 1965). PCO_2 of the mixture is conveniently measured by means of the PCO_2-sensitive electrode (see below). Calibration with sodium bicarbonate allows conversion of PCO_2 to CO_2 concentration.

Development of techniques for direct measurement of pH and PCO_2 removed much of the necessity for measurement of the carbon dioxide concentration of blood and plasma.

Blood PCO_2

Four methods of measurement have been described and each in its time has enjoyed widespread popularity.

Bubble tonometry was the first practical method (Pflüger, 1866). A tiny bubble of gas was equilibrated with blood at the patient's body temperature and then chemically analysed for the carbon dioxide concentration of the bubble, which was assumed to have the same PCO_2 as the blood. The technique was progressively refined over 100 years, culminating in the 'Riley bubble method' (Riley, Campbell and Shepard, 1957). However, the technique always remained very difficult to master and disappeared from use after 1960.

The indirect method. For many years PCO_2 was derived from the form of the Henderson–Hasselbalch equation given earlier in this chapter (equation 8, page 223). It was a most laborious procedure requiring measurements of both pH and CO_2 content, and there was always uncertainty of the value which should be taken for pK'. Nevertheless, tolerable accuracy was attainable (Thornton and Nunn, 1960).

The interpolation technique. The death knell of the methods described above was sounded by the development of the interpolation method by Siggaard-Andersen and Astrup in Copenhagen. In their approach, PCO_2 of blood is measured by interpolating the actual pH in a plot of log PCO_2 against pH derived from aliquots of the same blood sample. The plot is linear (Figures 10.5, and E.4 in Appendix E) and the whole operation became a practical proposition following the introduction of the microapparatus described by Siggaard-Andersen et al. (1960). A small error is introduced if the sample is desaturated. Minor refinements of technique and the level of accuracy were described by Kelman, Coleman and Nunn (1966). Accuracy is uninfluenced by the presence of anaesthetic gases. Between 1957 and 1960 the interpolation procedure was undertaken on separated plasma but this contained a conceptual source of error and the method was abandoned.

The PCO_2-sensitive electrode. All the above methods have finally given way to the PCO_2-sensitive electrode which, in its automated form, has removed the requirement for technical expertise. Analysis may now be satisfactorily performed by untrained staff on a do-it-yourself basis with results available within 5 minutes (Minty and Barrett, 1978).

PCO_2 of any gas or liquid may be determined directly by this technique (Severinghaus and Bradley, 1958; Severinghaus, 1965). The PCO_2 of a film of bicarbonate solution is allowed to come into equilibrium with the P_{CO_2} of a sample on the other side of a membrane permeable to carbon dioxide but not to hydrogen ions. The pH of the bicarbonate solution is constantly monitored by a glass electrode and the log of the P_{CO_2} is inversely proportional to the recorded pH. The accuracy obtainable is comparable to that of other techniques and is uninfluenced by the presence of anaesthetic gases.

The long and fascinating history of measurement of P_{CO_2} and acid–base has been recorded by Astrup and Severinghaus (1986) and Severinghaus and Astrup (1986).

Indirect measurement of arterial P_{CO_2}

Measurement of end-expiratory P_{CO_2} is of limited value due to the variable arterial end-expiratory P_{CO_2} gradient caused by lung disease or anaesthesia. However, the method is useful for recording changes. If a rapid carbon dioxide analyser is not available, end-expiratory samples may be collected (Rahn et al., 1946).

Measurement of mixed venous P_{CO_2} may be estimated indirectly with very simple apparatus, using the rebreathing technique of Campbell and Howell (1960). A modification of the technique for use in children was described by Sykes (1960).

It was originally recommended that 0.8 kPa (6 mmHg) should be subtracted from the mixed venous (rebreathing) P_{CO_2} to give the arterial P_{CO_2} since this is the normally accepted difference between mixed venous and arterial P_{CO_2}. However, many workers have found that the mixed venous P_{CO_2} measured by the rebreathing technique seems to give a higher value than would be expected. McEvoy, Jones and Campbell (1974) reconsidered the theoretical background of the method and drew attention to a number of factors which raise the rebreathing P_{CO_2}. Most important is the fact that the rebreathing method measures the P_{CO_2} of venous blood as it would be if fully oxygenated. The Haldane effect then raises the P_{CO_2} 0.5–1 kPa (3.8–7.5 mmHg) higher than the true mixed venous P_{CO_2} (see Figure 10.2). Furthermore, the mixed venous/arterial P_{CO_2} gradient will be increased in hypercapnia (due to the curvature of the carbon dioxide dissociation curve), as well as with arterial hypoxaemia, reduced cardiac output and anaemia. An additional factor is the finite time required for the physicochemical equilibration of carbon dioxide in the blood, the rate-limiting step being equation (2) on page 219. The P_{CO_2} of arterial blood when sampled and analysed may be different from the value when the blood left the pulmonary capillary where it was in equilibrium with alveolar gas. In general, the observed mixed venous P_{CO_2} (as measured by the rebreathing technique) is likely to exceed the arterial P_{CO_2} by 1–2 kPa (7.5–15 mmHg) in the normal resting subject, and it certainly does so in the author. Since this difference rises with increasing P_{CO_2}, McEvoy and his co-workers suggested that the indirect arterial P_{CO_2} should be calculated as 0.8 times the mixed venous P_{CO_2} measured by the rebreathing technique. Denison et al. (1971) and Godfrey and Wolf (1972) described the use of the method in exercise. However, nowadays it is usually simpler to measure arterial P_{CO_2} directly.

Transcutaneous P_{CO_2}. This technique uses a CO_2-sensitive electrode heated to about 44°C – which is, however, close to the temperature which burns the skin. Transcutaneous P_{CO_2} should be within about 0.5 kPa (3.8 mmHg) of the simultaneous arterial value, but it is necessary to apply a large correction factor for the difference in temperature between body and electrode (Severinghaus, 1981).

Venous P_{CO_2}. Blood draining skin has a very small arterial/venous P_{O_2} difference and results are quite acceptable for clinical purposes (Forster et al., 1972). However, it is surprisingly difficult to collect a good sample of blood anaerobically from the veins on the back of the hand. Cooper and Smith (1961) found that agreement between arterial and cutaneous venous P_{CO_2} was good in the majority of a series of anaesthetized patients, but considerable discrepancies appeared in a minority of patients, thought to have circulatory disturbances. Blood from veins draining muscles (e.g. the median cubital vein) has a P_{CO_2} much higher than the arterial level and is useless as an indication of the arterial P_{CO_2}.

Capillary P_{CO_2}. Blood obtained from a skin prick suffers from the same uncertainties which surround cutaneous venous P_{CO_2}. However, the technique is clearly useful in neonates. The likely error (say, 0.6 kPa or 4.5 mmHg) is seldom of much consequence in the management of a patient.

Handling of blood samples

It is important that samples be preserved from contact with air or oil, to which they may lose carbon dioxide. Analysis should be undertaken quickly, as the P_{CO_2} of blood *in vitro* rises by about 0.013 kPa/min (0.1 mmHg/min) at 37°C. If analysis is not carried out at the patient's body temperature, a correction factor should be applied, as the P_{CO_2} of an anaerobic blood sample falls by about 4% for each degree Celsius cooling. Nomograms for correction for both these errors were prepared by Kelman and Nunn (1966b) and are to be found in Appendix E (Figures E.1 and E.2).

Chapter 11

Oxygen

The appearance of oxygen in the atmosphere of this planet has played a crucial role in the development of life (see Chapter 1). The whole of the animal kingdom is totally dependent on oxygen, not only for function, but also for survival. This is notwithstanding the fact that oxygen is extremely toxic in the absence of elaborate defence mechanisms (see Chapter 32).

The role of oxygen in the cell

Dissolved molecular oxygen (dioxygen) enters into many metabolic processes in the mammalian body (Fisher and Forman, 1985). Quantitatively much the most important is the cytochrome c oxidase system which is responsible for about 90% of the total oxygen consumption of the body. However, cytochrome c oxidase is but one of more than 200 oxidases which may be classified as follows.

Electron transfer oxidases. As a group these oxidases involve the reduction of oxygen to superoxide anion, hydrogen peroxide or water, the last being the fully reduced state (see Chapter 32, Figure 32.2). The most familiar of this group of enzymes is cytochrome c oxidase. This is located in the mitochondria and is concerned in the production of the high energy phosphate bond in adenosine triphosphate (ATP) which is the main source of biological energy. This process is described in greater detail below under the heading 'Oxidative phosphorylation'. Another member of this group of oxidases is NADPH oxidase which is concerned in the generation of superoxide anion in phagocytes. While the superoxide anion and its derivatives are potentially toxic, they play a major role in bacterial killing (see Chapter 32). Other electron transfer oxidases are responsible for the conversion of 5-hydroxytryptamine to 5-hydroxyindoleacetaldehyde and urate to allantoin.

Oxygen transferases (dioxygenases). This group of oxygenases incorporates oxygen into substrates without the formation of any reduced oxygen product. Familiar examples are cyclo-oxygenase and lipoxygenase which are concerned in the first stage of conversion of arachidonic acid into prostaglandins and leukotrienes (see Chapter 12, page 314). A dioxygenase is also concerned in the conversion of tryptophan to formylkynurenine.

Mixed function oxidases. These oxidases result in oxidation of both a substrate and a co-substrate, which is most commonly NADPH. Well known examples are the cytochrome P-450 hydroxylases, which play an important role in detoxification and are considered further on page 254. Mixed function oxidases are also concerned in the conversion of phenylalanine to tyrosine and of dopamine to noradrenaline, the co-substrate being NADPH for the former and ascorbate for the latter.

Oxidative phosphorylation

Most of the energy deployed in the mammalian body is derived from the oxidation of food fuels, of which the most important is glucose:

$$C_6H_{12}O_6 + 6O_2 = 6CO_2 + 6H_2O + energy$$

The equation accurately describes the combustion of glucose *in vitro*, but is only a crude, overall representation of the oxidation of glucose in the body. The direct reaction would not produce energy in a form in which it could be utilized by the body. The biological oxidation proceeds by a large number of stages, with phased production of energy. This energy is not all immediately released but is partly stored by means of the reaction of adenosine diphosphate (ADP) with inorganic phosphate ion to form adenosine triphosphate (ATP):

$$ADP + inorganic\ phosphate\ ion + energy \rightleftharpoons ATP$$

The third phosphate group in ATP is held by a high energy bond which releases its energy when ATP is split back into ADP and inorganic phosphate ion. ADP is thus recycled indefinitely, with ATP acting as a short-term store of energy available in a form which may be used directly for work such as muscle contraction, ion pumping, protein synthesis and secretion. ATP is commonly transported short distances between the sites of synthesis and utilization. For example, in voluntary muscles, it is formed in the mitochondria and used in the myofibrils.

There is no large store of ATP in the body and it must be synthesized continuously as it is being used. The ATP/ADP ratio is an indication of the level of energy which is currently carried in the ADP/ATP system, and the ratio is normally related to the state of oxidation of the cell. The ADP/ATP system is not the only short-term energy store in the body but it is the most important.

The uses of ATP in the body lie outside the scope of this book, but its production from ADP is highly relevant to this chapter since the most efficient methods of production of ATP require the consumption of oxygen. However, the anaerobic methods are of great biological importance and were universal before the atmospheric P_{O_2} was sufficiently high for aerobic pathways of metabolism (see Chapter 1). Anaerobic metabolism is still the rule in anaerobic bacteria and also in the mammalian body when energy requirements outstrip oxygen supply as, for example, during severe exercise and in hypoxia.

The aerobic pathway permits the release of far greater quantities of energy from the same amount of substrate and is therefore used whenever possible. In simplified form, the contrasting pathways can be shown as follows:

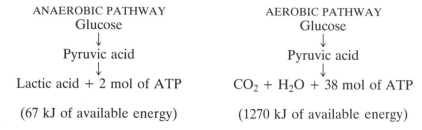

In vitro combustion of glucose liberates 2820 kJ/mol as heat. Thus, under conditions of oxidative metabolism, 45% of the total energy is made available for biological work and this compares favourably with most man-made machines.

Localization of oxidative phosphorylation in the cell. Oxygen consumption occurs in the mitochondria, where it combines with hydrogen to form water. The hydrogen has previously been removed from a variety of substrates by nicotinamide adenine dinucleotide (NAD), and then passed along a chain of hydrogen carriers to combine with oxygen at cytochrome a$_3$ which is the end of the chain. Figure 11.1 shows the transport of hydrogen along the chain, which consists of structural entities just visible under the electron microscope and arranged in rows along the cristae of the mitochondria. Three molecules of ATP are formed at various stages of the chain during the transfer of two atoms of hydrogen. The process is not associated directly with the production of carbon dioxide, which is formed by entirely different metabolic pathways. Oxidative phosphorylation can take place only when the PO_2 within the mitochondrion is above a critical level, thought to be of the order of 0.1 kPa. When the PO_2 falls below this level, metabolism reverts to anaerobic pathways. The reduction of oxygen to water by cytochrome a$_3$ is inhibited by cyanide.

The role of oxidative phosphorylation in the aerobic degradation of glucose is illustrated in Figure 11.2. One molecule of glucose is converted into two molecules of glyceraldehyde-3-phosphate in the cytoplasm of the cell. The latter then diffuses into the mitochondria where it is converted into 3-phosphoglyceric acid when hydrogen is removed by NAD and oxidized after transport along the chain shown in Figure 11.1. The next reactions can take place in the cytoplasm down to the point where pyruvic acid is formed. The oxidation of pyruvic acid, however, can take place only in the mitochondria where hydrogen is removed and oxidized at successive stages of Krebs' citric acid cycle. It will be seen that the production of carbon dioxide also occurs within the mitochondria but that it is not directly associated with oxygen consumption. The scheme shown in Figure 11.2 also accounts for the consumption of oxygen in the metabolism of fat. After hydrolysis, glycerol is converted into pyruvic acid while the fatty acids shed a series of 2-carbon molecules in the form of acetyl CoA. Pyruvic acid and acetyl CoA enter the citric acid cycle and are then degraded in the same manner as though they had been derived from glucose. Amino acids are dealt with in similar manner after deamination.

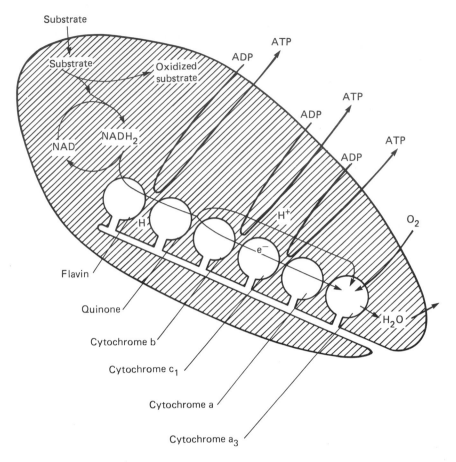

Figure 11.1 Diagrammatic representation of oxidation within the mitochondrion. The substrate diffuses from the cytoplasm into the mitochondrion where hydrogen is removed under the influence of the appropriate dehydrogenase enzyme. The hydrogen is carried by intramitochondrial NAD to the first of the chain of hydrogen carriers which are attached to the cristae of the mitochondria. When the hydrogen reaches the cytochromes, ionization occurs; the proton passes into the lumen of the mitochondrion while the electron is passed along the cytochromes where it converts ferric iron to the ferrous form. The final stage is at cytchrome a_3 where the proton and the electron combine with oxygen to form water. Three molecules of ADP are converted to ATP at the stages shown in the diagram. ADP and ATP can cross the mitchondrial membrane freely while there are separate pools of intra- and extramitochondrial NAD which cannot interchange.

Figure 11.3 gives further detail of the glycolytic pathway and the conversion of pyruvate to lactate. The whole comprises the Embden–Meyerhof pathway for the anaerobic metabolism of glucose. This is followed either when the PO_2 falls below its critical level or, in the case of erythrocytes, when there is an absence of the respiratory enzymes located in the mitochondria. Two molecules of ATP are consumed in the priming stages prior to the formation of fructose-1,6-diphosphate, 6-phosphofructokinase being the rate-limiting enzyme. These ATP molecules are regenerated in the conversion of two molecules of 1,3-diphosphoglyceric acid to two of 3-phosphoglyceric acid, but there is generation of a further two molecules

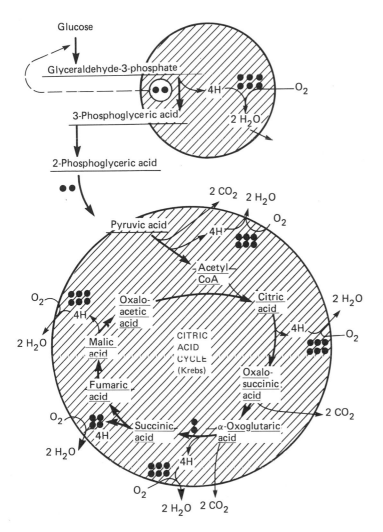

Figure 11.2 Successive stages in the principal oxidative metabolic pathway of glucose by the citric acid cycle. Many stages have been omitted for clarity. The two shaded circles represent mitochondria and indicate the reactions which can only take place within them. The names of substances which cross the membranes show those which are capable of diffusion into and out of the mitochondria. Underlining indicates that two molecules are formed from one of glucose. Black dots show where ATP is formed (the first two to be produced are offset by two which are required for the conversion of glucose to glyceraldehyde-3-phosphate). Note the dissociation between O_2 consumption and CO_2 production. The conversion of glyceraldehyde-3-phosphate to 3-phosphoglyceric acid can also take place in the cytoplasm as shown in Figure 11.3 but, in that case, it is not possible for the liberated hydrogen to be oxidized to water, because the $NADH_2$ cannot diffuse into the mitochondria.

of ATP (from one molecule of glucose) at the conversion of phosphoenolpyruvic acid to pyruvic acid. The conversion of glyceraldehyde-3-phosphate to 3-phospho-glyceric acid can take place in the cytoplasm with hydrogen released as in the aerobic pathway but, in this case, to extramitochondrial NAD. This hydrogen

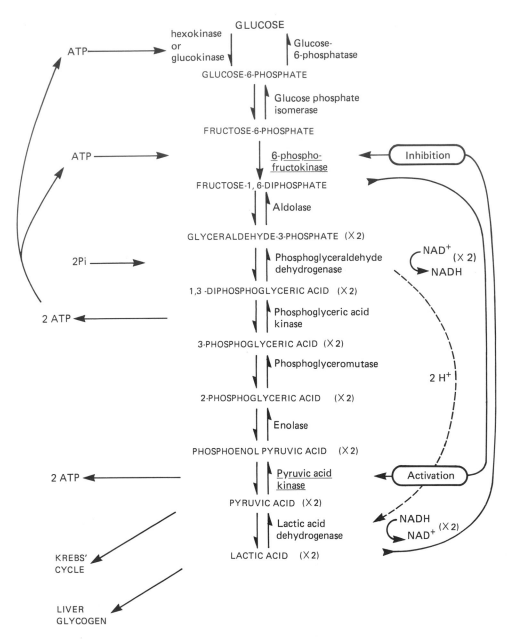

Figure 11.3 The Embden–Meyerhof pathway for anaerobic metabolism of glucose. From glyceraldehyde-3-phosphate downwards, two molecules of each intermediate are formed from one of glucose. Note the consumption of two molecules of ATP in the first three steps. These must be set against the total production of four molecules of ATP, leaving a net gain of two molecules of ATP from the consumption of one molecule of glucose. The hydrogen ions produced at the fifth step are used in the reduction of pyruvic acid to lactic acid. All the acids are largely ionized at tissue pH.

cannot be oxidized but it is taken up lower down the pathway by the reduction of pyruvic acid to lactic acid.

This series of changes is associated with the net formation of only two molecules of ATP from one of glucose, in contrast to the 38 produced in the course of aerobic metabolism.

$$\text{Glucose} + 2Pi + 2ADP \rightarrow 2\text{Lactic acid} + 2ATP + 2H_2O$$
$$(Pi = \text{inorganic phosphate})$$

However, considerable chemical energy remains in the lactic acid which, in the presence of oxygen, can be reconverted to pyruvic acid and then oxidized in the citric acid cycle, producing the balance of 36 molecules of ATP. Alternatively, lactic acid may be converted into liver glycogen to await more favourable conditions for oxidation. Conversion of glucose to ethyl alcohol (fermentation) provides energy without the consumption of oxygen in certain organisms but not in animals. This pathway also yields two molecules of ATP for one of glucose.

All the acids shown in Figure 11.3 are highly ionized at body pH, and the anaerobic pathway inevitably results in the release of hydrogen ions. It is now clear that 6-phosphofructokinase is inhibited by lactacidosis and this limits the generation of ATP. Fructose-1,6-diphosphate bypasses both the rate-limiting stage of 6-phosphofructokinase and also the requirement for two molecules of ATP for priming. It therefore increases the yield of ATP compared with glucose, and is not subject to rate limitation from acidosis.

Significance of oxidative phosphorylation. The production of a high yield of ATP requires oxygen. The alternative anaerobic pathways must either consume very much larger quantities of glucose or, alternatively, yield less ATP. In high energy consuming organs such as brain, kidney and liver it is not, in fact, possible to transfer the increased quantities of glucose and therefore these organs suffer ATP depletion under hypoxic conditions. In contrast, voluntary muscle is able to function satisfactorily on anaerobic metabolism during short periods of time and this is normal in the diving mammals.

Anaerobic metabolism carries not only the penalty of ATP depletion but also the serious disadvantage of production of two moles of lactic acid from one of glucose (Figure 11.3). At normal intracellular pH, the lactic acid so formed is almost entirely ionized. In most organs both hydrogen and lactate ions escape into the circulation, producing 'lactacidosis'. However, the situation in the brain is quite different. The blood/brain barrier is relatively impermeable to charged ions and both hydrogen and lactate ions are largely retained within the neuron, lowering the intracellular pH. The biochemical and physiological consequences of hypoxia are discussed in Chapter 31.

The critical oxygen tension for aerobic metabolism. When the mitochondrial PO_2 is reduced, oxidative phosphorylation continues normally down to a level of about 0.3 kPa (2 mmHg). Below this level, oxygen consumption falls and the various members of the electron transport chain tend to revert to the reduced state. $NADH/NAD^+$ and lactate/pyruvate ratios rise and the ATP/ADP ratio falls. The critical PO_2 varies between different organs and different species but, as an approximation, a mitochondrial PO_2 of about 0.13 kPa (1 mmHg) may be taken as the level below which there is serious impairment of oxidative phosphorylation and a switch to anaerobic metabolism. This level is, of course, far below the critical arterial PO_2, because there normally exists a large gradient of PO_2 between arterial blood and the site of utilization of oxygen in the mitochondria. This gradient is discussed in the oxygen cascade, below.

The critical PO_2 for oxidative phosphorylation is also known as the Pasteur point and has applications beyond the pathophysiology of hypoxia in man. In particular, it has a powerful bearing on putrefaction, many forms of which are anaerobic metabolism resulting from a fall of PO_2 below the Pasteur point in, for example, polluted rivers.

Cytochrome P-450

The cytochrome P-450 enzymes are the terminal oxidases for many mixed function oxidase systems, the typical hydroxylation reaction being:

$$RH + NADPH + H^+ + O_2 \rightarrow ROH + NADP^+ + H_2O$$

Cytochrome P-450 enzymes are at the end of an electron transport chain in a position analogous to cytochrome a_3 (see Figure 11.1) but there are very important differences. Firstly, these enzymes are bound to the membrane of the smooth endoplasmic reticulum (microsomes in homogenized and centrifuged preparations). Secondly, they are not concerned with energy production by synthesis of ATP, but with hydroxylation of a wide range of substrates, including many foreign substances and drugs. They are thus very important not only in detoxification but also in the formation of biotransformation products which may be more toxic than the original substance. These functions are largely carried out in the liver but also in other tissues, including the lung. It is generally possible to demonstrate that the substrate for hydroxylation is bound to cytochrome P-450 *in vitro* with characteristic changes of its spectral properties.

The cytochrome P-450 enzymes derive their name from the difference spectrum between preparations treated with nitrogen and carbon monoxide. The difference spectrum shows a strong band at a wavelength of 450 nm. It is likely that a number of mixed function oxidases share this property, and they are known collectively as cytochrome P-450.

The hepatic smooth endoplasmic reticulum hypertrophies as a result of *in vivo* treatment with enzyme inducers such as phenobarbitone. There is also an increased level of cytochrome P-450 with enhanced activity towards a wide variety of substrates. Induction with 3-methylcholanthrene causes synthesis of different structural forms of cytochrome with the peak of the difference spectrum at 448 nm (cytochrome P-448).

A likely scheme of action of cytochrome P-450 is shown in Figure 11.4. Biotransformation by the P-450 system does not only detoxify compounds but may

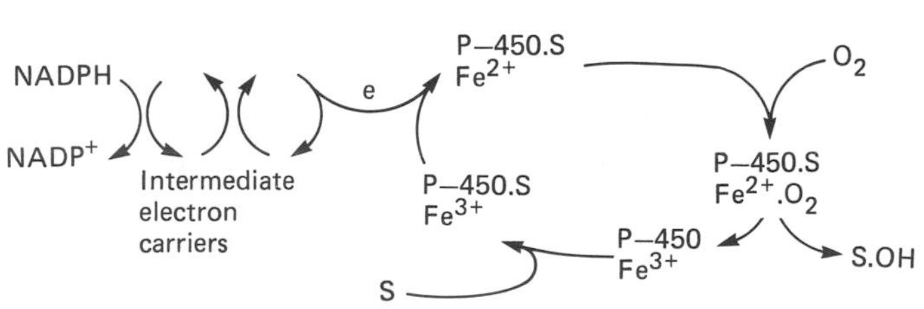

Figure 11.4 The likely scheme of action of cytochrome P-450. S indicates the substrate: both C- and N-oxygenations can occur.

also actually convert an inert molecule into a toxic moiety. A classic example is the anaesthetic fluroxene. Enzyme induction with phenobarbitone increases conversion to trifluoroethanol and thereby the toxicity of fluroxene in animals but not man (Cascorbi and Singh-Amaranath, 1972).

Cytochromes have a range of different P_{50} values and it has been suggested that herein lie the mechanisms for PO_2 sensors in the carotid body (page 102) and the pulmonary circulation (page 145).

The oxygen cascade

The PO_2 of dry air at sea level is 21.2 kPa (159 mmHg). Oxygen moves down a partial pressure gradient from air, through the respiratory tract, the alveolar gas, the arterial blood, the systemic capillaries and the cell. It finally reaches its lowest level within the mitochondria where it is consumed (Figure 11.5). At this point, the

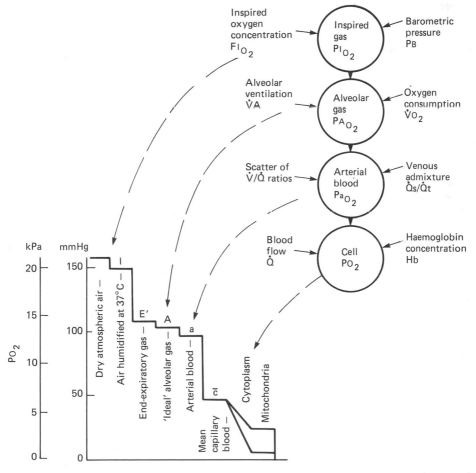

Figure 11.5 On the left is shown the oxygen cascade with PO_2 falling from the level in the ambient air down to the level in mitochondria, which is the site of utilization. On the right is shown a summary of the factors influencing oxygenation at different levels in the cascade.

PO_2 is probably within the range 0.5–3 kPa (3.8–22.5 mmHg) varying from one tissue to another, from one cell to another, and from one part of a cell to another.

The steps by which the PO_2 decreases from air to the mitochondria are known as the oxygen cascade and are of great practical importance. Any one step in the cascade may be increased under pathological circumstances and this may result in hypoxia. The steps will now be considered *seriatim*.

Dilution of inspired oxygen by water vapour

Analysis with the Haldane apparatus indicates the true fractional concentration of oxygen in a dry gas mixture. If the gas sample is humified, the added water vapour is ignored and the indicated fractional concentration of oxygen is still that of the dry part of the mixture. Thus the normal value for the concentration of atmospheric oxygen (20.94% or 0.2094 fractional concentration) indicates the concentration of oxygen in the dry gas phase, regardless of whether the gas is humidified or not. As gas is inhaled through the respiratory tract, it becomes humidified at body temperature and the added water vapour dilutes the oxygen and so reduces the PO_2 below its level in the ambient air. The process is similar to the reduction in PO_2 which occurs when ether is vaporized in air (Scott, 1847).

When dry gas kept at normal barometric pressure is humidified with water vaporized at 37°C, 100 volumes of the dry gas take up about 6 volumes of water vapour, giving a total gas volume of 106 units but containing the same number of molecules of oxygen. The PO_2 is thus reduced by the fraction 6/106. It follows from Boyle's law that PO_2 after humidification is indicated by the following expression:

$$\begin{array}{c} \text{fractional concentration of oxygen} \\ \text{in the dry gas phase} \\ \text{(Haldane value)} \end{array} \times \left(\begin{array}{c} \text{barometric} \\ \text{pressure} \end{array} - \begin{array}{c} \text{saturated water} \\ \text{vapour pressure} \end{array} \right)$$

(the quantity in parentheses is known as the dry barometric pressure)

Therefore the effective PO_2 of inspired air at a body temperature of 37°C is:

$$0.2094 \times (101.3 - 6.3) = 0.2094 \times 95$$
$$= 19.9 \text{ kPa}$$

or, in old units:

$$0.2094 \times (760 - 47) = 0.2094 \times 713$$
$$= 149 \text{ mmHg}$$

As a rough approximation, the partial pressure in kPa is close to the percentage concentration at normal barometric pressure. Partial pressure in mmHg may be approximately derived by multiplying the percentage concentration by 7; for example, the PO_2 of air is approximately $21 \times 7 = 147$ mmHg and the tension of 5% carbon dioxide is approximately $5 \times 7 = 35$ mmHg.

In respiratory physiology, gas tensions are almost always considered as being exerted by gas humidified at body temperature. This applies to inspired gas because it cannot participate in gas exchange until after it has been humidified in the upper respiratory tract. Therefore calculations almost always employ the dry barometric pressure whether considering inspired, alveolar or expired gas.

Primary factors influencing alveolar oxygen tension

The general equation for the calculation of the alveolar tension of a gas has been stated on pages 128 et seq. In the case of oxygen:

$$\text{alveolar } PO_2 \doteq \frac{\text{dry}}{\text{barometric}} \left(\frac{\text{inspired}}{\text{oxygen}} - \frac{\text{oxygen uptake}}{\text{alveolar ventilation}} \right) \qquad ...(1)$$

This equation is only approximate and does not include the second order correction factor due to the small difference in volume between the inspired and the expired gas. Normally this factor is small but, during the exchange of a soluble gas such as nitrous oxide, the difference may be quite large.

Various forms of the alveolar air equation may be used to correct for this difference (pages 195 et seq.). The commonest forms assume that the number of molecules of nitrogen inhaled equals the number exhaled. This is not the case when the composition of the inspired gas has been changed, as for example, during anaesthesia and intensive care. Therefore, under these circumstances it is necessary to use a special form of the equation introduced by Filley, MacIntosh and Wright (1954), which makes no assumptions of inert gas equilibrium, and is appropriate to most of the varied conditions likely to be encountered in clinical practice:

$$PA_{O_2} = PI_{O_2} - PA_{CO_2} \left(\frac{PI_{O_2} - P\bar{E}_{O_2}}{P\bar{E}_{CO_2}} \right) \qquad ...(2)$$

Applications of the equation were discussed by Nunn (1963). A further modification was described by Kelman and Prys-Roberts (1967) which allows for the addition of carbon dioxide to the inspired gas of the patient.

In its more accurate forms (e.g. equation 2), the alveolar air equation is used principally for calculation of the 'ideal' alveolar PO_2, a theoretical entity which was introduced on page 169 and explained in greater detail on pages 195 et seq. 'Ideal' alveolar gas has the same composition as gas from an imaginary alveolus with the ventilation/perfusion ratio of the lungs as a whole. In practice, it is defined as having a PCO_2 equal to that of arterial blood and a respiratory exchange ratio equal to that of mixed expired gas. Comparison of 'ideal' alveolar PO_2 with arterial PO_2 is the basis of quantification of 'venous admixture' (pages 194 et seq.).

In its simplified form (equation 1), the alveolar air equation is particularly useful for consideration of the important quantitative relationships between alveolar PO_2 and those factors which directly influence it, which will now be considered.

Dry barometric pressure. If other factors remain constant, the alveolar PO_2 will be directly proportional to the dry barometric pressure, which falls with increasing altitude to become zero at 19 kilometres where the actual barometric pressure equals the saturated vapour pressure of water at body temperature (see Table 15.1). The effect of increased pressure is complex (see Chapter 16, page 354). For example, a pressure of 10 atmospheres (absolute) increases the alveolar PO_2 by a factor of about 15 if other factors remain constant (see Table 16.2).

Inspired oxygen concentration. The alveolar PO_2 will be raised or lowered by an amount equal to the change in the inspired gas PO_2, provided that other factors remain constant. Since the concentration of oxygen in the inspired gas should always be under control, it is a most important therapeutic tool which may be used to counteract a number of different factors which may impair oxygenation.

Figure 11.6 shows the effect of an increase in the inspired oxygen concentration from 21 to 30% on the relationship between alveolar PO_2 and alveolar ventilation.

For any alveolar ventilation, the improvement of alveolar P_{O_2} will be 8.5 kPa (64 mmHg). This will be of great importance if, for example, hypoventilation while breathing air has reduced the alveolar P_{O_2} to 4 kPa (30 mmHg), a value which is close to the lowest level compatible with life. Oxygen enrichment of inspired gas to 30% will then increase the alveolar P_{O_2} to 12.5 kPa (94 mmHg), which is almost within the normal range. However, at this level of hypoventilation, P_{CO_2} would be about 13 kPa (98 mmHg) and might well have risen further on withdrawal of the hypoxic drive to ventilation. In fact, 30% is the maximum concentration of oxygen in the inspired gas which should be required to correct the alveolar P_{O_2} of a patient breathing air, who has become hypoxaemic as a result of hypoventilation. This problem is discussed at some length in Chapter 20 (pages 427 et seq.). Figure 6.8 shows ventilation/alveolar P_{O_2} curves for a wide range of inspired oxygen concentrations, indicating the protection against hypoxaemia (due to hypoventilation) which is afforded by different concentrations of oxygen in the inspired gas.

An entirely different problem is hypoxaemia due to venous admixture. This results in an increased alveolar/arterial P_{O_2} difference which, within limits, can be offset by increasing the alveolar P_{O_2}. Quantitative aspects are quite different from the problem of hypoventilation and are considered later in this chapter (page 268).

For completeness, it should be mentioned that high concentrations of oxygen may also be used for clearing as loculi (page 538) and also to provide an increase in the body stores of oxygen (page 288).

Oxygen consumption. The importance of oxygen consumption is only now belatedly receiving due attention. In the past there has been an unfortunate tendency to

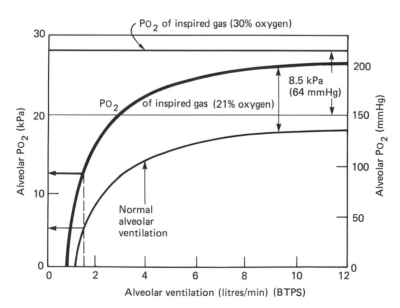

Figure 11.6 The effect on alveolar P_{O_2} of increasing the inspired oxygen concentration from 21% (thin curve) to 30% (heavy curve). The patient is assumed to have an oxygen consumption of 200 ml/min (STPD). In this example, the alveolar P_{O_2} is reduced to a dangerously low level when breathing air at an alveolar ventilation of 1.5 l/min. At this point, oxygen enrichment of the inspired gas to 30% is sufficient to raise the alveolar P_{O_2} almost to within the normal range. All points on the heavy curve are 8.5 kPa (64 mmHg) above the corresponding points on the thin curve at the same ventilation.

consider that all patients consume 250 ml of oxygen per minute under all circumstances. Oxygen consumption must, of course, be raised by exercise but is often well above basal in a patient supposedly 'at rest'. This may be due to restlessness, pain, increased work of breathing or the formation of oxygen-derived free radicals (page 542). These factors may well coexist with failure of other factors controlling the arterial P_{O_2}. Thus, for example, a patient may be caught by the pincers of a falling ventilatory capacity and a rising ventilatory requirement (see Figure 21.5).

Weaning from artificial ventilation may be unexpectedly difficult because of a high oxygen consumption. This may be measured directly but is not easy in the circumstances of intensive therapy unit (page 301). Thyrotoxicosis, convulsions and, to a lesser extent, shivering (Bay, Nunn and Prys-Roberts, 1968) cause a very marked rise in oxygen consumption and should, of course, be controlled. The value of measurement of oxygen consumption in the management of tetanus was stressed by Femi-Pearse et al. (1976).

Oxygen consumption is usually less than basal during anaesthesia, hypothermia and with hypothyroidism. Oxygen consumption during anaesthesia tends to be about 15% below basal on the usual standards. This tends to reduce the ventilatory requirement during anaesthesia, but the benefit in terms of gaseous homoeostasis is more than offset by other factors which are usually less favourable during anaesthesia (Chapter 20). Hypothermia causes a marked reduction in oxygen consumption with values of about 50% of basal at 31°C. Artificial ventilation of hypothermic patients may result in gross hypocapnia unless a conscious effort is made to reduce the minute volume or increase the apparatus dead space. Figure 11.7 shows the effect of different values for oxygen consumption on the relationship between alveolar ventilation and alveolar P_{O_2} for a patient breathing air.

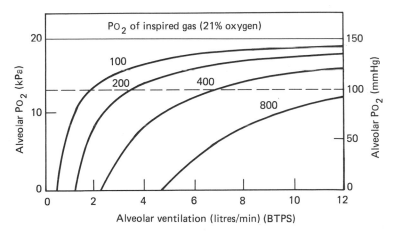

Figure 11.7 The relationship between alveolar ventilation and alveolar P_{O_2} for different values of oxygen consumption for a patient breathing air at normal barometric pressure. The figures on the curves indicate the oxygen consumption in ml/min (STPD). Alveolar ventilation is in l/min (BTPS). A typical value for oxygen consumption of a well rested or anaesthetized patient would be 200 ml/min; 100 ml/min would be an average value for hypothermia at 30°C. Higher values are related to exercise in Figure 13.1. Note that the alveolar ventilation required to maintain any particular alveolar P_{O_2} is directly proportional to the oxygen consumption. (In calculations of this type it is important to make the correction required by the fact that oxygen consumption and alveolar ventilation values are commonly expressed at different temperatures and pressures – see Appendix C.)

Alveolar ventilation. The alveolar air equation for oxygen (1) in the form given on page 257 implies a hyperbolic relationship between alveolar P_{O_2} and alveolar ventilation. This relationship, which is considered in Appendix F, has very important clinical relevance. As ventilation is increased, the alveolar P_{O_2} rises asymptomatically towards (but never reaches) the P_{O_2} of the inspired gas (see Figure 11.6). It will be seen from the shape of the curves that changes in ventilation above normal level have comparatively little effect upon alveolar P_{O_2}. In contrast, changes in ventilation below the normal level may have a very marked effect. At very low levels of ventilation, the alveolar ventilation becomes critical and small changes may precipitate gross hypoxia. Note that there is a finite alveolar ventilation at which alveolar P_{O_2} becomes zero.

Secondary factors influencing alveolar oxygen tension

Cardiac output. In the short term, cardiac output can influence the alveolar P_{O_2}. For example, if other factors remain constant, a sudden reduction in cardiac output will temporarily increase the alveolar P_{O_2}, since less blood passes through the lungs to remove oxygen from the alveolar gas. However, the reduced cardiac output also causes increased oxygen extraction in the tissues supplied by the systemic circulation, and before long the mixed venous oxygen level is decreased. When that has happened, the removal of oxygen from the alveolar gas returns to its original level as the reduction in blood flow rate is compensated by the greater amount of oxygen which is taken up per unit volume of blood flowing through the lungs. Thus, in the long term, cardiac output does not directly influence the alveolar P_{O_2}, and therefore it does not appear in equation (1).

The 'concentration', third gas or Fink effect. The above diagrams and equations have ignored a factor which influences alveolar P_{O_2} during exchanges of large quantities of soluble gases such as nitrous oxide. This effect was mentioned briefly in connection with carbon dioxide on page 236. Its effect on oxygen is probably more important.

During the early part of the administration of nitrous oxide, large quantities of the more soluble gas replace smaller quantities of the less soluble nitrogen previously dissolved in body fluids. There is thus a net transfer of 'inert' gas from the alveoli into the body, causing a *temporary* increase in the concentration of both oxygen and carbon dioxide, which will thus *temporarily* exert a higher tension than would otherwise be expected. Conversely, during recovery from nitrous oxide anaesthesia, large quantities of nitrous oxide leave the body to be replaced with smaller quantities of nitrogen. There is thus a net outpouring of 'inert' gas from the body into the alveoli, causing dilution of oxygen and carbon dioxide, both of which will *temporarily* exert a lower tension than would otherwise be expected. There may then be *temporary* hypoxia, the direct reduction of alveolar P_{O_2} sometimes being exacerbated by ventilatory depression due to decreased alveolar P_{CO_2}. Fortunately such effects last only a few minutes and hypoxia can easily be avoided by increasing the inspired oxygen concentration.

The alveolar/arterial P_{O_2} difference

The next step in the oxygen cascade is of great clinical relevance. In the healthy young adult breathing air, the alveolar/arterial P_{O_2} difference does not exceed 2 kPa (15 mmHg) but it may rise to above 5 kPa (37.5 mmHg) in aged but healthy subjects. These values may be exceeded in a patient with any lung disease which causes shunting or mismatching of ventilation to perfusion. Typical examples are pulmonary collapse, consolidation, neoplasm or infection. Extrapulmonary shunting (e.g. Fallot's tetralogy) will also increase the difference. An increased alveolar/arterial PO_2 difference is the commonest cause of arterial hypoxaemia in clinical practice and it is therefore a very important step in the oxygen cascade.

Unlike the alveolar PO_2, the alveolar/arterial PO_2 difference cannot be predicted from other more easily measured quantities, and there is no simple means of knowing the magnitude of the alveolar/arterial PO_2 difference in a particular patient other than by measurement of the arterial blood gas tensions. Therefore it is particularly important to understand the factors which influence the difference, and the principles of restoration of arterial PO_2 by increasing the inspired oxygen concentration when hypoxia is due to an increased alveolar/arterial PO_2 difference.

Factors influencing the magnitude of the alveolar/arterial PO_2 difference

In Chapter 8 it was explained how the alveolar/arterial PO_2 difference results from venous admixture (or physiological shunt) which consists of two components: (1) shunted venous blood which mingles with the oxygenated blood leaving the pulmonary capillaries; (2) a component due to scatter of ventilation/perfusion ratios in different parts of the lungs. Any component due to impaired diffusion across the alveolar/capillary membrane is likely to be very small and can probably be ignored (page 206).

Figure 8.9 shows the derivation of the following axiomatic relationship for the first component:

$$\frac{\dot{Q}s}{\dot{Q}t} = \frac{Cc'_{O_2} - Ca_{O_2}}{Cc'_{O_2} - C\bar{v}_{O_2}}$$

Two points should be noted.

1. The equation gives a slightly false impression of precision because it assumes that all the shunted blood has the same oxygen content as mixed venous blood. This is not the case, thebesian and bronchial venous blood being obvious exceptions (see Figure 7.2).
2. Oxygen content of pulmonary end-capillary blood (Cc'_{O_2}) is, in practice, calculated on the basis of the end-capillary oxygen tension (Pc'_{O_2}) being equal to the 'ideal' alveolar PO_2 which is derived by means of the alveolar air equation (see page 195).

The equation may be cleared and solved for the pulmonary end-capillary/arterial oxygen content difference as follows:

$$Cc'_{O_2} - Ca_{O_2} = \frac{\dfrac{\dot{Q}s}{\dot{Q}t}(Ca_{O_2} - C\bar{v}_{O_2})}{\left(1 - \dfrac{\dot{Q}s}{\dot{Q}t}\right)} \qquad \ldots(3)$$

(scaling factors are required to correct for the inconsistency of the units which are customarily used for the quantities in this equation).

$Ca_{O_2} - C\bar{v}_{O_2}$ is the arterial/mixed venous oxygen content difference and is a function of the oxygen consumption and the cardiac output thus:

$$\dot{Q}t(Ca_{O_2} - C\bar{v}_{O_2}) = \dot{V}O_2 \text{ (Fick equation)} \qquad \ldots(4)$$

Substituting for $(Ca_{O_2} - C\bar{v}_{O_2})$ in equation (3), we have:

$$Cc'_{O_2} - Ca_{O_2} = \frac{\dot{V}O_2\dfrac{\dot{Q}s}{\dot{Q}t}}{\dot{Q}t\left(1 - \dfrac{\dot{Q}s}{\dot{Q}t}\right)} \qquad \ldots(5)$$

This equation shows the content difference in terms of oxygen consumption ($\dot{V}O_2$), the venous admixture ($\dot{Q}s/\dot{Q}t$) and the cardiac output ($\dot{Q}t$).

The final stage in the calculation is to convert the end-capillary/arterial oxygen *content* difference to the *tension* difference. The oxygen content of blood is the sum of the oxygen in physical solution and that which is combined with haemoglobin:

$$\text{oxygen content of blood} = \alpha PO_2 + (SO_2 \times [Hb] \times 1.31)$$

where: α is the solubility coefficient of oxygen in blood (not plasma); SO_2 is the saturation, and varies with PO_2 according to the oxygen dissociation curve, which itself is influenced by temperature, pH and base excess (Bohr effect); [Hb] is the haemoglobin concentration (g/dl); 1.31 is the volume of oxygen (ml) which has been found to combine with 1 g of haemoglobin (page 271). Carriage of oxygen in the blood is discussed in detail on pages 269 et seq.

Derivation of the oxygen content from the PO_2 is laborious if due acccount is taken of pH, base excess, temperature and haemoglobin concentration. Derivation of PO_2 from content is even more laborious, as an iterative approach is required. Tables of tension/content relationships are particularly useful and Table 11.1 is an extract from Kelman and Nunn (1968) to show the format and general influence of the several variables.

The principal factors influencing the magnitude of the alveolar/arterial PO_2 difference caused by venous admixture may be summarized as follows.

The magnitude of the venous admixture increases the alveolar/arterial PO_2 difference with direct proportionality for small shunts, although this is lost with larger shunts (Figure 11.8). The resultant effect on arterial PO_2 is shown in Figure 8.10. Different forms of venous admixture are considered on pages 180 et seq.

$\dot{V}/\dot{Q}$ *scatter.* It was explained in Chapter 8 that scatter in ventilation/perfusion ratios produces an alveolar/arterial PO_2 difference for the following reasons.

1. More blood flows through the underventilated overperfused alveoli, and the mixed arterial blood is therefore heavily weighted in the direction of the suboxygenated blood from areas of low $\dot{V}/\dot{Q}$ ratio. The smaller amount of blood flowing through areas of high $\dot{V}/\dot{Q}$ ratio cannot compensate for this (see Figure 8.11).
2. Due to the bend in the dissociation curve around 8 kPa PO_2, the fall in saturation in blood from areas of low $\dot{V}/\dot{Q}$ ratio tends to be greater than the rise in saturation in blood from areas of correspondingly high $\dot{V}/\dot{Q}$ (see Figure 8.12).

Table 11.1 Oxygen content of human blood (ml/100 ml) as a function of PO_2 and other variables

	Haemoglobin concentration (g/dl)		
	10	14	18
PO_2 at pH 7.4, 37°Ch, base excess zero			
6.7 kPa (50 mmHg)	11.99	16.72	21.45
9.3 kPa (70 mmHg)	13.29	18.53	23.76
13.3 kPa (100 mmHg)	13.85	19.27	24.69
20.0 kPa (150 mmHg)	14.20	19.70	25.20
26.7 kPa (200 mmHg)	14.41	19.94	25.47
PO_2 at pH 7.2, 37°C, base excess zero			
6.7 kPa (50 mmHg)	10.45	14.57	18.69
9.3 kPa (70 mmHg)	12.60	17.56	22.52
13.3 kPa (100 mmHg)	13.62	18.94	24.27
20 kPa (150 mmHg)	14.11	19.58	25.04
26.7 kPa (200 mmHg)	14.37	19.87	25.38
PO_2 at pH 7.4, 34°C, base excess zero			
6.7 kPa (50 mmHg)	12.81	17.87	22.93
9.3 kPa (70 mmHg)	13.59	18.94	24.30
13.3 kPa (100 mmHg)	13.96	19.43	24.89
20 kPa (150 mmHg)	14.24	19.76	25.28
26.7 kPa (200 mmHg)	14.44	19.98	25.51

The fourth significant figure is not of clinical importance but is useful for interpolation.
(Values from the computer-written tables of Kelman and Nunn, 1968)

These two reasons in combination explain why blood from alveoli with a high $\dot{V}/\dot{Q}$ ratio cannot compensate for blood from alveoli with a low $\dot{V}/\dot{Q}$ ratio.

The actual alveolar PO_2 has a profound but complex and non-linear effect on the alveolar/arterial PO_2 gradient (see Figure 11.8). The alveolar/arterial oxygen *content* difference for a given shunt is uninfluenced by the alveolar PO_2 (equation 5), and the effect on the *tension* difference arises entirely in conversion from content to tension: it is thus a function of the slope of the dissociation curve at the PO_2 of the alveolar gas. For example, a loss of 1 ml/100 ml of oxygen from blood with a PO_2 of 93 kPa (700 mmHg) causes a fall of PO_2 of about 43 kPa (325 mmHg), most of the oxygen being lost from physical solution. However, if the initial PO_2 were 13 kPa (100 mmHg), a loss of 1 ml/100 ml would cause a fall of PO_2 of only 4.6 kPa (35 mmHg), most of the oxygen being lost from combination with haemoglobin. Should the initial PO_2 be only 6.7 kPa (50 mmHg), a loss of 1 ml/100 ml would cause a very small change in PO_2 of the order of 0.7 kPa (5 mmHg), drawn almost entirely from combination with haemoglobin at a point where the dissociation curve is steep.

The quantitative considerations outlined in the previous paragraph have most important clinical implications. Figure 11.8 clearly shows that, for the same degree of shunt, the alveolar/arterial PO_2 difference will be greatest when the alveolar PO_2 is highest. If the alveolar PO_2 be reduced (e.g. by underventilation), then the alveolar/arterial PO_2 gradient will also be diminished if other factors remain the

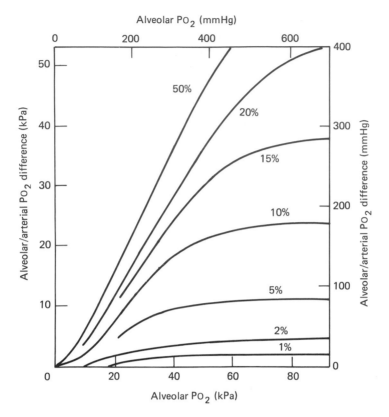

Figure 11.8 Influence of shunt on alveolar/arterial P_{O_2} difference at different levels of alveolar P_{O_2}. For small shunts, the difference (at constant alveolar P_{O_2}) is roughly proportional to the magnitude of the shunt. For a given shunt, the alveolar/arterial P_{O_2} difference increases with alveolar P_{O_2} in non-linear manner governed by the oxygen dissociation curve. At high alveolar P_{O_2}, a plateau of alveolar/arterial P_{O_2} difference is reached but the alveolar P_{O_2} at which the plateau is reached is higher with larger shunts. Note that, with a 50% shunt, an increase in alveolar P_{O_2} produces an almost equal increase in alveolar/arterial P_{O_2} difference. Therefore, the arterial P_{O_2} is virtually independent of changes in alveolar P_{O_2}, if other factors remain constant. Constants incorporated in this diagram: arterial/venous oxygen content differ- ence, 5 ml/100 ml; Hb concentration, 14 g/dl; temperature of blood, 37°C; pH of blood, 7.40; base excess, zero. Figures in the graph indicate shunt as percentage of total pulmonary blood flow.

same. The arterial P_{O_2} thus falls less than the alveolar P_{O_2}. This is fortunate and may be considered as one of the many benefits deriving from the shape of the oxygen dissociation curve. With a 50% venous admixture, changes in the alveolar P_{O_2} are almost exactly equal to the resultant changes in the alveolar/arterial P_{O_2} difference (Figure 11.8). Therefore the arterial P_{O_2} is almost independent of changes in alveolar P_{O_2} and administration of oxygen will do little to relieve cyanosis (see Figure 8.10).

Cardiac output changes have extremely complex effects on the alveolar/arterial P_{O_2} difference. The Fick relationship (equation 4, page 262) tells us that a reduced cardiac output *per se* must increase the arterial/mixed venous oxygen content difference if the oxygen consumption remains the same. This means that the shunted blood will be more desaturated, and will therefore cause a greater decrease in the arterial oxygen level than would less desaturated blood flowing through a shunt of the same magnitude. Equation (5) shows an inverse relationship between the cardiac output and the alveolar/arterial oxygen content difference if the venous admixture is constant (Figure 11.9b). However, when the content difference is converted to tension difference, the relationship to cardiac output is no longer truly inverse, but assumes a complex non-linear form in consequence of the shape of the oxygen dissociation curve. An example of the relationship between cardiac output and alveolar/arterial PO_2 difference is shown in Figure 11.9a but this applies only to the conditions specified, with an alveolar PO_2 of 24 kPa (180 mmHg).

Unfortunately the influence of cardiac output is even more complicated because it has been observed that a reduction in cardiac output is almost always associated with a reduction in the shunt fraction (Cheney and Colley, 1980). Conversely an increase in cardiac output usually results in an increased shunt fraction. This approximately counteracts the effect on mixed venous desaturation, so that arterial

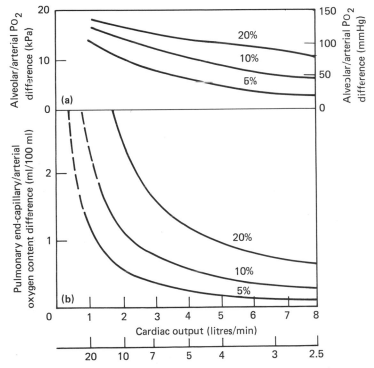

Figure 11.9 Influence of cardiac output on the alveolar/arterial PO_2 difference in the presence of shunts (values indicated for each curve). In this example it is assumed that the patient has an oxygen consumption of 200 ml/min and an alveolar PCO_2 of 24 kPa (180 mmHg). Changes in cardiac output produce an inverse change in the pulmonary end-capillary/arterial oxygen content difference (graph b). When converted to tension differences, the inverse relationship is distorted by the effect of the oxygen dissociation curve in a manner which is applicable only to the particular alveolar PO_2 of the patient (graph a). (Alveolar PO_2 is assumed equal to pulmonary end-capillary PO_2.)

PO$_2$ tends to be relatively little influenced by changes in cardiac output (see Chapter 8, page 181). Nevertheless, it must be remembered that, even if the arterial PO$_2$ is unchanged, the oxygen delivery (flux) will be reduced in proportion to the change in cardiac output.

Temperature, pH and base excess of the patient's blood influence the dissociation curve (page 274). In addition, temperature affects the solubility coefficient of oxygen in blood. Thus all three factors influence the relationship between tension and content (see Table 11.1), and therefore the effect of venous admixture on the alveolar/arterial PO$_2$ difference, although the effect is not usually important except in extreme deviations from normal.

Haemoglobin concentration influences the partition of oxygen between physical solution and chemical combination. While the haemoglobin concentration does not influence the pulmonary end-capillary/arterial oxygen *content* difference (equation 5), it does alter the *tension* difference. An increased haemoglobin concentration causes a small decrease in the alveolar/arterial PO$_2$ difference. Table 11.2 shows an example with a cardiac output of 5 l/min, oxygen consumption of 200 ml/min and a venous admixture of 20%. This would result in a pulmonary end-capillary/arterial oxygen content difference of 0.5 ml/100 ml. Assuming an alveolar PO$_2$ of 24 kPa (180 mmHg), the alveolar/arterial PO$_2$ difference is influenced by haemoglobin concentration as shown in Table 11.2. (Different figures would be obtained by selection of a different value for alveolar PO$_2$.)

Alveolar ventilation. The overall effect of changes in alveolar ventilation on the arterial PO$_2$ presents an interesting problem and serves to illustrate the integration of the separate aspects of the factors discussed above. An increase in the alveolar ventilation may be expected to have the following results.

1. *The alveolar PO$_2$* must be raised provided the barometric pressure, inspired oxygen concentration and oxygen consumption remain the same (equation 1 on page 257 and Figure 11.6).
2. *The alveolar/arterial PO$_2$ difference* is increased for the following reasons.
   a. The increase in the alveolar PO$_2$ will increase the alveolar/arterial PO$_2$ difference if other factors remain the same (see Figure 11.8).

Table 11.2 Effect of different haemoglobin concentrations on the arterial Po$_2$ under venous admixture conditions defined in text

Haemoglobin concentration	Alveolar/arterial Po$_2$ difference		Arterial Po$_2$	
(g/dl)	*kPa*	*mmHg*	*kPa*	*mmHg*
8	15.0	113	9.0	67
10	14.5	109	9.5	71
12	14.0	105	10.0	75
14	13.5	101	10.5	79
16	13.0	98	11.0	82

b. Under many conditions it has been demonstrated that a fall of P_{CO_2} (resulting from an increase in alveolar ventilation) reduces the cardiac output, with the consequent changes which have been outlined above.

c. The change in arterial pH resulting from the reduction in P_{CO_2} causes a small, unimportant increase in alveolar/arterial P_{O_2} difference.

Thus an increase in alveolar ventilation may be expected to increase both the alveolar P_{O_2} and the alveolar/arterial P_{O_2} difference. The resultant change in arterial P_{O_2} will depend upon the relative magnitude of the two changes. Figure 11.10 shows the changes in arterial P_{O_2} caused by variations of alveolar ventilation at an inspired oxygen concentration of 30% in the presence of varying degrees of venous admixture, assuming that cardiac output is influenced by P_{CO_2} as described in the legend. Up to an alveolar ventilation of 1.5 l/min, an increase in ventilation will always raise the arterial P_{O_2}. Beyond that, in the example cited, further increases in alveolar ventilation will increase the arterial P_{O_2} only if the venous admixture is less than 3%. For larger values of venous admixture, the increase in the alveolar/arterial P_{O_2} difference exceeds the increase in the alveolar P_{O_2} and the arterial P_{O_2} is thus decreased.

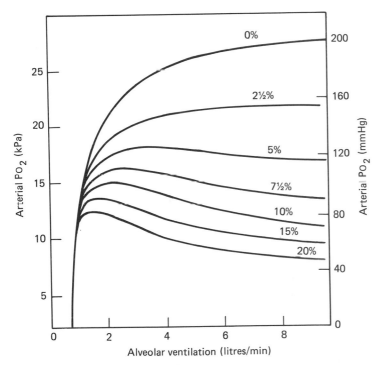

Figure 11.10 The effect of alveolar ventilation on arterial P_{O_2} is the algebraic sum of the effect upon the alveolar P_{O_2} (Figure 11.6) and the consequent change in alveolar/arterial P_{O_2} difference (Figure 11.8). When the increase in the latter exceeds the increase in the former, the arterial P_{O_2} will be diminished. The figures in the diagram indicate the percentage venous admixture. The curve corresponding to 0% venous admixture will indicate the alveolar P_{O_2}. Constants incorporated in the design of this figure: inspired O_2 concentration, 30%; O_2 consumption, 200 ml/min; respiratory exchange ratio, 0.8. It has been assumed that the cardiac output is influenced by the P_{CO_2} according to the equation: $\dot{Q} = 0.039 \times P_{CO_2}$ (mmHg) + 2.23. (Reproduced from Kelman and his colleagues (1967) by permission of the Editor of the British Journal of Anaesthesia)

Compensation for increased alveolar/arterial P_{O_2} difference by raising the inspired oxygen concentration

Many patients with severe respiratory dysfunction are hypoxaemic while breathing air. The main objective of treatment is clearly to remove the cause of the hypoxaemia but, when this is not immediately possible, it is often possible to relieve the hypoxaemia by increasing the inspired oxygen concentration. The principles for doing so depend upon the cause of the hypoxaemia. As a broad classification, hypoxaemia may be due to hypoventilation or to venous admixture or to a combination of the two. When hypoxaemia is primarily due to hypoventilation, and when it is not appropriate or possible to restore the normal ventilation, then the arterial P_{O_2} can usually be restored by elevation of the inspired oxygen within the range 21–30% as explained above (page 257 and Figure 11.6) and also in Chapter 21 (pages 427 et seq.).

Quantitatively, the situation is entirely different when hypoxaemia is primarily due to venous admixture. It is then only possible to restore the arterial P_{O_2} by oxygen enrichment of the inspired gas when the venous admixture does not exceed the equivalent of a shunt of 30% of the cardiac output, and this may require up to 100% inspired oxygen (page 183). The quantitative aspects of the relationship are best considered in relation to the iso-shunt diagram (see Figure 8.10).

Selection of the optimal arterial P_{O_2} is important to prevent hypoxia on the one hand and pulmonary oxygen toxicity on the other (see Chapter 32). In general, one is reluctant to use concentrations higher than 60–70% for more than a short period. This is sufficient to restore arterial P_{O_2} only when the shunt is less than about 22%, and it is therefore important to ensure that pulmonary function is optimized by careful attention to control of secretions, infection and expansion of areas of collapse. Positive end-expiratory pressure is a particularly valuable method of decreasing the virtual shunt (see page 451).

There is little point in deciding what is the optimal inspired oxygen concentration unless efficient means are available for delivery of the selected oxygen concentration to the patient. This important topic is considered below (page 290).

The 'normal' arterial oxygen tension

In contrast to the arterial P_{CO_2}, the arterial P_{O_2} shows a progressive decrease with age. Marshall and Whyche (1972) analysed 12 studies of healthy subjects and from the pooled results suggested the following relationship in subjects breathing air:

$$\text{mean arterial } P_{O_2} = 13.6 - 0.044 \text{ (age in years) kPa}$$

or $102 - 0.33$ (age in years) mmHg

About this regression line there are 95% confidence limits (2 s.d.) of ± 1.33 kPa (10 mmHg) (Table 11.3). Five per cent of normal patients will lie outside these limits and it is therefore preferable to refer to this as the reference range rather than the normal range.

It seems likely that some of the scatter of values for P_{O_2} is due to transient changes in ventilation, perhaps associated with arterial puncture. Because of the meagre body oxygen stores, such changes have a greater effect on P_{O_2} than on P_{CO_2}.

Table 11.3 Normal values for arterial Po₂

| Age (years) | Mean and range | |
	kPa	mmHg
20–29	12.5 (11.2–13.9)	94 (84–104)
30–39	12.1 (10.8–13.5)	91 (81–101)
40–49	11.7 (10.4–13.1)	88 (78–98)
50–59	11.2 (9.9–12.5)	84 (74–94)
60–69	10.8 (9.5–12.1)	81 (71–91)

When breathing oxygen the most important factor causing scatter of values for arterial Po₂ is failure to exclude air from the breathing system. Provided that great care is taken to prevent dilution with air, very high values of arterial Po₂ may be obtained in the healthy subject. A number of studies of normal conscious subjects were reviewed by Raine and Bishop (1963) and by Laver and Seifen (1965). Mean values for arterial Po₂ in these studies range from 80 to 86.7 kPa (600 to 650 mmHg), but individual values range from 73.3 kPa (550 mmHg) to values which are (no doubt erroneously) in excess of the alveolar Po₂.

Reports of 'abnormalities' of oxygenation must be interpreted against the high degree of scatter in normal subjects under normal conditions.

The carriage of oxygen in the blood

The preceding sections have considered at some length the factors which influence the Po₂ of the arterial blood and the normal values which may be expected. It is now necessary to consider how oxygen is carried in the blood and, in particular, the relationship between the Po₂ and the quantity of oxygen which is carried. The latter is crucially important to the delivery of oxygen and is no less important than the partial pressure at which it becomes available to the tissue. The all-important quantitative aspects of oxygen delivery are considered on pages 283 and 477.

Oxygen is carried in the blood in two forms. Much the greater part is in reversible chemical combination with haemoglobin, while a smaller part is in physical solution in plasma and intracellular fluid. The ability to carry large quantities of oxygen in the blood is of great importance to the organism. Without haemoglobin the amount carried would be so small that the cardiac output would need to be increased by a factor of about 20 to give an adequate delivery of oxygen. Under such a handicap, animals could not have developed to their present extent. The biological significance of the haemoglobin-like compounds is thus immense. It is interesting that the tetrapyrrole ring which contains iron in haemoglobin is also a constituent of chlorophyll which has magnesium in place of iron. The cytochromes also have iron in a tetrapyrrole ring and this structure is thus concerned with production, transport and utilization of oxygen.

Haemoglobin

Haemoglobin was the subject of many years of detailed X-ray crystallographic analysis by the team led by Perutz in Cambridge. Its structure is now well understood and this provides the molecular basis for its remarkable properties (Roughton, 1964; Lehmann and Huntsman, 1966; Perutz, 1969).

The haemoglobin molecule consists of four protein chains, each of which carries a haem group (Figure 11.11a, the total molecular weight being 64 458.5 (Braunitzer, 1963). The amino acids comprising the chains have been identified and it is known that, in the commonest type of adult human haemoglobin (HbA), there are

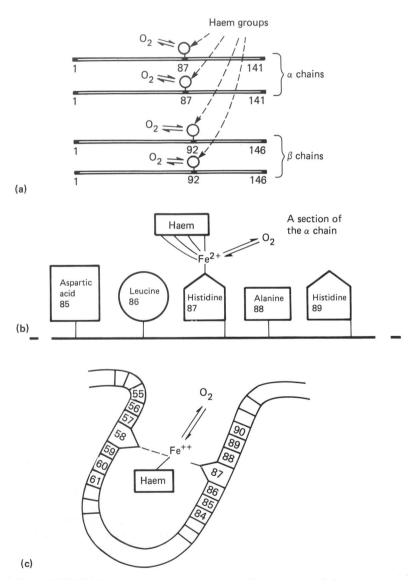

(a)

(b)

(c)

Figure 11.11 The haemoglobin molecule consists of four amino acid chains, each carrying a haem group. (a) Two chains are identical, each with 141 amino acid residues (alpha chains); the other two are also identical and have 146 amino acid residues (beta chains). (b) The attachment of the haem group to the alpha chain. (c) The crevice which contains the haem group.

two types of chain, two of each occurring in each molecule. The two alpha chains each have 141 amino acid residues, with the haem attached to a histidine residue (formula on page 226) occupying position 87. The two beta chains each have 146 amino acid residues, with the haem attached to a histidine residue occupying position 92. Figure 11.11b shows details of the point of attachment of the haem in the alpha chain. Similar information for the 'beta' chain is given on page 226.

The four chains of the haemoglobin molecule lie in a ball like a crumpled necklace. However, the form is not random and the actual shape (the quaternary structure) is of critical importance and governs the reaction with oxygen. The shape is maintained by loose bonds between certain amino acids on different chains and also between some amino acids on the same chain. One consequence of these bonds is that the haem groups lie in crevices formed by weak bonds between the haem groups and histidine residues, other than those to which they are attached by normal valency linkages. For example, Figure 11.11c shows a section of an alpha chain with the haem group attached to the iron atom which is bound to the histidine residue in position 87. However, the haem group is also attached by a loose bond to the histidine residue in position 58 and also by non-polar bonds to many other amino acids. This forms a loop and places the haem group in a crevice which limits and controls the ease of access for oxygen molecules.

Structural basis of the Bohr effect (page 274). The precise shape of the haemoglobin molecules is altered by factors which influence the strength of the loose bonds; such factors include temperature, pH, ionic strength and carbon dioxide binding to the *N*-terminal amino acid residues as carbamate (Kilmartin and Rossi-Bernardi, 1973). This alters the accessibility of the haem groups to oxygen and is believed to be the basis of the mechanism by which the affinity of haemoglobin for oxygen is altered by these factors, an effect which is generally considered in terms of its influence upon the dissociation curve (see Figure 11.14 below).

Structural basis of the Haldane effect (page 223). The quaternary structure of the haemoglobin molecule is also altered by the uptake of oxygen to form oxyhaemoglobin. It is believed that this increases the ionization of certain $-NH_2$ or $=NH$ groups and so reduces their ability to undertake carbamino carriage of carbon dioxide (see Figure 10.1).

Oxygen-combining capacity of haemoglobin. There is still confusion over the oxygen-combining capacity of haemoglobin. Until 1963 the value was taken to be 1.34 ml/g. Following the precise determination of the molecular weight of haemoglobin, the theoretical value of 1.39 ml/g was derived and passed into general use. However, it gradually became clear that this value was not obtained when direct measurements of haemoglobin concentration and oxygen capacity were compared. After an exhaustive study of the subject, Gregory (1974) proposed the values of 1.306 ml/g for human adult blood and 1.312 ml/g for fetal blood. Haemoglobin concentrations are ultimately compared with the International Cyan-methaemoglobin Standard, which is based on iron content and not on oxygen-combining capacity. Since some of the iron is likely to be in the form of haemochromogens, it is not altogether surprising that the observed oxygen-combining capacity is less than the theoretical value of 1.39.

Kinetics of the reaction of oxygen with haemoglobin

In 1925, Adair first proposed that the oxidation of haemoglobin proceeds in four separate stages. If the whole haemoglobin molecule, with its four haem groups, is designated as 'Hb$_4$', the reactions may be presented as follows:

$$\text{Hb}_4 + \text{O}_2 \underset{k_1}{\overset{k_1'}{\rightleftharpoons}} \text{Hb}_4\text{O}_2 \qquad K_1 = \frac{k_1'}{k_1}$$

$$\text{Hb}_4\text{O}_2 + \text{O}_2 \underset{k_2}{\overset{k_2'}{\rightleftharpoons}} \text{Hb}_4\text{O}_4 \qquad K_2 = \frac{k_2'}{k_2}$$

$$\text{Hb}_4\text{O}_4 + \text{O}_2 \underset{k_3}{\overset{k_3'}{\rightleftharpoons}} \text{Hb}_4\text{O}_6 \qquad K_3 = \frac{k_3'}{k_3}$$

$$\text{Hb}_4\text{O}_6 + \text{O}_2 \underset{k_4}{\overset{k_4'}{\rightleftharpoons}} \text{Hb}_4\text{O}_8 \qquad K_4 = \frac{k_4'}{k_4}$$

The velocity constant of each dissociation is indicated by a small k, while the addition of a prime ($'$) indicates the velocity constant of the corresponding forward reaction. k_3' is thus the velocity constant of the reaction of Hb$_4$O$_4$ with O$_2$ to yield Hb$_4$O$_6$. The ratio of the forward velocity constant to the reverse velocity constant equals the equilibrium constant of each reaction in the series (represented by capital K).

The separate velocity constants have been measured and it is now known that the last reaction has a forward velocity constant (k_4') which is much higher then that of the other reactions. During the saturation of the last 75% of reduced haemoglobin, the last reaction will predominate and the high velocity constant counteracts the effect of the ever-diminishing number of oxygen receptors which would otherwise slow the reaction rate by the law of mass action (Staub, Bishop and Forster, 1961). In fact, the reaction proceeds at much the same rate until saturation is completed. The significance of this to oxygen transfer in the lung was presented by Staub (1963a), and its importance in the concept of 'diffusing capacity' is discussed on page 205.

The velocity of the dissociation of oxyhaemoglobin is somewhat slower than its formation. The velocity constant of the combination of carbon monoxide with haemoglobin is of the same order, but the rate of dissociation of carboxyhaemoglobin is extremely slow by comparison.

The oxyhaemoglobin dissociation curve

The relationship between Po$_2$ and percentage saturation of haemoglobin with oxygen is non-linear and the precise form of the non-linearity is of fundamental biological importance. It is shown, under standard conditions, in graphical form for adult and fetal haemoglobin and also for myoglobin and carboxyhaemoglobin in Figure 11.12. It is displayed as a line chart in Figure 11.13.

Equations to represent the dissociation curve. Adair (1925) was the first to develop an equation which would reproduce the observed oxygen dissociation curve. This was modified by Kelman (1966) who used seven coefficients, each determined to eight significant figures. His equation generates a curve indistinguishable from the

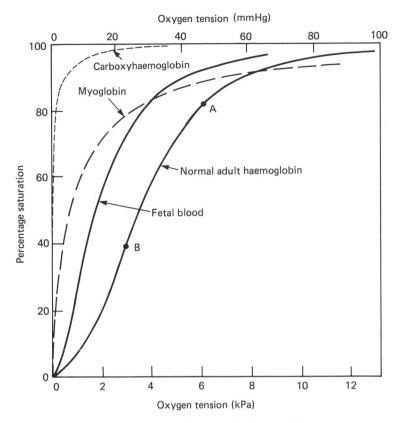

Figure 11.12 Dissociation curves of normal adult haemoglobin compared with fetal blood. Curves for myoglobin and carboxyhaemoglobin are shown for comparison. Note: (1) Fetal blood is adapted to operate at a lower Po_2 than adult blood. (2) Myoglobin approaches full saturation of Po_2 levels pertaining in voluntary muscle 2–4 kPa (15–30 mmHg); the bulk of its oxygen can be released only at very low oxygen tension. (3) Carboxyhaemoglobin can be dissociated only by the maintenance of very low levels of Pco_2. After birth, fetal haemoglobin is progressively replaced with adult haemoglobin and the dissociation curve gradually moves across to the position of the adult curve. In a patient with a normal circulation and haemoglobin concentration, point A represents serious hypoxia which requires urgent treatment. Arterial blood corresponding to point B is at the threshold of loss of consciousness from hypoxia.

true curve above a Po_2 of about 1 kPa (7.5 mm Hg) and this has remained the standard. Saturation may be conveniently determined from Po_2 by a computer subroutine but calculation of Po_2 from saturation requires an iterative approach. Severinghaus, Stafford and Thunstrom (1978) have described the following equation which is far more convenient to use, and agrees well with the Kelman equation at Po_2 values above 4 kPa (30 mmHg):

$$So_2 = \frac{100(Po_2^3 + 2.667 \times Po_2)}{Po_2^3 + 2.667 \times Po_2 + 55.47}$$

(Po_2 values are here in kilopascals; sat. is %)

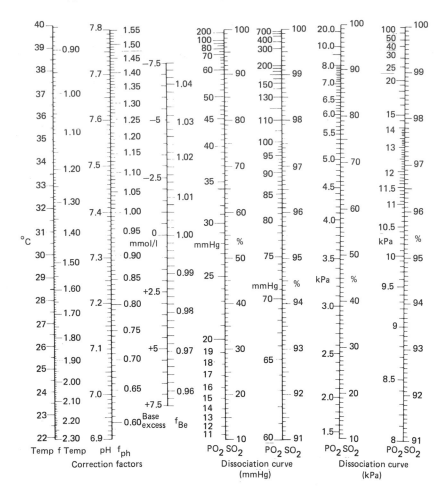

Figure 11.13 The standard oxyhaemoglobin dissociation curve with factors which displace it. The two right-hand line charts give corresponding values of P_{O_2} and saturation for standard conditions (temperature, 37°C; pH, 7.40; base excess, zero). The remaining lines indicate the factors by which the actual measured P_{O_2} should be multiplied before entering the standard dissociation curve to determine the saturation. When more than one factor is required, they should be multiplied together as in the example given in the text. (Reproduced from Kelman and Nunn (1966b) by permission of the Editor of the Journal of Applied Physiology, *modified in accord with data of Roughton and Severinghaus (1973) and with the addition of kPa scales)*

Displacement of the dissociation curve by the Bohr effect. Various factors displace the dissociation curve sideways, and the familiar effect of pH (the Bohr effect) is shown in Figure 11.14. Shifts may be defined as the ratio of the P_{O_2} which produces a particular saturation under standard conditions, to the P_{O_2} which produces the same saturation with a particular shift of the curve. Standard conditions include pH 7.4, temperature 37°C and zero base excess. In Figure 11.14, a saturation of 80% is produced by P_{O_2} 6 kPa (45 mmHg) at pH 7.4 (standard). At pH 7.0 the P_{O_2} required for 80% saturation is 9.4 kPa (70.5 mmHg). The ratio is 0.64 and this

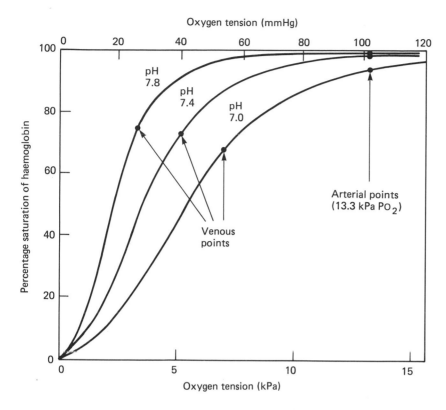

Figure 11.14 The Bohr effect and its effect upon oxygen tension. The centre curve is the normal curve under standard conditions; the other two curves shows the displacement caused by the indicated changes in pH, other factors remaining constant. The venous points have been determined on the basis of a fixed arterial/venous oxygen saturation difference of 25% in each case. They are thus 25% saturation less than the corresponding arterial saturation which is equivalent to a Po_2 of 13.3 kPa (100 mmHg) in each case. Under the conditions shown, alkalosis lowers venous Po_2 and acidosis raises venous Po_2. This effect is reversed in severe arterial hypoxaemia. Tissue Po_2 is related to venous Po_2. Temperature, 37°C; base excess, zero.

applies to all saturations at pH 7.0. The ratio is indicated on the line chart in Figure 11.13, which also shows the ratios (or correction factors) for different values of temperature and base excess.

Since the effects of temperature, pH and base excess are all similar, their influence on the dissociation curve may be considered simultaneously. The usual practice is to derive a factor for the influence of each and then to multiply them together. This combined factor is then multiplied by the observed Po_2 to give the apparent Po_2 which may be entered into the standard dissociation curve to indicate the saturation. The factors may be determined from the line charts in Figure 11.13; its use is illustrated by the following example.

	Factor
Blood temperature 33.7°C	1.20
Blood pH 7.08	0.70

Blood base excess -7 mmol/l	1.04
Combined factor $= 1.20 \times 0.70 \times 1.04 =$	0.87
Observed $P_{O_2} =$	9.3 kPa (70 mmHg)
Apparent $P_{O_2} =$ observed $P_{O_2} \times 0.87 \ =$	8.1 kPa (61 mmHg)
Calculated saturation (from line chart) $=$	91.3%

This calculation may be expeditiously performed on the slide rule as described by Severinghaus (1966). The factors are also incorporated in the digital computer subroutine described by Kelman (1966) and feature in the tables produced by Kelman and Nunn (1968).

A convenient approach to quantifying a shift of the dissociation curve is to indicate the P_{O_2} required for 50% saturation. This is known as the P_{50} and, under the standard conditions shown in Figure 11.13, is 3.5 kPa (26.6 mmHg). This is the usual method of reporting shift of the dissociation curve.

Clinical significance of the Bohr effect. The important effect is on tissue P_{O_2}, and the consequences of a shift in the dissociation curve are not intuitively obvious. It is essential to think quantitatively. For example, a shift to the right (caused by low pH) impairs oxygenation in the lungs but aids release of oxygen in the tissue. Do these effects in combination increase or decrease tissue P_{O_2}? An illustrative example is set out in Figure 11.14. The arterial P_{O_2} is assumed to be 13.3 kPa (100 mmHg) and arterial saturation is decreased by a reduction of pH. However, the effect is relatively small at normal arterial P_{O_2}, unless the pH falls to extremely low values as in a case reported by Prys-Roberts, Smith and Nunn (1967).

At the venous point the position is quite different, and the examples in Figure 11.14 show the venous oxygen tensions to be very markedly affected. Assuming that the arterial/venous oxygen saturation difference is constant at 25% it will be seen that at low pH the venous P_{O_2} is raised to 6.9 kPa (52 mmHg), while at high pH the venous P_{O_2} is reduced to 3.5 kPa (26 mmHg). This is important as the tissue P_{O_2} is closer to the venous P_{O_2} than to the arterial P_{O_2}. Thus, in the example shown, the shift to the right is beneficial. It should also be stressed that acidosis is likely to increase perfusion, particularly cerebral blood flow, and this will further increase tissue and venous P_{O_2}. Therefore, far from being universally harmful as is so often assumed, respiratory acidosis will usually increase the tissue P_{O_2}, particularly in the brain.

It is a general rule that a shift to the right (increased P_{50}) will benefit venous P_{O_2}, provided that the arterial P_{O_2} is not critically reduced. Below an arterial P_{O_2} of about 5 kPa (38 mmHg), the arterial point is on the steep part of the dissociation curve, and the deficiency in oxygenation of the arterial blood would outweigh the improved off-loading of oxygen in the tissues. Thus, with severe arterial hypoxaemia, the venous P_{O_2} would tend to be reduced by a shift to the right and a *leftward* shift would then be advantageous. It is therefore of great interest that a spontaneous leftward shift occurs at extreme altitude when arterial P_{O_2} is critically reduced (see below).

Other factors which shift the dissociation curve. In addition to the well known effects of pH, P_{CO_2} and temperature, described above, certain abnormal haemoglobins (such as San Diego and Chesapeake) have a high P_{50} while others (such as sickle and Kansas) have a low P_{50}. In 1967 it was found independently by Benesch and Benesch and by Chanutin and Curnish that the presence of certain organic phosphates in the erythrocyte has a pronounced effect on the P_{50}. The most important of these compounds is 2,3-diphosphoglycerate (2,3-DPG), one molecule of which is able to bind preferentially to the beta chains of one tetramer of deoxyhaemoglobin, resulting in a conformational change which reduces oxygen affinity (Arnone, 1972). The percentage occupancy of the 2,3-DPG binding sites governs the overall P_{50} of a blood sample within the range 2–4.5 kPa (15–34 mmHg).

2,3-DPG is formed in the Rapoport–Luebering shunt off the glycolytic pathway (see Figure 11.3) and its level is determined by the balance between synthesis and degradation (Figure 11.15). Activity of DPG mutase is enhanced and DPG phosphatase diminished at high pH which thus increases the level of 2,3-DPG.

The relationship between 2,3-DPG levels and P_{50} suggested that 2,3-DPG levels would have a most important bearing on clinical practice and therefore much research effort was devoted to determining those conditions which might result in substantial changes in 2,3-DPG levels.

Storage of bank blood with acid–citrate–dextrose (ACD) preservative results in depletion of all 2,3-DPG within the usual period of 3 weeks' storage, P_{50} being reduced to about 2 kPa (15 mmHg) (McConn and Derrick, 1972). A massive transfusion of old blood therefore shifts the patient's dissociation curve to the left but restoration is usually well advanced within a few hours (see review by Valeri, 1975). Changes in P_{50} of a patient do not usually exceed 0.5 kPa (3.8 mmHg). Storage of blood with citrate–phosphate–dextrose (CPD) substantially reduces the rate of 2,3-DPG depletion (Shafer et al., 1971).

Anaemia results in a raised 2,3-DPG level, with P_{50} of the order of 0.5 kPa (3.8 mmHg) higher than control levels (Torrance et al., 1970). This must raise the partial pressure of oxygen at its point of delivery to the tissues, and supplements the effect of increased tissue perfusion. The problem of oxygen delivery in anaemia is considered in Chapter 25.

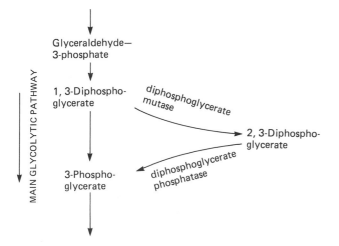

Figure 11.15 Rapoport–Luebering shunt for synthesis of 2,3-diphosphoglycerate.

Altitude. There is good evidence of an increased red cell concentration of 2,3-DPG at altitude (Ward, Milledge and West, 1989). However, there is a progressive respiratory alkalosis with increasing altitude, which has an opposite and much more pronounced effect on displacement of the dissociation curve. There is now a firm consensus that there is a *leftward* displacement at high altitude, which plays a major role in survival when the environmental PO_2 is critically reduced (see Chapter 15).

Ventilatory failure does not appear to cause any significant change in either 2,3-DPG levels or the P_{50}. Fairweather, Walker and Flenley (1974) and Flenley et al. (1975) studied a total of 71 patients with arterial PCO_2 ranging from 6.7 to 10.7 kPa (50 to 80 mmHg) and PO_2 4.3–8.7 kPa (32–65 mmHg). P_{50} values (at pH 7.4) ranged from 3 to 4 kPa (22.5–30 mmHg) and did not appear to differ from the normal value by more than the experimental error of determination. 2,3-DPG levels were widely scattered about the normal value.

Haemorrhagic and endotoxic shock do not appear to be associated with any significant changes of 2,3-DPG or 2,3-DPG-mediated changes in P_{50} (Naylor et al., 1972).

In general it may be said that subsequent research has failed to substantiate the earlier suggestions that 2,3-DPG was of major importance in clinical problems of oxygen delivery. In fact, the likely effects of changes in P_{50} mediated by 2,3-DPG seem to be of marginal significance in comparison with changes in arterial PO_2, acid–base balance and tissue perfusion. Similarly, there has been little application of the suggestions that drug-induced shifts of the dissociation curve would have a major therapeutic role. A valuable review of the subject was presented in its heyday by Shappell and Lenfant (1972).

Binding of anaesthetics to haemoglobin. It has long been known that anaesthetics bind to haemoglobin and this accounts for a substantial part of their carriage in blood (Featherstone et al., 1961). Barker et al. (1975) identified specific changes in the nuclear magnetic resonance spectrum for haemoglobin in equilibrium with halothane, methoxyflurane and diethyl ether, suggesting different binding sites for each agent. It is clearly a possibility that hydrophobic binding of anaesthetics, or indeed other compounds, to haemoglobin might result in a conformational change which would alter the P_{50}, and certain preliminary reports sugested this possibility. However, a series of carefully controlled studies have established that, even with high concentrations of methoxyflurane, halothane, enflurane, cyclopropane and nitrous oxide, there is no significant change in P_{50} (Cohen and Behar, 1970; Millar, Beard and Hulands, 1971; Weiskopf, Nishimura and Severinghaus, 1971; Lanza, Mercadante and Pignataro, 1988).

Carbon monoxide. The effect of carbon monoxide on the affinity of reduced haemoglobin for oxygen is considered below (page 279 and Figure 11.16).

Abnormal forms of haemoglobin

There are a great number of alternative amino acid sequences in the haemoglobin molecule. Most animal species have their own peculiar haemoglobins while, in man, gamma and delta chains occur in addition to the alpha and beta monomers already mentioned. Gamma and delta chains occur normally in combination with alpha chains. The combination of two gamma chains with two alpha chains constitutes fetal haemoglobin (HbF), which has a dissociation curve well to the left of adult haemoglobin (Figure 11.12). The combination of two delta chains with two alpha chains constitutes A_2 haemoglobin (HbA$_2$), which forms 2% of the total haemoglobin in normal adults. Other variations in the amino acid chains can be considered abnormal, and a large number have been reported and named. Many are associated with disordered oxygen carriage or impaired solubility.

Sickle cell anaemia is caused by the presence of HbS in which valine replaces glutamic acid in position 6 on the beta chains. This apparently trivial substitution is sufficient to cause critical loss of solubility of reduced haemoglobin. It is a hereditary condition and in the homozygous state is a grave abnormality.

Thalassaemia is another hereditary disorder of haemoglobin. It consists of a suppression of formation of HbA with a compensatory production of fetal haemoglobin (HbF), which persists throughout life instead of falling to low levels after birth. The functional disorder thus includes a shift of the dissociation curve to the left (Figure 11.12).

Methaemoglobin consists of haemoglobin in which the iron has assumed the trivalent ferric form. Methaemoglobin is unable to combine with oxygen but is slowly reconverted to haemoglobin in the normal subject by the action of enzymes which are deficient in familial methaemoglobinaemia (Lehmann and Huntsman, 1966). Alternatively, conversion may be brought about by reducing agents such as ascorbic acid or methylene blue. The nitrite ion is a potent cause of methaemoglobin formation and is a major factor in poisoning by higher oxides of nitrogen (see symposium in the May 1967 issue of *British Journal of Anaesthesia*). Conversely, haemoglobin provides a potent mechanism for scavenging nitric oxide in its probable role as the endothelium-derived relaxing factor (see page 311). Methaemoglobin and sulphaemoglobin are a brownish colour and produce a slate-grey colouring of the patient which may be confused with cyanosis.

Abnormal ligands

The iron in haemoglobin is able to combine with other inorganic molecules apart from oxygen. The compounds so formed are, in general, more stable than oxyhaemoglobin and therefore block the combination of haemoglobin with oxygen. The most important of these abnormal compounds is carboxyhaemoglobin but ligands may also be formed with nitric oxide, cyanide, ammonia and a number of other substances. Apart from the loss of oxygen-carrying power, there is often a shift of the dissociation curve to the left (see below), so that the remaining oxygen is released only at lower tensions of oxygen. This may cause tissue hypoxia when the arterial PO$_2$ and oxygen content would otherwise appear to be at a safe level.

Carbon monoxide in combination with haemoglobin. Carbon monoxide is well known to displace oxygen from combination with haemoglobin, the affinity being approximately 300 times greater than the affinity for oxygen (see above). However, the presence of carboxyhaemoglobin also causes a leftward shift of the dissociation curve of the remaining oxyhaemoglobin (Roughton and Darling, 1944), partly mediated by a reduction in 2,3-DPG levels. This is conveniently shown on a plot of

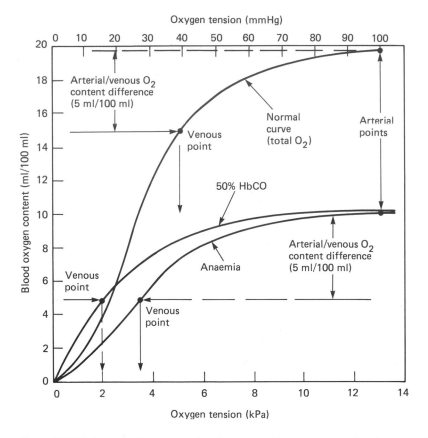

Figure 11.16 Influences of anaemia and carbon monoxide poisoning on the relationship between oxygen tension and content. The normal curve is constructed for a haemoglobin concentration of 14.4 g/dl. Assuming an arterial/venous oxygen content difference of 5 ml/100 ml, the venous P_{O_2} is about 5.3 kPa (40 mmHg). The curve of anaemic blood is constructed for a haemoglobin concentration of 7.2 g/dl. If the arterial/venous oxygen content difference remains unchanged, the venous P_{O_2} will fall to 3.6 kPa (27 mmHg), a level which is low but not dangerously so. The curve of 50% carboxyhaemoglobin is based on a total haemoglobin (incl. carboxyhaemoglobin) of 14.4 g/dl. The curve is interplotted from Roughton (1964). Assuming an arterial/venous oxygen content difference of 5 ml/100 ml, the venous P_{O_2} is only 1.9 kPa (14 mmHg), a level which is dangerously low as it must be associated with a greatly reduced tissue P_{O_2}. Arterial P_{O_2} is assumed to be 13.3 kPa (100 mmHg) in all cases.

oxygen content against P_{O_2} (Figure 11.16), the values on the ordinate being the sum of dissolved and combined oxygen. The upper curve is for the normal concentration of haemoglobin without carbon monoxide. The lowest of the three curves applies to a patient with haemoglobin at half the normal concentration. At each P_{O_2}, the oxygen content is approximately half that of the patient with a normal concentration of haemoglobin. The intermediate curve applies to blood with normal total haemoglobin concentration, but with half of the haemoglobin bound to carbon monoxide. This has the dual effect of halving the bound oxygen capacity and also displacing the dissociation curve of the remaining haemoglobin to the left. It will be seen that, in comparison with the anaemic blood, the displacement of the curve has little effect on the oxygen content of the arterial blood, provided that it is in excess of about 8 kPa (60 mmHg). However, the effect on the venous PO_2, after unloading of oxygen in the tissues, is very great. Assuming an arterial PO_2 of 13.3 kPa (100 mmHg) and an arterial venous oxygen content difference of 5 ml/100 ml, the venous points are as follows:

Normal haemoglobin concentration	5.3 kPa (40 mmHg)
Half normal haemoglobin concentration	3.6 kPa (27 mmHg)
50% carboxyhacmoglobin	1.9 kPa (14 mmHg)

The disappearance of coal gas from domestic use in many countries has decreased the popularity of carbon monoxide for attempted suicide. However, carbon monoxide is still to be found in the blood of patients, in trace concentrations as a result of its production in the body, but mainly as a result of the internal combustion engine and smoking. Jones, Commins and Cernik (1972) reported levels of 0.4–9.7% in London taxi drivers but the highest level in a non-smoking driver was 3.0%. Levels up to 10% of carboxyhaemoglobin were also found in smokers by Castleden and Cole (1974). Maternal smoking results in appreciable levels of carboxyhaemoglobin in fetal blood (Longo, 1970), and smoking prior to blood donation may result in levels of carboxyhaemoglobin up to 10% in the blood. This level appears to persist throughout the usual 3 weeks of storage (Millar and Gregory, 1972). Smoking is considered in Chapter 19.

Physical solution of oxygen in blood

In addition to combination with haemoglobin, oxygen is carried in physical solution in both erythrocytes and plasma. There does not appear to have been any recent determination of the solubility coefficient, and we tend to rely on earlier studies indicating that the amount carried in normal blood in solution at 37°C is about 0.0225 ml/dl per kPa or 0.003/dl per mmHg. At normal arterial PO_2, the oxygen in physical solution is thus about 0.25–0.3 ml/dl or rather more than 1% of the total oxygen carried in all forms. However, when breathing 100% oxygen, the level rises to about 2 ml/dl. Breathing 100% oxygen at 3 atmospheres pressure absolute (303 kPa), the amount of oxygen in physical solution rises to about 6 ml/dl, which is sufficient for the arteriovenous extraction. The amount of oxygen in physical solution rises with decreasing temperature for the same PO_2.

Physical solution in artificial blood substitutes

There are obvious military and civilian advantages in the provision of an artificial haemoglobin substitute, which would carry oxygen in a synthetic fluid to be used instead of blood.

Fluorocarbons. Oxygen is highly soluble in these hydrophobic compounds, which are above the critical molecular size to act as anaesthetics (Faithfull, 1987). Fluosol DA20 is a 20% emulsion, which will carry about 5 ml of oxygen per 100 ml on equilibration with 100% oxygen. The use of fluorocarbons thus requires the patient to breathe a very high concentration of oxygen, which will just provide sufficient oxygen in physical solution to satisfy the normal mean arteriovenous extraction of 5 ml/dl. Since oxygen is in physical solution in fluorocarbons, its 'dissociation curve' is a straight line, with PO_2 directly proportional to the quantity of dissolved oxygen.

If, for example, the arterial PO_2 is 80 kPa (600 mmHg) and half of the oxygen is extracted in the systemic circulation, the mixed venous PO_2 would be 40 kPa (300 mmHg). Even with 90% extraction, mixed venous PO_2 would still be well above the normal mixed venous level. When fluorocarbons function alongside the recipient's remaining blood, the overall relationship between tension and content would depend upon their relative proportions.

Fluorocarbons dissolve gases solely in accord with their solubility coefficients. Thus there is no preferential bonding to carbon monoxide, and nitrogen is effectively removed in bends. However, they are cleared from the circulation into the reticuloendothelial system, particularly in the liver. Being volatile they are eventually cleared through the lungs.

Fluosol DA20 will sustain life in animals which are virtually free of erythrocytes. However, experience at the maximum permitted dose (only 40 ml/kg), in grossly anaemic patients who were unwilling to receive transfusion, has been less satisfactory. Perfluoroctobromide has five times the oxygen carrying capacity of Fluosol DA20 and may be more effective (Urbaniak, 1991).

Droplet size in the emulsion is of the order of 0.1 μm, compared with the 5 μm diameter of an erythrocyte. The flow resistance is considerably less than that of blood, and as it is virtually unaffected by shear rate, the rheological properties are particularly favourable at low flow rates. Fluorocarbons may therefore be useful in partial obstruction of the circulation, for example in myocardial infarction and during percutaneous transluminal coronary angioplasty (Faithfull, 1987; Lowe, 1991).

Stroma-free haemoglobin solutions. Early attempts at using erythrocyte haemolysates resulted in acute renal failure. However, this was due to the stroma rather than the free haemoglobin: interest in the subject has been reawakened by the development of stroma-free haemoglobin solutions. Although relatively stable *in vitro*, the haemoglobin tetramer dissociates in the body into dimers, which are excreted in the urine. This results in a half-life of only 2–4 hours (Urbaniak, 1991). Further problems relate to oxidation to methaemoglobin during storage, and loss of 2,3-DPG which reduces the P_{50}. In his review, Urbaniak considers the potential scope for polymerization of the haemoglobin molecule with glutaraldehyde, the use of bovine haemoglobin and artificial encapsulation in liposomes.

Recombinant human haemoglobin has now been prepared by expression in *E. coli* and the alpha and beta chains associate into tetramers with a full complement of haem groups (Hoffman et al., 1990). There is, however, an additional methionine residue at the amino terminal, which reduces the Bohr effect. Clearly this approach offers possibilities for producing large quantities of blood without using donors, and also modifying the properties of the haemoglobin.

Transport of oxygen from the lungs to the cell

The concept of oxygen delivery

The most important function of the respiratory and circulatory systems is the supply of oxygen to the cells of the body in adequate quantity and at a satisfactory partial pressure. The quantity of oxygen made available to the body in 1 minute is known as oxygen delivery ($\dot{D}o_2$) or oxygen flux, and is equal to cardiac output $\times$ arterial oxygen content.

At rest, the numerical values are (in round figures):

5000 ml blood/min $\times$ 20 ml O_2/100 ml blood   = 1000 ml O_2/min
(cardiac output)   (arterial oxygen content)   (oxygen delivery)

Of this 1000 ml/min, approximately 250 ml/min are utilized by the conscious resting subject. The circulating blood thus loses 25% of its oxygen and the mixed venous blood is approximately 70% saturated (i.e. 95 − 25). The 70% of unextracted oxygen forms an important reserve which may be drawn upon under the stress of such conditions as exercise, to which additional extraction forms one of the integrated adaptations (see Figure 13.2).

Oxygen consumption must clearly depend upon delivery but the relationship is non-linear. Modest reduction of oxygen delivery is well tolerated by the body which is, within limits, able to draw on the reserve of unextracted venous oxygen without reduction of oxygen consumption. However, below a critical value for delivery, consumption is decreased and the subject shows signs of hypoxia. The important quantitative aspects of the relationship between oxygen consumption and delivery are considered below.

Quantification of oxygen delivery

The arterial oxygen content consists predominantly of oxygen in combination with haemoglobin and this fraction is given by the following expression:

$$Ca_{O_2} = Sa_{O_2} \times [Hb] \times 1.31$$

where Ca_{O_2} is the arterial oxygen content
    Sa_{O_2} is the arterial oxygen saturation (as a fraction)
    [Hb] is the haemoglobin concentration of the blood

1.31 is the volume of oxygen (ml) which has been found to combine with 1 g of haemoglobin (see above, page 271).

To the combined oxygen must be added the oxygen in physical solution which will be of the order of 0.3 ml/dl, and the expression for total arterial oxygen concentration may now be expanded thus:

$$Ca_{O_2} = (Sa_{O_2} \times [Hb] \times 1.31) + 0.3 \qquad \qquad ...(6)$$

ml/dl   %/100 g/dl   ml/g   ml/dl

e.g.   19 = (0.97 $\times$ 14.7 $\times$ 1.31) + 0.3

Since oxygen delivery is the product of cardiac output and arterial oxygen content:

$$\dot{D}o_2 \quad = \quad \dot{Q} \quad \times \quad Ca_{O_2} \qquad \qquad ...(7)$$

ml/min   l/min   ml/dl

e.g.   1000 =   5.25 $\times$ 19

(right-hand side is multiplied by a scaling factor of 10)

$\dot{Q}$ is cardiac output

By combining equations (6) and (7) the full expression for oxygen delivery is as follows:

$$\dot{D}O_2 \;=\; \dot{Q} \;\times\; \{(Sa_{O_2} \;\times\; [Hb] \;\times\; 1.31) + 0.3\} \qquad \ldots(8)$$

$\dot{D}O_2$	$\dot{Q}$	Sa_{O_2}	[Hb]		
ml/min	l/min	%/100	g/dl	ml/g	ml/dl

e.g. $1000 \;=\; 5.25 \;\times\; \{(0.97 \;\times\; 14.7 \;\times\; 1.31) + 0.3\}$

(right-hand side is multiplied by a scaling factor of 10)

Interaction of the variable factors governing oxygen delivery

Equation (8) contains, on the right-hand side, three variable factors which govern oxygen delivery.

1. *Cardiac output (or, for a particular organ, the regional blood flow).* Failure of this factor has been termed 'stagnant anoxia'.
2. *Arterial oxygen saturation.* Failure of this (for whatever reason) has been termed 'anoxic anoxia'.
3. Haemoglobin concentration. Reduction as a cause of tissue hypoxia has been termed 'anaemic anoxia'.

The classification of 'anoxia' into 'stagnant', 'anoxic' and 'anaemic' was proposed by Barcroft in 1920 and has stood the test of time. The three types of 'anoxia' may be conveniently displayed on a Venn diagram (Figure 11.17) which shows the possibility of combinations of any two types of anoxia or all three together. For example, the combination of anaemia and low cardiac output, which occurs in untreated haemorrhage, would be indicated by the overlapping area of the stagnant and anaemic circles (indicated by X). If the patient also suffered from lung injury, he might then move into the central area, indicating the addition of anoxic anoxia. On a more cheerful note, compensations are more usual. Patients with anaemia normally have a high cardiac output; subjects resident at altitude have polycythaemia, and so on. Such considerations provide a classic example of the importance of viewing a patient as a whole. For example, the question of the lowest permissible haemoglobin concentration for major surgery can be answered only after consideration of the actual and projected cardiac output during surgery, the pulmonary function and so on. Clinical implications of oxygen delivery are considered in Chapter 31.

It is important to note that oxygen delivery equals the product of three variables and one constant. If one variable is halved, delivery is halved; but if all three variables are simultaneously halved, then delivery is reduced to one-eighth of the original value. One-eighth of 1000 is 125 ml/min, and this is a value which, if maintained for any length of time, is incompatible with life, although the reduction of each individual variable is not in itself lethal. The minimum value of oxygen delivery compatible with survival at rest must vary with circumstances but appears to be of the order of 300–400 ml/min.

The relationship between oxygen delivery and consumption

The relationship between oxygen delivery ($\dot{D}O_2$) and consumption ($\dot{V}O_2$) is best illustrated on the coordinates shown in Figure 11.18. The abscissa shows oxygen delivery as defined above, while consumption is shown on the ordinate. The fan of

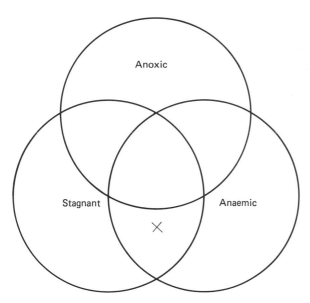

Figure 11.17 Barcroft's classification of causes of hypoxia displayed on a Venn diagram to illustrate the possibility of combinations of more than one type of hypoxia. The lowest area of overlap, marked with a cross, shows coexistent anaemia and low cardiac output. The central area illustrates a combination of all three types of hypoxia (e.g. a patient with haemorrhage and 'shock lung').

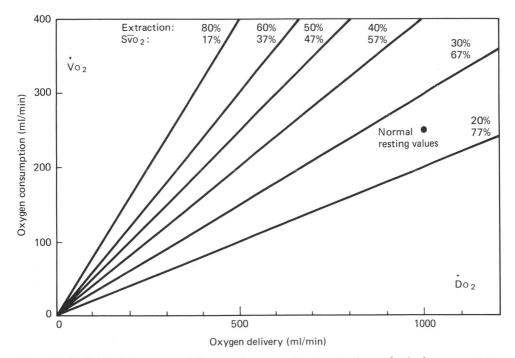

Figure 11.18 Grid relating oxygen delivery and consumption to extraction and mixed venous oxygen saturation, on the assumption of 97% saturation for arterial blood. The spot marks the normal resting values.

lines originating from the zero point indicate different values for oxygen extraction ($\dot{V}O_2/\dot{D}O_2$) expressed as a percentage. Since the mixed venous oxygen saturation is the arterial saturation less the extraction, it is a simple matter to indicate the mixed venous saturation which corresponds to a particular value for extraction. The black dot indicates a typical normal resting point, with delivery of 1000 ml/min, consumption of 250 ml/min and extraction 25%. With an arterial saturation of 97%, the mixed venous saturation will therefore be about 72%.

When oxygen delivery is moderately reduced, for whatever reason, oxygen consumption tends to be maintained at its normal value, by increasing oxygen extraction and therefore decreasing mixed venous saturation. There should be no evidence of additional anaerobic metabolism, such as increased lactate production. This is termed 'supply-independent oxygenation', a condition which applies provided that delivery remains above a critical value. This is shown by the horizontal line in Figure 11.19. Below the critical level of oxygen delivery, oxygen consumption decreases as a linear function of delivery. This is termed 'supply-dependent oxygenation' and is usually accompanied by evidence of hypoxia, such as increased lactate in peripheral blood. This is clearly an undesirable situation and,

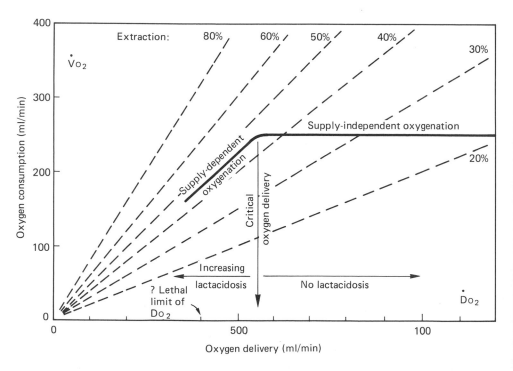

Figure 11.19 This diagram is based on the grid shown in Figure 11.18. For an otherwise healthy subject, the thick horizontal line shows the extent to which oxygen delivery can be reduced without reducing oxygen consumption and causing signs of hypoxia (supply-independent oxygenation). Below the postulated critical delivery, oxygen consumption becomes supply-dependent and there are signs of hypoxia. There is uncertainty of the precise values for critical delivery and the lethal limit of delivery in otherwise healthy subjects.

under conditions of intensive therapy, has been shown to be a strong predictor of an unfavourable prognosis (Shoemaker, Bland and Appel, 1985).

Much attention is currently being devoted to determination of the critical value for oxygen delivery under various pathological circumstances. There are obvious difficulties in assessing the critical value by deliberately reducing oxygen delivery in patients. However, in cases of anaemia or reduced cardiac output, it is possible to measure oxygen consumption before and after taking measures to improve oxygen delivery. If consumption is unchanged it is presumed that the original delivery was above the critical level. If, on the other hand, consumption improves, then it suggests that delivery was less than critical and oxygen consumption was supply-dependent. It is still uncertain to what extent induced increases in cardiac output are themselves responsible for increased total oxygen consumption as a result of increased cardiac work.

In uncomplicated anaemia, the critical delivery seems to less than 500 ml/min (see Chapter 25, Figure 25.2). However, it should be noted that increasing the haemoglobin concentration tends to reduce cardiac output and perhaps the myocardial oxygen consumption. The situation is less clear in many of the complex clinical situations which arise during intensive care, where there is still uncertainty about the critical level of oxygen delivery. Although baseline values for oxygen consumption are often high, it is a common finding in intensive care units that oxygen consumption continues to increase when delivery is increased within the range $600-900$ ml min^{-1} m^{-2} (Wolf et al., 1987; Edwards et al., 1989). It has generally been difficult to demonstrate in this situation that oxygen delivery ever reaches levels compatible with supply-independent oxygenation. It should, however, be stressed that oxygen consumption in these studies has been measured by the reversed Fick technique which excludes the very large component found in patients with infected lungs (page 510). Furthermore, therapeutic measures such as the administration of inotropic drugs must increase the myocardial oxygen consumption. Also the comparison of delivery and consumption may be compromised by there being two shared variables (cardiac output and arterial oxygen content) in the measurement of oxygen delivery and consumption (by the reversed Fick technique).

Tissue PO_2

The ultimate goal of improving oxygen delivery by manipulation of the factors discussed above is to increase the tissue PO_2. However, it is almost impossible to quantify tissue PO_2. It is evident that there are differences between different organs, with the tissue PO_2 influenced not only by arterial PO_2 but also by the ratio of tissue oxygen consumption to perfusion. However, even greater difficulties arise from the regional variations in tissue PO_2 in different parts of the same organ. They are presumably caused by regional variations in tissue perfusion and oxygen consumption. Nor is this the whole story. An advancing PO_2-sensitive microelectrode detects variations in PO_2 which can be interpreted in relation to the proximity of the electrode to small vessels (see Figure 9.4). Very large variations have been demonstrated with exploring electrodes in the brain (Cater et al., 1961). Tissue PO_2 is thus an unsatisfactory quantitative index of the state of oxygenation of an organ. Functional or metabolic indicators, such as lactate production, are more useful.

Oxygen stores and the steady state

In spite of its great biological importance, oxygen is a very difficult gas to store in a biological system. There is no satisfactory method of physical storage in the body. Haemoglobin is the most efficient chemical carrier, but more than 0.5 kg is required to carry 1 g of oxygen. The concentration of haemoglobin in blood far exceeds the concentration of any other protein in any body fluid. Even so the quantity of oxygen in the blood is barely sufficient for 3 minutes' metabolism in the resting state. It is a fact of great clinical importance that the body oxygen stores are so small and, if replenishment ceases, they are normally insufficient to sustain life for more than a few minutes. The principal stores are shown in Table 11.4.

While breathing air, not only are the total oxygen stores very small but also, to make matters worse, only part of the stores can be released without an unacceptable reduction in P_{O_2}. Half of the oxygen in blood is still retained when the P_{O_2} is reduced to 3.5 kPa (26 mmHg). Myoglobin is even more reluctant to part with its oxygen and very little can be released above a P_{O_2} of 2.7 kPa (20 mmHg).

Breathing oxygen causes a substantial increase in total oxygen stores. Most of the additional oxygen is accommodated in the alveolar gas from which 80% may be withdrawn without causing the P_{O_2} to fall below the normal value. With 2400 ml of easily available oxygen after breathing oxygen, there is no difficulty in breath holding for as long as 8 minutes without becoming hypoxic. Clinical relevance of preoxygenation is considered below.

The small size of the oxygen stores means that changes in factors affecting the alveolar or arterial P_{O_2} will produce their full effects very quickly after the change. This is in contrast to carbon dioxide where the size of the stores buffers the body against rapid changes (page 238). Figure 11.20 compares the time course of changes in P_{O_2} and P_{CO_2} produced by the same changes in ventilation. Figure 10.11 showed how the time course of changes of P_{CO_2} is different for falling and rising P_{CO_2}.

Factors which reduce the P_{O_2} always act, rapidly, but the following is the order of rapidity of changes which produce anoxia.

1. Circulatory arrest. When the circulation is arrested, hypoxia supervenes as soon as the oxygen in the tissues and stagnant capillaries has been exhausted. In the case of the brain, with its high rate of oxygen consumption, there is only about 10 seconds before consciousness is lost. If the eyeball is gently compressed with a finger to occlude its vessels, vision commences to be lost at the periphery within about 6 seconds (a convincing experiment suggested by Rahn in 1964). Circulatory

Table 11.4 Principal stores of body oxygen

	While breathing air	While breathing 100% oxygen	
In the lungs (FRC)	450 ml		3 000 ml
In the blood	850 ml		950 ml
Dissolved in tissue fluids	50 ml	?	100 ml
In combination with myoglobin	? 200 ml	?	200 ml
Total	1 550 ml		4 250 ml

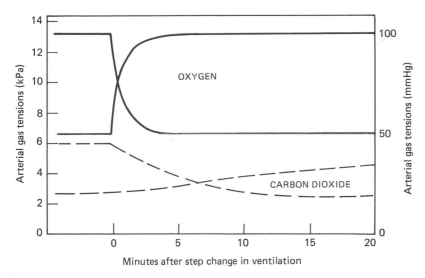

Figure 11.20 *The upper pair of curves indicate the rate of change of arterial P_{O_2} following step changes in ventilation. Half of the total change occurs in about 30 seconds. The rising curve could be produced by an increase of alveolar ventilation from 2 to 4 l/min while breathing air (see Figure 11.6). The falling curve could result from the corresponding reduction of alveolar ventilation from 4 to 2 l/min. The lower pair of curves indicate the time course of changes in P_{CO_2} which are very much slower than for oxygen. These changes are shown in greater detail in Figure 10.11.*

arrest also differs from other forms of hypoxia in the failure of clearance of products of anaerobic metabolism (e.g. lactic acid) which, with the exception of the brain, should not occur in arterial hypoxaemia.

2. Exposure to a barometric pressure of less than 6.3 kPa (47 mmHg). At a pressure of less than 6.3 kPa (47 mmHg), body fluids boil and alveolar gas is replaced with 100% water vapour (page 338). Oxygen and other gases are then displaced from the lungs, and the P_{O_2} rapidly falls to zero. Consciousness is lost within one circulation time, which is of the order of 15 seconds (Ernsting and McHardy, 1960).

3. Inhalation of nitrogen. Washing out the alveolar oxygen by hyperventilation with nitrogen results in a very rapid fall of arterial P_{O_2}, which reached 4 kPa (30 mmHg) in 30 seconds in a series of dogs (Cater et al., 1963). Even more rapid changes were obtained in human volunteers by Ernsting (1963).

4. Inhalation of nitrous oxide. Alveolar wash-out with a soluble gas such as nitrous oxide causes a slower fall of P_{O_2} because of the loss of the flushing gas into the tissues. This delays the decrease in alveolar P_{O_2} (page 260).

5. Apnoea. The rate of onset of anoxia is dependent upon the initial alveolar P_{O_2}, the lung volume and the rate of oxygen consumption. It is, for example, more rapid while swimming underwater than while breath holding at rest in the laboratory. Generally speaking, after breathing air, 90 seconds of apnoea results in a substantial fall of P_{O_2} to a level which threatens loss of consciousness. If a patient has previously inhaled a few breaths of oxygen, the arterial P_{O_2} should remain above 13.3 kPa (100 mmHg) for at least 3 minutes of apnoea (Heller and Watson, 1961), and this is the basis of the usual method of protection against hypoxia during any deliberate interference with ventilation, as for example during tracheal intubation. If a patient breathes 100% oxygen for a few minutes and is then connected to a supply of oxygen while apnoeic, the arterial P_{O_2} is well maintained for a long time by the process of apnoeic mass-movement oxygenation (see pages 241 et seq.)

In view of the rapid changes shown in Figure 11.20, it follows that, for a patient breathing air, a pulse oximeter will probably give an earlier indication of underventilation than will a carbon dioxide analyser. However, if the patient is protected from hypoxia by the inhalation of a gas mixture enriched with oxygen, then the carbon dioxide will give the earlier indication of hypoventilation. It should be remembered that oxgyen levels change quickly and are potentially much more dangerous. Carbon dioxide levels change only slowly (in response to a change in ventilation) and are usually less dangerous.

Since a steady state for oxygen is very rapidly attained, it follows that oxygen uptake is seldom appreciably different from consumption in the tissues. Therefore, measurement of oxygen uptake usually gives a satisfactory estimate of the oxygen consumption. In contrast, measured values of carbon dioxide output may be very different from the simultaneous level of metabolic production of carbon dioxide production when the ventilation has just changed. Thus the respiratory exchange ratio may be very low during acute underventilation, and well above unity during a brief period of hyperventilation (page 239). During the irregular and depressed breathing of anaesthesia with spontaneous respiration, values for carbon dioxide output (and therefore the respiratory exchange ratio) may range widely, while values for oxygen consumption are reasonably steady (Nunn and Matthews, 1959; Nunn, 1964).

Control of the inspired oxygen concentration

Much of this chapter has been concerned with the theoretical basis for selection of the optimal inspired oxygen concentration for a particular pathophysiological state. It now remains to be considered how this should be put into effect.

Interface with the patient's airway

A crucial factor in oxygen therapy is the nature of the seal between the patient's airway and the external breathing apparatus. Airtight seals may be obtained with cuffed tracheal or tracheostomy tubes or with the recently introduced laryngeal mask (page 386). These devices should give complete control over the composition of the inspired gas. An anaesthetic facemask will usually provide an airtight seal with the face, but it must be held by a trained person and is at best a temporary measure. Various patterns of masks intended for use by aircrew can give an excellent seal, but there is no mask generally available for clinical use which can be guaranteed to provide an airtight fit to a patient's face, unless it is actually held onto the face by trained staff. Most disposable oxygen masks do not attempt to provide an airtight fit. Physiological mouthpieces with a noseclip are satisfactory for short-term use with co-operative or trained subjects but cannot be tolerated for long periods. An alternative solution to the problem of the airtight seal is to provide a high flow of gas which can vent to the atmosphere between the mask and the face, thus preventing the inflow of air (see below).

Gas mixing

The most satisfactory technique for delivery of a designated inspired oxygen concentration is to mix the required proportions of air and oxygen. Gas mixtures are conveniently obtained from air and oxygen pipeline installations with appropriate humidification. A pair of rotameters may be used, and Figure E.7 in Appendix E shows a wall chart to facilitate the calculation of flow rates. A simpler arrangement is to employ a mixing device such as the Quantiflex with separate controls for total flow rate and oxygen concentration. It is a valuable safety feature if such devices have a visible indication of oxygen flow (Richardson, Chinn and Nunn, 1976).

Air/oxygen mixtures can be delivered to ventilators, passed over a T-piece for patients breathing spontaneously with a cuffed endotracheal tube or delivered to the patient by means of a non-rebreathing gas delivery system. They can also be passed to loose-fitting disposable masks but, under these circumstances, high flow rates are required, preferably in excess of the peak inspiratory flow rate (page 84). A small inspiratory reservoir will store fresh gas during expiration for use during inspiration: this will greatly reduce the fresh gas flow requirement.

Use of venturi devices

Oxygen may be passed through the jet of a venturi to entrain air. This is a convenient and highly economical method of preparing oxygen mixtures in the range 25–40% concentration. For example, 1 l/min of oxygen passed through the jet of a venturi with an entrainment ratio of 8:1 will deliver 9 l/min of 30% oxygen. Higher oxygen concentrations require a lower entrainment ratio and therefore a higher oxygen flow in order to maintain an adequate total delivered flow rate. The familiar venturi mask was introduced by Campbell (1960b) on the suggestion of the author who had used a venturi to provide the oxygen-enriched carrier gas for an anaesthetic apparatus designed for use in the Antarctic (Nunn, 1961b).

With an adequate flow rate of the air/oxygen mixture, the venturi mask need not fit the face with an airtight junction. The high flow rate escapes round the cheeks as well as through the holes in the mask, and room air is effectively excluded. Numerous studies have indicated that the venturi mask gives excellent control over the inspired oxygen concentration with an accuracy of ±1% unaffected by variations in the ventilation of the patient (Leigh, 1973). There is no doubt that this is the most satisfactory method of controlling the inspired oxygen concentration of a patient who is breathing spontaneously without tracheal intubation.

Control of the patient's gaseous environment

The popularityy of oxygen tents declined because of their large volume and high rate of leakage, which made it difficult to attain and maintain a high oxygen concentration, unless the volume was reduced and a high gas flow rate was used (Wayne and Chamney, 1969). In addition, the fire hazard cannot be ignored. These problems are minimized when the patient is an infant, and oxygen control within an incubator is a satisfactory method of administering a precise oxygen concentration. Largely because of the danger of retrolental fibroplasia (page 554), it is mandatory to monitor the oxygen concentration in the incubator.

Spectacles, nasal catheters, simple disposable oxygen masks, etc.

These simple devices aim to blow oxygen at or into the air passages. This oxygen is mixed with inspired air to give an inspired oxygen concentration which is a complex function of the geometry of the device, the oxygen flow rate, the patient's ventilation and whether the patient is breathing through his mouth or nose. The effective inspired oxygen concentration is impossible to predict and may vary within very wide limits (Leigh, 1973). These devices cannot be used for oxygen therapy when the exact inspired oxygen concentration is critical (e.g. ventilatory failure), but may be useful in less critical situations such as recovery from routine anaesthesia. Nasal prongs are the preferred method for delivering 'sleeping oxygen' (Flenley, 1985b). Fairly high oxygen concentrations may be obtained with a combination of two techniques such as nasal catheters used under a simple mask, an arrangement with which Down and Castleden (1975) obtained an arterial P_{O_2} of 51.7 kPa (388 mmHg). Administration by transtracheal catheter appears to be effective at about half the flow rate required for nasal catheters (Banner and Govan, 1986).

With a device such as a nasal catheter or prongs, the lower the ventilation, the greater will be the fractional contribution of the fixed flow of oxygen to the inspired gas mixture. There is thus an approximate compensation for hypoventilation, with greater oxygen concentrations being delivered at lower levels of ventilation. Arterial P_{O_2} may then be maintained in spite of a progressively falling ventilation. However, this will do nothing to prevent the rise in P_{CO_2}, which may reach a dangerous level without the appearance of cyanosis to warn that all is not well (Davies and Hopkin, 1989).

Hyperbaric oxygenation

Two systems are in use. One-man chambers are filled with 100% oxygen and the patient is entirely exposed to 100% oxygen at high pressure, no mask being required. Larger chambers are pressurized with air which is breathed by staff: 100% oxygen is made available to the patient by means of a well fitting facemask. The quality of the airtight fit is obviously crucial and has caused considerable difficulties in the past.

Monitoring oxygen concentrations

When the inspired gas has a fixed composition (e.g. in oxygen tents and with venturi masks), there is no problem in sampling inspired gas and measuring the oxygen concentration with devices such as paramagnetic analysers (see below). With variable performance devices (e.g. oxygen spectacles, nasal catheters, simple masks, etc.), it is extremely difficult to determine the inspired oxygen, which may not be constant throughout the duration of inspiration. Furthermore, the measured oxygen concentration may be highly dependent on the point from which the sample is taken and whether the patient is breathing through his nose or his mouth. In the face of these difficulties, it may be preferable to measure the end-expiratory oxygen concentration or even the arterial blood P_{O_2}. However, if such measures are necessary it would be wiser to use a device with a fixed performance.

Supply of oxygen

Choice of the best method for supplying oxygen depends on consumption and convenience. For a large hospital, the most economical provision of oxygen is by bulk deliveries of liquid oxygen with the evaporated oxygen distributed by a pipeline, usually at 4 atmospheres pressure. For a smaller hospital it may be more economical to use a bank of cylinders of oxygen, also distributed by pipeline. With only occasional and small scale use of oxygen, it may be cheaper to use cylinders at the point of consumption. This avoids the cost of installing a pipeline but the logistic costs are considerable and there is always the fear of a cylinder running empty unnoticed. Domestic pipelines can be installed for provision of oxygen in the home. The patient then plugs into various strategically located outlets as required. Small cylinders are available which are suitable for 'walking oxygen'. Miniature liquid oxygen dispensers are used in military aircraft.

An entirely different approach is the oxygen concentrator which removes most of the nitrogen from air, providing an oxygen concentration in the range 90–95%, the remainder being a mixture of argon and residual nitrogen. Nitrogen is removed at high pressure by zeolite acting as a molecular sieve with pore size of 0.5 nm (5 Å). Its activity is regenerated by exposure to vacuum or by purging with air at atmospheric pressure. Thus a pair of sieves can be used alternately to provide a continuous supply. It is difficult to imagine any clinical condition which requires administration of 100% oxygen rather than the 90–95% oxygen provided by an oxygen concentrator and the contaminating argon is harmless.

It appears that oxygen concentrators can compete economically with traditional methods of oxygen supply for both large and small levels of consumption. However, the method would seem to have outstanding advantages in remote locations (Ezi-Ashi, Papworth and Nunn, 1983) and small units are now extensively used for domestic oxygen.

Cyanosis

The commonest method of detection of hypoxia is by the appearance of cyanosis, and the change in colour of haemoglobin on desaturation affords the patient a safeguard of immense value. There must have been countless occasions in which the appearance of cyanosis has given warning of hypoventilation, pulmonary shunting, stagnant circulation or decreased oxygen concentration of inspired gas. Indeed, it is interesting to speculate on the additional hazards to life if gross arterial hypoxaemia could occur without overt changes in the colour of the blood.

Central and peripheral cyanosis

If shed arterial blood is seen to be purple, this is a reliable indication of arterial desaturation. However, when skin or mucous membrane is inspected, most of the blood which colours the tissue is lying in veins (i.e. subpapillary venous plexuses) and its oxygen content is related to the arterial oxygen content as follows:

$$\frac{\text{venous oxygen}}{\text{content}} = \frac{\text{arterial oxygen}}{\text{content}} - \frac{\text{arterial/venous oxygen}}{\text{content difference}}$$

The last term may be expanded in terms of the tissue metabolism and perfusion:

$$\frac{\text{venous oxygen}}{\text{content}} = \frac{\text{arterial oxygen}}{\text{content}} - \frac{\text{tissue oxygen consumption}}{\text{tissue blood flow}}$$

The oxygen consumption by the skin is usually low in relation to its circulation, so the second term on the right-hand side of the second equation is generally small. Therefore the cutaneous venous oxygen content is close to that of the arterial blood and inspection of the skin usually gives a reasonable indication of arterial oxygen content. However, when circulation is reduced in relation to skin oxygen consumption, cyanosis may occur in the presence of normal arterial oxygen levels. This occurs typically in patients with low cardiac output, in cold weather and in the face of a patient in the Trendelenburg position.

The influence of anaemia

Lundsgaard and Van Slyke (1923) stressed the importance of anaemia in appearance of cyanosis. Much credence is attached to their statement that cyanosis is apparent when there are 5 g of reduced haemoglobin per dl of capillary blood. They defined capillary blood as having a desaturation equal to the mean of the levels in arterial and venous blood. If, for example, the arterial blood contained 3 g/dl of reduced haemoglobin (80% saturation at normal haemoglobin concentration) and the arterial/venous difference for the skin were 2 ml/100 ml of oxygen (corresponding to the reduction of a further 1.5 g/dl of haemoglobin), the 'capillary' blood would contain only 3.75 g/dl of reduced haemoglobin, well below the threshold at which cyanosis should be evident. This seems improbable for an arterial So_2 of 80%. In cases of severe anaemia, it might be impossible for the reduced haemoglobin concentration of the capillary blood to attain the level of 5 g/dl, which is said to be required for the appearance of cyanosis and, clearly, cyanosis could never occur if the haemoglobin concentration were only 5 g/dl.

There seems little doubt that Lundsgaard and Van Slyke were right to stress the importance of the total haemoglobin concentration, although there has been little confirmation of 5 g of reduced haemoglobin being the critical value for detection. It is generally found that cyanosis can be detected at an arterial oxygen saturation of about 85% although there is much variation (Comroe and Botelho, 1947). Such a level would probably correspond to a 'capillary' saturation of more than 80% and a reduced haemoglobin of about 3 g/dl.

Sites for detection of cyanosis

Kelman and Nunn (1966a) carried out a comparison of the appearance of cyanosis in different sites with various biochemical indices of hypoxaemia of arterial blood. Best correlations were obtained with cyanosis observed in the buccal mucosa and lips, but there was no significant correlation between the oxygenation of the arterial blood and the appearance of cyanosis in the ear lobes, nail bed or conjunctivae.

The importance of colour-rendering properties of source of illumination

Kelman and Nunn also compared the use of five types of fluorescent lighting in use in hospitals. There was no significant difference in the correlation between hypoxaemia and cyanosis for the different lights. Nevertheless, although none was more reliable than the others for the detection of hypoxaemia, the degree of bias was strikingly different. Some lamps tended to make the patient look pinker and others imparted a bluer tinge to the patients. The former gave false negatives (no cyanosis in the presence of hypoxaemia), while the latter gave false positives (cyanosis in the absence of hypoxaemia). However, the total number of false results was approximately the same with all tubes.

It is potentially dangerous for patients to be inspected under lamps of different colour-rendering properties, particularly if the medical and nursing staff do not know the characteristics of each type of lamp. It would be too much to suggest that the staff should calibrate their impressions of cyanosis for a particular lamp by relation to arterial oxygen levels, but it is not too much to expect that hospitals will standardize their lighting and acquaint staff with the colour-rendering properties of the type which is finally chosen.

Sensitivity of cyanosis as an indication of hypoxaemia

It has been stressed above that the appearance of cyanosis is considerably influenced by the circulation, haemoglobin concentration and lighting conditions. Even when all these are optimal, cyanosis is by no means a precise indication of the arterial oxygen level and it should be regarded as a warning sign rather than a measurement. Kelman and Nunn (1966a) detected cyanosis in about 50% of patients who had a saturation of 93%. Cyanosis was detected in about 95% of patients who had a saturation of 89%. It should be remembered that 89% saturation corresponds to about 7.5 kPa (56 mmHg) PO_2, a level which most would consider unacceptable. Cyanosis was not seen in 5% of patients at or below this level of arterial PO_2. It is quite clear that absence of cyanosis does not necessarily mean normal arterial oxygen levels.

Principles of measurement of oxygen levels

Oxygen concentration in gas samples

For many years the use of the Haldane apparatus, or its modification by Lloyd (Cormack, 1972), has been the standard method of measurement of oxygen concentrations in physiological gas samples. However, analysers working on the paramagnetic properties of oxygen (Pauling, Wood and Sturdivant, 1946) many years ago attained a degree of accuracy and reliability which enabled them to supplant the older chemical methods of analysis (Nunn et al., 1964; Ellis and Nunn, 1968). A particularly attractive feature of the method is that interference by other gases likely to be present does not cause major inaccuracies and, if particularly high accuracy is required, correction factors may be employed. Fuel cells and polarographs may also be used and are particularly suitable as monitors.

Measurement of breath-to-breath changes in oxygen concentrations of respired gases requires an instrument with a response time of less than about 300 ms.

Formerly the only suitable technique for oxygen measurement was the mass spectrometer (Fowler and Hugh-Jones, 1957). However, a number of alternative methods have been described, although their use has remained limited. The first of these was a modification of the polarograph (Severinghaus, 1963), followed by a fast-response version of the Servomex DCL 83 paramagnetic oxygen analyser (Cunningham, Kay and Young, 1965). A previously unapplied principle was employed in the oxygen-sensitive solid electrochemical cell described by Elliot, Segger and Osborn (1966).

Oxygen content of blood samples

The classic chemical methods are those of Haldane (1920) and Van Slyke and Neill (1924), the latter remaining the standard for many years. Gregory (1973) described a technique for assessment of the accuracy of the Van Slyke apparatus against hydrogen peroxide. There was no significant systematic error, but random error was in the range of ± 0.3 ml/100 ml.

Intended substitutes for the Van Slyke have included the Natelson apparatus (1951) and a polarographic method based on the liberation of oxygen from haemoglobin by saponin-ferricyanide solution. The PO_2 of the resultant solution is proportional to the oxygen content of the blood sample (Linden, Ledsome and Norman, 1965). This method is uninfluenced by the presence of inhalational anaesthetic agents, and has proved to be simple, accurate and reliable. The favoured technique at present uses a fuel cell for measurement of oxygen evolved from blood. However, the reliability and simplicity of measurements of PO_2 and saturation have decreased the demand for measurement of oxygen content, which is now often derived from saturation and haemoglobin concentration.

Blood oxygen saturation

The classic method of measurement of saturation is as the ratio of content to capacity (with dissolved oxygen subtracted from each):

$$\text{saturation} = HbO_2/(Hb + HbO_2)$$

$$= \frac{\text{oxygen content} - \text{dissolved oxygen}}{\text{oxygen capacity} - \text{dissolved oxygen}}$$

Oxygen capacity is determined as the content after saturation of the blood by exposure to 100% oxygen at room temperature. Both content and capacity can be measured by the methods described above, classically with the Van Slyke apparatus.

Nowadays, it is more usual to measure saturation photometrically. Methods are based on the fact that the absorption of monochromatic light of certain wavelengths (e.g. 805 nm) is the same (isobestic) for reduced and oxygenated haemoglobin. At other wavelengths (particularly 650 nm) there is a marked difference between the absorption of transmitted or reflected light by the two forms of haemoglobin (Zijlstra, 1958). Various devices are marketed which depend upon the simultaneous absorption of light at two wavelengths and so indicate the saturation directly. Depending on the wavelengths which are selected, carboxyhaemoglobin may be seen as though it were either oxygenated or reduced haemoglobin. If it is seen as though it were oxygenated haemoglobin, this will lead to a substantial error in a patient with appreciable carboxyhaemoglobinaemia. These instruments tend to be used uncritically. Their calibration is seldom checked, for the simple reason that such a check is a difficult and time-consuming operation, requiring technical skills which have been lost in the face of modern self-calibratting equipment.

Saturation may be derived from PO_2. This is reasonably accurate above a PO_2 of about 7.3 kPa (55 mmHg) where the dissociation curve is flat. However, it is inaccurate at lower tensions since, on the steep part of the curve, the saturation changes by 3% for a PO_2 change of only 0.13 kPa (1 mmHg).

Blood PO_2

Four methods of measurement are available.

The Riley bubble method. A tiny bubble of gas may be equilibrated with blood at the patient's body temperature and then analysed quantitatively for oxygen (Riley, Campbell and Shepard, 1957). PO_2 is derived from the oxygen concentration of the bubble. The technique is difficult and inaccurate when the PO_2 is more than 12.7 kPa (95 mmHg). It cannot be used in the presence of anaesthetic gases.

Derivation from saturation. If the dissociation curve is known, the PO_2 may be derived from the saturation (see above). This method is quite accurate on the steep part of the dissociation curve, but is of limited value when the PO_2 is greater than about 10 kPa (75 mmHg).

Derivation from oxygen concentration in plasma. PO_2 of blood is directly proportional to the oxygen content of the plasma. This relationship may be used for deriving PO_2 from content, provided that blood can be separated anaerobically without change in the distribution of oxygen between plasma and erythrocytes. The solubility of oxygen in the patient's plasma must be accurately known. The method is difficult because of the small quantities of oxygen dissolved in plasma. However, Stark and Smith (1960) successfully used the method of Smith and Pask (1959) for measuring plasma oxygen content and derived values for blood PO_2 in a pioneer study.

Polarography. Since 1960, polarography has virtually displaced all other methods of measurement of blood PO_2. This technique is now widely used both for research and for the management of patients who present problems of oxygenation. It has been of immense value in anaesthesia since it is uninfluenced by the presence of anaesthetic agents. The apparatus consists essentially of a cell formed by a silver anode and a platinum cathode, both in contact with an electrolyte in dilute solution. If a potential difference of about 700 mV is applied to the cell, a current is passed which is directly proportional to the PO_2 of the electrolyte in the region of the cathode. In use, the electrolyte is separated from the sample by a thin membrane which is permeable to oxygen. The electrolyte rapidly attains the same PO_2 as the sample and the current passed by the cell is proportional to the PO_2 of the sample, which may be gas, blood or other liquids.

Gas mixtures are normally used for calibration of polarographs and an important source of error is the difference in reading between blood and gas of the same PO_2. Estimates of the ratio vary between 1.0 and 1.17 but it may change unexpectedly due to changes in the position of the membrane. This source of error has been greatly reduced in modern microelectrodes which consume much less oxygen at the cathode. The error may be detected and avoided by calibration with tonometer-equilibrated blood which is not difficult. It is possible to calibrate with a solution of 30% glycerol in water which gives the same reading as blood of the same PO_2. Additional errors arise from a current due to the polarographic reduction of anaesthetic gases at the cathode. This may be minimized by selection of the appropriate polarizing voltage. Automated blood gas analysers are used extensively and should give satisfactory results even when used by untrained staff (Minty and Barrett, 1978).

Common errors in measuring oxygen levels

The major errors in the measurement of blood oxygen levels usually arise from faulty sampling and handling of the sample (Nunn, 1962b), and from failure to correct for differences in temperature between the patient and the measurement system. The blood sample must be collected without exposure to air, and blood previously lying in the sampling line must be discarded.

The effect of delayed analysis. Oxygen is consumed by blood *in vitro* (Greenbaum et al., 1967b), and this may in part be due to formation of free radicals (Nunn et al., 1979). Avoidance of error due to the consequent fall in PO_2 after sampling requires one of the following courses of action. The best solution is immediate analysis after sampling. If this is not possibble the blood should be stored at 0°C. As a final resort there is a correction factor for oxygen consumed during the interval between sampling and analysis (see Appendix E, Figure E.1).

The effect of temperature. If blood PO_2 is measured at a lower temperature than the patient, the measured PO_2 will be less than the PO_2 of the blood while it was in the patient. It is not usual to maintain the measuring apparatus at the patient's body temperature, and significant error results from a temperature difference of more than about 1°C. Correction is possible but the factor is variable depending upon the saturation (Nunn et al., 1965a). A convenient nomogram was described by Kelman and Nunn (1966b) and is included in Appendix E as Figure E.2.

Cutaneous oximetry

Saturation may be measured photometrically *in vivo* as well as *in vitro* as described above for blood. Light at the appropriate wavelengths is either transmitted through a finger or an ear lobe or else is reflected from the skin, usually on the forehead. With the original techniques, most of the blood which was visualized was venous or capillary rather than arterial and the result therefore depended on there being a brisk cutaneous blood flow to minimize the arterial/venous oxygen difference (see above in relation to cyanosis).

Pulse oximetry (see review by Severinghaus and Kelleher, 1992). The older techniques have now been completely replaced by pulse oximeters, which relate the optical densities (at different wavelengths) to the pulse wave detected by the same sensor. The signal between the pulse waves is subtracted from the signal at the height of the pulse wave, the difference being due to the inflowing arterial blood and so reflecting the saturation of the arterial blood. Thus, after many decades of development, oximetry has now become a practical clinical monitor, considered essential in many clinical fields such as anaesthesia.

Instruments currently available continued to function down to levels of gross arterial hypotension and failure of finger circulation, although there was usually a delayed indication of changes in saturation (Severinghaus and Spellman, 1990). Anaemia tends to exaggerate desaturation readings. At a haemoglobin concentration 8 g/dl, normal saturations were correctly recorded, but there was a mean bias of -15% at a true saturation of 53.6% (Severinghaus and Koh, 1990). The problem was only clinically important below a saturation of about 75%. Pulse oximeters cannot distinguish between carboxy- and oxyhaemoglobin (Severinghaus and Kelleher, 1992). Methaemoglobin is read as though it were half oxyhaemoglobin and half reduced haemoglobin up to about 20% methaemoglobin. At higher levels of methaemoglobin, pulse oximeter readings tend to become fixed at about 85%.

As with blood oximetry, calibration of cutaneous oximeters presents a problem. Optical filters may be used for routine calibration, but the gold standard is calibration against arterial blood PO_2 or saturation. This is seldom undertaken. An indirect method of calibration suggested by Campbell (unpublished) was described by Nunn et al. (1965b). It involves rebreathing air and relating the decreasing alveolar PO_2 to the saturation simultaneously displayed. When oxygenation is critical, there is no substitute for direct measurement of arterial PO_2.

Measurement of mixed venous PO_2

The usual method of measurement of mixed venous PO_2 (or oxygen content) is to sample blood from the right ventricle or pulmonary artery and analyse it according to the methods described above. With the current widespread use of the Swan–Ganz catheter, this has become very simple and is widely used for measurement of oxygen consumption by the reversed Fick technique (see below). It has, however, been suggested that a rebreathing technique might be used to derive mixed venous PO_2 indirectly, along the same lines as the Campbell and Howell technique for measurement of mixed venous PCO_2 (page 245). The technique for oxygen was described by Cerretelli et al. (1966) and requires the rebreathing of a mixture of carbon dioxide in nitrogen. This procedure causes a reduction of the arterial PO_2 to the level of the mixed venous blood PO_2, which is about 5.3 kPa or 40 mm Hg in normal subjects, but often much lower in patients. Although the technique is of short duration, it is clearly unacceptable for some patients. There is, however, a more serious objection to the method. Calculations show that the cardiac output in most patients will not be sufficiently high for the alveolar PO_2 to be brought into equilibrium with the mixed venous PO_2 in one circulation time (Spence and Ellis, 1971). Furthermore, the change in alveolar PO_2 is likely to be so slow that there may be a false impression that equilibrium has been attained.

Indirect methods of measurement of arterial PO_2

Unfortunately, indirect methods of measurement of arterial PO_2 are of limited value. The arterial/venous PO_2 difference is so large that any rebreathing method of measurement of mixed venous PO_2 (see above) must be useless for indirect assessment of the arterial PO_2. The end-expiratory PO_2 differs from arterial PO_2 by important components due to both alveolar dead space and shunting. End-expiratory PO_2 is not, therefore, a reliable indicator of arterial PO_2, particularly in the presence of respiratory disease, although it may give some indication of changes.

Cutaneous venous or capillary blood PO_2 may, under ideal conditions, be close to the arterial PO_2, but a modest reduction in skin perfusion will cause a substantial fall in PO_2 since the oxygen is consumed at the flat part of the dissociation curve, where small changes in content correspond to large changes in PO_2. Unsatisfactory correlation between arterial and 'arterialized' venous PO_2 was formally demonstrated by Forster et al. (1972).

Tissue PO_2

Clearly the tissue PO_2 is of greater significance than the PO_2 at various intermediate stages higher in the oxygen cascade. It would therefore appear logical to attempt the measurement of PO_2 in the tissues, but this has proved difficult both in technique and in interpretation.

Needle electrodes. Polarographic electrodes may be inserted directly into tissue on the tip of a needle. Difficulties of interpretation arise from the fact that PO_2 varies from one cell to another and from one part of a cell to another, the most important factor being the relation of the electrode to the capillaries (see Figure 9.4). Thus the significance of measurements of tissue PO_2 depends upon the precise location of the electrode and the degree of damage caused by its insertion. Resolution of these difficulties can be achieved only by meticulous attention to detail. Cater et al. (1961) inserted electrodes by a stereotaxic technique, fixed the tissues before removal and then examined serial sections cut along the track of the electrode to determine its position in relation to blood vessels and to exclude the possibility of a haematoma around the tip of the electrode.

Tissue surface electrodes. A miniaturized polarographic electrode may be placed on or attached to the surface of an organ to indicate the PO_2. Interpretation of the reading is subject to many of the same limitations as with the needle electrode, described in the previous paragraph. Nevertheless, tissue surface PO_2 may provide the surgeon with useful information regarding perfusion and viability in cases of organ ischaemia. Changes in PO_2 may also provide useful information on the efficacy of surgical techniques to improve circulation (Kram and Shoemaker, 1984).

Near infrared spectroscopy. The biochemical state of tissue oxidation may be determined by the use of transmission spectroscopy in the near infrared (700–1000 nm), where tissues are relatively translucent. The state of relative oxidation of haemoglobin and cytochome a_3 may be determined within this wave band. At present it is feasible to study transmission over a path length up to about 9 cm, although there is much scattering of light. Fortunately this is sufficient to permit monitoring the brain of newborn infants.

Organ venous PO_2. Such are the difficulties of measurement of tissue PO_2 that it may be preferable to measure the venous PO_2 of blood draining a particular tissue. Even the significance of this measurement is not entirely clear, but the venous PO_2 is roughly related to the mean pressure head of oxygen for diffusion into the cells of the area drained by the blood. Jugular bulb oximetry provides a real-time estimate of cerebral oxygenation.

Transcutaneous PO_2. Polarographic estimation of PO_2 of skin has been advocated as a non-invasive method of determination of PO_2. A polarographic electrode is applied to the skin which must be heated to at least 44°C to maximize cutaneous blood flow (Severinghaus, 1981). The resultant PO_2 does not equal arterial PO_2 in all circumstances but is nevertheless a useful indirect determination of the adequacy of the overall oxygenation of a patient, particularly infants. It has the special advantage of providing a continuous record. Transcutaneous PO_2 is probably best considered as a measurement in its own right and not as a substitute for arterial PO_2.

Measurement of oxygen consumption and delivery

Oxygen consumption

There are four main methods for the measurement of oxygen consumption:

1. Oxygen loss from (or replacement into) a closed breathing system.
2. Subtraction of the expired from the inspired volume of oxygen.
3. The ventilated hood.
4. Multiplication of cardiac output by arterial/mixed venous oxygen content difference.

Oxygen loss from (or replacement into) a closed breathing system. Probably the simplest method of measuring oxygen consumption is by observing the loss of volume from a closed-circuit spirometer, with expired carbon dioxide absorbed by soda lime. Alternatively, a known flow rate of oxygen may be added to maintain the volume of the spirometer and its oxygen concentration constant: under these conditions, the oxygen inflow rate must equal the oxygen consumption. It is essential that the spirometer should initially contain an oxygen enriched mixture so that the inspired oxygen concentration does not fall to a level which is dangerous for the subject or patient. The subject's nitrogen stores will exchange with the spirometer gas if the partial pressures are different and this may introduce a small error when the subject is first connected to the spirometer. The technique may be adapted to the conditions of artificial ventilation (Figure 11.21), but the technique, although accurate, is cumbersome (Nunn, Makita and Royston, 1989).

Subtraction of expired from inspired volume of oxygen. The essence of the technique is subtraction of (expired minute volume × mixed expired oxygen concentration) from (inspired minute volume × inspired oxygen concentration). The difference between the inspired and expired minute volumes is a very important factor in achieving accuracy with the method, particularly when a high concentration of oxygen is inhaled. Inspired and expired minute volumes differ as a result of the respiratory exchange ratio, and also any exchange of inert gas (e.g. nitrogen) which might occur. On the assumption that the patient is in equilibrium for nitrogen, and the mass of nitrogen inspired is the same as that expired, it follows that the ratio of inspired/expired minute volumes is inversely proportional to the respective ratios of nitrogen concentrations. Therefore:

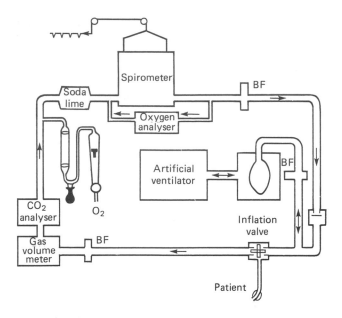

Figure 11.21 A closed-circuit spirometer system for measurement of oxygen consumption by a patient ventilated artificially by means of a box–bag system. When the system is in equilibrium, oxygen consumption is indicated by the oxygen added to the system (accurately measured with a soap film analyser) and carbon dioxide output is measured as the product of expired minute volume and mean carbon dioxide concentration in the mixed expired gas. BF, bacterial filter (Reproduced from Smithies et al. (1991) with permission of the Editor and publishers of Critical Care Medicine)

$$\text{insp. minute volume} = \text{exp. minute vol.} \times \frac{\text{exp. nitrogen conc.}}{\text{insp. nitrogen conc.}}$$

The ratio of the nitrogen concentrations is known as the Haldane transformation factor, which is used to calculate the inspired minute volume from the expired minute volume which is usually measured. Its reciprocal is used to calculate the expired minute volume, if the inspired minute volume has been measured. Use of the Haldane factor is valid only if the subject is in equilibrium with regard to nitrogen.

This is the basis of the classic Douglas bag technique, in which expired gas is measured for volume, and analysed for oxygen and carbon dioxide concentrations. The expired nitrogen concentration is determined by subtraction and the inspired minute volume derived. The approach has been automated by several manufacturers and their systems can be used satisfactorily during artificial ventilation (Makita, Nunn and Royston, 1990). The essential feature is the measurement of gas composition of inspired and expired gas by the same analysers under the same conditions of humidity, temperature and pressure, with a very high level of accuracy. The potential for error is theoretically increased when the inspired oxygen concentration and minute volume are increased (Nunn and Pouliot, 1962), but the manufacturers have had considerable success in overcoming the formidable practical problems.

The ventilated hood. In this approach, the subject's head is covered by a hood, through which is drawn a known high flow rate of air, sufficient to capture all the expired air. The gas drawn into the hood is expired air mixed with entrained air, and is treated in the calculations as though it were expired air. The surplus entrained air is like a very large dead space, but it does not alter the essential calculations. Clearly, the product of the air flow rate and the concentration of CO_2 in the gas drawn through the hood must equal the CO_2 output of the subject. Similarly it is possible to derive oxygen consumption and respiratory exchange ratio. The system is virtually non-invasive and potentially very accurate. However, it can be used only when the subject is breathing air.

Multiplication of cardiac output by arterial/mixed venous oxygen content difference. This approach is the reverse of using the Fick principle for measurement of cardiac output (see page 152) and is commonly known as the reversed Fick technique.

$$\dot{V}O_2 = \dot{Q}(Ca_{O_2} - C\bar{v}_{O_2})$$

where $\dot{V}O_2$ is the oxygen consumption
$\dot{Q}$ is the cardiac output
Ca_{O_2} is the arterial oxygen content
$C\bar{v}_{O_2}$ is the mixed venous oxygen content

The technique is essentially invasive as the cardiac output must be measured by an independent method (usually thermodilution), and it is also necessary to sample arterial and mixed venous blood, the latter preferably from the pulmonary artery. Nevertheless it is convenient in the intensive care situation where the necessary lines are commonly in place.

The method has a larger random error than the gasometric techniques described above (Smithies et al., 1991), but also has a systematic error as it excludes the oxygen consumption of the lungs (Figure 11.22). The difference is negligible in the case of healthy lungs but is substantial when the lungs are infected (Table 11.5). Conversely the Fick method of measurement of cardiac output must have a systematic error when there is appreciable pulmonary oxygen consumption.

Validation of methods of measurement of oxygen consumption. Meticulous attention to detail is required if oxygen consumption is to be measured with a satisfactory degree of accuracy. Various metabolic simulators have been described for validation of techniques under different circumstances of use. These include the combustion of known flow rates of an inflammable gas (see Figure 11.21) (Nunn, Makita and Royston, 1989; Svensson, Sonander and Stenqvist, 1990) and the preparation of a mock 'expired gas' by nitrogen dilution and addition of carbon dioxide (Braun et al., 1989; Takala et al., 1989).

Oxygen delivery

Oxygen delivery is measured as the product of cardiac output and arterial oxygen consumption. This excludes oxygen delivered for consumption within the lung. In the intensive care situation, cardiac output is now commonly measured by thermal

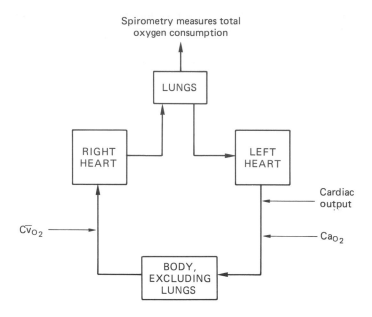

Oxygen delivery = cardiac output × Ca_{O_2}
Oxygen consumption (by reversed Fick technique)
= cardiac output $(Ca_{O_2} - C\bar{v}_{O_2})$

Figure 11.22 Schematic representation of the essential differences in measurement of oxygen consumption by spirometry and by the reversed Fick technique, which measures the oxygen consumption of the body excluding the lungs. The reversed Fick technique is very conveniently undertaken at the same time as measurement of oxygen delivery.

Table 11.5 Comparisons of oxygen consumption measured simultaneously by spirometry and the reversed Fick technique

Subjects	Spirometry	Reversed Fick technique	Reference
Healthy dogs	110 (4.78/kg)	114 (4.96/kg)	Light (1988)
Dogs with pneumonia	146 (5.74/kg)	127 (4.91/kg)	Light (1988)
Patients (IPPV)	319	298	Behrendt et al. (1987)
Patient (spont.)	321	243	Takala et al. (1989)
Patients (SIMV)	344	268	Takala et al. (1989)
Patients (IPPV)	294	247	Takala et al. (1989)
Patients (IPPV)	286	249	Smithies et al. (1991)

The difference is presumed to be due to the oxygen uptake of the lung. All values are expressed as ml/min. IPPV, intermittent positive pressure ventilation; SIMV, synchronized intermittent mandatory ventilation; spont., spontaneous breathing.

dilution and simultaneously an arterial sample is drawn for measurement of oxygen content by any of the methods described above. If oxygen delivery is determined at the same time as oxygen consumption is measured by the reversed Fick technique, it should be remembered that two of the variables (cardiac output and arterial oxygen content) are common to both measurements. This linking of data is a potential source of error in inferring the consequences of changes in one product on the other (Archie, 1981).

Chapter 12

Non-respiratory functions of the lung

The structure of the lungs and their location within the circulatory system are primarily adapted to subserve the purpose of gas exchange. Thus almost the entire circulation passes through the lungs during a single circulation, and the interface between gas and blood is very large, being of the order of 125 m^2 (Weibel, 1983). These characteristics are also ideally suited for the lungs to undertake many other important functions. The location of the lungs within the circulatory system is ideal for its role as a filter to protect the systemic circulation, not only from particulate matter but also from a wide range of chemical substances which undergo removal or biotransformation in the pulmonary circulation. The pulmonary arterial tree is well adapted for the reception of emboli without resultant infarction, and the very large area of endothelium gives the lung a metabolic role out of proportion to its total mass.

These non-respiratory functions were extensively reviewed in the *Handbook of Physiology* of the American Physiological Society, section 3, volume 1, edited by Fishman (1985). The relationship of pulmonary ultrastructure to non-respiratory function was reviewed by Ryan and Ryan (1977), Simionescu (1980), Ryan (1982) and Weibel (1985). More recent reviews of biochemistry and metabolism include Davidson (1990) and Bakhle (1990).

Filtration

Sitting astride the whole output of the right ventricle, the lung is ideally situated to filter out particulate matter from the venous return. Without such a filter, there would be a constant risk of particulate matter entering the arterial system where the coronary and cerebral circulations are particularly vulnerable. In this respect, the position and function of the lungs are closely analogous to the oil filter of the internal combustion engine. Desirable though this function appears at first sight, it cannot be essential to life, since it is bypassed in patients with a right-to-left intracardiac shunt.

Pulmonary capillaries have a diameter of about 7 μm, but this does not appear to be the effective pore size of the pulmonary circulation considered as a filter. There is no clear agreement on the maximal diameter of particles which can traverse the pulmonary circulation. Tobin and Zariquiey (1950) demonstrated the passage through perfused animal lungs of glass beads up to 500 μm. Niden and Aviado (1956) observed the passage of glass beads up to 420 μm following embolization of dog's lungs. It is well known that small quantities of gas and fat emboli may gain access to the systemic circulation in patients without intracardiac shunting. More extensive invasion of the systemic arteries may occur in the presence of an overt right-to-left intracardiac shunt. However, 20–35% of the population have a probe-patent foramen ovale which is normally kept closed by the left atrial pressure being slightly greater than the right (Edward, 1960). Paradoxical embolism may result from a relative increase in right atrial pressure (page 502). Furthermore, emboli may bypass the alveoli as a result of the opening of 'sperr' arteries (page 137).

So far as the survival of the lung is concerned, the geometry of the pulmonary microcirculation is particularly well adapted to maintaining perfusion in the face of microembolization (page 33). However, a significant degree of embolization inevitably blocks the circulation to parts of the lungs, disrupting ventilation/perfusion relationships. It is not surprising that the alveolar component of the physiological dead space is increased after pulmonary embolization and the end-expiratory PCO_2 is reduced (page 175).

Thrombi are cleared more rapidly from the lungs than from other organs. The lung possesses well developed proteolytic systems not confined to the removal of fibrin. Pulmonary endothelium is known to be rich in plasmin activator (Warren, 1963). This converts plasminogen into plasmin which itself converts fibrin into fibrin degradation products. However, the lung is also rich in thromboplastin which converts prothrombin to thrombin. To complicate the position further, the lung is a particularly rich source of heparin, and bovine lung is used in its commercial preparation. The lung can thus produce high concentrations of substances necessary to promote or delay blood clotting and also for fibrinolysis. Apart from the lung's ability to clear itself of thromboemboli, it may play a role in controlling the overall coagulability of the blood.

Oxidative metabolism of the lung

The oxygen consumption of the lung is included in measurement of whole body oxygen consumption by spirometry or indirect calorimetry. However, it is not included in measurement of oxygen consumption by the reversed Fick equation (i.e. as the product of the cardiac output and difference between the oxygen content of the arterial and mixed venous blood, see page 304). There are now several studies of oxgen consumption, measured simultaneously by the two methods, and large differences have been found when there is pulmonary pathology (see Table 11.5). It is still unclear to what extent the enhanced oxygen consumption of the infected lung reflects increased metabolism or the production of oxygen-derived free radicals (see below and Chapter 29).

It is less easy to measure the oxygen consumption of the normal healthy human lung, and estimates range from 3 to 15 ml/min. In relation to its weight of metabolically active tissue, the lung ranks below kidney, brain, heart and liver but above the average for the body as a whole (Fisher and Forman, 1985). Clearly the oxygen consumption of the lung constitutes a systematic error in the measurement of cardiac output by the direct Fick method (page 152).

Oxidative phosphorylation. The major part of the oxygen consumption by the normal lung is in the mitochondria for the production of high energy phosphate compounds by the process of oxidative phosphorylation (page 248). This is essentially the same process as in other tissues, except that the tissue PO_2 is higher in the lungs, being close to that of alveolar gas. However, when ventilation of parts of the lung fails (e.g. in consolidation or collapse), the PO_2 of the unventilated parts of lung tissue must then reflect the PO_2 of the mixed venous blood. Substrates consumed by the lungs include glucose, lactate, pyruvate and amino acids (Datta, Stubbs and Alberti, 1980; Tierney and Young, 1985).

Cytochrome P-450 systems. The lung is one of the major extrahepatic sites of mixed function oxidation by the cytochrome P-450 systems (see page 254). However, gram-for-gram the lung is considerably less active than the liver, and its weight of metabolically active tissue is much less than that of the liver. Therefore the total contribution of the lung is quite small in relation to the liver. Furthermore, the lung has only limited capacity for induction of the cytochrome P-450 enzymes.

The role of the cytochrome P-450 system in the lung is not immediately obvious. Biotransformation of drugs has been demonstrated, but the total contribution to the body cannot be large. Fisher and Forman (1985) do not think it likely to provide a mechanism for the active transport of oxygen (Gurtner and Burns, 1975), which was considered at some length in the second edition of this book. It has, however, been considered more recently as a possible mechanism in hypoxic pulmonary vasoconstriction. There may be a role in the metabolism of steroids or fatty acids, and pulmonary cytochrome P-450 systems may be well placed for the detoxification of inhaled substances.

Formation of oxygen-derived free radicals and related species. It has been mentioned above that enhanced oxygen consumption of the lung has been demonstrated in patients with pulmonary infection. For example, Smithies et al. (1991) demonstrated a mean difference of 36 ml/min, with values as high as 97 ml/min in some patients. It seems very unlikely that such changes are explained entirely by increased oxidative phosphorylation, and it is well established that neutrophils, macrophages and certain other cells, which can marginate on the pulmonary capillary endothelium, are active in the formation of oxygen-derived free radicals for bacterial killing. Fall-out from this process may play an important role in damaging the lung. Very substantial quantities of oxygen are consumed in the formation of free radicals and related species derived from molecular oxygen. The mechanisms is described elsewhere (page 542) in relation to oxygen toxicity.

Miscellaneous forms of oxygen consumption include inactivation of vasoactive amines and synthesis of eicosanoids which are considered below.

Protease transport system

The activity of neutrophils and other phagocytes in the lungs leads to the release of dangerous proteases, particularly elastase and trypsin. These enzymes may destroy the alveolar septa but there are at least two mechanisms to protect against this eventuality. Firstly, the proteases are swept towards the larynx by the flow of mucus. Secondly, they are conjugated by α_1-antitrypsin, present in plasma.

Conjugated proteases are then removed in the pulmonary circulation and lymph, and transferred to conjugation with α_2-macroglobulin, which is then destroyed in the liver.

In 1963 Laurell and Eriksson described patients whose plasma proteins were deficient in α_1-antitrypsin and who had developed emphysema. The enzyme deficiency is inherited as an autosomal recessive gene and the incidence of homozygous patients is about 1:3000 of the population, with perhaps a higher incidence in Scandinavia. Homozygotes form a higher proportion of patients with emphysema and estimates range from 3% to 26%. These patients tend to have basal emphysema, onset at a younger age and a severe form of the disease (Hutchison et al., 1971). It thus appears that α_1-antitrypsin deficiency is an aetiological factor in a small proportion of patients with emphysema. There may be a family history and heterozygotes may have a slightly increased incidence of the disease.

Synthesis of surfactant

The role of surfactant in the control of alveolar surface tension was considered in Chapter 3 (page 37). Surfactant is a complex mixture including neutral lipids, protein and carbohydrate, but the most important constituents are phospholipids of the general structure shown in Figure 12.1. The fatty acids are hydrophobic while the other end of the molecule is hydrophilic, the whole thus comprising a detergent. It is believed that the surfactant is concentrated on the surface of the alveolar lining fluid, with the fatty acid chains projecting into the alveolar gas, perpendicular to the interface, with the rest of the molecule in solution.

Lecithins are a series of phospholipids in which the nitrogenous base is choline. Dipalmitoyl lecithin is the most important constituent of the pulmonary surfactant. Palmitic acid is saturated and the fatty acid chains are therefore straight. Harlan and Said (1969) advanced the attractive theory that lipids with straight chain fatty acids will pack together more closely during lung deflation than would be the case with lipids with unsaturated fatty acids (e.g. oleic acid) which are bent at the double bond.

It seems likely that surfactant is both formed in and liberated from the alveolar epithelial type II cell (page 30). Pulmonary surfactant is formed relatively late in the process of maturation of the fetus.

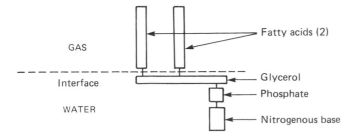

Figure 12.1 General structure of phospholipids.

Processing of hormones and other vasoactive compounds

As long ago as 1925, Starling and Verney observed that passage of blood through the lungs was essential for maintenance of adequate circulation through an isolated perfused kidney. It was later found that the 'detoxification of a serum vasoconstrictor substance' in the blood was due to removal of 5-hydroxytryptamine (serotonin) in the pulmonary circulation. Much recent research has now shown that certain hormones pass through the lung unchanged while others may be almost entirely removed from the blood during a single pass: some may be secreted in the lung while others are chemically changed during transit (Table 12.1). Vane (1969) suggested that substances with local vasomotor effects (e.g. noradrenaline, bradykinin and 5-hydroxytryptamine) are removed in the pulmonary circulation so that their effects are not broadcast by recirculation. In contrast, generally active circulating hormones, such as adrenaline, pass unchanged through the pulmonary circulation. Somewhat similar arguments have been adduced in relation to the highly selective removal of eicosanoids by the pulmonary circulation (Said, 1982). Teleological though this argument may be, it focuses the mind and the theme has been developed in many reviews.

Of the many types of cell in the lungs, it is the endothelium which is most active metabolically (page 27). The most important location is the pulmonary capillary but it must be stressed that endothelium from a very wide range of vessels has been shown to possess a very similar repertoire of metabolic processes (Ryan, 1982). This is fortunate because it is not possible to harvest pulmonary capillary endothelium, and so cultures must be prepared from vascular endothelial cells harvested from other sites, such as human umblical vein. However, there are some important differences in activity between endothelium from different vessels. For example, endothelium grown from various non-pulmonary vessels will not inactivate PGE_2, although this is well known to occur in the pulmonary circulation. The extensive metabolic activity of the pulmonary endothelium takes place in spite of

Table 12.1 Summary of metabolic changes in the lungs

Substances largely removed from the circulation
Noradrenaline
5-Hydroxytryptamine
Bradykinin
ATP, ADP, AMP
PGE_2, PGE_1, $PGF_{2\alpha}$
Leukotrienes

Substances largely unaffected by passage through the lung
Adrenaline
Angiotensin II
Vasopressin
Isoprenaline
Dopamine
Histamine
PGI_2, PGA_2

Substances biotransformed by the lung
Angiotensin I (into angiotensin II)

---

the paucity of organelles which are normally associated with metabolic activity, in particular mitochondria and smooth endoplasmic reticulum or microsomes (see Figure 2.8). Nevertheless, the caveolae result in a major increase in the already extensive surface area of these cells (about 126 m^2; Weibel, 1983). This is highly advantageous for membrane-bound enzymes.

Endogenous vasoactive compounds
(see reviews by Junod, 1985, and Bakhle, 1990)

Nitric oxide – endothelium-derived relaxing factor. Furchgott and Zawadzki (1980) demonstrated the obligatory role of endothelial cells for the relaxation of smooth muscle by acetylcholine. Their group later coined the term 'endothelium-derived relaxing factor' (EDRF) for the presumed second messenger. It was postulated that EDRF was synthesized in and released from endothelium in response to the action of certain known vasodilators, including acetylcholine and bradykinin. EDRF was then presumed to diffuse to the underlying smooth muscle to cause vasodilatation. Two groups showed that the free radical nitric oxide was released from endothelium and was indistinguishable from EDRF in its properties (Ignarro et al., 1987; Palmer, Ferrige and Moncada, 1987). It seems very likely that nitric oxide is EDRF, but there remains the possibility that there are other endothelium-derived vasodilator mediators, as yet undiscovered. Many new biological roles of nitric oxide have been found, not only in the circulation but also in immunological reactions and as a neurotransmitter in the central nervous system (Garthwaite, 1991; Moncada, Palmer and Higgs, 1991).

Nitric oxide (NO) is synthesized in endothelium from L-arginine, in response to several stimuli including histamine, bradykinin, adenosine triphosphate and acetylcholine (Bakhle, 1990; Ignarro, 1990). The enzyme NO synthase is activated by calmodulin and the reaction consumes oxygen and NADPH forming nitric oxide and L-citrulline (Figure 12.2). L-NMMA and a range of novel compounds are competitive inhibitors of the synthesis of nitric oxide (Moncada, Palmer and Higgs, 1991). Nitric oxide is a free radical which reacts with oxygen or the superoxide free radical to form nitrite or nitrate ions respectively. Its half-life is a few seconds and it is selectively inactivated by haemoglobin, myoglobin and methylene blue. Nevertheless, it is lipid soluble and so able to diffuse rapidly to underlying smooth muscle, where it causes relaxation by conversion of GTP to cyclic GMP. This is the common final pathway of action for the nitrate, nitrite and nitroprusside vasodilators which release nitric oxide in the smooth muscle without the requirement for intact endothelium. Endothelium-derived nitric oxide is functionally significant in local arterioles but, because of its short half-life, cannot act as a freely circulating vasoactive hormone.

It has been shown that nitric oxide is a potent vasodilator of the pulmonary circulation. Furthermore it has been shown that synthesis is attenuated at low Po_2 (Warren et al., 1989). Since pulmonary hypoxic vasoconstriction (see page 145) is known to be in large part dependent on the presence of a functioning endothelium, it appears possible that hypoxic suppression of synthesis of nitric oxide may have a role in its mechanism. This view is supported by studies of isolated pulmonary arterial segments (Rodman et al., 1990).

A major development in the area has been the therapeutic use of inhaled low concentrations of nitric oxide for the relief of pulmonary hypertension and as a

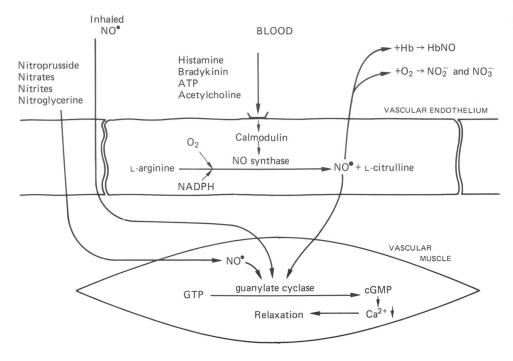

Figure 12.2 Scheme to show synthesis of nitric oxide in the vascular endothelium, with diffusion into the muscular coat where nitric oxide acts as a vasodilator. Nitrite and nitrate vasodilators are converted to nitric oxide in the muscle cells, where inhaled nitric oxide acts directly. Nitric oxide is rapidly removed from circulating blood by oxygenation and by formation of a ligand with haemoglobin, which is then converted to methaemoglobin. cGMP, cyclic guanosine monophosphate; GTP, guanosine triphosphate.

selective vasodilator of ventilated areas of the lung (see pages 146 and 516). It is also a bronchodilator. Inhibitors of nitric oxide synthesis may have a role as pressor agents, since there appears to be a standing vasodilator tone.

Various inhibitors of NO synthase have been developed and these compounds may well have an important clinical role in the management of intractable hypotension, as for example in septic shock.

Noradrenaline (norepinephrine,). There is a striking difference in the handling of noradrenaline and adrenaline. Although each catecholamine has a half-life of about 20 seconds in blood, some 30% of noradrenaline is removed in a single pass through the lungs in animals (Ginn and Vane, 1968) and also in man (Sole et al., 1979), while adrenaline (and isoprenaline and dopamine) is unaffected. Noradrenaline is taken up by the endothelium, mainly in the microcirculation, including arterioles and venules.

In contrast to neuronal uptake, noradrenaline is rapidly metabolized after uptake in the lung. Uptake is not inhibited by monoamine oxidase or catechol-*o*-methyl transferase inhibitors but has been reported to be inhibited by inhalational anaesthetics in laboratory animals (Naito and Gillis, 1973; Bakhle and Block, 1976). Extraneuronal uptake of noradrenaline is not confined to the endothelium of the lungs, but uptake by the pulmonary circulation differs in some respects from extraneuronal uptake (uptake 2) in other tissues (Junod, 1985).

5-Hydroxytryptamine (5-HT, serotonin) is very effectively removed by the lungs, up to 98% being removed in a single pass (Thomas and Vane, 1967). There are considerable similarities to the processing of noradrenaline. Uptake is in the endothelium, mainly in the capillaries (see Junod, 1985). Following uptake, 5-HT is rapidly metabolized by monoamine oxidase. Uptake is not blocked by monoamine oxidase inhibitors but unchanged 5-HT then accumulates in the lung (Alabaster, 1980). The half-life of 5-HT in blood is about 1–2 minutes and pulmonary clearance plays the major role in the prevention of its recirculation. If the uptake of 5-HT is inhibited (e.g. by cocaine or tricyclic antidepressant drugs), its pulmonary clearance is greatly reduced (Said, 1982).

Histamine is not removed from the pulmonary circulation although histamine is inactivated by chopped lung. It thus appears that removal of histamine from the circulation is limited by its transport mechanism across the blood/endothelium barrier. The lung is a major site of synthesis of histamine, and mechanisms for its release from mast cells are considered elsewhere (page 73).

Acetylcholine is rapidly hydrolysed in blood where it has a half-life of less than 2 seconds. This tends to overshadow any changes attributable to the lung, which nevertheless does contain acetylcholinesterases and pseudocholinesterases.

Angiotensin, bradykinin and other peptides. It has long been known that angiotensin I (a decapeptide formed by the action of renin on a plasma α_2-globulin) is converted into the vasoactive octapeptide angiotensin II by incubation with plasma (Figure 12.3). In 1967, Ng and Vane found greatly increased conversion in the pulmonary circulation, some 80% being converted in a single pass. Enhanced conversion of angiotensin is not peculiar to the pulmonary circulation but the lung is certainly a major site for angiotensin conversion. Angiotensin-converting enzyme (ACE) is free in the plasma but is also bound to the surface of endothelium. This appears to be a general property of endothelium but ACE is present in abundance on the vascular surface of pulmonary endothelial cells, also lining the inside of the caveolae and extending onto the projections into the lumen (Ryan, 1982).

Bradykinin, a vasoactive nonapeptide, is also very effectively removed during passage through the lung and other vascular beds. The half-life in blood is about 17 seconds but less than 4 seconds in various vascular beds (Ryan, 1985). Bakhle (1968) reported that bradykinin and angiotensin I were both cleaved by the same fraction of lung homogenate, and it transpired that ACE was the enzyme responsible in both cases. Thus angiotensin I may act as a competitive inhibitor of the bradykininase activity. There is evidence that other enzymes are capable of metabolizing both angiotensin I and bradykinin but they have not yet been characterized. It is likely that these other enzymes are also located on the endothelial surface.

ACE is inhibited by many substances, some of which (e.g. captopril and enalapril) have a clinical role in the treatment of hypertension. However, this also decreases the degradation of bradykinin by ACE, although other enzymes are capable of handling bradykinin. Even with total inhibition of ACE there is thought

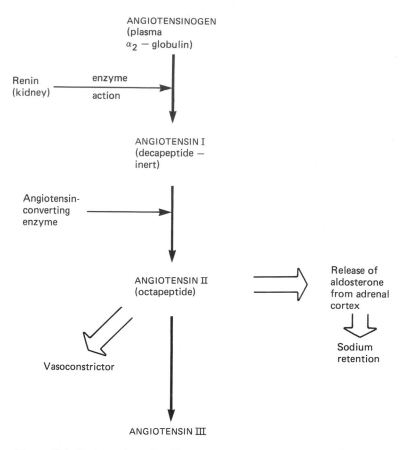

Figure 12.3 Renin–angiotensin–aldosterone axis. Angiotensin-converting enzyme is present on the vascular surface of the pulmonary endothelium.

to be an adequate reserve for bradykinin metabolism (Bakhle, 1980). Angiotensin II itself passes through the lung unchanged, as do vasopressin and oxytocin.

Atrial natriuretic peptide (ANP) is largely removed by the rabbit lung in a single pass but can then be released from what appears to be binding to a 'silent' receptor (Needleman et al., 1989).

Prostaglandins, thromboxanes and leukotrienes

The lung is a major site of synthesis, metabolism, uptake and release of arachidonic acid metabolites (see Bakhle and Ferreira, 1985). The group as a whole are 20-carbon carboxylic acids, generically known as eicosanoids. The initial stages of metabolism of arachidonic acid are oxygenations with two main pathways for which the enzymes are respectively cyclo-oxygenase and lipoxygenase. The cyclo-oxygenase pathway (Figure 12.4) commences with oxygenation and cyclization to form the prostaglandin PGG_2, the enzyme being microsomal and found in most

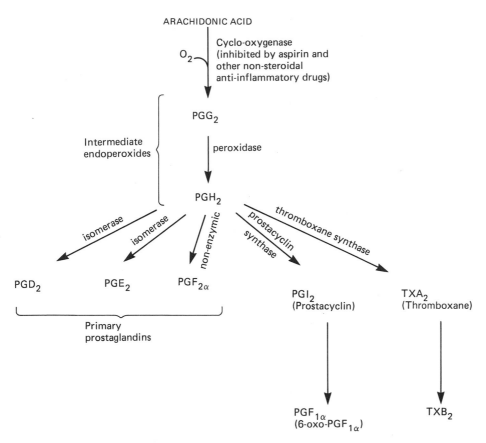

Figure 12.4 The cyclo-oxygenase pathway of metabolism of arachidonic acid to form the prostaglandins and thromboxane. See text for metabolism taking place in the lungs.

cells. (The subscript 2 indicates two double bonds in the carbon chain.) A non-specific peroxidase then converts PGG_2 to PGH_2, which is the parent compound for synthesis of many important derivatives shown in Figure 12.4.

$PGF_{2\alpha}$, PGD_2, PGG_2, PGH_2 and thromboxane TXA_2 are bronchial and tracheal constrictors, $PGF_{2\alpha}$ and PGD_2 being much more potent in asthmatics than in normal subjects. PGE_1 and PGE_2 are bronchodilators, particularly when administered by aerosol. Prostacyclin (PGI_2) has different effects in different species. In man, it has no effect on airway calibre in doses which have profound cardiovascular effects (Hardy et al., 1985). PGI_2 and PGE_1 are pulmonary vasodilators. PGH_2 and $PGF_{2\alpha}$ are pulmonary vasoconstrictors.

Eicosanoids are not stored preformed, but are synthesized as required by many cell types in the lung, including endothelium, airway smooth muscle, mast cells, epithelial cells and vascular muscle. Activation of the complement system is a potent stimulus to the metabolism of arachidonic acid. Synthesis from endogenous arachidonic acid in the lung appears to be limited by the rate of formation of arachidonic acid from parent lipids. Steroids decrease the availability of endogenous arachidonic acid. Infusion of exogenous arachidonic acid bypasses this stage and results in both bronchoconstriction and vasoconstriction, mediated by its metabolites and depending on the dose. This effect can be blocked by high dose aspirin and some other non-steroidal anti-inflammatory drugs which inhibit cyclo-oxygenase. Release of eicosanoids, particularly TXA_2, occurs in anaphylactic reactions in response to complement activation. However, release of cyclo-oxygenase products does not seem to be a major factor in allergic asthma, which is not significantly relieved by inhibition of cyclo-oxygenase. This may well be explained by increased availability of arachidonic acid for the lipoxygenase pathway (see below). PGI_2 appears to be continuously released from the lungs of certain anaesthetized laboratory animals. In anaesthetized man, blood levels of PGI_2 are subthreshold, but artificial ventilation or extracorporeal circulation causes a tenfold increase (Edlund et al., 1981).

Various specific enzymes in the lung are responsible for extensive metabolism of PGE_2, PGE_1 and $PGF_{2\alpha}$. However, PGA_2 and PGI_2 pass through the lung unchanged, but are metabolized on passing through the portal circulation (see review by Bakhle and Ferreira, 1985).

Leukotrienes are also eicosanoids derived from arachidonic acid but by the lipoxygenase pathway (Figure 12.5). The leukotrienes LTC_4 and LTD_4 are mainly responsible for the bronchoconstrictor effects of what was formerly known as slow-reacting substance A or SRS-A (Morris et al., 1980; Piper et al., 1981). SRS-A also contains LTB_4, which is a less powerful bronchoconstrictor but increases vascular permeability. These compounds, which are synthesized by the mast cell, could have an important role in asthma, and the mechanism of their release is discussed in Chapter 4 (page 75).

Handling of foreign substances by the lungs

The lungs have considerable ability to take up, store or detoxify foreign substances (Bend, Serabjit-Singh and Philpot, 1985). This includes a wide range of drugs which bind reversibly although most of them are not metabolized. Drugs which are taken up in the pulmonary circulation include propranolol (Geddes et al., 1979), lignocaine (Jorfeldt et al., 1979), chlorpromazine, imipramine and nortriptyline (Gillis, 1973). Basic drugs tend to be taken up in the pulmonary circulation while acidic drugs preferentially bind to plasma proteins (Bakhle, 1986, personal communication).

Accumulation of toxic substances in the lung may cause dangerous local toxicity, and paraquat is an outstanding example (page 548). Chronic exposure to a number of amphiphilic drugs may induce phospholipidosis (Philpot, Anderson and Eling, 1977).

The cytochrome P-450 system is active in the lung (see above) and Philpot, Anderson and Eling (1977) listed an impressive number of compounds which are detoxified in this manner. It is also known that certain anaesthetics undergo biotransformation (Blitt et al., 1979). Mixed function oxidase systems have been identified in the microsomes of alveolar macrophages and bronchial epithelium. As outlined at the beginning of this chapter, the microsomal systems of the lung cannot be induced as effectively as in the liver. It will be of special interest to know how well the lung can detoxify inhaled substances. Unfortunately, there is little information on this subject at present.

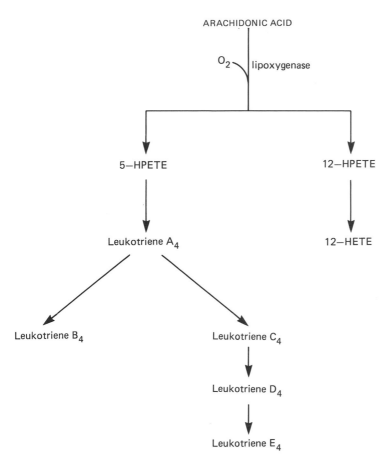

Figure 12.5 The lipoxygenase pathway of metabolism of arachidonic acid to form the leukotrienes. See text for metabolism taking place in the lungs.

Conclusion

Processing of substances in the lungs has many important implications. Firstly, there will be a substantial difference between arterial and venous plasma concentrations of various substances. Therefore analyses of such substances are meaningful only if the appropriate sampling site is used and specified. Secondly, processing of drugs in the lungs must influence the route of administration and dosage. Thirdly, bypassing the pulmonary circulation must have substantial effects on the levels of many substances which will then pass into the systemic circulation. It always seems to the author remarkable how well this is tolerated.

The last word should perhaps be by John Vane (1969): 'It is intriguing to think that venous blood may be full of noxious, as yet unidentified, chemicals released from the peripheral vascular beds, but removed by the lungs before they can cause effects in the arterial circulation'.

Part II

The Applications

Chapter 13

Respiratory aspects of exercise

Levels of exercise

The respiratory response to exercise depends on the level of exercise, which can be conveniently divided into three grades (Whipp, 1981):

1. *Moderate exercise* is below the subject's anaerobic threshold and the arterial blood lactate is not raised. He is able to transport all the oxygen required and remain in a steady state. This would correspond to work (more correctly 'power' – see below) levels up to about 100 watts (612 kg m min^{-1}).
2. *Heavy exercise* is above the anaerobic threshold. The arterial blood lactate is elevated but remains constant. This too may be regarded as a steady state.
3. *Severe exercise* is well above the anaerobic threshold and the arterial blood lactate continues to rise. This is an unsteady state and the level of work cannot long be continued.

Units of work and power. In the biomedical field, it is commonplace to use the term *work* when *power* is meant. Work is force × distance, and a kilopond is the force resulting from the action of normal gravity on a mass of 1 kg. The SI unit of work is the joule (newton metre). Power is work per unit time. Correct units of power are watts (joules/second) or kilopond metres minutes^{-1}. However, it is common practice, particularly in the USA, to express work (meaning power) as kilogram (actually kilopond) metres minutes^{-1}; 6.12 kg m min^{-1} = 1 watt (see Appendix A).

Oxygen consumption

There is a close relationship between the external power which is produced and the oxygen consumption of the subject (Figure 13.1). The oxygen consumption at rest (the basal metabolic rate) is of the order of 200–250 ml/min. As work is done, the oxygen consumption increases by about 12 ml/min per watt (approx 2 ml/min per kp m min^{-1}). A consumption of about 1 l/min is required for walking briskly on the level. About 3 l/min is needed to run at 12 km/hour (7.5 miles/hour). A fit and healthy young adult of 70 kg should be able to maintain a maximal oxygen consumption ($\dot{V}O_{2max}$) of about 3 l/min, but this decreases with age to about 2 l/min at the age of 70. A sedentary existence without exercise can reduce $\dot{V}O_{2max}$ to

50% of the expected value. Conversely, $\dot{V}O_{2max}$ can be increased by regular exercise, and athletes commonly achieve values of 5 l/min. The highest levels (over 6 l/min) are attained in rowers, who utilize a greater muscle mass than other athletes. Clark, Hagerman and Gelfand (1983) have reported an elite group of oarsmen who, for a brief period, attained a mean oxygen consumption of 6.6 l/min on the treadmill. This required a minute volume of 200 l/min (tidal volume 3.29 litres at a frequency of 62 b.p.m.).

Oxygen consumption rises rapidly to a steady level at the onset of a period of continuous light or moderate exercise. If the level of exercise exceeds 60% of the maximal oxygen consumption, there is usually a secondary slow increase in oxygen consumption which has been observed between the 5th and 20th minutes of exercise. This has been attributed to lactacidosis but Hagberg, Mullin and Nagle (1978) adduced evidence to suggest that it could be explained by increased temperature and the oxygen cost of breathing, which is disproportionately high as minute volume increases (Figure 13.1).

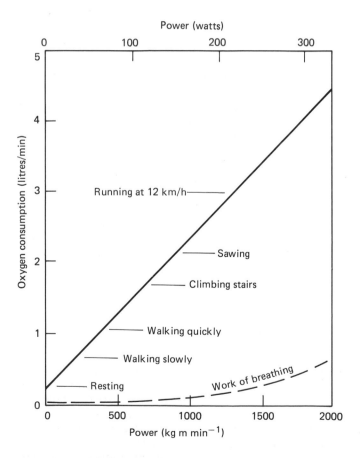

Figure 13.1 The continuous straight line denotes whole body oxygen consumption as a function of the level of power developed. The broken curve is an estimate of the oxygen cost of breathing for the increasing hyperventilation of exercise (Otis, 1964; Aaron et al., 1992).

At the end of moderate exercise below the anaerobic threshold, the oxygen consumption rapidly returns within a few minutes to the resting level. However, after heavy exercise there is a delay in the return of oxygen consumption to basal levels as the oxygen debt is discharged (see below).

Anaerobic metabolism

During heavy work, the total work exceeds the capacity for aerobic work, which is limited by oxygen transport (see below). The difference is made up by anaerobic metabolism, of which the principal product is lactic acid (see Figure 11.3) which is almost entirely ionized to lactate and hydrogen ions. An increase in blood lactate level is therefore taken as the indication that there is a significant anaerobic contribution to metabolism. This defines the anaerobic threshold, which depends not only on the power produced but also on many other factors including altitude, environmental temperature and the degree of training undertaken by the subject. An additional factor is the muscle groups which are used to accomplish the work. Thus it was found that lactate began to rise when oxygen consumption exceeded about 2 l/min during leg exercise but at less than 1 l/min during arm exercise (Asmussen and Neilsen, 1946). Lactacidosis probably provides part of the stimulus for the excess ventilation required for work in excess of the anaerobic threshold (see below).

During steady state heavy anaerobic exercise, the lactate level reaches a plateau within the first 5–10 minutes. The level is influenced by the factors described above in relation to the anaerobic threshold, but is of the order of 100 mg/dl at 200 watts (1200 kp m min^{-1}).

During severe exercise the lactate level continues to rise and begins to cause distress at levels above about 100 mg/dl, ten times the resting level. However, trained athletes can tolerate levels of 200 mg/dl. Lactate accumulation appears to be the limiting factor for sustained heavy work, and the progressive increase in blood lactate results in the level of work being inversely related to the time for which it can be maintained. Thus there is a reciprocal relationship between the record time for various distances and the speed at which they are run (Asmussen, 1965).

Oxygen debt

The difference between the total work and the aerobic work is achieved by anaerobic metabolism of carbohydrates to lactate, which is ultimately converted to citrate, enters the citric acid cycle and is then fully oxidized. Like glucose, lactate has a respiratory quotient of 1.0. Although this process continues during heavy exercise, lactate accumulates and the excess is oxidized in the early stages of recovery. Oxygen consumption remains above the resting level during recovery for this purpose. This constitutes the 'repayment of the oxygen debt' and is related to the lactate level attained by the end of exercise.

Repayment of the oxygen debt is especially well developed in the diving mammals such as seals and whales. During a dive, their circulation is largely diverted to heart and brain and the metabolism of the skeletal muscles is almost entirely anaerobic (page 360). On regaining the surface, very large quantities of lactate are suddenly released into the circulation and are rapidly metabolized while the animal is on the surface between dives.

There is considerable evidence that some of the early part of the repayment of the oxygen debt is not only concerned with clearing lactate. Apart from oxidation of other products of anaerobic metabolism, there is the restoration of both oxygen stores and levels of high energy phosphate compounds to their normal resting levels (Asmussen, 1965).

Response of the oxygen delivery system

A ten- or twentyfold increase in oxygen consumption requires a complex adaptation of both circulatory and respiratory systems.

Oxygen delivery or flux is the product of cardiac output and arterial oxygen content (page 283). The latter cannot be significantly increased and therefore an increase in

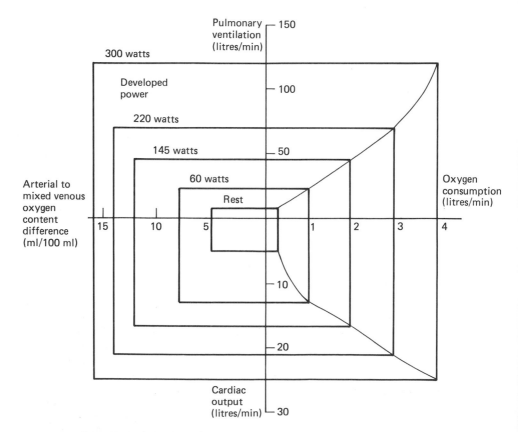

Figure 13.2 Changes in ventilation, oxygen consumption, cardiac output and oxygen extraction at different levels of power developed.

cardiac output is essential. However, the cardiac output does not, and indeed could not, increase in proportion to the oxygen consumption. For example, an oxygen consumption of 4 l/min is a 16-fold increase compared with the resting state. A typical cardiac output at this level of exercise would be only 25 l/min (Figure 13.2), which is only five times the resting value. Therefore, there must also be increased extraction of oxygen from the blood. Figure 13.2 shows that the largest relative increase in cardiac output occurs at mild levels of exercise. At an oxygen consumption of 1 l/min cardiac output is already close to 50% of its maximal value.

Oxygen extraction. In the resting state, blood returns to the right heart with haemoglobin 70% saturated. This provides a substantial reserve of available oxygen and the arterial to mixed venous oxygen content difference increases progressively as oxygen consumption is increased, particularly in heavy exercise when the mixed venous saturation may be as low as 20% (Figure 13.2). This decrease in mixed venous saturation covers the steep part of the oxygen dissociation curve (see Figure 11.12) and, therefore, the decrease in PO_2 is relatively less (5 to 2 kPa, or 37.5 to 15 mmHg. The additionally desaturated blood returning to the lungs and the greater volume of blood require that the respiratory system transport a larger quantity of oxygen to the alveoli. If there were no increased oxygen transport to the alveoli, the reserve oxygen in the mixed venous blood would be exhausted in one or two circulation times. Fortunately, the respiratory system normally responds rapidly to this requirement.

The ventilatory response to exercise

Time course. We have seen in the previous section that exercise without a rapid ventilatory response would be dangerous if not fatal. In fact, the respiratory system does respond with great rapidity (Figure 13.3). There is an instant increase in ventilation at, if not slightly before, the start of exercise (phase I). During moderate exercise, there is then a further increase (phase II) to reach an equilibrium level of ventilation (phase III) within about 3 minutes (Wasserman, 1978). With heavy exercise there is a secondary increase in ventilation which may reach a plateau, but ventilation continues to rise in severe work. At the end of exercise, the minute volume falls to resting levels within a few minutes. After heavy and severe exercise, return to the resting level of ventilation takes longer, as the oxygen debt is repaid and lactate levels return to normal.

The ventilation equivalent for oxygen. The respiratory minute volume is normally very well matched to the increased oxygen consumption, and the relationship between minute volume and oxygen consumption is approximately linear up to an oxygen consumption of about 2 l/min and more in the trained subject (Figure 13.4). The slope of the linear part is the ventilation equivalent for oxygen and is within the range 20–30 l/min ventilation per l/min of oxygen consumption (Cotes, 1979; Åstrand and Rodahl, 1986; Forster and Pan, 1991). The slope does not appear to change with training.

In heavy exercise, above a critical level of oxygen consumption (Owles point), the ventilation increases above the level predicted by an extrapolation of the linear

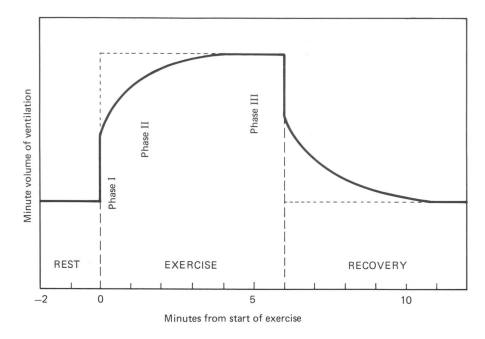

Figure 13.3 The time course of changes in ventilation in relation to a short period of moderate exercise. Note the instant increase in ventilation at the start of exercise before the metabolic consequences of exercise have had any effect.

part of the ventilation/oxygen consumption relationship (Figure 13.4). This is surplus to the requirement for gas exchange and is accompanied by hypocapnia with arterial P_{CO_2} decreasing by levels of the order of 1 kPa (7.5 mmHg). The excess ventilation is probably driven by lactacidosis. In the trained athlete, the break from linearity occurs at higher levels of oxygen consumption (Cotes, 1979). This together with improved tolerance of high minute volumes allows the trained athlete to increase his $\dot{V}O_{2max}$ as shown in Figure 13.4.

Minute volume and dyspnoea. It is generally believed that the ventilatory system does not limit exercise in normal subjects, although the evidence for this view is elusive (Bye, Farkas and Roussos, 1983). Shephard (1967) found that 50—60% of maximal breathing capacity (MBC) was required for work at 80% of aerobic capacity. However, Cotes (1979) took the view that the breaking point of exercise is usually determined by breathlessness, which occurs when the exercise ventilation utilizes a high proportion of the maximal breathing capacity (page 133). There is a close correlation between maximal ventilation and $\dot{V}O_{2max}$ (Åstrand and Rodahl, 1986). There can, of course, be no doubt that ventilation is the limiting factor in many patients with reduced ventilatory capacity.

Minute volumes as great as 200 l/min have been recorded during exercise although the normal subject cannot maintain a minute volume approaching his maximal breathing capacity (MBC) for more than a very short period. Tidal volume during maximal exercise is about half vital capacity (Åstrand and Rodahl, 1986), and 70–80% of the MBC can be maintained with difficulty for 15 minutes by fit young subjects (Shephard, 1967). Wasserman (1978) observed that ventilation

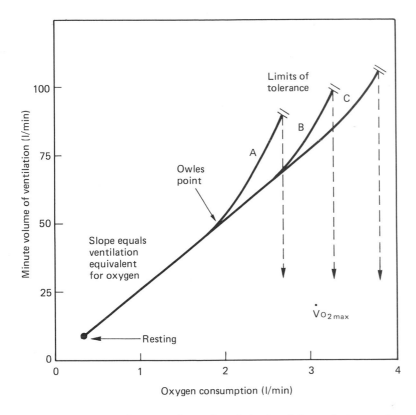

Figure 13.4 Changes of minute volume of ventilation in relation to the increased oxygen consumption of exercise. The break from linearity (Owles point) occurs at higher levels of oxygen consumption in trained athletes, who can also tolerate higher minute volumes. A to C shows progressive levels of training. Both mechanisms combine to enable the trained athlete to increase his maximum oxygen consumption.

approximates to 60% of MBC at maximal oxygen consumption. The usable fraction of the maximal breathing capacity can, however, be increased by training.

Diffusing capacity. Diffusion across the alveolar/capillary membrane does not limit the increased oxygen consumption at sea level but this is a limiting factor at altitude (see Chapters 9 and 15).

Control of ventilation

Elucidation of the mechanisms which underlie the remarkably efficient adaptation of ventilation to the demands of exercise has remained a challenge to generations of physiologists, and a complete explanation remains elusive at the time of writing (see reviews by Asmussen, 1965; Wasserman, 1978; Whipp, 1981; Forster and Pan, 1991).

Arterial blood gas tensions and the chemoreceptors

There is a large body of evidence that, during exercise at sea level with oxygen consumption up to about 3 l/min, there is no significant change in either P_{CO_2} or P_{O_2} of arterial blood. Asmussen and Neilsen (1960) found that even at the point of exhaustion for their subjects (oxygen consumption 3.5 l/min), the arterial P_{O_2} was the same as the resting value and P_{CO_2} was actually reduced. Blood gas tensions do not therefore appear at first sight to be the main factor governing the increased minute volume, although they are critically important at great altitude (see Chapter 15). Two caveats must be mentioned.

Inhalation of 100% oxygen during exercise reduces minute volume for a particular oxygen consumption (Cotes, 1979). The P_{O_2}/ventilation response curve is known to be steeper during exercise (see Figure 5.6), and therefore ventilation responds to small fluctuations in normal arterial P_{O_2} under these circumstances. Asthmatic patients after carotid body resection have shown a slowing of the rate of increase of ventilation during exercise (Wasserman, 1978). The second caveat is that during exercise there is an increased respiratory phasic variation in arterial P_{CO_2}, which is known to stimulate the carotid body (page 99). In spite of these caveats, it is difficult to avoid the conclusion that arterial blood gas tensions acting on the chemoreceptors cannot be the main factor in the increase of ventilation during exercise. This contrasts sharply with their dominant role in the control of resting ventilation.

Neural factors

It has long been evident that neural factors play an important role, particularly since ventilation normally increases at or even before the start of exercise (phase I), when no other physiological variable has changed except cardiac output (Figure 13.3). Kao (1963) and his colleagues showed that virtually all of the hyperventilation of exercise can be explained by afferents arising from the exercising muscles of anaesthetized dogs. This was convincingly shown in crossed-circulation studies. The essential observation was that an anaesthetized dog in neurological continuity with electrically stimulated limb muscles hyperventilated, while another dog receiving the venous drainage from the exercising muscles did not. It was established that afferent traffic from the stimulating electrode was not the explanation (Tibes, 1977).

Humoral mechanisms

Humoral factors play a comparatively minor role in moderate exercise but are more important in heavy and severe exercise when lactacidosis is an important factor. Exercise at high altitude is a special case when oxygen transport becomes a limiting factor (see Chapter 15).

Metabolic acidosis causes excess ventilation during heavy and severe exercise (Figure 13.4), causing a slight reduction in arterial P_{CO_2}. However, study of arterial pH may be misleading since the very short transit time from lungs to carotid body during exercise (of the order of 4–6 seconds) is insufficient for the change in P_{CO_2} in the lungs to result in an equilibrium change in plasma pH by the time the blood reaches the chemoreceptors. The limiting step is the dehydration of carbonic acid (equation 2 in Chapter 10), which takes an appreciable time even in the presence of carbonic anhydrase. However, there is ample time for equilibration to occur in arterial blood sampled for analysis. Therefore the peripheral chemoreceptors see a different pH from that indicated by the pH meter, and blood perfusing the carotid bodies may be 0.02–0.03 pH units more acid, and the P_{CO_2} slightly higher than indicated by analysis of an arterial blood sample by conventional methods (Crandall, Bidani and Forster, 1977). Slight additional respiratory drive may result from hyperthermia.

It has not escaped notice that the hyperventilation of exercise accords with the blood gas changes of the mixed venous blood. However, there is no evidence of any chemoreceptor in the great veins, the right heart or the input side of the lungs. There is some evidence that there may be metabolic chemoreceptors in the muscles (see review by Whipp, 1981). There is, however, no general agreement on the importance of this factor (Dejours, 1964).

The influence of training

Much is known about the effects of training on exercise performance, but it is far from clear how training can influence the respiratory aspects of exercise.

Minute volume of ventilation. Maximal expiratory flow rate is limited by flow-dependent airway closure (page 77), and is relatively unaffected by training (Shephard, 1967; Cotes, 1979). However, within the limits of maximal breathing capacity, it is possible to increase the strength and endurance of the respiratory muscles. It is therefore possible to improve the *fraction* of the maximal breathing capacity which can be sustained during exercise (Cotes, 1979). Highly trained athletes may be able to maintain ventilations at as much as 90% of their maximal breathing capacity.

Ventilation equivalent for oxygen. There is no evidence that training can alter the slope of the plot of ventilation against oxygen consumption (Figure 13.4). However, the upward inflection of the curve (Owles point) is further to the right in the trained subject. This permits the attainment of a higher oxygen consumption for the same minute volume. Prolongation of the straight part of the curve is achieved by improving metabolic processes in skeletal muscle to minimize the stimulant effect of lactacidosis. There is ample evidence that training can improve the aerobic performance of muscles by many adaptations including, for example, the increased density of the capillary network in the muscles. The consequent reduction in lactacidosis and therefore the excess ventilation, together with an increase in the tolerable minute volume, combine to increase the $\dot{V}_{O_2max}$ as shown in Figure 13.4. It would appear that the major factor in increasing the $\dot{V}_{O_2max}$ is improved performance of skeletal muscles, rather than any specific change in respiratory function.

Chapter 14

Respiratory aspects of sleep

Since about 1980, there has been a surge of interest in the danger of hypoxic episodes during sleep, especially in relation to snoring, obesity and in the post-operative period. The syndrome of obstructive sleep apnoea is now well rec-ognized, as are the deleterious effects of chronic intermittent hypoxia. The purpose of this chapter is to provide a general review of the effects of sleep on respiration in the normal and pathological states.

Normal sleep

Sleep is classified on the basis of the electroencephalogram (EEG) and electro-oculogram (EOG) into non-REM (stages 1–4) and REM (rapid eye movement) sleep.

Stage 1 is dozing from which arousal easily takes place. The EEG is low voltage and the frequency is mixed but predominantly fast. This progresses to stage 2 in which the background EEG is similar to stage 1 but with episodic sleep spindles (frequency 12–14 Hz) and K complexes (large biphasic waves of characteristic appearance). Slow, large amplitude (delta) waves start to appear in stage 2 but become more dominant in stage 3 in which spindles are less conspicuous and K complexes become difficult to distinguish. In stage 4, which is often referred to as deep sleep, the EEG is mainly high voltage (more than 75 μV and more than 50% slow (delta) frequency.

REM sleep has quite different characteristics. The EEG pattern is the same as in stage 1 but the EOG shows frequent rapid eye movements which are easily distinguished from the rolling eye movements of non-REM sleep. Other forms of activity are manifest in REM sleep and dreaming occurs.

The stage of sleep changes frequently during the night, and the pattern varies between different individuals and on different nights for the same individual (Figure 14.1). Sleep is entered in stage 1 and usually progresses through 2 to 3 and sometimes into 4. Episodes of REM sleep alternate with non-REM sleep through-out the night. On average there are four or five episodes of REM sleep per night, with a tendency for the duration of the episodes to increase towards morning. Conversely, stages 3 and 4 predominate in the early part of the night. The sleeper can pass from any stage to any other stage but it is unusual for him to pass from stage 1 or REM into either 3 or 4 or from stage 3 or 4 into REM. However, it is not uncommon for the sleeper to pass from any stage into stage 1 or full consciousness.

Respiratory changes

The metabolic rate decreases during sleep to about 10% below the conventional basal level. This corresponds to the basal level as defined by Robertson and Reid (1952) and is similar to levels encountered during anaesthesia (page 402). The oxygen consumption tends to be highest in REM sleep and lowest in stages 3 and 4.

Ventilation. Tidal volume decreases with deepening levels of non-REM sleep and is minimal in REM sleep, when it is about 25% less than in the awake state (Douglas et al., 1982). Respiratory frequency increases slightly in all stages of sleep but the minute volume is progressively reduced in parallel with the tidal volume. Arterial PCO_2 is usually slightly elevated by about 0.4 kPa (3 mmHg). In the young healthy adult, arterial PO_2 decreases by about the same amount as the PCO_2 is increased, and therefore the oxygen saturation remains reasonably steady, usually within the range 95–98%. Mean value for rib cage contribution to breathing (page 121) was found to be 54% in stage 1–2, decreasing slightly in stages 3–4 (Millman et al., 1988). However, in REM sleep, the value was reduced to 29%, which is close to the normal awake value in the supine position.

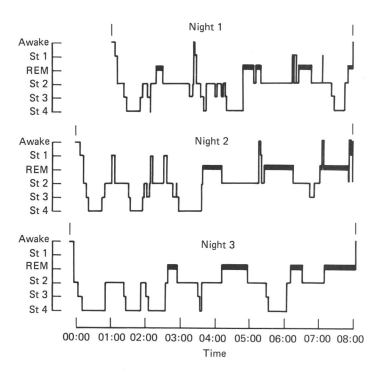

Figure 14.1 Patterns of sleep on three consecutive nights in a young fit man aged 20. The thick horizontal bars indicate rapid eye movement (REM) sleep. (Record kindly supplied by Dr Christine Thornton)

Pharyngeal airway resistance. The nasal airway is normally used during sleep, and upper airway resistance is consistently increased, especially in REM sleep. The main sites of increase are across the soft palate and in the hypopharynx (Hudgel and Hendricks, 1988). Tonic EMG activity in tensor palati was found to decrease progressively with deepening non-REM sleep, and this correlated very well with increased upper airway resistance (Tangel, Mezzanotte and White, 1991). These authors could not, however, detect any diminution of phasic or tonic EMG activity in genioglossus during sleep. Wiegand et al. (1989) reported a modest 24% decrease in the normal awake phasic inspiratory EMG activity of geniohyoid in non-REM sleep. It thus appears that the major effect is upon the nasopharynx and the increase in hypopharyngeal resistance seems to be due to secondary downstream collapse. This was clearly shown during application of external resistive loads in normal subjects during non-REM sleep (Wiegand, Zwillich and White, 1989). Schwartz et al. (1988) found that pharyngeal collapse occurred at a mean value of 1.3 kPa (13 cmH$_2$O) below atmospheric in normal sleeping subjects.

Upper airway dilator muscles are more markedly affected in REM sleep (Dempsey et al., 1991). Forced use of the oral airway during sleep causes an increased incidence of apnoeas and periods of hypoventilation (Surrat, Turner and Wilhoit, 1986).

Chemosensitivity. The slope of the P$_{CO_2}$/ventilation response curve is little different from the conscious state, but is markedly depressed in REM sleep in the dog (Phillipson, 1977). However, withdrawal of 'wakefulness' means that reduction of P$_{CO_2}$ below the apnoeic threshold may result in apnoea. The P$_{O_2}$/ventilation response remains present in all levels of sleep, in marked contrast to what happens during anaesthesia (page 390). Parisi, Santiago and Edelman (1988) showed a relatively normal diaphragmatic EMG response to hypoxia in non-REM sleep in goats. However, response was substantially reduced in REM sleep. Probably more important was the observation that activation of genioglossus EMG activity (normally seen in goats below arterial saturation of 80%) was abolished in REM sleep.

The ventilatory response to increased airway resistance is important in normal sleep because of the increased pharyngeal resistance. It is far more important in cases of abnormal increase in upper airway resistance (see below). Kuna and Smickley (1988) showed substantial and rapid increases in both diaphragmatic and genioglossal inspiratory activity following nasal occlusion in normal sleeping adults.

Effect of age. As age advances, episodes of transient hypoxaemia occur in subjects who are otherwise healthy. Saturation may fall to 75%, usually in association with hypoventilation and irregular breathing in REM sleep (Flenley, 1985b). Such changes must be regarded as a normal part of the ageing process.

Snoring

Snoring may occur at any age, but the incidence is bimodal, peaking in the first, fifth and sixth decades of life. It is more common in males than females, and obesity is an additional factor. It may occur in any stage of sleep, becoming more pronounced as non-REM sleep deepens, though usually attenuated in REM sleep

(Lugaresi et al., 1984). It has been suggested that about 25% of the population are habitual snorers, but there is a continuum from the occasional snorer (e.g. after alcohol or with an upper respiratory tract infection) to the habitual persistent and heavy snorer. Such patients may progress to the obstructive sleep apnoea syndrome (see below).

Snoring originates in the oropharynx and in its mildest form is due to vibration of the soft palate and posterior pillars of the fauces. However, in its more severe forms, the walls of the oropharynx collapse as a result of the subatmospheric pressure generated during inspiration against more upstream airway obstruction (Jennett, 1984). This may be at the level of the palate as described above or may be the result of nasal polyps, nasal infection or adenoids which are the commonest cause of snoring in children. The tongue may be drawn back during inspiration until it obstructs against the posterior pharyngeal wall although, in contrast to anaesthesia, the tone of the genioglossus is not normally lost during sleep (page 384). As obstruction develops, the inspiratory muscles greatly augment their action and intrathoracic pressure may fall as low as 7 kPa (70 cmH$_2$O). Rather surprisingly, formal investigation has not shown posture to be a major factor in the production of snoring (Sullivan, Berton-Jones and Issa, 1983). Nevertheless it is widely believed that snoring is worse in the supine position.

Apart from the annoyance to conjugal partners and others, there are strong associations between snoring and a wide range of pathological conditions, including hypertension, heart and chest disease, rheumatism, diabetes and depression (Norton and Dunn, 1985). In addition, these authors confirmed the association with obesity, smoking and alcoholism. However, perhaps the most serious aspect of snoring is that it may be a precursor of the obstructive sleep apnoea syndrome.

The sleep apnoea syndrome

This syndrome is characterized by periods of apnoea lasting more than 10 seconds and recurring at least 11 times per hour during sleep (Guilleminault, van der Hoed and Mitler, 1978). In fact, durations of apnoea may be as long as 90 seconds and the frequency of the episodes as high as 160 hour. Typically, 50% of sleep time may be spent without tidal exchange. Apnoea may be central (absence of all respiratory movements, as in Figure 14.2a) or obstructive. Both types may occur in the same patient. Differentiation between central and obstructive apnoea is conveniently made by continuous recording of rib cage and abdominal movements. Inductance plethysmography permits calculation of the tidal volume attributable to each component and, if these are equal but opposite in phase, there is total obstructive apnoea (Figure 14.2b). Obstructive apnoea may occur in REM or non-REM sleep but the longest periods of apnoea tend to occur in REM sleep. The syndrome can occur at any age but is commonest in obese male snorers. The condition is well recognized in children, when it usually associated with enlarged tonsils and adenoids.

The effects of the sleep apnoea syndrome are not trivial. Disrupted sleep leads to daytime somnolence with decrement of performance in many fields. The repeated hypoxic episodes (Figure 14.3) appear to be responsible for both intellectual deterioration and pulmonary hypertension which, in due course, becomes irreversible.

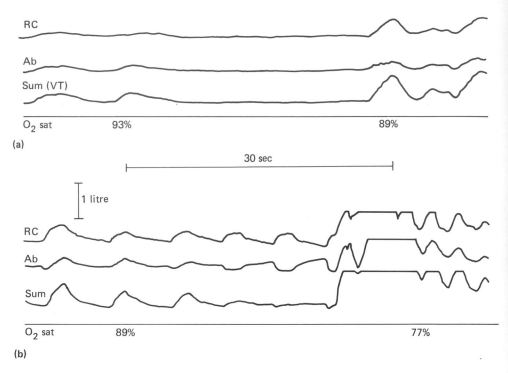

RC

Ab

Sum (VT)

O$_2$ sat   93%   89%

(a)

|⟵————— 30 sec —————⟶|

1 litre

RC

Ab

Sum

O$_2$ sat   89%   77%

(b)

Figure 14.2 Continuous records of breathing showing a central (a) and an obstructive (b) apnoea in a patient sleeping after surgery. 'RC' indicates the cross-sectional area of rib cage and 'Ab' that of the abdomen. 'Sum' indicates the arithmetic sum of RC and Ab. Note the absence of all movement in (a) and out-of-phase movements in (b), indicating obstruction. Note that the desaturation is much greater in the obstructive apnoea. (Record kindly supplied by C. Jordan)

The mechanism of obstructive sleep apnoea

The obstructive sleep apnoea syndrome is the extreme form of pharyngeal airway obstruction as described above for normal sleep. The primary cause is increased upstream resistance. This results in secondary downstream collapse which is a function of the compliance (collapsibility) of the hypopharyngeal walls and attenuation of the action of the pharyngeal dilator muscles (page 16).

Upstream obstruction may become excessive at the nares, within the nasal cavity (e.g. because of polyps or adenoids) or, most commonly, behind the soft palate (Horner et al., 1989b). Computed tomography has shown pharyngeal narrowing in patients with obstructive sleep apnoea, even while awake (Haponik et al., 1983; Horner et al., 1989b). Yildrim et al. (1991) used cephalometric radiography to show that subjects with the sleep apnoea/hypopnoea syndrome had a significant decrease in anteroposterior diameter of both nasopharynx and oropharynx, when changing from upright to supine position. This did not occur in their normal subjects, and absolute values in the supine position were substantially less in the patients. Interference with tonic activity of tensor palati may well be the precipitating factor during sleep (see above). In the case of oral breathing, there may be obstruction at the lips, or by the tongue falling against the palate.

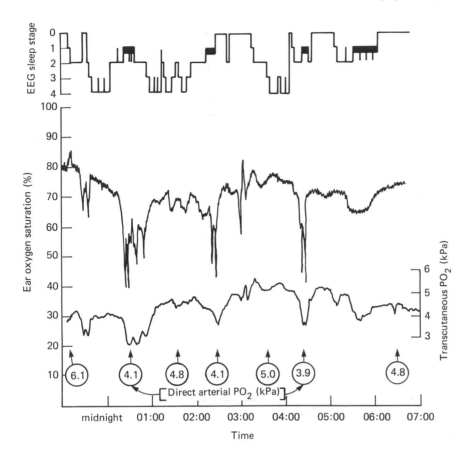

Figure 14.3 EEG sleep stage, ear oximetry and transcutaneous Po_2 and arterial Po_2 in a 'blue bloater' throughout a night while breathing air. Note that the worst episodes of desaturation occur during REM sleep (indicated by closed bars in the EEG record). (Reproduced from Flenley (1985c) by permission of the author and the publishers)

Downstream collapse occurs more easily when pharyngeal compliance is high and particularly when there is increased submucosal fat (Horner et al., 1989a). This explains the correlation with neck circumference (Davies and Stradling, 1990). The tendency to collapse is counteracted by the pharyngeal dilator muscles and their response is probably attenuated to some extent in all forms of sleep, but especially in REM sleep. Severe collapse of the hypopharynx occurs with the combination of enhanced diaphragmatic contraction, depressed pharyngeal dilator muscle activity and upstream obstruction (Horner et al., 1989b). Bonora et al. (1984) showed that alcohol induced a significant reduction in hypoglossal and recurrent nerve activities in doses which had little or no effect on phrenic nerve activity. This appears to be relevant to the well known effect of alcohol on both snoring and obstructive sleep apnoea.

Arousal

Obstruction normally results in arousal, followed by clearance of the pharyngeal airway, and this is crucially important for survival. Hypoxia is a major factor in arousal, and studies in dogs have demonstrated a normal threshold for arousal at about 85% saturation in non-REM sleep and 70% in REM sleep (Bowes and Phillipson, 1984). This mechanism appears to be dependent on the peripheral chemoreceptors and the arousal thresholds are significantly reduced by carotid body denervation. It is not entirely clear whether mechanical obstruction can result in arousal other than as a result of hypoxaemia. In the postoperative period arousal was observed following obstruction when hypoxaemia had been prevented by administration of oxygen (Catley et al., 1985). Arousal is accompanied by massive sympathetic discharge.

The postoperative period
(see pages 416 et seq.)

Continuous monitoring has shown that transient apnoeas occur very frequently during sleep in the postoperative period (Catley et al., 1985). Both central and obstructive apnoeas occur but hypoxaemia is more pronounced in the obstructive type (see Figure 14.2). Stage 3 and 4 and REM sleep were not observed in the first 24 hours after operation and apnoeas were therefore restricted to stages 1 and 2. Patients tend to catch up on REM sleep on the second and third postoperative nights and obstructive episodes are often more common at that time. Avoidance of opiates greatly reduced the incidence of episodes of hypoxia, which were seldom seen in patients whose postoperative pain was controlled only with regional analgesia.

Chronic bronchitis

Transient nocturnal hypoxaemia is particularly dangerous in patients with chronic bronchitis who have lost much of their chemosensitive drive to respiration (Douglas and Flenley, 1990). These patients ('blue bloaters') fare very much worse than 'pink puffers' and tend to have more frequent and more severe episodes of desaturation, particularly during REM sleep (Wynne, 1984). Although the prognosis is grave in such patients, the condition can be ameliorated by the administration of sleeping oxygen. Almitrine has also been found effective in preventing transient hypoxaemia in these patients (Connaughton et al., 1985). Combination of chronic bronchitis and the obstructive sleep apnoea syndrome in the same patient has been termed the 'overlap' syndrome (see Flenley, 1985b, c).

Treatment of obstructive sleep apnoea and snoring

Surgical relief of obstruction

The first approach is the removal of any pathological obstruction such as nasal polyps which cause downstream collapse. A more radical approach is uvulo-palatopharyngoplasty (Fujita et al., 1980), which corrects anatomical abnormalities in the oropharynx and dampens palatal oscillations. This is usually very effective in the relief of snoring (Sharp et al., 1990), but its value in obstructive sleep apnoea is less clear. Tracheotomy (opened only at night) has been used in some cases as a last resort. If obstruction is at the external nares, relief may be obtained by inserts which hold the external nares open.

Continuous positive airway pressure (CPAP)

The physiological basis of CPAP is to prevent the development of a subatmospheric pharyngeal pressure sufficient to cause downstream pharyngeal collapse (Sullivan, Berton-Jones and Issa, 1983). It has proved to be highly effective in the relief of obstructive sleep apnoea. It requires a well-fitting nasal mask or soft plastic tubes which fit inside the external nares. Compressed air must then be provided at the requisite flow rate and with humidification. CPAP serves no useful purpose during expiration and systems have been developed to return airway pressure to atmospheric during expiration. In effect this provides a modest level of intermittent positive pressure ventilation.

Oxygen

Hypoxaemia may be prevented by nocturnal administration of oxygen through nasal catheters or prongs. This method has the advantage of increasing the inspired oxygen concentration as minute volume decreases. In fact, oxygen does not decrease the incidence of sleep apnoea, but it does reduce the desaturation which results. It does not appear to delay arousal from obstruction and neither does it result in hypercapnia. Provision of sleeping oxygen is important for preventing the sequelae of the recurrent bouts of hypoxaemia, particularly pulmonary hypertension and intellectual deterioration.

Relationship to sudden infant death syndrome (SIDS)

Healthy infants do not have apnoeic episodes exceeding 15 seconds during sleep. However, severe attacks of hypoxaemia (PO_2 2–4 kPa, 15–30 mmHg) have been described by Southall et al. (1985), predominantly during sleeping and feeding in infants under 2 months old. The hypoxaemia developed very rapidly, usually within about 20 seconds of the start of apnoea. The attacks were characterized by expiratory muscle activity and reduced lung volume. Although there appeared to be glottic closure, episodes continued after tracheostomy in two children. Apnoea terminated spontaneously even when administration of oxygen prevented hypoxaemia.

Apnoeic episodes have also been observed in infants with relatively mild illnesses such as upper respiratory tract infections, stridor, metabolic alkalosis and also in infants who have had a 'near miss' from SIDS (Abreu e Silva et al., 1985). It seems very likely that something resembling the classic obstructive sleep apnoea syndrome may account for at least some cases of SIDS, but it is unlikely to be the sole cause. There is a substantial body of agreement that the prone sleeping position is more common in infants dying of SIDS (Southall and Samuels, 1992), and a reduction in prone sleeping paralleled a reduced mortality from SIDS in a recent study (Wigfield et al., 1992). It is difficult to see how the supine position could be advantageous in the mechanisms of obstruction described above.

Chapter 15

Respiratory aspects of high altitude and space

With increasing altitude, the barometric pressure falls, but the fractional concentration of oxygen in the air (0.21) and the saturated vapour pressure of water at body temperature remain constant (6.3 kPa or 47 mmHg). The PO_2 of the inspired air is related to the barometric pressure as follows:

Inspired gas PO_2 = 0.21 (Barometric pressure − 6.3) kPa
Inspired gas PO_2 = 0.21 (Barometric pressure − 47) mmHg

The influence of the saturated vapour pressure of water becomes relatively more important until, at an altitude of approximately 19 000 metres or 63 000 feet, the barometric pressure equals the water vapour pressure, and alveolar PO_2 and PCO_2 become zero.

Table 15.1 is based on the standard table relating altitude and barometric pressure. However, there are important deviations from the predicted barometric pressure under certain circumstances, particularly at low latitudes. At the summit of Everest, the actual barometric pressure was found to be 2.4 kPa (18 mmHg) greater than predicted, and this was crucial to reaching the summit without oxygen. The uppermost curve in Figure 15.1 shows the expected PO_2 of air as a function of altitude, while the crosses indicate observed values which have been consistently higher than expected in the Himalayas.

Equivalent oxygen concentration

The acute effect of altitude on inspired PO_2 may be simulated by reduction of the oxygen concentration of gas inspired at sea level (Table 15.1). This provides the basis for much experimental work. Conversely, up to 10 000 metres (33 000 ft), it is possible to restore the inspired PO_2 to sea level value by an appropriate increase in the oxygen concentration of the inspired gas (also shown in Table 15.1). Lower inspired PO_2 values may be obtained between 10 000 and 19 000 metres, above which body fluids boil.

Acute exposure to altitude

Transport technology permits altitude to be attained quickly and without the exertion of climbing. This results in effects which are quite different from classic mountain sickness, which is discussed below. Rail, cable car or motor transport

Table 15.1 Barometric pressure relative to altitude

Altitude		Barometric pressure		Inspired gas P_{O_2}		Equivalent oxygen % at sea level	Percentage oxygen required to give sea level value of inspired gas P_{O_2}
feet	metres	kPa	mm Hg	kPa	mm Hg		
0	0	101	760	19.9	149	20.9	20.9
2 000	610	94.3	707	18.4	138	19.4	22.6
4 000	1 220	87.8	659	16.9	127	17.8	24.5
6 000	1 830	81.2	609	15.7	118	16.6	26.5
8 000	2 440	75.2	564	14.4	108	15.1	28.8
10 000	3 050	69.7	523	13.3	100	14.0	31.3
12 000	3 660	64.4	483	12.1	91	12.8	34.2
14 000	4 270	59.5	446	11.1	83	11.6	37.3
16 000	4 880	54.9	412	10.1	76	10.7	40.8
18 000	5 490	50.5	379	9.2	69	9.7	44.8
20 000	6 100	46.5	349	8.4	63	8.8	49.3
22 000	6 710	42.8	321	7.6	57	8.0	54.3
24 000	7 320	39.2	294	6.9	52	7.3	60.3
26 000	7 930	36.0	270	6.3	47	6.6	66.8
28 000	8 540	32.9	247	5.6	42	5.9	74.5
30 000	9 150	30.1	226	4.9	37	5.2	83.2
35 000	10 700	23.7	178	3.7	27	3.8	—
40 000	12 200	18.8	141	2.7	20	2.8	—
45 000	13 700	14.8	111	1.8	13	1.9	—
50 000	15 300	11.6	87	1.1	8	1.1	—
63 000	19 200	6.3	47	0	0	0	—

100% oxygen restores sea level inspired P_{O_2} at 10 000 metres (33 000 ft)

may take a passenger within a few hours from near sea level to as high as 4000 metres (13 100 ft), or 5000 metres (16 400 ft) in certain exceptional locations. Aircraft, helicopters and balloons can take the traveller very much higher and faster, but passengers in unpressurized commercial aircraft are not normally exposed to altitudes exceeding 3700 metres (12 000 ft). Pressurized aircraft normally maintain the cabin pressure equivalent to about 2000–2500 metres (6500–8200 ft), but only 1500 metres (5000 ft) in Concorde. The most acute exposure to altitude occurs after rupture of the pressurized hull of an aircraft. Subsonic jet airliners have an operational ceiling of 13 000 metres (43 000 ft) but Concorde operates up to 18 300 metres (60 000 ft). Military aircraft can fly very much higher with an external pressure well below that at which body fluids boil.

Ventilatory changes. At high altitude the decrease in inspired gas P_{O_2} reduces alveolar and therefore arterial P_{O_2}. The actual decrease in alveolar P_{O_2} is mitigated by hyperventilation caused by the hypoxic drive to ventilation (see Figure 5.6). However, on acute exposure to altitude, the ventilatory response to hypoxia is rapidly antagonized by the resultant hypocapnia. During the first few days of acclimatization, this disadvantageous negative feedback is nullified by bicarbonate shifts in the cerebrospinal fluid (CSF), causing a further increase in ventilation and P_{O_2}, and a decrease in P_{CO_2} (Figure 15.2).

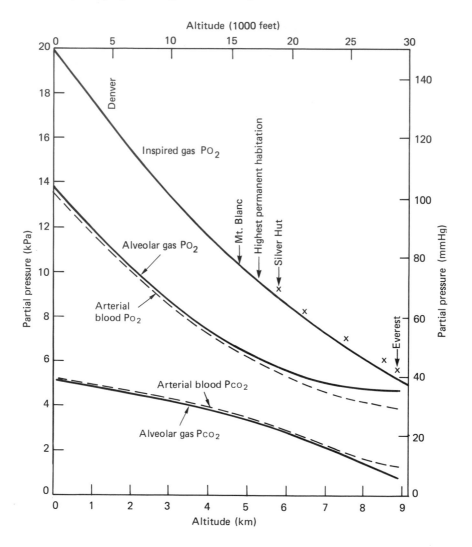

Figure 15.1 Inspired, alveolar and arterial gas tensions at rest, as a function of altitude. The curve for inspired gas PO_2 is taken from standard data in Table 15.1, but the crosses show actual measurements in the Himalayas. The alveolar gas data are from West et al. (1983b), and agree remarkably well with the arterial blood data from the simulated ascent of Everest (Sutton et al., 1988).

Signs and symptoms. Impairment of night vision is the earliest sign of hypoxia, and may be detected as low as 1200 metres (4000 ft). However, the most serious aspect of acute exposure to altitude is impairment of mental performance, culminating in loss of consciousness, which usually occurs on acute exposure to altitudes in excess of 6000 metres (about 20 000 ft). The time to loss of consciousness varies with altitude and is of great practical importance to pilots in the event of loss of pressurization (Figure 15.3). The shortest possible time to loss of consciousness (about 15 seconds) is governed by lung-to-brain circulation time and the capacity of

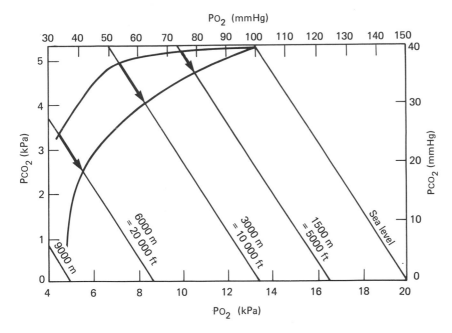

Figure 15.2 Straight lines representing the respiratory exchange ratio (R) have been drawn for various altitudes through the inspired gas points at the bottom of the graph. Intersections between the R lines and the upper curve indicate alveolar gas tensions on acute exposure to altitude. Early acclimatization results in the alveolar points moving down the R lines (as shown by the arrows) until they lie on the lower curve, thus decreasing P_{CO_2} and improving P_{O_2}. (Data from Rahn and Otis, 1949; and West et al., 1983b)

high energy phosphate stores in the brain (page 529). This applies above about 16 000 metres (52 000 ft).

The use of oxygen

Oxygen must be provided for passengers if unpressurized aircraft operate above 3700 metres (12 000 ft), while the pilots are required to use oxygen above 3000 metres (10 000 ft) to ensure proper handling of the aircraft; 100% oxygen provides adequate protection from loss of consciousness up to an altitude of about 12 000 metres (40 000 ft), where the atmospheric pressure is roughly equal to the sea level atmospheric P_{O_2}. This covers the maximal cruising altitude of subsonic transports. Concorde, however, operates above the altitude at which oxygen would be effective, and has therefore been designed to minimize the rate at which accidental depressurization would be likely to occur in the event of, for example, breakage of a window (Mills and Harding, 1983a). Precautions include the small size of the windows, reserve capacity for pressurization and pressure breathing equipment for the flight crew. This equipment supplies oxygen at 4 kPa (40 cmH$_2$O) and is essential equipment for all pilots flying above 12 200 metres (40 000 ft) (*Medical Aspects of Supersonic Flight*, published by British Airways Medical Services).

Manned spacecraft rely on a sealed closed-circuit environment. The American Gemini and Mercury projects used 100% oxygen at a total pressure of 34.5 kPa (259 mmHg). Because of the tragic fire in 1967, the composition was first changed to 64% oxygen/36% nitrogen at the same pressure, which still gave an inspired P_{O_2}

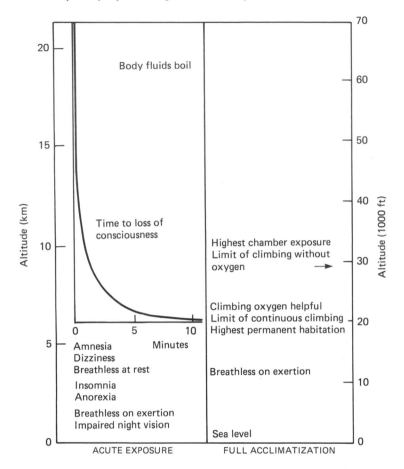

Figure 15.3 Symptomatology of acute and chronic exposure to altitude.

in excess of the normal sea level value. Current designs use normal air at sea level pressure (West, 1991), as was always used by cosmonauts of the USSR (Mills and Harding, 1983b). Extravehicular activity in space presents a particular problem. Flexibility of the space suit in the vacuum of space requires an internal pressure of only 28 kPa (212 mmHg). This entails the use of 100% oxygen after careful decompression.

Acute mountain sickness

The mountaineer is affected by altitude in a manner which differs from that of the aviator because his physical exertion is much greater and the time course of exposure is different. Rate of ascent seldom exceeds 2000 metres (6500 ft) per day from sea level, decreasing to only 300 metres (1000 ft) per day at very high altitude.

Acute mountain sickness has been categorized into benign and malignant forms (Dickinson, 1985; Ward, Milledge and West, 1989), but the relationship between the two forms is not clear. Benign manifestations may progress to the malignant forms, pulmonary, cerebral and mixed.

The unacclimatized mountaineer usually first becomes aware of increased breathlessness on exertion at about 2000 metres (6600 ft); above that level, new arrivals at altitude often have headache, nausea, anorexia, difficulty in sleeping and their climbing performance may be impaired (Figure 15.3). At about 5000 metres (or approximately 16 000 ft), there are feelings of unreality (often enhanced by the environment!), amnesia and dizziness. The unacclimatized person has extreme dyspnoea on exertion at this level and usually has dyspnoea at rest.

Sleep apnoea is common above about 4000 metres (13 000 ft) and may take many forms. The commonest is classic Cheyne–Stokes breathing with periodic apnoeas and a cycle time of about 20 seconds. Apnoeas may result in considerable additional hypoxaemia at high altitude, saturation changing by a mean value of 10% at 6300 metres (21 000 ft) (West et al., 1986; Ward, Milledge and West, 1989). The incidence of Cheyne–Stokes breathing was found by Lahiri (1984) to be related to the strength of the subject's hypoxic ventilatory drive, and it is seldom seen in high altitude residents who have a much attenuated hypoxic drive.

Pulmonary oedema may occur during acute exposure to altitudes in excess of about 3000 metres (10 000 ft). It is most commonly seen in the unacclimatized but overambitious climber. However, it is difficult to predict who will be affected and it may occur in subjects who have previously attained higher altitudes without mishap. Several fatalities have been recorded, the first being on Mont Blanc in 1891.

The aetiology of high altitude pulmonary oedema is far from clear. Various theories have been advanced and the condition may well be multifactorial (Ward, Milledge and West, 1989). Fluid retention probably occurs in susceptible subjects when exercise is taken at altitude (Milledge, 1985a) but this is unlikely to be the only cause. Many different theories are discussed by Hultgren (1978) but the most credible are based on pulmonary hypertension caused by hypoxic pulmonary vasoconstriction with pulmonary vascular pressures exacerbated by exercise. It is postulated that hypertension results in capillary stress failure (page 490) or an opening of the tight endothelial junctions in the pulmonary arterial tree allowing transudation to occur. Groves et al. (1987) recorded a resting mean pulmonary arterial pressure of 34 mmHg in acclimatized subjects at a barometric pressure of 282 mmHg (equivalent to 7620 metres). This increased to 54 mmHg during exercise. However, pulmonary venous (wedge) pressures were generally less than 10 mmHg during exercise at altitude and it is difficult to say whether pulmonary capillary pressures would have been sufficient for appreciable capillary stress failure to have occurred. Very high pulmonary arterial pressures (81/49 mmHg) have been reported in patients with high altitude pulmonary oedema, although the wedge pressures were subnormal (Antezana et al., 1982). High altitude pulomary oedema is typically patchy, and regional failure of vasoconstriction in some parts of the lung could lead to a localized hyperdynamic circulation with high upstream pressure resulting in transudation. Dickinson et al. (1983) have stressed that in some cases oedema has been found to be associated with bronchopneumonia, pulmonary thrombosis and infarction.

Cerebral oedema is also potentially lethal and is manifest in the early stages by ataxia, irritability and irrational behaviour. It may progress to hallucinations, drowsiness and coma; papilloedema has been observed. Postmortem studies have shown that cerebral oedema may be accompanied by intracranial thrombosis and haemorrhage (Dickinson et al., 1983; Ward, Milledge and West, 1989). Pulmonary and cerebral forms of malignant acute mountain sickness may both be present in the same patient.

Treatment of the malignant forms of mountain sickness includes relief of hypoxaemia and dehydration. Administration of oxygen and descent to a lower altitude are the first essentials. Diuretics may be used, and acetazolamide may improve the arterial P_{O_2} (see below). Administration of oxygen at altitude reduces pulmonary arterial pressure but not pulmonary vascular resistance (Groves et al., 1987). Other studies have shown a reduction in pulmonary vascular resistance, but not a return to normal (West, 1992, personal communication),

Acclimatization and adaptation to altitude

'Acclimatization' refers to the processes by which tolerance and performance are improved over a period of hours to months at altitude. 'Adaptation' refers to physiological and genetic changes which occur over a period of years to generations by those who have taken up permanent residence at high altitude. There are qualitative as well as quantitative differences between acclimatization and adaptation but each is remarkably effective. Everest has been climbed without oxygen by well-acclimatized lowlanders, although the barometric pressure on the summit would cause rapid loss of consciousness without acclimatization (Figure 15.3). High altitude residents, Sherpas in particular, have remarkable ability to exercise under grossly hypoxic conditions, but their adaptations show many striking differences from those in acclimatized lowlanders.

Acclimatization

Data obtained on Himalayan scientific expeditions have now been amplified by a simulated ascent in decompression chambers over 32 days to the equivalent altitude of Everest (Operation Everest II; Houston et al., 1987). These conditions permitted sophisticated observations including arterial and Swan–Ganz catheterization at rest and at exercise.

Ventilatory control. The initial hypoxic drive to ventilation on acute exposure to altitude undergoes complex subsequent changes if hypoxia is maintained (Severinghaus, 1992). There is a rapid initial decline due mainly to the resultant respiratory alkalosis. However, in the course of a few days, ventilation returns towards its initial value. Michel and Milledge (1963) suggested that the restoration of cerebrospinal fluid (CSF) pH, by means of bicarbonate transport, might explain this acclimatization of ventilation to altitude, on the basis of observations by Merwarth and Sieker (1961). Later in 1963, Severinghaus and his colleagues measured their own CSF pH during acclimatization to altitude and showed that it did indeed tend to return towards its initial value of 7.2. The improvement in P_{O_2} is substantial (Figure 15.2) and a similar effect may be achieved by the administration of acetazolamide during acute exposure to altitude. This carbonic anhydrase inhibitor interferes with the transport of carbon dioxide out of cells, causing an intracellular acidosis which includes the cells of the medullary chemoreceptors and so drives respiration (Cotev, Lee and Severinghaus, 1968; Milledge, 1985a). The mechanism of the shift in CSF bicarbonate is considered on page 105. In addition to changes influencing the central chemoreceptors, the hypoxic ventilatory response is itself increased during the first few days of hypoxia (page 107).

The initial ventilatory response to hypoxia is also opposed by the resultant respiratory alkalaemia of the arterial blood. This is counteracted over the course of a few days by renal excretion of bicarbonate, resulting in a metabolic acidosis which increases respiratory drive (see Figure 5.8). This was formerly thought to be the main factor in the ventilatory adaptation to altitude but it now appears to be of secondary importance to the change in CSF pH.

With prolonged residence at altitude there is a progressive blunting of the hypoxic ventilatory response which is considered below under adaptation.

Blood gas tensions. Figure 15.1 shows changes in alveolar gas tensions with altitude in acclimatized mountaineers at rest. Alveolar PO_2 was found to be unexpectedly well preserved at extreme altitude (West et al., 1983b) and above 8000 metres (26 000 ft) tended to remain close to 4.8 kPa (36 mmHg). Operation Everest II found a mean arterial PO_2 of 4 kPa (30 mmHg) at a pressure equivalent to the summit of Everest (32 kPa or 240 mmHg) (Table 15.2, from data of Groves et al., 1987), with an alveolar/arterial PO_2 difference of less than 0.3 kPa (2 mmHg) at rest (Wagner et al., 1987). Operation Everest II fully confirmed the observation of West et al. (1983b) of extreme hypocapnia both at rest and during exercise at the equivalent altitude of the summit of Everest (Table 15.2).

Haemoglobin concentration and oxygen affintity. An increase in haemoglobin concentration was the earliest adaptation to altitude to be demonstrated. Operation Everest II reported an increase from 13.5 to 17 g/dl which, at the resting value of 58% saturation, maintained an arterial oxygen content of 12 ml/dl (Sutton et al., 1988). Plasma erythropoietin levels begin to increase within a few hours at altitude, reaching a maximum at 24–48 hours and then declining (Ward, Milledge and West, 1989). Haemoglobin concentrations may also be influenced by changes in plasma volume. Increases in haemoglobin concentration above about 18 g/dl are probably detrimental because of the increased viscosity of the blood.

The haemoglobin dissociation curve at altitude is affected by changes in both pH and 2,3-diphosphoglycerate (2,3-DPG) concentration (page 276). 2,3-DPG concentrations increased from 1.7 to 3.8 mmol/l on Operation Everest II (Sutton et al., 1988). It has been estimated that the resultant effect is a leftward shift at extreme altitude, where oxygen loading in the lung takes priority over maintaining PO_2 at the point of release (Ward, Milledge and West, 1989; West, 1992b).

Circulation and anaerobic metabolism. Resting cardiac output is unchanged at moderate altitude and only slightly increased at extreme altitude. For a given power expenditure, cardiac output at altitude is the same as at sea level (Sutton et al., 1988). Surprisingly, exercise at altitude (up to 70% of $\dot{V}O_{2max}$) results in no higher blood lactate levels than at sea level (Cerretelli, 1980; Sutton et al., 1988), possibly due to inhibition of phosphofructokinase (West, 1992b).

Table 15.2 Cardiorespiratory data obtained at rest and exercise at extreme reduction of ambient pressure during the simulated ascent of Everest in a low pressure chamber

	Sea level equivalent		Extreme high altitude	
Ambient pressure (kPa)	101		33.7	
(mmHg)	760		253	
Mean body weight (kg)	79.2		75.9	
Haemoglobin concentration (g/dl)	13.5		17.0	
Haematocrit	40		52	
$\dot{V}O_{2max}$ (ml/min, STPD)	3980		1170	

State	Rest	Exercise	Rest	Exercise
Exercise intensity (watts)	0	281	0	90
Ventilation (l/min, BTPS)	11	107	42.3	157.5
$\dot{V}O_2$ (ml/min, STPD)	350	3380	386	1002
Ventilation equivalent	31	32	110	157
Arterial PO_2 (kPa)	13.2	12.0	4.0	3.7
(mmHg)	99.3	90.0	30.3	27.7
Arterial PCO_2 (kPa)	4.5	4.7	1.5	1.3
(mmHg)	33.9	35.0	11.2	10.1
(a–v) oxygen content diff. (ml/dl)	5.7	15.0	4.6	6.7
Mixed venous PO_2 (kPa)	4.7	2.6	2.9	1.9
(mmHg)	35.1	19.7	22.1	14.3
Cardiac output (l/min)	6.7	27.2	8.4	15.7
Pulm. mean arterial pressure (mmHg)	15	33	33	48

Data from Groves et al. (1987), Sutton et al. (1988) and Cymerman et al. (1989).
Notes
1. Actual ambient pressure at simulated high altitude was 32 kPa (240 mmHg) but leakage of oxygen from masks worn by investigators had caused the oxygen concentration to rise to 22%, the equivalent of 33.7 kPa at 21%, which is equivalent to the summit of Everest.
2. Groves et al. (1987) reported cardiovascular data for a mean exercise intensity of 90 watts at the highest altitude. Data from the other papers have been interpolated to give values corresponding to the same exercise intensity in order to achieve overall compatibility.

High altitude deterioration

The major mechanisms of acclimatization have their maximal effect within 6 weeks. As the beneficial changes described above develop, they are increasingly offset by the processes of deterioration, to which dehydration, anorexia, insomnia and polycythaemia all contribute. However, there was a mean weight loss of 7.44 kg on Operation Everest II, without the stress of cold, inadequate supplies or exhausting exercise (Houston et al., 1987). A wide range of circulatory disorders has occurred on mountaineering expeditions including cerebral and coronary thromboses, thrombophlebitis and haemoptysis (Pugh, 1962; Ward, Milledge and West, 1989). Climbing to very high altitudes requires a careful balance between acclimatization and deterioration.

Polycythaemia. During the Himalayan Scientific and Mountaineering Expedition of 1960/61 (Pugh et al., 1964), residence in the Silver Hut (500 metres or 19 000 ft), resulted in an increase in haemoglobin concentration from 14.1 to 19.6 g/dl after 4 weeks. Haematocrit values reached 55.8% (sea level controls were 43.2%), and blood viscosity would inevitably have been increased.

Pulmonary hypertension. Pulmonary hypoxic vasoconstriction results in increased pulmonary arterial pressure, which does not appear to be beneficial. On Operation Everest II, mean pulmonary arterial pressure increased from 15 to 33 mmHg at a pressure of 240 mmHg (Groves et al., 1987). Administration of oxygen reduced pulmonary arterial pressure and cardiac output, but not pulmonary vascular resistance.

Cerebral function. Investigations up to 30 days after expeditions to very high altitudes have shown a variety of impairments, including visual long-term memory (Hornbein et al., 1989). Changes were more marked in those with a vigorous hypoxic ventilatory response, perhaps because of hypocapnic decrease in cerebral blood flow. Some defects persisted for years after high altitude expeditions (West, 1992b).

Adaptation and its limits

It is at first surprising that high altitude residents develop a blunted hypoxic ventilatory response over a period of decades. However, hypoxic pulmonary vasoconstriction is preserved, with chronic pulmonary hypertension and right ventricular hypertrophy (Ward, Milledge and West, 1989). This does not seem beneficial and has been lost by the yak. Polycythaemia is normal and the highest levels (haemoglobin concentrations of 22.9 g/dl) occur in Andean miners living at 5300 metres (17 500 ft). Lower haemoglobin concentrations have more recently been found in residents of the Himalayas and the Tibetan plateau (Ward, Milledge and West, 1989).

The major adaptation to altitude by long-term residents appears to be increased vascularity of heart and striated muscles, a change which is also important for the trained athlete. For the high altitude resident, increased perfusion appears to compensate very effectively for the reduced oxygen content of the arterial blood. Their capacity for work is usually superior to that of acclimatized lowlanders.

Limits for residence and work. The upper limit for sustained work seems to be 5950 metres (19 500 ft) at the Aucanquilcha sulphur mine in the Andes. The upper limit for elective permanent habitation is lower, and the Andean miners declined to live in accommodation built for them near the mine, preferring to live at 5330 metres (17 500 ft) and climb every day to their work. However, some caretakers now live at the mine indefinitely (West, 1986).

The Himalayan Scientific and Mountaineering Expedition of 1960/61 (Pugh et al., 1964) set up temporary residence in the 'Silver Hut' at 5800 metres (19 000 ft), the same altitude as the highest Andean mine. Several members of the expedition completed 3 months' residence but this was generally agreed to be close to the limits of tolerance.

Monge's disease. A small minority of those who dwell permanently at very high altitude in certain locations develop a characteristic condition known as Monge's syndrome or chronic mountain sickness. The condition is well recognized in miners living above 4000 metres in the Andes. It is characterized by an exceptionally poor ventilatory response to hypoxia, resulting in low arterial PO_2 and high PCO_2. There is cyanosis, high haematocrit, finger clubbing, pulmonary hypertension, dyspnoea and lethargy.

Exercise at high altitude

The summit of Everest was attained without the use of oxygen in 1978 by Messner and Habeler, and by many other climbers since that date. Studies of exercise have been made at various altitudes up to and including the summit, and on the simulated ascent in Operation Everest II. Of necessity these observations are largely confined to very fit subjects.

Capacity for work performed. There is a progressive decline in the external work which can be performed as altitude increases (Figure 15.4). On Operation Everest II, 300–360 watts was attained at sea level, 240−270 at 440 mmHg pressure, 180–210 watts at 350 mmHg, and 120 watts at 280 and 250 mmHg, very close to the results obtained by West et al. (1983a). $\dot{V}O_{2max}$ declined in accord with altitude to 1177 ml/min at 240 mmHg pressure (Cymerman et al., 1989).

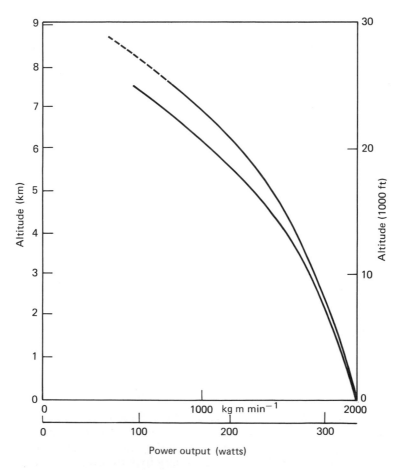

Figure 15.4 Maximal power output by acclimatized mountaineers at different altitudes.

Oxygen cost of work performed. Figure 13.1 shows the linear relationship between oxygen uptake and work performed. This relationship is relatively constant, but Operation Everest II found a reduction in the ratio of oxygen consumption/power output below a pressure of 438 mmHg. At a pressure of 250 mmHg (equivalent to the summit of Everest), $\dot{V}O_2$ for a work level of 120 watts was 1177 ml/min compared with 1796 at sea level (Sutton et al., 1988).

Ventilation equivalent of oxygen consumption. Figure 13.4 shows that ventilation as a function of $\dot{V}O_2$ is comparatively constant. The length of the line increases with training but the slope of the linear portion remains the same. With increasing altitude, the slope and intercept are both dramatically increased up to four times the sea level value (Sutton et al., 1988; Cymerman et al., 1989) with maximal ventilation approaching 200 l/min (Figure 15.5). This is because ventilation is reported at body temperature and pressure saturated (BTPS) and oxygen consumption at standard temperature and pressure dry (STPD) – see Appendix C. Fortunately, the density of air is reduced in proportion to the barometric pressure at altitude. Resistance to turbulent flow is decreased and therefore the work of breathing at a particular minute volume of respiration is less. Maximum breathing capacity is increased by about 40% at an altitude of 8200 metres (27 000 ft) (Miles, 1957).

PCO_2 and PO_2. During exercise at altitude, alveolar PCO_2 falls and PO_2 rises (Pugh et al., 1964; Sutton et al., 1988) (Figure 15.6). Arterial PCO_2 falls with alveolar PCO_2 but oxygenation of the pulmonary end-capillary blood is diffusion-limited during exercise at high altitude (West et al., 1962). The alveolar/arterial PO_2 difference increases more than the alveolar PO_2 rises (Pugh et al., 1964) and there is a consistent decrease in arterial PO_2 during exercise at altitude. The lowest measured value was 2.7 kPa (20 mmHg) in the case of John West himself (Figure 15.6).

Space and zero gravity
(see review by West, 1992c)

Chapter 8 contains numerous references to the effect of gravity on the topography of the lung and the distribution of blood and gas. Space travel no longer imposes an abnormal gaseous environment (page 555) but the loss of gravity provides an opportunity to examine the influence of gravity on pulmonary function. The first studies with microgravity used a Lear jet flying in keplerian arcs, which gave 20–25 seconds of weightlessness. In June 1991 a more extended series of studies was undertaken in Spacelab SLS-1 which was carried into orbit for a 9-day mission by the space shuttle. Only preliminary information was available at the time of writing (West, 1992a).

Lung shape and size. Radiography in the sitting position (Lear jet studies) showed no striking changes other than a tendency for the diaphragm to be slightly higher in some of the subjects at functional residual capacity (FRC) (Michels, Friedman and West, 1979). This accords with a 413 ml reduction in FRC also measured in keplerian arc on seated subjects (Paiva, Estenne and Engel, 1989). In the Spacelab

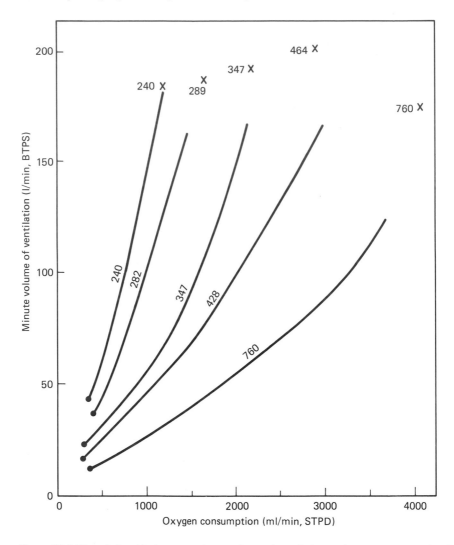

Figure 15.5 The relationship between minute volume of ventilation and oxygen consumption is radically changed at altitude, primarily because ventilation is reported at body temperature and pressure (saturated), whereas oxygen consumption is reported at standard temperature and pressure (dry). Numbers in the Figure indicate barometric pressure (mmHg) x: $\dot{V}_{O_{2max}}$ and ventilation data from Cymerman et al. (1989). •: resting points. Curves are derived from Sutton et al. (1988).

studies, FRC was intermediate between the sitting and supine volumes at normal gravity (West, 1992, personal communication). Abdominal contribution to tidal excursion was increased at microgravity in the seated position, probably because of loss of tone in the abdominal muscles (Paiva, Estenne and Engel, 1989).

Topographical inequality of ventilation and perfusion. Early results in the Lear jet, using single-breath nitrogen washout, indicated a substantial reduction in topographical inequality of ventilation and perfusion disappeared during weightlessness as expected (Michels and West, 1978). However, the more detailed studies in

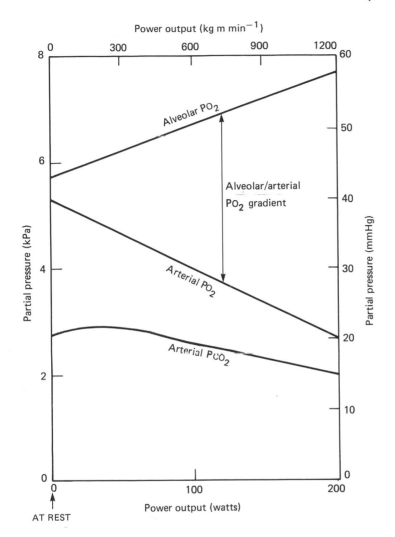

Figure 15.6 PO₂ and PCO₂ changes during exercise in a single subject (John West) at 5800 metres (19 000 feet). (Data from Pugh et al., 1964).

Spacelab showed that a surprising degree of residual inequality of blood flow and ventilation persisted in spite of the major improvement at zero gravity (Guy et al., 1992; West, 1992).

Diffusing capacity. Spacelab studies have shown progressive increases in carbon monoxide diffusing capacity, the membrane component and the pulmonary capillary blood volume (page 210) all reaching 33% more than control by the ninth day in orbit (Prisk et al., 1992).

Chapter 16

Respiratory aspects of high pressure and diving

Man has sojourned temporarily in high pressure environments since the introduction of the diving bell. The origin of this development is lost in antiquity but Alexander the Great was said to have been lowered to the sea bed in a diving bell in 320 BC.

The environment of the diver is often, but not invariably, aqueous. Saturation divers spend most of their time in a gaseous environment in chambers which are held at a pressure close to that of the depth of water at which they will be working. Tunnel and caisson workers may also be at high pressure in a gaseous environment. Workers in both environments share the physiological problems associated with increased pressures and partial pressures of respired gases. However, those in an aqueous environment also have the additional effect of different gravitational forces applied to their trunks, which influence the mechanics of breathing and other systems of the body. Further problems arise as a result of any change in the composition of the inspired gas, which is standard practice at pressures of more than about 6 atmospheres.

The aim of this chapter is to review the salient features of those aspects of high pressure which concern the respiratory system, together with an outline of the effects of inhalation of the various inspired gas mixtures which are used at high pressure. In this field, as in others, we cannot escape from the multiplicity of units, and some of these are set out in Table 16.1. Note particularly that 'atmosphere gauge' is relative to ambient pressure. Thus 2 atmospheres absolute (ATA) equals 1 atmosphere gauge relative to sea level. Throughout this chapter atmospheres of pressure mean absolute and not gauge.

Exchange of oxygen and carbon dioxide

Oxygen consumption

The relationship between power output and oxygen consumption at pressures up to 66 ATA, whether under water or dry, is not significantly different from the relationship at normal pressure shown in Figure 13.1 (Lundgren, 1984; Salzano et al., 1984). Oxygen consumption is expressed under standard conditions of temperature and pressure, dry (STPD, Appendix C) and therefore represents an absolute quantity of oxygen. However, this volume, when expressed at the diver's environmental pressure, is inversely related to the pressure. Thus, an oxygen consumption

Table 16.1 Pressures and Po₂ values at various depths of sea water

Depth of sea water		Pressure (absolute)		Po₂ (breathing air)				Percentage oxygen to give sea level inspired Po₂
				inspired		alveolar		
metres	feet	atm.	kPa	kPa	mmHg	kPa	mmHg	
0	0	1	101	19.9	149	13.9	104	20.9
10	32.8	2	203	41.2	309	35.2	264	10.1
20	65.6	3	304	62.3	467	56.3	422	6.69
50	164	6	608	126	945	120	900	3.31
		Usual limit for breathing air						
100	328	11	1 110					1.80
200	656	21	2 130					0.94
		Usual limit for saturation dives						
		Threshold for high pressure nervous syndrome						
500	1 640	51	5 170					0.39
1000	3 280	101	10 200					0.20
		Depth reached by sperm whale						
2000	6 560	201	20 400					0.098
2500	8 200	251	25 400					0.078
		Pressure reached by non-aquatic mammals with pharmacological amelioration of the high pressure nervous syndrome						

Notes
1 metre = 3.28 feet; 10 metres sea water = 1 atmosphere (gauge); 1 atmosphere = 101.3 kPa = 760 mmHg; air is 20.94% oxygen.
Alveolar Po₂ is assumed to be 6 kPa (45 mmHg) less than inspired Po₂.
Saturated water vapour pressure at body temperature assumed to be 6.3 kPa (47 mmHg).
All values are rounded to three significant figures.

of 1 l/min (STPD) at a pressure of 10 atmospheres would be only 100 l/min when expressed at the pressure to which the diver was exposed. Similar considerations apply to carbon dioxide output.

Oxygen consumption may reach very high values during free swimming and are of the order of 2–3 l/min (STPD) for a swimming speed of only 2 km/h (Lanphier and Camporesi, 1982). Maximal oxygen consumptions in the range 2.4–3.3 l/min have been attained at pressures of 66 atmospheres (Salzano et al., 1984).

Ventilatory requirement

The ventilatory requirement for a given oxygen consumption at increased pressure is also not greatly different from the normal relationship shown in Figure 13.4 provided that the oxygen consumption is expressed at STPD, and minute volume is expressed at body temperature, saturated with water vapour, and at the pressure to which the diver is exposed (BTPS, Appendix C). Considerable confusion is possible as a result of the different methods of expressing gas volumes. Differences are trivial at sea level but become very important at high pressures. As an example, specimen calculations are set out in Table 16.2 comparing certain respiratory

Table 16.2 Respiratory variables at sea level and pressure

		Sea level		10 ATA	
		Rest	Exercise 220 watts	Rest	Exercise 220 watts
Oxygen consumption (ml/min)	STPD	250	3000	250	3000
	BTPS	303	3630	28.5	342
Minute volume (l/min)	BTPS	7	70	7	70
Inspired oxygen concentration (%)		20.9	20.9	20.9	20.9
Inspired P_{O_2}	kPa	19.9	19.9	210	210
	mmHg	149	149	1575	1575
Alveolar oxygen concentration (%)		14.3	14.4	20.2	20.1
Alveolar P_{O_2}	kPa	13.6	13.7	203	202
	mmHg	102	103	1523	1515
Carbon dioxide output (ml/min)	STPD	200	2400	200	2400
	BTPS	242	2904	22.8	274
Alveolar ventilation (l/min)	BTPS	4.55	56.0	4.06	42.0
Alveolar carbon dioxide concentration (%)		5.3	5.2	0.56	0.65
Alveolar P_{CO_2}	kPa	5.1	4.9	5.6	6.5
	mmHg	38	37	42	49

Assumptions are listed in the text.
This Table is for illustrative purposes only and is not a recommendation to expose divers to 10 atmospheres pressure of air.

volumes and gas tensions at sea level and at 10 atmospheres while breathing air. Oxygen consumptions, minute volume and dead space/tidal volume ratios are taken from the data of Salzano et al. (1984). Conversions of gas volumes for different pressures are described in Appendix B. Although it clarifies the problem to consider conditions at 10 atmospheres, air would not nowadays be considered an appropriate inspired gas at this pressure, for reasons which are discussed below.

Effect of pressure on alveolar P_{CO_2} and P_{O_2}

Pressure has complicated and very important effects on P_{CO_2} and P_{O_2}. The alveolar concentration of CO_2 equals its rate of production divided by the alveolar ventilation (page 232). However, both gas volumes must be measured under the same conditions of temperature and pressure. Table 16.2 shows that alveolar CO_2 concentration at 10 ATA will be about one-tenth of sea level values, i.e. 0.56% compared with 5.3% at sea level. When these concentrations are multiplied by pressure to give P_{CO_2}, values are similar at sea level and 10 atmospheres. Thus, as a rough approximation, alveolar CO_2 concentration decreases inversely to the environmental pressure, but the P_{CO_2} remains near its sea level value.

Effects on the P_{O_2} are slightly more complicated but no less important. The difference between the inspired and alveolar oxygen *concentrations* equals the ratio of oxygen uptake to inspired alveolar ventilation (see the universal alveolar air equation, page 128). This fraction, like the alveolar concentration of carbon dioxide, decreases inversely with the increased pressure. However, the corresponding *partial pressure* will remain close to the sea level value, as does the alveolar P_{CO_2}. Therefore the difference between the inspired and alveolar P_{O_2} will remain roughly constant, and the alveolar P_{O_2}, to a first approximation, increases by the same amount as the inspired P_{O_2} (Figure 16.1). However, these considerations only take into account the direct effect of pressure on gas tensions. There are other and more subtle effects on respiratory mechanics and gas exchange which must now be considered.

Effect on mechanics of breathing

Two main factors must be considered. Firstly, there is the increased density of gases at pressure, although this can be reduced by changing the composition of the inspired gas. The second factor is the pressure of water on the body, which alters the gravitational effects to which the respiratory system is normally exposed.

Gas density is increased in direct proportion to pressure. Thus air at 10 atmospheres has ten times the density of air at sea level, which increases the resistance to

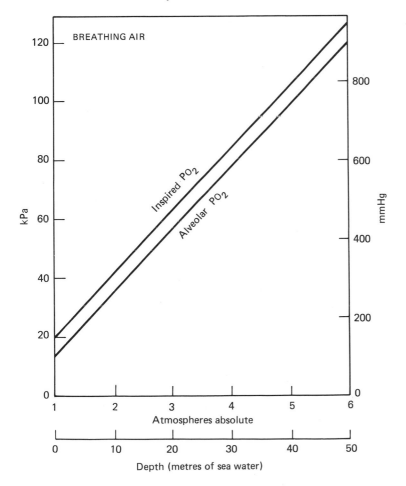

Figure 16.1 Inspired and alveolar P_{O_2} values as a function of increasing pressure, while breathing air at rest.

turbulent gas flow (page 64). Lanphier and Camporesi (1982) found that the maximal breathing capacity (MBC) of a subject breathing air was 200 l/min at sea level, 100 l/min at 5 atmospheres and 50 l/min at 15 atmospheres. In fact, it is usual to breathe a helium/oxygen mixture at pressures in excess of about 6 atmospheres because of nitrogen narcosis (see below). Helium has only one-seventh of the density of air and so is easier to breathe. Furthermore, lower inspired oxygen concentrations are both permissible and indeed desirable as the pressure increases (see Table 16.1). Therefore, at 15 atmospheres it would be reasonable to breathe a mixture of 98% helium and 2% oxygen. This would more than double the MBC which the diver could attain while breathing air at that pressure (Lanphier and Camporesi, 1982).

The effect of immersion is additional to any change in the density of the respired gases. In open-tube snorkel breathing, the alveolar gas is close to normal atmospheric pressure but the trunk is exposed to a pressure depending on the depth of the subject, which is limited by the length of the snorkel tube. This is equivalent to a standing subatmospheric pressure applied to the mouth and it is difficult to inhale against a 'negative' pressure loading of more than about 5 kPa (50 cmH$_2$O). This corresponds to a mean depth of immersion of only 50 cm. It is virtually impossible to use a snorkel tube at a depth of 1 metre. An additional problem with an extended snorkel tube is the imbalance of the absolute increase in circulatory pressures in relation to the normal alveolar pressure (Lundgren, 1991). However, the normal length of a snorkel tube assures that the swimmer is barely more than awash, and so these problems should not arise.

Derion et al. (1992) have shown that head-out water immersion causes reductions in expiratory reserve volume of the order of 1 litre, and this may result in airway closure, particularly in older subjects, in whom there may be a small increase in shunt.

'Negative' pressure loading is avoided by supplying gas at a pressure which is close to the hydrostatic pressure surrounding the diver. This may be achieved by providing an excess flow of gas with a pressure relief valve controlled by the surrounding water pressure. Such an arrangement was used for the traditional helmeted diver supplied by an air pump on the surface. Free-swimming divers carrying their own compressed gas supply rely on inspiratory demand valves, which are also balanced by the surrounding water pressure.

These arrangements supply gas which is close to the hydrostatic pressure surrounding the trunk. However, the precise 'static lung loading' depends on the location of the pressure-controlling device in relation to the geometry of the chest. Minor differences also result from the various postures which the diver may assume. Thus, if he is 'head-up', the pressure surrounding the trunk is higher than the airway pressure by a mean value of about 3 kPa (30 cmH$_2$O). If he is 'head-down', airway pressure is greater than the pressure to which the trunk is exposed. The 'head-down' position thus corresponds to positive pressure breathing and the 'head-up' position to 'negative pressure' breathing (Lundgren, 1984). The latter causes a reduction of functional residual capacity (FRC) of about 20–30% but breathing is considered to be easier head-up than head-down (Lanphier and Camporesi, 1982). The 'head-up' position under water is similar in effect to head-out immersion with the body vertical, which may result in a small reduction of arterial PO$_2$ (Lundgren, 1991). Apart from these considerations, immersion has relatively little effect on respiratory function, and the additional work of moving extracorporeal water does not seem to add appreciably to the work of breathing.

Effect on efficiency of gas exchange

The efficiency of gas exchange can be assessed only by measurement of arterial blood gas tensions and this presents formidable technical difficulties at high pressures. Salzano and his colleagues (1984) found the dead space/tidal volume ratio (page 169) increased from 35% at sea level to 42% at 47 and 66 atmospheres. However, during exercise at depth, values remained close to 40%, in contrast to a decrease to 20% during exercise at sea level. Therefore, for the same minute volume, alveolar ventilation would be less at depth in comparison with sea level. This factor has been taken into account in the preparation of Table 16.2, although data at 10 atmospheres are not currently available.

The best measure of the efficiency of oxygenation of the arterial blood is the alveolar/arterial PO_2 gradient, and this has not been rigorously quantified at high pressures. However, Salzano and his colleagues (1984) reported arterial PO_2 values in the range 33–41 kPa (248–308 mmHg) at pressures of 47 and 66 atmospheres, both at rest and at work when inspired oxygen tensions were in the range 47–50 kPa (353–375 mmHg). Intrapulmonary shunting did not thus appear to exceed about 5% (Figure E.6).

Arterial blood gas tensions

Since it is customary to supply deep divers with an inspired oxygen tension of at least 0.5 atmosphere, arterial hypoxaemia is unlikely to occur either from hypoventilation or from maldistribution of pulmonary ventilation and perfusion, and this was confirmed by the study of Salzano et al. (1984).

The position as regards arterial PCO_2 is less satisfactory. Salzano et al. (1984) found values within the normal range at pressures of 47 and 66 atmospheres when the subjects were at rest and performing exercise up to about 200 watts in one of his subjects. However, the remaining four subjects, although normocapnic at rest, became hypercapnic at exercise levels ranging from 100 to 200 watts. Maximal values of arterial PCO_2 during exercise at pressure were in the range 6.2–8.3 kPa (46.7–62.2 mmHg). This cannot be regarded as satisfactory since 9 kPa is approaching the level at which there may be some clouding of consciousness, and that is potentially dangerous at depth. It seems likely that the increased dead space during exercise at pressure compared with the value at sea level plays a significant role by reducing the alveolar ventilation. Hypocapnia is a well recognized complication, and divers are known to have a blunted PCO_2/ventilation response (Lundgren, 1991).

In addition to hypercapnia, some of Salzano's subjects showed a metabolic acidosis in association with an increased arterial lactate concentration. Lactate levels were consistently higher at pressure than at sea level, not only at all rates of exercise but also at rest.

Effects attributable to the composition of the inspired gas

Air

Up to about 55 years ago, helmeted divers worked up to pressures of about 10 atmospheres breathing air. Nowadays, with the increased use of helium, it is unusual to breathe air at pressures of more than 6 atmospheres (depths of 50 metres of sea water). The effects of increased partial pressures of oxygen and nitrogen will be considered separately.

Oxygen. When breathing air at a pressure of 6 atmospheres, the inspired P_{O_2} will be about 126 kPa (945 mmHg) and the alveolar P_{O_2} about 120 kPa (900 mmHg). This is below the threshold for oxygen convulsions (see below), but probably above the threshold for pulmonary oxygen toxicity if exposure is continued for more than a few hours (see Chapter 32).

Nitrogen. It is actually nitrogen which limits the depth to which air should be breathed. It has three separate undesirable effects.

Nitrogen is an anaesthetic and, in accord with its lipid solubility, can cause full surgical anaesthesia at a partial pressure of about 30 atmospheres. The narcotic effect of nitrogen is first detectable when breathing air at about 4 ATA and there is usually serious impairment of performance at 10 atmospheres (Bennett, 1982a). This effect is known as nitrogen narcosis or 'the rapture of the deep'. It is believed that there is some cross-tolerance with alcohol and it has been suggested that divers accustomed to regular alcohol intake are capable of better performance under these conditions. It is a general rule that nitrogen narcosis precludes the use of air at depths greater than 100 metres of sea water (11 ATA pressure) and, in fact, air is not used today at pressures greater than 6 atmospheres. Helium is the preferred substitute at higher pressures and has no detectable narcotic properties up to at least 100 atmospheres.

The second problem attributable to nitrogen is increased solution of the gas in body tissues at high pressures. This creates no problem during compression but, if decompression is too rapid, gas bubbles may be evolved causing a range of disabilities variously known as 'bends', 'chokes' or caisson disease (Vann, 1982). Detailed and elaborate tables have been prepared to indicate the safe rate of decompression depending on the pressure and time of exposure. Other inert gases, particularly helium, are less soluble in body tissues and this is the second reason for the use of helium at high pressures.

The third problem with nitrogen at high pressures is its density, which causes greatly increased hindrance to breathing at high pressure (see above). Helium has only one-seventh of the density of nitrogen and this is the third reason for its choice.

Helium/oxygen mixtures (Heliox)

For the three reasons outlined in the previous section, helium is the preferred diluent inert gas at pressures above about 6 atmospheres. The concentration of oxygen required to give the same inspired gas P_{O_2} as at sea level is shown in Table 16.1. In fact, it is usual practice to provide an inspired P_{O_2} of about 0.5 atmosphere (50 kPa or 375 mmHg) to give a safety margin in the event of error in gas mixing and to provide protection against hypoventilation or defective gas exchange. This level of P_{O_2} appears to be below the threshold for pulmonary oxygen toxicity, even during prolonged saturation dives.

With an inspired P_{O_2} of 0.5 atmosphere, the *concentration* of oxygen in the gas mixture is very low at high pressures (e.g. 2.5% oxygen at 20 atmospheres pressure). Clearly such a mixture would be lethal if breathed at sea level. Therefore the inspired oxygen concentration must be very carefully monitored as it is changed during compression and decompression.

A special problem of helium is its very high thermal conductivity, which tends to cause hypothermia unless the diver's environment is heated. It is usual for chambers to be maintained at temperatures as high as 30–32°C during saturation dives on helium/oxygen mixtures. The low density of helium causes a considerable increase in the pitch of the voice, sometimes resulting in difficulty in communication.

Helium/oxygen/nitrogen mixtures (Trimix)

The pressure which can be attained while breathing helium/oxygen mixtures is currently limited by the high pressure nervous syndrome (Halsey, 1982). This is a hyperexcitable state of the central nervous system which appears to be due to hydrostatic pressure *per se* and not to any changes in gas tensions. It becomes a serious problem for divers at pressures in excess of about 50 atmospheres, but is first apparent at about 20 atmospheres.

Various treatments can mitigate this effect and so increase the depth at which a diver can safely operate. At the time of writing, the most practicable is the use of partial nitrogen narcosis. Not only does the nitrogen mitigate the high pressure nervous syndrome but also the high pressure reverses the narcosis which would be caused by the nitrogen (Halsey, Wardley-Smith and Green, 1978). Various concentrations of nitrogen have been used in the range 4–10% (Bennett, 1982b).

Oxygen

The use of oxygen as inspired gas permits the use of closed circuit apparatus, which does not leave a trail of bubbles to reveal the presence of a clandestine diver. While this requirement may be of overwhelming importance in warfare, sabotage and espionage, it carries the grave hazard of oxygen convulsions (page 552). The lowest threshold for convulsions in man is a PO_2 of 2 ATA and this limits diving on oxygen to a depth of 10 metres (Donald, 1947).

Special circumstances of exposure to pressure

Breath-hold dives on air

The simplest method of diving is by breath holding and this is still used for collecting pearls, sponge and various edibles from the sea bed. After breathing air, breath holding time is normally limited to 60–75 seconds, and the changes in alveolar gas tensions are shown in Figure 5.9. Astonishingly, the depth record is 112 metres requiring 3 minutes of submersion (Lundgren, 1991). Many remarkable mechanisms interact to make this possible.

Lung volume. As pressure increases, lung volume decreases by Boyle's law (page 562). Thus at 10 ATA, an initial lung volume of 6 litres would be reduced to about 600 ml, well below residual volume (RV), and with the loss of 5.4 kg of buoyancy. During descent a point is reached when the body attains neutral buoyancy and the body will sink below that depth. Craig (1968) showed that transthoracic pressure remained roughly constant when pressure was increased by 4 atmospheres after the lung volume was already reduced to RV. He explained this by transfer of blood into the thorax to replace the gas volume lost by compression.

Alveolar PO_2 increases with depth as the alveolar gas is compressed, a PO_2 of approximately 90 kPa being attained during a dive to a depth of 100 metres (Lundgren, 1991). More of the alveolar oxygen is therefore available at depth. Conversely, during ascent, alveolar PO_2 decreases due to oxygen consumption, but mainly to decreasing pressure. There is thus danger of hypoxia just before reaching the surface. However, when the alveolar PO_2 falls below the mixed venous PO_2, there is a paradoxical transfer of oxygen from mixed venous blood to alveolar gas, and the arterial PO_2 is maintained. This may be an important factor in preventing loss of consciousness in the final stages of ascent.

Alveolar PCO_2. By a similar mechanism, alveolar PCO_2 is greater during a breath-holding dive than during a simple breath hold at sea level. At an environmental pressure of only 12 kPa (90 mmHg), the alveolar PCO_2 will be increased above the mixed venous PCO_2, and there will be a paradoxical transfer of carbon dioxide from alveolus to arterial blood (Lundgren, 1991). Fortunately there is a limited quantity of carbon dioxide in the alveolar gas, and the process is reversed during ascent. Duration of breath hold can be increased by previous hyperventilation, but this carries the danger of syncope from hypoxia before the breaking point is reached. Duration can be more safely increased by preliminary oxygen breathing, and a time of 14 minutes has been attained (page 113).

Adaptations in the diving mammals. The diving mammals rely on breath holding for dives and have adaptations which permit remarkably long times under water and the attainment of great depths. Sperm whales, for example, can attain depths of 1000 metres (Halsey, 1982). Weddell seals can reach 500 metres and remain submerged for 70 minutes (Zapol, 1987). Such feats depend on a variety of biochemical and physiological adaptations. It seems likely that the lungs of the Weddell seal collapse completely at depths between 25 and 50 metres, thus preventing the partial pressure of nitrogen increasing above the level of 320 kPa (2400 mmHg) which has been recorded at depths between 40 and 80 metres (Falke et al., 1985). In the same species, splenic contraction is the probable cause of an increase of haemoglobin concentration from 15 to 25 g/dl during long dives (Qvist et al., 1986). Furthermore, these animals have twice the blood volume per kilogram body weight relative to man, so oxygen stored in blood for a dive is proportionately about three times that of humans.

During a dive the circulation is directed almost exclusively through heart and brain (Hempleman and Lockwood, 1978), which rely on the oxygen stores in the lungs and the blood. With a smaller brain, total cerebral oxygen consumption is much less than in man. Intense vasoconstriction severely limits flow through other organs and also the voluntary muscles. Muscle contraction is based on anaerobic metabolism and there is extreme lactacidosis which is confined to the muscle beds and so is not sensed by the peripheral chemoreceptors. After surfacing, the vasoconstriction is relaxed and there is generalized acidaemia. While on the surface, the excess lactate is metabolized and the arterial PCO_2 returns to normal. This process takes only a few minutes and the animal is then ready for another dive.

The diving reflex in man. The diving reflex is less well developed in man than in the diving mammals, but it may nevertheless be detected. The primary stimulus is immersion of the face in water, the most effective temperature being 10–20°C (Gooden, 1982). Breath holding seems to be an essential adjunct. It is possible to demonstrate vasoconstriction in skin, muscle, kidney and intestines but the main effect in man is bradycardia. The latter effect has been proposed for treatment of paroxysmal tachycardia.

Limited duration dives

Most dives are of relatively brief duration and involve a rapid descent to operating depth, a period spent at depth, followed by an ascent, the rate of which is governed by the requirement to prevent release of inert gas dissolved in the tissues. The profile and the duration of the ascent are governed by the depth attained, the time spent at depth and the nature of the diluent inert gas.

The diving bell. The simplest and oldest technique was the diving bell. Air was trapped on the surface but the internal water level rose as the air was compressed at depth. Useful time at depth was generally no more than 20–30 minutes. Crude though this technology appears, it was used to recover most of the guns from the Wasa in Stockholm harbour in 1663 and 1664 from a depth of 34 metres. It seems unlikely that the salvage operators left the bell. At a later date, additional air was introduced into the bell under pressure from the surface and divers could leave the bell.

The helmeted diver. From about 1820 until recent times, the standard method of diving down to 100 metres has been by a helmeted diver supplied with air pumped from the surface into the helmet and escaping from a relief valve controlled by the water pressure. This gave much greater mobility than the old diving bell and permitted the execution of complex tasks. The system was used with helium/oxygen mixtures in 1939 for the salvage of the United States submarine *Squalus* from a depth of 74 metres.

SCUBA diving. Since about 1930 there has been a progressive move towards free-swimming divers carrying their own gas supply (SCUBA – self-contained underwater breathing apparatus). The system is based on a demand valve which is controlled by both the ambient pressure and the inspiration of the diver. Air-breathing SCUBA dives are usually restricted to depths of 30 metres. Greater depths are possible but special precautions must then be taken to prevent 'bends'. SCUBA divers are far more mobile than helmeted divers and can also work in any body position. They also avoid the hazard of suit inflation, which was caused by a helmeted diver lowering his head below the rest of his body. This resulted in a rapid ascent to the surface and the danger of 'bends'.

Caisson and tunnel working

Since 1839, tunnel and bridge foundations have been constructed by pressurizing the work environment to exclude water. This does not normally require a pressure greater than 4 ATA and air is usually breathed. The work environment is maintained at pressure with staff entering and leaving by air locks. Shifts normally last 8 hours. Entry is rapid but exit requires adherence to the appropriate decompression schedule if the working pressure is in excess of 2 ATA. Workers can be rapidly transferred from the working pressure to atmosphere and then, within 5 minutes, transferred to a separate chamber where they are rapidly recompressed to the working pressure and then follow the decompression schedule (Walder, 1982). This process, known as decanting, has obvious logistic advantages. Apart from the danger of 'bends', working in compressed air carries the additional hazard of bone necrosis for which the aetiological factors are not yet clearly established (Walder, 1982).

Saturation dives

When prolonged and repeated work is required at great depths, it is more convenient to hold the divers in a dry chamber, kept on board a ship or oil rig, and held at a pressure close to the pressure of their intended working depth. Divers transfer to a smaller chamber at the same pressure which is lowered to depth as and when required. The divers then leave the chamber for work, without any major change in pressure, but remaining linked to the chamber by an umbilical. On return to the chamber, they can be raised to the surface where they wait, still at pressure, until they are next required. A normal tour of duty is about 3 weeks, the whole of which is spent at operating pressure, currently up to about 20 atmospheres breathing helium/oxygen mixtures.

During the long period at pressure, tissues are fully saturated with inert gas at the chamber pressure and prolonged decompression is then required which may last for several days.

Free submarine escape

It is possible to escape from a submarine by free ascent from depths down to about 100 metres. The submariner first enters an escape chamber which is then pressurized to equal the external water pressure. He then opens a hatch communicating with the exterior and leaves the chamber. His natural buoyancy is sufficient to take him to the surface but he may be helped with additional buoyancy or an apron which traps gas leaving the escape chamber. During the ascent, the gas in his lungs expands according to Boyle's law. It is therefore imperative that he keeps his glottis and mouth open, allowing gas to escape in a continuous stream. If gas is not allowed to escape, lung rupture is almost certain to occur. Buoyancy is not changed by the loss of gas during ascent. In an uneventful escape, the time spent at pressure is too short for there to be any danger of 'bends'. Thorough training is necessary and all submariners are trained in a vertical tank of 100 feet depth. Free escape has also taken place from aircraft which have ditched from aircraft carriers and then sunk rapidly. The normal ejection procedure is followed, but it is essential for the cabin pressure to increase sufficiently for the canopy to open against the water pressure. Timing during the descent is therefore crucial (Coles, 1992, personal communication).

Avoidance of exposure of man to pressure

The maintenance of a diver at great depths is both very expensive and potentially dangerous, although the economic importance of his work is very great. The future may well lie either with remotely controlled unmanned devices, such as were used for the discovery of the *Titanic*, or with solutions which maintain man underwater at a pressure of 1 atmosphere, under so-called 'shirt sleeve conditions'. There are three possibilities for exploiting the last option. Firstly, there are armoured diving suits (manufactured under the names JIM or WASP) with an internal pressure of 1 atmosphere and capable of operating down to 700 metres of sea water. It is possible for a diver in a JIM to walk short distances and carry out very simple manipulations by means of pincers mounted on the arms. Secondly, there is the minisubmarine, capable of free movement but severely limited in the manipulations which can be carried out by the crew. Thirdly, a habitat can be constructed at the base of an oil rig which encompasses the working area and is maintained at 1 atmosphere and can be entered as the work schedule requires.

All of these solutions have their limitations. None has yet achieved the dexterity and adaptability of the free-swimming diver, although they are constantly being improved. While the habitat is an attractive option for pipeline tie-ins and work on the well head, it is clearly useless for structural work on underwater parts of the rig itself or for attention to a pipeline at some distance from the rig. The future position is by no means clear at the time of writing, but it is beginning to appear unlikely that the free-swimming diver will be employed at very great depths in the foreseeable future.

Chapter 17

Drowning

In many countries, drowning is a major cause of accidental death, many victims being under 20 years and unable to swim. Alcohol is an important aetiological factor, particularly in older victims (Mackie, 1979). In addition to death by drowning, there are substantial numbers who are resuscitated and others who recover spontaneously. Death from pulmonary complications ('secondary drowning') may occur a considerable time after the accident. There may be residual brain damage but this is happily rare (Modell, Graves and Ketover, 1976).

The essential feature of drowning is asphyxia, but many of the physiological responses depend on whether aspiration of water occurs and upon the substances which are dissolved or suspended in the water. The temperature of the water is crucially important, and hypothermia following drowning in very cold water is a major factor influencing survival. In addition, much depends on the state of the victim at the time of the accident. Important factors include his state of health, his gastric contents, blood alcohol, exhaustion and lung volume at the time of immersion. Although comparatively little water is directly inhaled by human victims, a great deal is swallowed. Vomiting occurs in over 50% of resuscitation procedures (Harries, 1981) and inhalation may occur as a result. Drowning may be murder, accident or suicide.

Drowning without aspiration

The larynx is firmly closed during submersion and some victims will lose consciousness before water is aspirated. Modell (1984) has cited the evidence for believing that this applies in approximately 10% of cases. It is particularly likely to occur if there has been previous hyperventilation (Craig, 1961). The breaking point then occurs at lower values of both P_{O_2} and P_{CO_2} (see Figure 5.9). Because of the difference in alveolar/mixed venous gas tension gradients, arterial P_{O_2} falls initially at almost ten times the rate of rise of arterial P_{CO_2}. The subsequent rate of decrease is mainly dependent on the lung volume and the oxygen consumption. Oxygen stored in the alveolar gas after a maximal inspiration is unlikely to exceed 1 litre and an oxygen consumption of 2 l/ min would not be unusual in a subject either swimming or struggling (page 353). Loss of consciousness from decreased alveolar

PO$_2$ usually occurs very suddenly and without warning. The critical level is probably in the range 4–6 kPa (30–45 mmHg). The diving reflex is probably not a major factor in human drowning and is considered on page 361.

If a swimmer who has lost consciousness from hypoxia can be removed from the water before aspiration occurs, the situation is no different from other forms of simple asphyxia and restoration of pulmonary ventilation (spontaneous or artificial) should result in a near-normal arterial PO$_2$. The outcome will then depend upon the intensity and duration of hypoxia. Apart from the extremes of full recovery and death, there may be any degree of residual cerebral damage, and details of assessment have been described by Conn and Barker (1984).

Drowning with aspiration of water

Fresh water

Two-thirds of all fatal immersion incidents in the USA, Britain, Australia, Canada and New Zealand occur on inland waters (Harries, 1981). This contributes to the belief that fresh water is inherently more dangerous. However, it seems likely that a major factor is the relative lack of rescue services in inland locations. This contrasts with the very high success rate of the rescue services on beaches used for surfing (Simcock, 1986).

Most victims will eventually aspirate water either before or after the loss of consciousness, although the quantity of water is usually much less than in experimental studies of anaesthetized laboratory animals. Aspiration of fresh water results in a temporary reflex bronchospasm and, in addition, there is a loss of compliance due to effects on the pulmonary surfactant (Giammona and Modell, 1967).

In fresh water drowning, almost none of the water which enters the lungs can be recovered by suction, because it rapidly enters the circulation (Modell and Moya, 1966). Nevertheless, there is always a significant shunt which responds favourably to positive end-expiratory pressure (PEEP) or continuous positive airway pressure (CPAP). This may be compared with the effect of these measures in pulmonary oedema. Modell and Spohr (1989) drew attention to the possibility that neurogenic pulmonary oedema caused by cerebral hypoxia might coexist with alveolar flooding due to aspirated water. The distinction would clearly be difficult. Modell (1984) cited a patient with severe pulmonary oedema thought to be a near-drowned victim but who, on careful enquiry, was found to have fractured his skull in a misjudged dive without having actually entered the water. The pulmonary changes caused by immersion appear to be reversible, with good prospects of return to normal pulmonary function in those who survive near-drowning (Butt et al., 1970).

Absorption of fresh water from the lungs results in haemodilution. This becomes significant when the aspirated water approaches 800 ml for a 70 kg man (Modell and Moya, 1966). However, redistribution rapidly corrects the blood volume and there may even be hypovolaemia if pulmonary oedema supervenes. Haemodilution can theoretically result in haemolysis but dangerous changes in plasma electrolytes and the appearance of free haemoglobin are unusual, probably because most human victims inhale only small quantities of water (Modell and Spohr, 1989). Nevertheless, profound hyponatraemia (less than 100 mmol/l) may occur in infants drowned in fresh water.

Sea water

Sea water, like fresh water, causes reflex bronchospasm after aspiration. However, there are major differences on other aspects of lung function, which are attributable to the tonicity of the water which enters the lungs. Sea water is hypertonic, having more than three times the osmolarity of blood. Consequently, sea water in the lungs is not initially absorbed and, on the contrary, draws fluid from the circulation into the alveoli. Thus, in laboratory animals that have aspirated sea water, it is possible to recover from the lungs 50% more than the original volume which was inhaled (Modell et al., 1974). This clearly maintains the proportion of flooded alveoli and results in a persistent shunt with reduction in arterial P_{O_2}. However, surprisingly, sea water has less effect than fresh water on the surfactant which remains (Giammona and Modell, 1967). Haemoconcentration and hypernatraemia seldom occur to any significant extent in human victims.

Other material contaminating the lungs

It is not unusual for drowning persons to swallow large quantities of water and then to regurgitate or vomit. Material aspirated into the lungs may then be contaminated with gastric contents and the drowning syndrome complicated with features of the acid-aspiration syndrome. Aspiration of solid foreign bodies is a frequent complication of near-drowning in shallow rivers and lakes.

Tests of drowning

There appears to be no conclusive test for aspiration of either fresh or sea water. Modell (1984) reviewed and dismissed the use of tests based on differences in specific gravity and chloride content of plasma from the right and left chambers of the heart. He was also unimpressed by the value of demonstration of diatoms in the tissues and concluded that there is still no definitive test.

The role of hypothermia

Some degree of hypothermia is usual in near-drowned victims and body temperature is usually in the range 33–36°C (Pearn, 1985). In cold water, temperature may fall very rapidly under drowning conditions and rates of 1°C/min have been reported (Conn and Barker, 1984). Reduction in cerebral metabolism is protective (Conn, Edmonds and Barker, 1978) but, on the other hand, consciousness is lost at about 32°C and ventricular fibrillation may occur at temperatures below 28°C. There have been reports of survival of near-drowned children trapped for periods as long as 40 minutes beneath ice. Current practice is to rewarm the patient over a few hours and then to maintain normal temperature, except when hypothermia is indicated for treatment of brain damage.

Principles of treatment of near-drowning

There is a high measure of agreement on general principles of treatment (Conn and Barker, 1984; Pearn, 1985; Modell and Spohr, 1989).

Immediate treatment

At the scene of the drowning, it can be very difficult to determine whether there has been cardiac or even respiratory arrest. However, there are many records of apparently dead victims who have recovered without evidence of brain damage after long periods of total immersion. It is therefore essential that cardiopulmonary resuscitation be undertaken in all victims until fully assessed in hospital, no matter how hopeless the outlook may appear.

Early treatment of near-drowning is crucial and this requires efficient instruction in resuscitation for those who may be available in locations where drowning is likely to occur. The normal priorities of airway clearance, artificial ventilation and chest compression (cardiac massage) should be observed. Mouth-to-mouth ventilation is the method of choice, but high inflation pressures are usually required when there has been flooding of the lungs. In sea water drowning it may be possible to drain water from the lungs by gravity but this is less important than the prompt institution of ventilation (Modell, 1984). Many authorities do not believe that it is practicable to drain water from the lungs. Abdominal thrust (the Heimlich manoeuvre) may expel some water from the lungs, but is not generally recommended because of the risk of squeezing swallowed water out of the stomach, which may then be inhaled. Oxygen is clearly valuable if available and should be continued until hospital is reached. Most survivors will breathe spontaneously within 1–5 minutes after removal from the water. The decision to discontinue resuscitation should not be taken until assessment in hospital, particularly if the state of consciousness is confused by hypothermia.

Circulatory failure and loss of consciousness may occur when a patient is lifted from the water in a vertical position, as for example by a helicopter winch. This is probably due to the loss of water pressure resulting in relative redistribution of blood volume into the legs.

Hospital treatment

On arrival at the accident and emergency department of a hospital, patients should be triaged into the following categories:

1. Awake.
2. Blunted (but conscious).
3. Comatose.

There should be better than 90% survival in the first two categories, but they should be admitted for observation and followed up after discharge. Patients who are comatose will require admission to intensive care. Treatment follows the general principles for hypoxic cerebral damage and aspiration lung injury. Pulmonary shunting may be as high as 70% of pulmonary blood flow and this may only slowly resolve. Late deterioration of pulmonary function may occur and is known as 'secondary drowning', which is a form of the adult respiratory distress syndrome (see Chapter 29). If spontaneous breathing does not result in satisfactory levels of P_{O_2} and P_{CO_2}, continuous positive airway pressure (CPAP) may be tried, but it is more usual to institute artificial ventilation with or without positive end-expiratory pressure (PEEP) (Simcock, 1986). If severe, metabolic acidosis should be corrected, as should abnormal electrolyte levels. Steroids have been used in high dosage but there is no clear evidence for their efficacy (Modell, Graves and Ketover, 1976; Simcock, 1986).

Chapter 18

Pregnancy, neonates and children

Respiratory function in pregnancy

Lung volumes. Vital capacity is either unchanged or actually increases during pregnancy (de Swiet, 1980). However, the residual volume is decreased, by about 20% (200–300 ml). Expiratory reserve volume is also reduced, and functional residual capacity (FRC) is decreased by about 500 ml.

Oxygen consumption. Oxygen consumption is increased by about 16% above normal at full term (Pernoll et al., 1975), mainly attributable to the demands of the fetus, uterus and placenta. The increase is negligible at the 20th week of gestation (de Swiet, 1980).

Ventilation. Tidal volume and minute volume of ventilation increase in parallel up to 40% above normal at full term. There is no reduction in ventilatory capacity (Nørregaard et al., 1989). In the third trimester, $FEV_{1.0}$ was close to, and maximal breathing capacity actually exceeded, the postpartum values, particularly in the supine position when the diaphragm is high in the chest. The hyperventilation appears to be attributable to progesterone levels, and is accompanied by a threefold increase in slope of PCO_2/ventilation response curve (de Swiet, 1980). The hypoxic ventilatory response is increased twofold, most of the change occurring before the mid-point of gestation, at which time oxygen consumption has hardly begun to increase (Moore, McCullough and Weil, 1987). Hyperventilation may be very uncomfortable for the mother.

PCO_2 and PO_2. The increase in ventilation is beyond the requirements of the enhanced oxygen uptake, and alveolar and arterial PCO_2 are reduced to about 4 kPa (30 mmHg). This must facilitate clearance of carbon dioxide by the fetus. There must also be an increase in alveolar PO_2 of about 1 kPa (7.5 mmHg) and mean values for oxygen saturation (by pulse oximetry) in the last 4 weeks of pregnancy were 97.3% sitting and 96.9 % supine (Nørregaard et al., 1989)

The lungs before birth

Embryologically, the lungs develop as an outgrowth from the foregut and first appear about the 24th day of gestation. The lungs begin to contain surfactant and are first capable of function by approximately 24–26 weeks, this being a major factor in the viability of premature infants. At full term all major elements of the lungs are fully formed but the respiratory tract is filled with some 40 ml of fluid replenished by a transudate of plasma of some 500 ml/day (Bland, 1991). Its volume corresponds approximately with the FRC after breathing is established (Strang, 1965). There is a net flow of fluid up the trachea to be swallowed or discharged into the amniotic fluid.

Fetal breathing movements. There is excellent evidence that respiratory movements are present *in utero* for about 40% of the time in the last third of gestation in the lamb (Dawes et al., 1972). These movements occur predominantly during rapid eye movement (REM) sleep (see Chapter 14). Harding (1991) has reviewed the evidence supporting similar respiratory activity in the human fetus, in whom it occurs in episodes at a frequency of about 45 breaths per minute. The diaphragm seems to be the main muscle concerned and it is estimated that there is a fluid shift of about 2 ml at each 'breath'.

The fetal circulation

The fetal circulation differs radically from the postnatal circulation (Figure 18.1). Blood from the right heart is deflected away from the lungs, partly through the foramen ovale and partly through the ductus arteriosus. Less than 10% of the output of the right ventricle reaches the lungs (Tod and Cassin, 1991) the remainder passing to the systemic circulation and the placenta. Right atrial pressure exceeds left atrial pressure and this maintains the patency of the foramen ovale. Furthermore, since the vascular resistance of the pulmonary circulation exceeds that of the systemic circulation before birth, pressure in the right ventricle exceeds that in the left ventricle and these factors control the direction of flow through the ductus arteriosus. The direction may be reversed in abnormal circumstances if the pressure gradient between the ventricles is reversed.

The umbilical veins drain via the ductus venosus into the inferior vena cava which therefore contains better oxygenated blood than the superior vena cava. The anatomy of the atria and the foramen ovale is such that the better oxygenated blood from the inferior vena cava passes preferentially into the left atrium and thence to the left ventricle and so to the brain. (This is not shown in Figure 18.1.) Overall gas tensions in the fetus are of the order of 6.4 kPa (48 mmHg) for P_{CO_2} and 4 kPa (30 mmHg) for P_{O_2} (Longo, 1991). The fact that the fetus remains apnoeic for most of the time *in utero* with these blood gas levels is probably in part attributable to central hypoxic ventilatory depression (page 106, and Edelman and Neubauer, 1991).

Events at birth

Oxygen stores in the fetus are small and it is therefore essential that air breathing and oxygen uptake be established within a few minutes of birth. This requires radical changes in the function of both lungs and circulation.

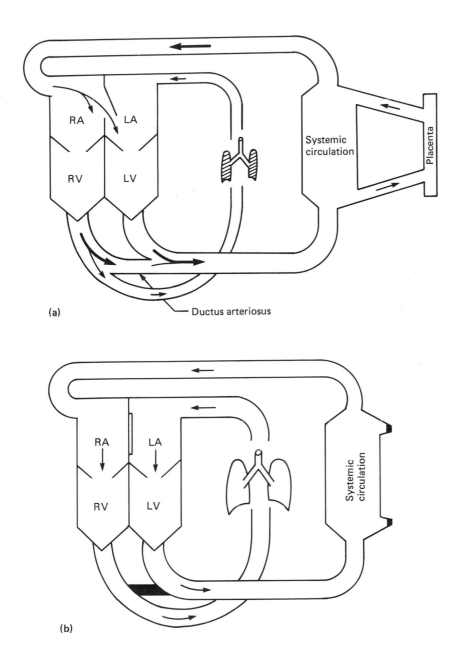

(a)

Ductus arteriosus

(b)

Figure 18.1 Fetal circulation (a) compared with adult circulation (b). The foramen ovale is between right atrium (RA) and left atrium (LA). RV and LV, right and left ventricles.

Factors in the initiation of breathing

Most normal infants take their first breath within the first 20 seconds after delivery, and rhythmic respiration is usually established within 90 seconds. Following thoracic compression during delivery, the recoil of the rib cage tends to cause air to be drawn passively into the lungs (Rees, 1980). However, the major stimuli to breathing are probably the cooling of the skin and mechanical stimulation (Hodson, 1991). Hypoxaemia, resulting from apnoea or clamping of the cord, is unlikely to be a reliable respiratory stimulus at this time because of central hypoxic ventilatory depression (see above). Ceruti (1966) found that inhalation of 12% oxygen in a warm environment induced only transient hyperventilation lasting barely a minute, and this was followed by respiratory depression. However, reduced environmental temperature increased ventilation by about 30%. A ventilatory response to 3% carbon dioxide of about 15% was observed which was not related to temperature. There was limited evidence to suggest that the hypoxic drive to ventilation became more sustained by the seventh day of life.

Fate of the fetal lung fluid

The volume of intraluminal fluid decreases just before and during labour. Some of the residual fluid may be expressed during a vaginal delivery but this is not thought to be a major factor (Bland, 1991). After the first breath, most of the fluid passes into distensible perivascular spaces around blood vessels and bronchi, forming cuffs as in pulmonary oedema (page 485). These spaces are then cleared in the first few hours after delivery.

Changes in the circulation

The geometry of the circulation changes radically and quickly at birth. The establishment of spontaneous breathing causes a massive decrease in the vascular resistance of the pulmonary circulation, due partly to mechanical factors and partly to reduction of hypoxic pulmonary vasoconstriction following the first breath. Simultaneously there is an increase in the resistance of the systemic circulation, due partly to vasoconstriction and partly to cessation of the placental circulation. As a result, the right atrial pressure falls below the left atrial pressure, to give the relationship which is then maintained throughout life. This normally results in closure of the foramen ovale (Figure 18.1), which is followed by closure of the ductus arteriosus as a result of active vasoconstriction of its smooth muscle layer. The circulation is thus converted from the fetal mode, in which the lungs and the systemic circulation are essentially in parallel, to the adult mode in which they are in series.

The Apgar score

The scoring system devised many years ago by Virginia Apgar is still widely accepted as an assessment of the overall condition of the neonate. This is based on scoring of a scale of 0–2 for five attributes, two of which are related to respiration (Table 18.1). The total score is the sum of each of the five constituent scores and is best undertaken 1 and 5 minutes after delivery. Scores of 8–10 are regarded as normal.

Table 18.1 The Apgar scoring system

Score	0	1	2
Heart rate	Absent	Less than 100/min	More than 100/min
Respiratory effort	Absent	Slow, irregular	Good, crying
Colour	Blue, pale	Body pink, extremities blue	Completely pink
Reflex irritability	Absent	Grimace	Cough, sneeze
Muscle tone	Limp	Some flexion of extremities	Active motion

Add together scores for each section (maximum possible 10).
Score at 1 and 5 minutes after delivery.
(After Gregory, 1981)

Neonatal asphyxia

Asphyxia may occur *in utero* from partial detachment of the placenta, maternal hypoxia or any reduction in uterine perfusion. After delivery, it has been reported in various studies that 13% of infants were still apnoeic 2 minutes after birth and 4.7% after 3 minutes (Davenport and Valman, 1980). This constitutes primary apnoea and, if prolonged for 5–10 minutes, characteristically leads to a gasp which is then followed by secondary or terminal apnoea (Dawes, 1968). Brain damage commences after about 10 minutes of apnoea. Various stimuli may initiate breathing and usually do so during primary apnoea. However, in secondary apnoea, only artificial ventilation is effective. There are many causes of fetal asphyxia and these include the administration of respiratory depressant drugs to the mother before delivery.

In view of the short time scale of events, active measures should be instituted if breathing has not commenced by 30 seconds after delivery, and intermittent positive pressure ventilation (IPPV) may be started with oxygen using a well-fitting facemask. If there is no response after 1 minute, the trachea should be intubated, since this permits more effective suction to remove mucus and also more effective IPPV.

Neonatal lung function

Mechanics of breathing

Functional residual capacity is about 30 ml/kg and total respiratory compliance 50 ml/kPa (5 ml/cmH$_2$O). Most of the impedance to expansion is due to the lung and depends primarily on the presence of surfactant in the alveoli. The chest wall of the neonate is highly compliant. This contrasts with the adult where compliance of lung and chest wall are approximately equal. Total respiratory resistance is of the order of 7 kPa l^{-1} s (70 cmH$_2$O l^{-1} s), most of which is in the bronchial tree. Compliance is about one-twentieth that of an adult and resistance about 15 times greater. The time constant (product of compliance and resistance – see page 437) is thus rather less than in the adult and is about 0.3 second. At the first breath the infant is capable of generating a subatmospheric intrathoracic pressure of the order of 7 kPa (70 cmH$_2$O).

Ventilation and gas exchange

For a 3.5 kg neonate, the minute volume is about 0.8 litre, with a high respiratory frequency of about 40 b.p.m. (Longo, 1991). Dead space is variously reported as between a third and a half of tidal volume, giving a mean alveolar ventilation of about 0.5 l/min for a neonate of average size. There is a shunt of about 10% immediately after birth. However, distribution of gas is better than in the adult and there is, of course, a negligible hydrostatic pressure gradient in the vertical axis of the tiny lungs of an infant. Diffusing capacity for carbon monoxide per square metre of body area is about half the corresponding value in the adult (Nelson, 1966).

Oxygen consumption is of the order of 20–30 ml/min depending on weight in the range 2–4 kg. Arterial P_{CO_2} is close to 4.5 kPa (34 mmHg) and P_{O_2} 9 kPa (68 mmHg). Due to the shunt of 10 per cent, there is an alveolar/arterial P_{O_2} gradient of about 3.3 kPa (25 mmHg) compared with less than half of this in a young adult. Arterial pH is within the normal adult range.

Control of breathing (see reviews by Chernick, 1981; Fleming and Ponte, 1983; Lagerkrantz, Milerad and Walker, 1991). After birth, there is a very rapid transition towards the adult pattern of respiratory control. Central hypoxic ventilatory depression gives way to hypoxic respiratory stimulation and, soon after birth, ventilation is depressed by the inhalation of 100% oxygen (Brady, Cotton and Tooley, 1964), indicating a tonic drive from the peripheral chemoreceptors. Chemoreceptor drive is probably the mechanism of the periodic breathing which is often seen in infants. Ventilatory response to carbon dioxide appears to be similar to that in the adult if allowance is made for body size, although depressed in REM sleep (Cohen, Xu and Henderson-Smart, 1991).

Haemoglobin

Children are normally born polycythaemic with a mean haemoglobin of about 18 g/dl and a haematocrit of 53% (Delivoria-Papadopoulos, Roncevic and Oski, 1971). Seventy per cent of the haemoglobin is HbF and the resultant P_{50} is well below the normal adult value (see Figure 11.12). Arterial oxygen content is close to the normal adult value in spite of the low arterial P_{O_2}. The haemoglobin concentration decreases rapidly to become less than the normal adult value by 3 weeks of life. HbF gradually disappears from the circulation to reach negligible values by 6 months, by which time the P_{50} has already attained the normal adult value.

Development of lung function during childhood

The lungs continue to develop during childhood. Between birth and adult life, there is an approximately tenfold increase in the number of airways. Cotes (1979) has provided tables and graphs showing the gradual assumption of adult values of lung volumes and various indices of ventilatory capacity in relation to the height of the subject. Ventilatory capacity at the age of 7–8 years was studied by Strang

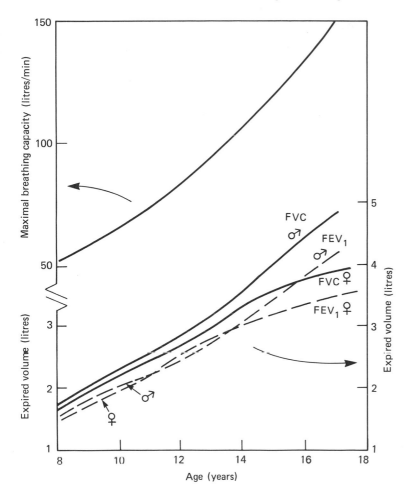

Figure 18.2 Indices of ventilatory capacity as a function of age. FVC, forced vital capacity; FEV₁, forced expiratory volume (1 second). (Drawn from data of Strang, 1959).

(1959), and Figure 18.2 summarizes some of his results. It is not practicable to determine ventilatory capacity in very young children.

Various indices of respiratory function are independent of age and body size, so adult values can be used. These include forced expiratory volume (1 second) as a fraction of vital capacity, FRC and peak expiratory flow rate as a fraction of total lung capacity, specific airway conductance and compliance divided by FRC and probably dead space/tidal volume ratio (Cotes, 1979).

Arterial PCO_2 and alveolar PO_2 do not change appreciably during childhood but arterial PO_2 increases from the neonatal value to reach a maximum of about 13 kPa (98 mmHg) at young adulthood. Much of this increase occurs during the first year of life (Mansell, Bryan and Levison, 1972). There are obvious difficulties in determining the normal arterial PO_2 in children.

Respiratory distress syndrome (RDS)

The essential lesion is a deficiency of surfactant and it occurs in 1% of all live births, but with a greatly increased incidence in premature infants. Surfactant is first detectable in the fetal lung at 20–24 weeks of gestation but the concentration increases rapidly after the 30th week. Therefore, prematurity is a major factor in the aetiology of RDS.

The disease presents with difficulty in inspiration against the decreased compliance due to the high surface tension of the alveolar lining fluid deficient in surfactant. This progresses to ventilatory failure, alveolar collapse, hyaline membrane deposit and interference with gas exchange resulting in severe hypoxaemia. Increased pulmonary vascular resistance may raise right atrial pressure and reopen the foramen ovale, so increasing the shunt.

Physiological principles of treatment of RDS

The physiological basis of therapy is to supplement surfactant activity and employ artificial ventilation as a temporary expedient to spare the infant the excessive work of breathing against stiff lungs. Results have improved over the years and most infants with a birth weight greater than 1 kg should survive (Jobe and Ikegami, 1987). Overall treatment is very complex and outside the scope of this book.

Surfactant replacement therapy. Natural surfactant may be obtained from alveolar lavage or amniotic fluid and may be modified in its composition. Alternatively, synthetic surfactant may be used, and colfosceril palmitate (Exosurf) is currently marketed in the UK. Apart from the phospholipids (see pages 39 et seq.), preparations have included the surfactant proteins which are soluble in chloroform/methanol. Their particular value is in the improvement of spreading following administration by intratracheal instillation (Whitsett, 1991). Clearance of exogenous surfactant is fortunately very slow (Jobe and Ikegami, 1987). It appears to be taken up in type II cells and recycled.

Artificial ventilation. Surfactant replacement therapy has reduced the necessity to ventilate infants with RDS, particularly if used before the start of ventilation. Artificial ventilation is considered in Chapter 22. For neonates, the usual choice is a time-cycled square-wave pressure generator (page 436), but operating at much higher respiratory frequencies than for the adult. Inspiratory and expiratory durations may be as little as 0.3 second, but inflation pressures are of the same order as those used in adults and do not usually exceed 3 kPa (30 cmH$_2$O). Positive end-expiratory pressure (PEEP) is widely used, and spontaneous respiration is often supported with continuous positive airway pressure (CPAP). Bronchopulmonary dysplasia appears to be a form of pulmonary barotrauma in the ventilated infant and is considered on page 456. Normal humidification and monitoring of airway pressure are important.

Both the compressible volume of the ventilator circuit and the apparatus dead space tend to be large in relation to the size of very small children. It is for this reason that pressure generators are preferable to volume generators. Furthermore, there is considerable practical difficulty in measuring the very small imposed tidal volumes or minute volumes. For this reason, close monitoring of Po$_2$ and Pco$_2$ is essential. Use of infrared gas analysis is very difficult at high respiratory frequencies and transcutaneous Pco_2 is a useful monitor. High frequency ventilation (page 444) may well have a place here but has not yet been fully evaluated. Detailed management of ventilation of neonates has been described by Llewellyn and Swyer (1975).

Treatment by CPAP with preservation of spontaneous respiration was described by Gregory et al. (1971). Much thought has been given to the possibility of raising airway pressure without the necessity of tracheal intubation. Gastight facemasks have been described by Llewellyn and Swyer, and it is also possible to obtain a seal around the head. However, these techniques are not generally used as a first line of treatment, although they may have some role in weaning from artificial ventilation.

Chapter 19

Smoking

Smoking and lung function

Smoking was introduced from the New World into Europe in the sixteenth century. Although first used for supposedly medicinal purposes, Sir Walter Raleigh made it an essential fashionable activity of every gentleman. Thereafter the practice steadily increased in popularity until the explosive growth of the habit following the First World War (1914–1918). Particularly in the Second World War (1939–1945), large numbers of women adopted the habit and, more recently, there seems to have been a relative increase in young smokers.

There have always been those opposed to smoking and King James I (1603–1625) described it as 'a custom loathsome to the eye, hateful to the nose, harmful to the brain and dangerous to the lungs'. However, firm evidence to support his last conclusion was delayed by some 350 years. Only relatively recently did it become clear that smokers had a higher mortality (Doll and Peto, 1976) and that the causes of the excess mortality included lung cancer (Doll and Hill, 1950), chronic bronchitis, emphysema and cor pulmonale (Anderson and Ferris, 1962).

Constituents of tobacco smoke

More than 2000 potentially noxious constituents have been identified in tobacco smoke, some in the gaseous phase and others in the particulate or tar phase. The particulate phase is defined as the fraction eliminated by passing smoke through a Cambridge filter of pore size 0.1 μm. This is not to be confused with the 'filter tip' which allows passage of considerable quantities of particulate matter.

The quantities of the various compounds yielded by a burning cigarette are determined by the use of a smoking machine. This simulates a typical human smoking pattern and normally draws air through the cigarette in a series of 'puffs' of 35 ml, each lasting 2 seconds and repeated every minute until the cigarette is reduced to a length of 2 cm from the butt. Constituents are then expressed in units of milligrams per cigarette. Values so obtained exclude components of 'side-stream smoke' which escape from the smouldering cigarette between puffs. This is somewhat in excess of half of the total products of the burning cigarette.

There is great variation in the yields of the various constituents between different brands and different types of cigarettes. This is achieved by using leaves of different species of plants, varying the conditions of curing and cultivation, and by the use of filter tips. Ventilated filters have a ring of small holes in the paper between the filter tip and the tobacco. These holes admit air during a puff and dilute all constituents of the smoke. By these various means, it is possible to have wide variations in the different constituents of smoke, which do not bear a fixed relationship to one another. Quantities of constituents retained by the smoker are influenced by the pattern of smoking (see below).

The gaseous phase

Yields of carbon monoxide generally vary from 15 to 25 mg (12–20 ml) (Borland et al., 1983) but levels as low as 1.8 mg have been achieved. The concentration issuing from the butt of the cigarette during a puff is in the range 1–5%, which is far into the toxic range. A better indication of the extent of carbon monoxide exposure is the percentage of carboxyhaemoglobin in blood. For non-smokers, the value is normally less than 1.5% but is influenced by exposure to traffic because automobile exhaust contains carbon monoxide. Typical values for smokers range from 2 to 12%. The value is influenced by the number of cigarettes smoked, the type of cigarette and the pattern of inhalation of smoke. Nevertheless, it remains the most reliable objective indication of smoke exposure and correlates well with most of the harmful effects of smoking (see below).

Tobacco smoke also contains very high concentrations (about 400 p.p.m.) of the relatively inactive free radical nitric oxide (Church and Pryor, 1991) and trace concentrations of nitrogen dioxide, the former being slowly oxidized to the latter in the presence of oxygen. The toxicity of these compounds is well known. Nitrogen dioxide hydrates in alveolar lining fluid to form an equimolecular mixture of nitrous and nitric acids. Both acids ionize, forming hydrogen ions. In addition, the nitrite ion converts haemoglobin to methaemoglobin. These higher oxides of nitrogen may be lethal in concentrations above 1000 p.p.m. (Greenbaum et al., 1967a). Industrial environmental contamination is limited in the UK to 25 p.p.m. of nitric oxide and 3 p.p.m. of nitrogen dioxide for long-term exposure.

Other constituents of the gaseous phase include hydrocyanic acid, cyanogen, aldehydes, ketones and volatile polycyclic aromatic hydrocarbons and nitrosamines which have been shown to be carcinogenic and mutagenic in animals.

The particulate phase

The material removed by a Cambridge filter is known as the 'total particulate matter', with aerosol particle size in the range 0.2−1 μm. The particulate phase comprises water, nicotine and 'tar'. Nicotine ranges from 0.05 to 2.5 mg per cigarette and 'tar' from 0.5 to 35 mg per cigarette. The means of both levels declined progressively by about 50% between 1954 and 1980 (Report of the US Surgeon General, 1981). The tar phase also contains quinone, the semiquinone free radical and hydroquinone in a polymeric matrix. Church and Pryor (1991) have proposed that these compounds can reduce oxygen in the body to yield the superoxide free radical and thence the highly damaging hydroxyl free radical (see Figure 32.3). Yields of the main constituents of cigarette smoke are currently classified in the UK as set out in Table 19.1.

Table 19.1 Classification of tar content of British cigarettes (Department of Health and Social Security, 1982) (yields in mg per cigarette)

	Tar	*Nicotine*	*Carbon monoxide*
Low tar	<4–10	<0.3–1	<3–14
Low to medium tar	11–16	0.6–1.6	10–19
Medium tar	17–22	1.1–1.9	10–19
Medium to high tar	24–26	1.3–2.6	14–19

Individual smoke exposure

Individual smoke exposure is a complex function of the quantity of cigarettes which are smoked and the pattern of inhalation.

The quantity of cigarettes smoked

Exposure is usually quantified in 'pack years'. This equals the product of the number of packs (20 cigarettes) smoked per day, multiplied by the number of years that that pattern was maintained. The totals for each period are then summated for the lifetime of the subject.

There is good evidence that the habituated smoker adjusts his smoking pattern to maintain a particular blood level of nicotine (Russell et al., 1975; Ashton, Stepney and Thompson, 1979). For example, after changing to a brand with a lower nicotine yield, it is common practice to modify the pattern of inhalation to maximize nicotine absorption.

The pattern of inhalation

There are very wide variations in patterns of smoking. Air is normally drawn through the cigarette in a series of 'puffs' with a volume of about 25–50 ml per puff. The puff may be simply drawn into the mouth and rapidly expelled without appreciable inhalation. However, the habituated smoker will either inhale the puff directly into the lungs or, more commonly, pass the puff from the mouth to the lungs by inhaling air either through the mouth or else through the nose while passing the smoke from the mouth into the pharynx by apposing the tongue against the palate and so obliterating the gas space in the mouth. The inspiration is often especially deep, to flush into the lung any smoke remaining in the dead space.

It will be clear that the quantity of nicotine, 'tar' and carbon monoxide obtainable from a single cigarette is highly variable and the number and type of cigarettes smoked are not the sole determinants of effective exposure. Furthermore, retention is different for different constituents, being about 60% for carbon monoxide but as much as 90% for nicotine.

Passive smoking

The non-smoker is exposed to all constituents of smoke when he is indoors in the presence of smokers (Report of the US Surgeon General, 1984). Exposure varies with many factors, including size and ventilation of the room, number of people smoking and absorption of smoke constituents on soft furnishings and clothing. Carbon monoxide concentrations of 20 p.p.m. have been reported, which is above the recommended environmental concentration (9 p.p.m. in the USA). It has been estimated that non-smokers are exposed to quantities of 'tar' ranging from zero to 14 mg/day (Rapace and Lowrey, 1982). 'Side-stream smoke' from a smouldering cigarette stub produces greater quantities of potentially noxious substances than 'main-stream smoke' produced when a cigarette burns in a stream of air drawn through it during a puff. On average, 'side-stream smoke' is generated during 58 seconds in each minute and this is not included in the measured yield of a cigarette. There is conflicting evidence as to whether passive smoking increases the incidence of smoking-related diseases.

Respiratory effects of smoking

Cigarette smoking has most extensive effects on respiratory function and is clearly implicated in the aetiology of a number of respiratory diseases, particularly emphysema, chronic bronchitis and bronchial carcinoma. The progress of emphysema is usually accelerated in smokers, who also have an increased susceptibility to respiratory infection.

Ventilatory capacity

The Report of the US Surgeon General (1984) reviews a large number of publications indicating that there is a greater decline in indices of ventilatory capacity with increasing age in smokers, compared with non-smokers. For example, $FEV_{1.0}$ reached a mean value of 2.22 litres in American male smokers at the age of 65–74, compared with 2.86 in a comparable group of non-smokers. Somewhat larger differences were found for the mean expiratory flow rate at 25 per cent of a forced vital capacity. The Report of the US Surgeon General (1984) concluded that cigarette smoking was the major cause of morbidity in chronic obstructive lung disease in the USA, and that 80–90% of cases were attributable to cigarette smoking.

Oxidative injury

Church and Pryor (1991) discuss the compelling evidence for believing that oxidative injury, including peroxidation of membrane lipids, is an important component of the pulmonary damage caused by cigarette smoking. The antioxidants glutathione, vitamin C and vitamin E are all depleted in smokers. Church and Pryor attribute this to the quinones in the tar phase and also to the nitric oxide in the gaseous phase, exacerbated by iron deposits which could catalyse the Fenton reaction (page 545). Vitamin E protects the lungs of rats from cigarette smoke exposure.

Alveolar/capillary barrier function

The integrity of the alveolar/capillary barrier is readily impaired by lipid peroxidation. Horseradish peroxidase (molecular weight 40 000 daltons) penetrates the alveolar epithelium in guinea-pigs exposed to cigarette smoke (Simani, Inoue and Hogg, 1974). However, the most sensitive indication of impaired respiratory function in smokers is the clearance of ^{99m}Tc-DTPA from the alveoli into the blood (Jones et al., 1980). The mean half-time of clearance was 59 minutes in non-smokers but only 20 minutes in smokers, with almost total separation of the two groups. This change occurs in all smokers, including young and asymptomatic smokers in whom all other pulmonary function tests are normal. Clearance is increased within days of starting smoking and returns to a plateau value about 70% of normal within a week of cessation of smoking (Minty, Jordan and Jones, 1981). This contrasts with changes of other pulmonary function tests which tend to be irreversible.

Clearance of DTPA is closely related to carboxyhaemoglobin levels in the blood (Jones et al., 1983) but filtration of the particulate matter prevented the change in rats, despite the development of very high levels of carboxyhaemoglobin (Minty and Royston, 1985).

Bronchoalveolar lavage in man has shown that smokers have larger numbers of intra-alveolar macrophages and also significant numbers of neutrophils which are not normally present in non-smokers (Hunninghake and Crystal, 1983). These authors have also demonstrated that it is the particulate component of smoke which is responsible for the recruitment and activation of the neutrophils in the alveoli. This suggests that the interaction of particulate matter and alveolar macrophages releases a neutrophil chemattractant and neutrophils are subsequently activated to release either proteases or oxygen-derived free radicals (page 542). Either of these could impair the integrity of the alveolar/epithelial barrier.

Other effects on respiratory function
(see editorial by Samet, 1990)

Distribution of inspired gas as indicated by the single-breath nitrogen test (page 188) is often abnormal in asymptomatic smokers but there is no good evidence that this is predictive of the development of chronic obstructive airway disease. There is usually increased production of mucus in smokers, and there is also impairment of the normal mechanisms of mucus clearance, such as ciliary activity (Dalhamn and Rylander, 1965). There is almost always increased coughing which is often productive.

Reference has been made above to the accelerated decline in indices of ventilatory capacity with age in smokers. This change is attributable to narrowing of small airways and there is usually increased reactivity of the airways. The concentration of inhaled histamine required to reduce specific airway conductance by 35% is, in smokers, less than 40% of that required in non-smokers (Gerrard et al., 1980). Carbon monoxide diffusing capacity is slightly reduced in heavy smokers (Tockman et al., 1976).

An inverse relationship between smoking and body weight has been widely observed, and this is a factor which may encourage smoking. However, resting metabolic rate is not appreciably different between smokers and non-smokers (see review by Perkins, 1992), and there is only a slight and inconsistent decrease on cessation of smoking. However, a small but significant increase in metabolic rate (less than 11%) has been observed immediately after smoking. This has been attributed to sympathoadrenal activation by nicotine.

Postoperative respiratory complications

There is ample evidence that smokers have an increased incidence of postoperative respiratory complications (see review by Pearce and Jones, 1984). This is attributable both to increased secretion of mucus and impaired clearance and to small airway narrowing. Apart from changes in respiratory function considered above, there is an impairment of many aspects of the response to infection in smokers, and this may contribute further to postoperative morbidity.

Chapter 20

Respiratory aspects of anaesthesia

It has long been recognized that anaesthesia has profound effects upon the respiratory system. However, these effects are diverse and highly specific, some aspects of respiratory function being profoundly modified while others are scarcely affected at all.

Much of this chapter is concerned with anaesthesia without paralysis and with spontaneous breathing preserved. However, it will also describe the effects of the combination of anaesthesia, paralysis and artificial ventilation.

Pattern of contraction of respiratory muscles

One of the most remarkable examples of the specificity of anaesthetic actions is upon certain muscles associated with respiration. Many of these effects could hardly have been predicted but, nevertheless, have great clinical importance and underlie many of the secondary effects described later in this chapter.

The pharynx

Anaesthesia usually causes obstruction of the pharyngeal airway unless measures are taken for its protection. Figure 20.1 shows changes in the sagittal geometry of the pharynx immediately after induction of anaesthesia in the supine position (Nandi et al., 1991a). The soft palate fell against the posterior pharyngeal wall, occluding the nasopharynx in almost every patient, presumably due to interference with the action of some or all of tensor palati, palatoglossus or palatopharyngeus (page 13). There was considerable posterior movement of tongue and epiglottis, but usually not sufficient to occlude the oral or hypopharyngeal airway. Genioglossus and probably geniohyoid have both tonic and inspiratory phasic activity (page 16). In the cat, there is well marked interference with genioglossus activity during anaesthesia (Nishino et al., 1984; Ochiai, Guthrie and Motoyama, 1989). Human observations have shown that thiopentone decreases the EMG activity of genioglossus and the strap muscles (Drummond, 1989a). Nevertheless, Nandi et al. showed that the posterior movement of the palate was not caused by pressure from the tongue. The changes shown in Figure 20.1 are very similar to those observed with anaesthesia and *paralysis* (Morikawa, Safar and DeCarlo, 1961).

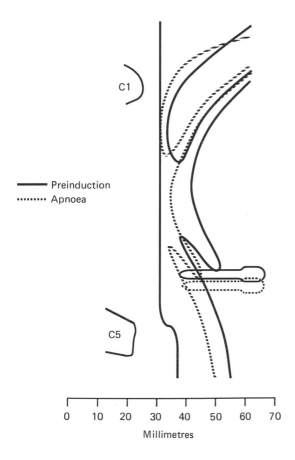

C1

— Preinduction

········ Apnoea

C5

```
 0    10   20   30   40   50   60   70
```
Millimetres

Figure 20.1 Median sagittal section of the pharynx to show changes between the conscious state (continuous lines) and following induction of anaesthesia (broken lines). The most consistent change was occlusion of the nasopharynx. (Reproduced from Nandi et al. (1991a) with permission of the Editors and publishers of the British Journal of Anaesthesia)

Secondary changes occur when the patient attempts to breathe. Upstream obstruction then often causes major passive downstream collapse of the entire pharynx (Figure 20.2), a mechanism with features in common with obstructive sleep apnoea (pages 16 and 335). This secondary collapse of the pharynx is due to interference with the normal action of pharyngeal dilator muscles, particularly genioglossus. Boidin (1985) noted that the epiglottis may be involved in hypopharyngeal obstruction during anaesthesia, and posterior movement is clearly shown in Figures 20.1 and 20.2.

Protection of the pharyngeal airway. In many countries, the changes described above are countered by the universal use of a tracheal tube, and management of the difficult airway has recently been reviewed by Benumof (1991) and Cobley and Vaughan (1992). However, there are effective alternatives to tracheal intubation which are useful for relatively minor procedures, particularly when spontaneous breathing is preserved. Extension of the neck moves the origin of genioglossus

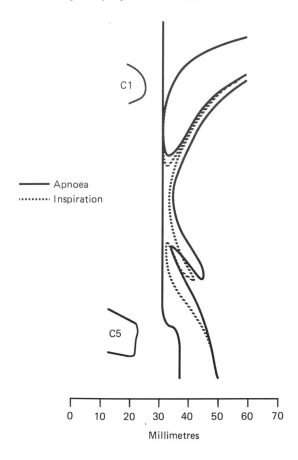

C1

——— Apnoea
·········· Inspiration

C5

| 0 | 10 | 20 | 30 | 40 | 50 | 60 | 70 |

Millimetres

Figure 20.2 Median sagittal section of the pharynx during anaesthesia to show changes between the apnoeic state (continuous lines, corresponding to the broken lines in Figure 20.1) *and following attempted inspiration (broken lines). Upstream obstruction in the nasopharynx results in downstream collapse of the oro- and hypopharynx. (Reproduced from Nandi et al. (1991a) with permission of the Editors and publishers of the* British Journal of Anaesthesia)

anteriorly by 1–2 cm and usually clears the hypopharyngeal airway (Morikawa, Safar and DeCarlo, 1961). Protrusion of the mandible moves the origin of genioglossus still further forward and this manoeuvre was proposed by Heiberg in 1874. The use of a pharyngeal airway, such as that of Guedel, is frequently helpful, but the tip may become lodged in the vallecula, or the tongue may be pushed downwards and backwards to obstruct the tip of the airway (Marsh et al., 1991). Therefore successful use of a pharyngeal airway usually requires neck extension and often jaw protrusion as well (the Esmarch–Heiberg manoeuvre). However, this increases the pharyngeal volume (and anatomical dead space) by as much as 70 ml (Nunn, Campbell and Peckett, 1959).

The laryngeal mask is a revolutionary new approach to airway management (Brain, 1983). This device provides an airtight seal around the laryngeal perimeter, with a leak pressure of about 1.7 kPa (17 cmH$_2$O). Intermittent positive pressure ventilation is therefore entirely feasible, but it is especially suitable for use with preserved spontaneous breathing. In the form available at the time of writing, the laryngeal mask does not prevent regurgitated gastric contents gaining access to the larynx. However, there should be no problem in the normally prepared surgical patient. Nandi et al. (1991b) have described the normal and abnormal anatomical locations of the mask.

Placement of the laryngeal mask does not require laryngoscopy or neuromuscular block, and the technique is rapidly and easily learned (Broderick, Webster and Nunn, 1989; Davies et al., 1990). It has also been possible to pass a laryngeal mask in many situations where conventional tracheal intubation has failed. However, its most important application is in routine anaesthesia with spontaneous breathing, where it gives a clear airway and frees the hands of the anaesthetist from the Esmarch–Heiberg manoeuvre, so facilitating monitoring and record keeping. The laryngeal mask is still under active development.

The inspiratory muscles
(see reviews by Drummond, 1989b, and Nunn, 1990)

In the very early days of anaesthesia John Snow (1858) observed that deepening anaesthesia was associated with a decrease in thoracic respiratory excursion and this has been used as a sign of deepening anaesthesia. The effect was quantified by Miller (1925) and more precisely related to depth of anaesthesia with halothane by Jones and his colleagues (1979). However, isoflurane at minimal alveolar concentration for anaesthesia (MAC = 1) showed no such changes (Lumb, Petros and Nunn, 1991). Neither did methohexitone (Bickler, Dueck and Prutow, 1987) nor ketamine (Mankikian et al., 1986). It seems that this change should not be regarded as an invariable feature of anaesthesia and there is certainly an increased thoracic component of ventilation during IPPV of the anaesthetized paralysed patient (Vellody et al., 1978).

Diaphragmatic function appears to be well preserved during anaesthesia but there may be a change in its pattern of contraction. Muller et al. (1979) showed evidence of residual end-expiratory tone during normal breathing by the conscious subject in the supine position. This might well be to prevent the weight of the viscera pushing the diaphragm too far into the chest in the supine position. They showed that this diaphragmatic end-expiratory tone was lost during anaesthesia with halothane. Such a change would result in the diaphragm moving cephalad during anaesthesia, which has been reported by Froese and Bryan (1974) and Hedenstierna et al. (1985). However, other investigators have not found the diaphragm to move consistently cephalad during anaesthesia (Drummond, Allan and Logan, 1986; Krayer et al., 1989). Drummond (1989a) observed thiopentone to decrease the EMG activity of sternothyroid, sternohyoid and the scalene muscles.

The expiratory muscles

Freund, Roos and Dodd (1964) demonstrated that general anaesthesia caused expiratory phasic activity of the abdominal muscles which are normally silent in the conscious supine subject. The observations were extended by Kaul, Heath and Nunn (1973) who found that it was very difficult to abolish this activity as long as spontaneous breathing persisted. This activation of expiratory muscles seems to serve no useful purpose and does not appear to have any significant effect on the change in functional residual capacity (Hewlett et al., 1974b).

Control of breathing
(see reviews by Pavlin and Hornbein, 1986; Nunn, 1990)

Anaesthesia may diminish pulmonary ventilation, and hypercapnia is commonplace if spontaneous breathing is preserved. The first aspect of the problem to be elucidated was the effect of anaesthetics on the P_{CO_2}/ventilation response curve.

Effect on P_{CO_2}/ventilation response curve
(see page 107)

It has long been known that progressive increases in the alveolar concentration of all inhalational anaesthetic agents decrease the slope of the P_{CO_2}/ventilation response curve and, at deep levels of anaesthesia, there may be no response at all to P_{CO_2}. Furthermore, the anaesthetized patient, as opposed to the awake subject, always becomes apnoeic if the P_{CO_2} is reduced below this intercept which is known as the apnoeic threshold P_{CO_2} (page 108). In Figure 20.3, the flat curve rising to the left represents the starting points for various P_{CO_2}/ventilation response curves. Without added carbon dioxide in the inspired gas, deepening anaesthesia is associated with a decreasing ventilation and a rising P_{CO_2} points moving progressively down and to the right. At intervals along this curve are shown P_{CO_2}/ventilation response curves resulting from adding carbon dioxide to the inspired gas.

Anaesthetics differ quantitatively in their capacity to depress the response of ventilation to P_{CO_2}. This is conveniently shown by plotting the slope of the P_{CO_2}/ventilation response curve against equi-anaesthetic concentrations of different anaesthetics, shown as multiples of MAC (Figure 20.4), although the validity of using MAC multiples in this way has been questioned. The halogenated agents do not differ greatly from one another but diethyl ether is exceptional in having little effect up to 1.0 MAC. Thereafter the effect increases markedly with increasing concentrations until, at 2.5 MAC, the extrapolated value appears to be comparable to the halogenated agents. Anaesthesia with diethyl ether causes an increase in the level of circulating catecholamines which may counteract the depressant effect of the anaesthetic (Cunningham et al., 1963).

Surgical stimulation antagonizes the effect of anaesthesia on the P_{CO_2}/ventilation response curve (Figure 20.5). It may easily be observed that a surgical incision increases the ventilation whatever the depth of anaesthesia, provided that spontaneous breathing is still present. During prolonged anaesthesia without surgical stimulation, there is no progressive change in the response curve up to 3 hours, but partial return towards the preanaesthetic position has been reported after 6 hours (Fourcade et al., 1972). Depression of ventilation by anaesthesia is relatively greater in patients with chronic obstructive airway disease (Pietak et al., 1975). Barbiturates have little effect on ventilation in sedative or light sleep dosage. However, anaesthetic doses have effects similar to the inhalational anaesthetics

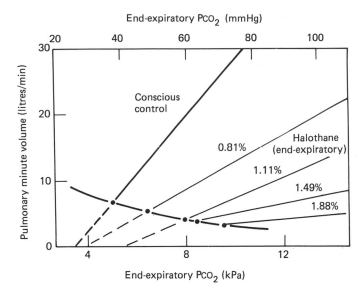

Figure 20.3 Displacement of Pco₂/ventilation response curve with different end-expiratory concentrations of halothane. The curve sloping down to the right indicates the pathway of Pco₂ and ventilation change resulting from depression without the challenge of exogenous carbon dioxide. The broken lines indicate extrapolation to apnoeic threshold Pco₂. The curves have been constructed from the data of Munson et al. (1966). A rather similar set of curves was obtained for methoxyflurane by Dunbar, Ovassapian and Smith (1967) except that these workers did not observe the same degree of displacement to the right of the initial Pco₂ at different depths of anaesthesia before the carbon dioxide challenge. Roughly similar changes in slope were reported for equipotent concentrations of the two agents.

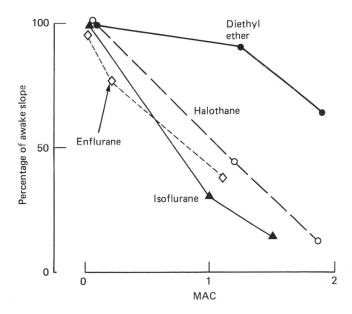

Figure 20.4 Relative respiratory depression of different anaesthetics as a function of multiples of minimal alveolar concentration (MAC) required for anaesthesia. (Based on a review by Eger, 1981)

(Bellville and Seed, 1960). Ketamine is exceptional in having little effect. Opiates are well known to depress ventilation, and a reduction in respiratory frequency is often observed. Small doses have been reported to increase the intercept of the PCO_2/ventilation response curve on the PCO_2 axis without changing the slope (Loeschcke et al., 1953), but there is certainly a marked change in slope at higher dosage. With very large doses (of the order of 2 mg/kg) there is a plateau of effect on slope, with a reduction to about 20% of the value in the conscious state. Apnoea does not normally occur when doses of this order are given to the conscious subject.

Effect on PO_2/ventilation response curve

The normal relationship between PO_2 and ventilation has been described on pages 98 et seq. It was long believed that this reflex was the *ultima moriens* and, unlike the PCO_2/ventilation response curve, unaffected by anaesthesia. This doctrine was a source of comfort to many generations of anaesthetists in the past. No one seemed to notice the observation of Gordh in 1945 that ether anaesthesia nearly abolished the ventilatory response to hypoxaemia while the response to carbon dioxide was still present.

Nearly 30 years later Weiskopf, Raymond and Severinghaus (1974) showed depression of the PO_2/ventilation response curve in anaesthetized dogs. Then Duffin, Triscott and Whitwam (1976) showed that halothane anaesthesia reduced the ventilatory response to oxygen in man. Shortly afterwards, Knill and Gelb (1978) showed that not only was the hypoxic response affected by inhalational anaesthetics but it was also, in fact, exquisitely sensitive (Figure 20.6). Hypoxic drive was markedly attenuated at 0.1 MAC, a level of anaesthesia which would not be reached for a considerable time during recovery from anaesthesia. This effect

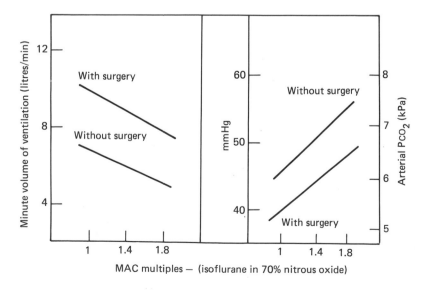

Figure 20.5 Respiratory depression of isoflurane with and without surgery at different multiples of minimal alveolar concentration (MAC) required for anaesthesia. (Drawn from data of Eger et al., 1972)

has now been amply confirmed and shown to occur with at least six inhalational anaesthetics including even nitrous oxide (Knill and Clement, 1982). The responses to halothane and isoflurane are very similar. It seems likely that the effect is on the carotid body chemoreceptor itself (Davies, Edwards and Lahiri, 1982; Knill and Clement, 1984) and there is evidence that the effect can be reversed with almitrine (Clergue et al., 1984). Anaesthesia also impairs the ventilatory response to doxapram, which acts on the peripheral chemoreceptors (Knill and Gelb, 1978).

There are four important practical implications of the loss of the hypoxic ventilatory response in anaesthesia. Firstly, the patient cannot act as his own hypoxia alarm by responding with hyperventilation. Secondly, the patient who has already lost his sensitivity to PCO_2 (e.g. 'the blue bloater' category of patient with chronic bronchitis) may stop breathing after induction of anaesthesia has abolished his hypoxic drive. This effect was, in fact, well known in the past but the cause was not understood at the time. Thirdly, anaesthesia may be dangerous at very high altitude or in other situations where survival depends on hyperventilation in response to hypoxia (Nunn, 1989). In contrast to anaesthesia, sleep has no effect on the hypoxic drive and this is important for survival of high-altitude mountaineers. Finally, since the hypoxic drive is obtunded at subanaesthetic concentrations, this effect will persist into the early postoperative period after the patient has regained consciousness and is apparently able to fend for himself.

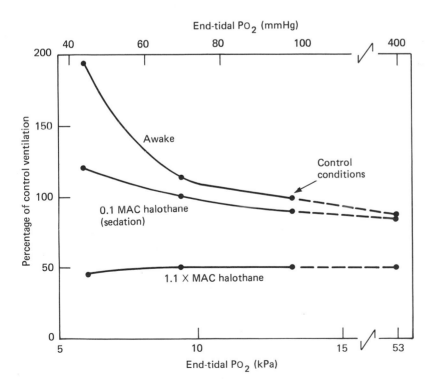

Figure 20.6 Effect of halothane anaesthesia on ventilatory response to hypoxia. MAC is the minimal alveolar concentration required for anaesthesia. (Redrawn from data of Knill and Gelb, 1978)

Response to metabolic acidaemia

The ventilatory response to non-respiratory changes in arterial P_{CO_2} has been described on page 109. This response is also obtunded by anaesthesia and even by subanaesthetic concentrations of anaesthetics (Knill and Clement, 1985). The sensitivity of this response to anaesthesia is no less than that of the hypoxia response (Figure 20.7).

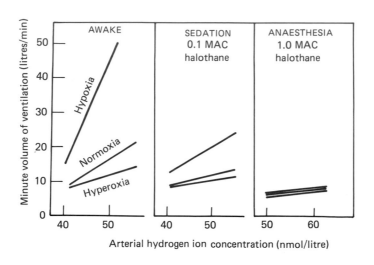

Figure 20.7 Effect of halothane anaesthesia on the ventilatory response to acidaemia. MAC is the minimal alveolar concentration required for anaesthesia. (Redrawn, with permission, from data of Knill and Clement, 1985)

Response to added resistance

The paragraphs above would lead one to expect that anaesthesia would cause grave impairment of the ability of a patient to increase his work of breathing in the face of added resistance. Surprisingly, this is not the case and anaesthetized patients preserve a remarkable ability to overcome added resistance (Nunn and Ezi-Ashi, 1961). The anaesthetized patient responds to inspiratory loading in two phases. Firstly, there is an instant augmentation of the force of contraction of the inspiratory muscles, mainly the diaphragm, during the first loaded breath (Muller et al., 1979). This has the appearance of a typical spindle reflex, and the same authors have reported the existence of spindles in the human diaphragm. The second response is much slower and overshoots when the loading is removed (Nunn and Ezi-Ashi, 1961). The time course suggests that this is mediated by an increase in P_{CO_2}. In combination, these two mechanisms enable the anaesthetized patient to achieve good compensation with inspiratory loading up to about 0.8 kPa (8 cmH$_2$O). Moote, Knill and Clement (1986) have confirmed the ability of the anaesthetized patient to compensate for respiratory loading. Even more remarkable is the preservation of the elaborate response to expiratory resistance (see Figure 4.14).

Anaesthetics and pulmonary stretch receptors

It has been shown in cats that the common inhalational anaesthetics, particularly trichloroethylene, sensitize the pulmonary stretch receptors and so would be expected to cause an enhancement of the inflation reflex (Whitteridge and Bulbring, 1944). This is in contrast to Head's conclusion (1889) that ether and chloroform paralysed vagal endings. Whitteridge and Bulbring concluded that the sensitization of the stretch receptor was largely responsible for the shallow breathing seen in trichloroethylene anaesthesia, but observed that trichloro-ethylene and cyclopropane could have opposite effects on respiratory rate while both agents were causing sensitization of stretch receptors. They further stated that these agents 'must exert another action on a second set of pulmonary endings, or on the respiratory centre, or on extrapulmonary endings'. Ngai, Katz and Farhi (1965) showed that, in midcollicular decerebrate cats, the marked tachypnoea produced by trichloroethylene was not prevented by bilateral vagotomy and carotid denerva-tion. It would therefore seem that there is no solid foundation for the oft repeated view that trichloroethylene causes tachypnoea as a result of sensitization of the pulmonary stretch receptors.

Change in functional residual capacity
(see reviews by Froese, 1985; Rehder, 1985; Wahba, 1991)

Bergman (1963) was the first to report a decrease of functional residual capacity (FRC) during anaesthesia. This was followed by many studies which have established the following characteristics of the change.

1. FRC is reduced during anaesthesia with all anaesthetic drugs which have been investigated, by a mean value of about 16–20% of the FRC (in the supine position). However, there is considerable individual variation and changes range from about +19% to −50%.
2. FRC does not seem to fall progressively during anaesthesia and appears to reach its final value within the first few minutes of anaesthesia. It does not return to normal until some hours after the end of anaesthesia.
3. Inhalation of high concentrations of oxygen does not appear to be a factor in the change and does not usually result in progressive changes.
4. FRC is reduced to the same extent during anaesthesia whether the patient is paralysed or not (Table 20.1).
5. Expiratory muscle activity has no significant effect on the change in FRC.
6. The reduction in FRC has a weak but significant correlation with the age of the patient.
7. Artificial ventilation of the conscious subject causes only a small reduction in FRC.
8. Anaesthesia does not change FRC in the sitting position.
(References: Don et al., 1970; Rehder et al., 1971; Don, Wahba and Craig, 1972; Hewlett et al., 1974b, c; Rehder and Marsh, 1987.)

The cause of the reduction in FRC

This is still not entirely clear. There is agreement that there is a reduction in the cross-sectional area of the rib cage corresponding to a decrease in lung volume of

Table 20.1 Values for functional residual capacity

Conscious subjects

Seated	3.0 litres	(normalized for body height of 170 cm; mean of normal values from Cotes, 1975, and Bates, Macklem and Christie, 1971)
Supine mean	2.2 litres	(mean of 125 values in volunteers and patients prior to
s.d.	0.64 litre	surgery, reported in studies cited in this chapter)

Anaesthetized patients (supine) mean percentage reductions in FRC following induction of anaesthesia

Spontaneous breathing	31.4%	(Don et al., 1970)
	19.0%	(Don, Wahba and Craig, 1972)
	23.3%*	(Westbrook et al., 1973)
	12.6%	(Hickey et al., 1973)
	16.1%	(Hewlett et al., 1974b)
Mean	20.5%	
Artificial ventilation	9.0%	(Laws, 1968)
	14.0%*	(Rehder et al., 1971)
	25.0%*	(Westbrook et al., 1973)
	15.4%	(Hewlett et al., 1974c)
	17.0%	(Hedenstierna et al., 1985b)
	22.0%†	(Bickler, Dueck and Prutow, 1987)
	20.0%*	(Krayer et al., 1987)
Mean	17.5%	

*These studies were of healthy volunteers and not patients.
†These patients had tracheal intubation. There was no significant change in patients who were not intubated.

about 200 ml (Hedenstierna et al., 1985; Krayer et al., 1987; Gunnarsson et al., 1991). Following induction of anaesthesia and paralysis in the supine position, there is a small decrease in the anteroposterior and a small increase in the lateral diameter of the chest wall (Vellody et al., 1978). Earlier in this chapter, we have outlined the substantial measure of disagreement on whether or not anaesthesia causes cephalad movement of the diaphragm. There is also no agreement on whether anaesthesia causes movement of blood into or out of the chest (Hedenstierna et al., 1985; Krayer et al., 1987). Drummond et al. (1988) found no change in distribution of blood volume in relation to anaesthesia. Bickler, Dueck and Prutow (1987) have made the novel observation that reduction in FRC occurs only when a tracheal tube has been inserted, possibly due to increased trapping of gas behind airways constricted in response to the stimulus of the tracheal tube.

In summary, it appears that loss of tone in some of the inspiratory muscles must be the main factor (Wahba, 1991). Possible additional mechanisms include gas trapping behind closed airways, shift of blood volume and the effect of tracheal intubation. Increased elastic recoil of the lungs seems an unlikely cause.

The effect of reduction in FRC on airway closure

In the supine position, the expiratory reserve volume has a mean value of only 1 litre in males and 600 ml in females (Whitfield, Waterhouse and Arnott, 1950). Therefore, the reduction in FRC following the induction of anaesthesia will bring the lung volume close to residual volume. This will tend to reduce the end-expiratory lung volume below the closing capacity (CC), particularly in older patients (see Figure 3.13), and so result in airway closure, collapse of lung and shunting. Pulmonary collapse can easily be demonstrated in conscious subjects who voluntarily breathe oxygen close to residual volume (Nunn et al., 1965b, 1978), and Figure 20.8 shows the effect on arterial PO_2 of simulating the reduction in lung volume which occurs during anaesthesia. 'Miliary atelectasis' was put forward by Bendixen, Hedley-Whyte and Laver (1963) as an explanation of the increased alveolar/arterial PO_2 difference during anaesthesia. Conventional radiography, however, failed to show any appreciable areas of collapse, except in the dependent lung in the lateral position (Potgieter, 1959).

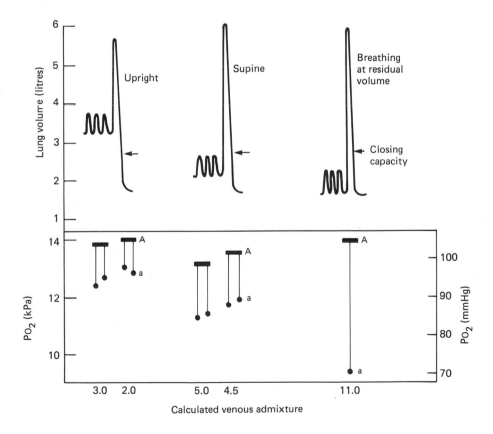

Figure 20.8 Changes in tidal excursion relative to vital capacity in the author when aged 45: arrows indicate the closing capacity. Ideal alveolar (A) PO_2 is shown by the horizontal bar and arterial (a) PO_2 by the black circles. Venous admixture was calculated on the assumption of an arterial/mixed venous oxygen content difference of 5 ml/100 ml. (Reproduced from Nunn (1978) by permission of the Editors of Acta Anaesthesiologica Scandinavica*)*

A brilliant series of investigations from Hedenstierna's laboratory (see review by Hedenstierna, 1990) used computed tomography to show that anaesthesia caused what they termed 'compression atelectasis' in dependent lung areas (Figure 20.9). For technical reasons, it would be extremely difficult to define these areas with conventional radiography. The opacities disappeared during the application of positive end-expiratory pressure (Brismar et al., 1985), and their extent correlated very strongly with the calculated intrapulmonary shunt (Tokics et al., 1987; Gunnarsson et al., 1991). Areas of opacity showed typical histological appearance of total collapse with only moderate vascular congestion and no clear interstitial oedema (Hedenstierna et al., 1989). There can be little doubt that this was the explanation of much of the intrapulmonary shunt, demonstrated 20 years previously. It also vindicated Bendixen, Hedley-Whyte and Laver (1963) to the extent that there was indeed atelectasis during anaesthesia, even though it was not 'miliary' as these workers had suggested.

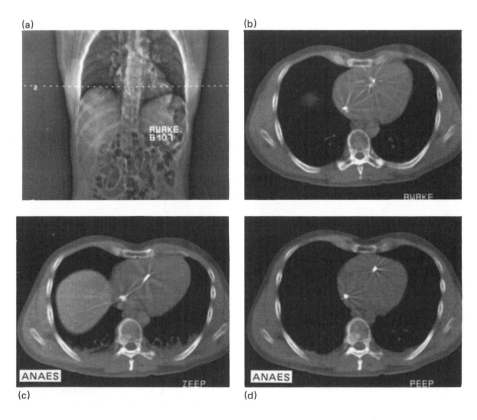

Figure 20.9 Computed tomography of transverse sections of the thoracic cage (supine position) at the level shown in the scout view (a). (b) The control awake view. (c) Anaesthesia with zero end-expiratory pressure (ZEEP). Note the development of opacities in the dependent parts of the lung and the ascent of the right dome of the diaphragm. (d) The same patient with positive end-expiratory pressure (PEEP), which causes the opacities to disappear. This is patient no. 6 from the study of Hedenstierna et al. (1986), where further details are given. (The transverse scans while awake and anaesthetized (ZEEP) are reproduced with the permission of the authors and the Editors and publishers of Acta Anaesthesiologica Scandinavica. *I am indebted to the authors for supplying the other two scans)*

An important aspect of this problem is whether CC remains constant during anaesthesia or whether it changes with FRC. Earlier studies suggested that CC remained constant (Hedenstierna, McCarthy and Bergstrom, 1976). However, Juno et al. (1978) provided convincing evidence that FRC and CC are both reduced during anaesthesia. Bergman and Tien (1983) obtained very similar results and concluded that CC had decreased in parallel with FRC following the induction of anaesthesia. It is possible that bronchodilatation caused by the anaesthetic counteracts the reduction in airway calibre which would be expected to result from the reduction in FRC (see below). The results of the last two studies suggest that there should be no increased tendency towards airway closure during anaesthesia, but this is clearly at variance with Hedenstierna's studies.

Respiratory mechanics
(see review by Milic-Emili, Robatto and Bates, 1990)

Calibre of the lower airways
(see review by Hirshman and Bergman, 1990)

Effect of reduced FRC. Figure 20.10 shows the hyperbolic relationship between lung volume and airway resistance. This is due to the fact that the airways participate in the overall change in lung volume and, other things being equal, as the lung volume decreases, the airway calibre is reduced and the airway resistance increased. Figure 20.10 clearly shows that the curve is steep in the region of FRC in the supine position and therefore the reduction in FRC which occurs during anaesthesia might be expected to result in a marked increase in airway resistance. However, most anaesthetics are bronchodilators as outlined in the following paragraphs and, at least with halothane, this effect almost exactly offsets the effect of reduction in lung volume (Joyner, Warner and Rehder, 1992). Airway resistance during anaesthesia (below the carina) is normally not greatly different from that of the whole respiratory tract with the subject awake and supine (Table 20.2, Figure 20.10). D'Angelo et al. (1991) clearly showed resistance to increase with increasing flow rate and to decrease with increasing inflation volume as would be expected. They also found that the resistance to *flow* due to the chest wall was negligible.

Table 20.2 Pulmonary resistance studies in healthy anaesthetized patients

	$kPa\ l^{-1}\ s^{-1}$	$cmH_2O/l/sec$
Newman, Campbell and Dinnick (1959)	0.05–0.3	0.5–3.0
Bodman (1963)*	0.12–0.32	1.2–3.2
Bergman (1966)	0.55–0.60	5.5–6.0
Bergman (1969)* at 1.5 l/s	0.50–0.57	5.0–5.7
at 1.0 l/s	0.44–0.49	4.4–4.9
at 0.5 l/s	0.36–0.39	3.6–3.9
Hedenstierna and McCarthy (1975)	0.4–0.6	4.0–6.0
Bergman and Waltemath (1974)	0.4–0.6	4.0–6.0

Values exclude apparatus resistance.
  *These series also report patients with physical and radiographic evidence of pulmonary disease, who showed much greater levels of resistance.

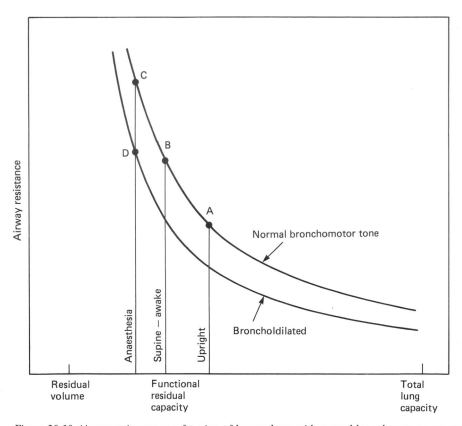

Figure 20.10 Airway resistance as a function of lung volume with normal bronchomotor tone and when bronchodilated. A = upright and awake; B = supine and awake; C = supine and anaesthetized without bronchodilatation; D = supine, anaesthetized and with the degree of bronchodilatation which normally occurs during anaesthesia. Note that the airway resistance is similar at B and D bronchodilatation approximately compensating for the decrease in FRC.

Inhalational anaesthetics. All inhalational anaesthetics investigated have shown bronchodilator effects. Suppression of airway vagal reflexes, direct relaxation of airway smooth muscle and inhibition of release of bronchoconstrictor mediators combine to cause an increase in specific airway conductance (Lehane, Jordan and Jones, 1980; Heneghan et al., 1986). In clinical concentrations, halothane reduces the amount of acetylcholine released from nerve terminals in response to nerve stimulation (Korenaga, Takeda and Ito, 1984), and suppresses the increase in both airway and tissue resistance following vagal stimulation (Joyner, Warner and Redher, 1992). This appears to be more important than the direct effect of clinical concentrations of halothaane on airway smooth muscle or histamine release from mast cells (Hirshman and Bergman, 1990). Diethyl ether has been used in the treatment of status asthmaticus.

Barbiturates. Deep barbiturate anaesthesia has generally similar effects to the inhalational anaesthetics. However, there are many older reports of bronchospasm occurring in relation to the use of thiopentone, although others have found no such association (Hirshman and Bergman, 1990). Undoubtedly some instances were reflex bronchospasm due to stimuli such as the presence of a tracheal tube, with barbiturate levels too low to provide adequate protection.

Ketamine. The bronchodilator effects of ketamine appear to be largely due to catecholamine release and stimulation of β_2 receptors on airway smooth muscle (Hirshman et al., 1979).

Neuromuscular blockers. Tubocurarine and atracurium may cause histamine release, but there is usually no change in airway resistance in patients with normal lungs (Gerbershagen and Bergman, 1967). Due to chemical similarity to acetyl-choline, neuromuscular blockers interact with cholinesterases and, in common with cholinesterase inhibitors, potentiate the action of acetylchloline. However, as a general rule, it is only patients with hypersensitive airways in whom neuromuscular blocking drugs have any detectable effect on calibre of the lower airways.

Other sites of increased airway resistance

Breathing circuits. Excessive resistance or obstruction may arise in apparatus such as breathing circuits, valves, connectors and tracheal tubes. The tubes may be kinked, the lumen may be blocked or the cuff may herniate and obstruct the lower end, which may also abut against the carina or the side wall of the trachea. A reduction in diameter of a tracheal tube greatly increases its resistance, the pattern of flow being intermediate between laminar and turbulent for the conditions shown in Figure 20.11.

The pharynx and larynx. The pharynx is commonly obstructed during anaesthesia by the mechanisms described earlier in this chapter, unless active steps are taken to preserve patency. Reflex laryngospasm is still possible at depths of anaesthesia which suppress other airway protective reflexes. The resulting obstruction is usually total and may be life threatening. In most cases the spasm eventually resolves spontaneously, but is most reliably terminated by neuromuscular blockade.

Compliance
(see review by Rehder, Sessler and Marsh, 1975)

*Values for compliance during anaesthesia.*The reduction in total respiratory comp-liance during anaesthesia has been known for many years and Table 20.3 lists consensus values based on the review of Rehder, Sessler and Marsh (1975). Similar values were obtained for the lung by D'Angelo et al. (1991), while their values for chest wall averaged 1.3 l/kPa (130 ml/cmH$_2$O) for dynamic compliance and 1.6 l/kPa (160 ml/cmH$_2$O) for static. They analysed the effects of different inspiratory flow rates and volumes in terms of the spring and dashpot model (see Figure 4.6). Compliance appears to be reduced very early in anaesthesia and the change is not progressive.

Figure 20.12, based on the work of Westbrook et al. (1973) and Butler and Smith (1957), summarizes the effect of anaesthesia on the pressure/volume relationships of the lung and chest wall. The diagram shows the major differences between the conscious state and anaesthesia. There are only minor differences between anaesthesia with and without paralysis. The left-hand section shows the relation-

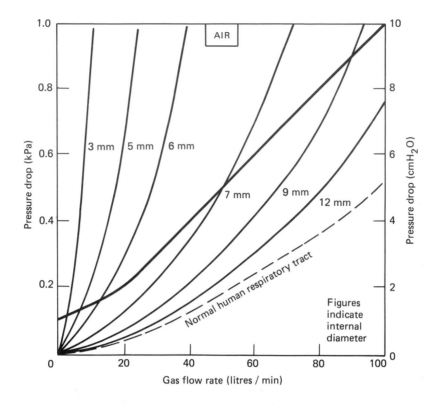

Figure 20.11 Flow rate/pressure drop plots of a range of tracheal tubes, with their connectors and catheter mounts. The heavy line is the author's suggested upper limit of acceptable resistance for an adult. Pressure drop does not quite increase according to the fourth power of the diameter (inverse) because the catheter mount offered the same resistance throughout the range of tubes. With 70% N_2O/30% O_2, the pressure drop is about 40% greater for the same gas flow rate when flow is turbulent, but little different when the flow is chiefly laminar

Table 20.3 Values for compliance in anaesthetized and paralysed subjects

		l/kPa	ml/cmH$_2$O
Lungs	static	1.5	150
	dynamic	1.0	100
Chest wall		2.0	200
Total compliance	static	0.85	85
	dynamic	0.6	60

These values represent a reasonable mean from a large number of studies in anaesthetized patients reviewed by Rehder, Sessler and Marsh (1975).

ship for the whole respiratory system comprising lungs plus chest wall. The curves obtained during anaesthesia clearly show the reduction in FRC (lung volume with zero pressure gradient from alveoli to ambient). The subatmospheric section of the curve also shows the very small volume change which can be achieved by

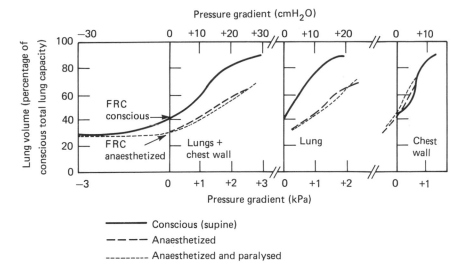

Figure 20.12 Pressure/volume relationships in supine volunteers before and after the induction of anaesthesia and paralysis. The first section shows the relationship for lungs plus chest wall where the relevant pressure gradient is alveolar minus ambient. The second section represents lungs alone where the pressure gradient is alveolar minus intrathoracic (transmural). The third section relates to chest wall alone for which the pressure gradient is intrathoracic minus ambient. There are only insignificant differences between observations during anaesthesia with and without paralysis. There are, however, major differences in pressure/volume relationships of the lung and whole system following the induction of anaesthesia. Arrows indicate the FRC which, during anaesthesia, is only slightly greater than residual volume. (Redrawn from the data of Westbrook et al. (1973), except that the subatmospheric extensions of the curves for the lungs plus chest wall have been derived from other sources)

application of a subatmospheric pressure to the airway of an anaesthetized patient. This implies a very low expiratory reserve volume. Application of a positive pressure as high as 3 kPa (30 cmH$_2$O) to the airways expands the lungs to barely 70% of the preoperative total lung capacity, which implies a reduced overall compliance. The two sections of Figure 20.12 on the right show that the major changes are in the lung rather than the chest wall.

Cause of the reduced compliance. The change appears to be mainly due to a reduction in pulmonary compliance, the cause of which has been difficult to explain. There is no general agreement on a direct effect of anaesthetics on the pulmonary surfactant. The study of Pattle, Schock and Battensby (1972) suggested that anaesthesia does not alter pulmonary compliance although Forrest (1972) demonstrated decreased surfactant activity in the lung of the hyperventilated guinea-pig. Woo, Berlin and Hedley-Whyte (1969) showed that ventilation of excised dogs' lungs with air containing 1.2% halothane produced small but significant decreases of compliance. They showed that no such changes occurred when the lungs were filled with liquid, and concluded that the anaesthetic might have altered surfactant function. Stanley, Zikria and Sullivan (1972) found that halothane and cyclopropane increased the minimal surface tension of tracheobronchial aspirations from a series of patients. None of this evidence is entirely convincing.

An alternative explanation is that the reduced lung compliance is simply the consequence of breathing at reduced lung volume (Schmidt and Rehder, 1981). Caro, Butler and DuBois (1960) and also Scheidt, Hyatt and Rehder (1981) strapped the chest of volunteers, thereby decreasing their lung volume, and found that this resulted in a decrease in pulmonary compliance which could be restored to normal by taking a maximal inspiration. This suggests that partial pulmonary atelectasis was the explanation, and the unequivocal demonstration of compression atelectasis during anaesthesia by Hedenstierna's group (see above) makes this the most likely cause of the reduced compliance.

Metabolic rate

During anaesthesia, the metabolic rate is reduced to about 15% below basal according to the conventional standards of Aub and DuBois (1917) and Boothby and Sandiford (1924). However, these standards do not stipulate sedation or any period of rest. Robertson and Reid proposed new standards for metabolic rate in 1952, based on 3 hours' rest, with or without sedation. Their values are about 15% below the conventional standards and so correspond fairly closely to those of the anaesthetized patient (Nunn and Matthews, 1959). Table 20.4 lists expected values for oxygen consumption and carbon dioxide output during uncomplicated

Table 20.4 Predicted values for oxygen consumption and carbon dioxide output during uncomplicated anaesthesia (ml/min) (STPD)

Age	Oxygen consumption			Carbon dioxide		
	Small patient	Average patient	Large patient	Small patient	Average patient	Large patient
Male						
14–15		190			152	
16–17		200			160	
18–19	168	210	252	134	168	202
20–29	162	203	243	130	162	194
30–39	162	203	243	130	162	194
40–49	158	198	237	126	158	190
50–59	155	194	233	124	155	186
60–69	150	187	224	120	159	179
Female						
14–15		174			139	
16–17		188			150	
18–19	156	194	233	125	155	186
20–29	152	190	228	122	152	182
30–39	150	187	224	120	150	179
40–49	148	184	221	118	147	177
50–59	144	180	216	115	144	173
60–69	140	175	210	112	140	168

Values for CO_2 output will apply only in a steady respiratory state.
Values are probably about 6% lower during artificial ventilation.
Figures are based on 85% of basal according to data of Aub and Dubois (1917) and Boothby and Sandiford (1924).

anaesthesia at normal body temperature (mean 36.5°C). In comparison with the conscious subject there are major reductions in cerebral and cardiac oxygen consumptions during anaesthesia.

Gas exchange

Almost every factor influencing gas exchange may be altered during anaesthesia. One fortunate exception is the oxyhaemoglobin dissociation curve which, despite early fears to the contrary, is now known to be substantially unchanged by the binding of anaesthetics to haemoglobin (page 278). However, there are many changes in respiratory function which can be considered as normal features of the anaesthetized state. These 'normal' changes usually pose no threat to the patient, since their effects can easily be overcome by such simple means as increasing the concentration of oxygen in the inspired gas and the minute volume. The 'normal' changes may be contrasted with a range of pathological alterations in gas exchange which may arisee during anaesthesia from such circumstances as tension pneumothorax or apnoea. These may be life threatening and require urgent action for their correction.

The major changes which adversely affect gas exchange during anaesthesia are reduced minute volume of ventilation, increased dead space and shunt (considered in terms of the three-compartment model) and altered distribution of ventilation and perfusion in relation to ventilation/perfusion ratios.

Minute volume of ventilation

Preserved spontaneous breathing. During anaesthesia with spontaneous breathing, the minute volume may remain normal but it is usually decreased. This is due partly to the reduction in metabolic demand but mainly to the interference with chemical control of breathing as described earlier in this chapter. In an uncomplicated anaesthetic, there should not be sufficient resistance to breathing to affect the minute volume. However, the minute volume may be much decreased if there is overt respiratory obstruction (see above).

Spontaneous minute volume may decrease to very low levels, particularly in the absence of surgical stimulation. Thus, for example, Nunn (1964) reported 3 patients out of 27 with a minute volume of less than 3 l/min. This will inevitably result in hypercapnia which, in the various studies of the author, has ranged up to 10 kPa (75 mmHg). Clearly there is no limit to the rise which may occur if the anaesthetist is prepared to tolerate gross hypoventilation, and Birt and Cole (1965) reported arterial P_{CO_2} values up to 20 kPa (150 mmHg) during closed-circuit halothane anaesthesia (not administered by the authors!).

There are anaesthetists in many parts of the world, including the UK, who do not believe that temporary hypercapnia during anaesthesia is harmful to a healthy patient. Under normal circumstances, arterial P_{CO_2} rapidly returns to normal in the postoperative period (Nunn and Payne, 1962). Many hundreds of millions of patients must have been subjected to this transient physiological trespass since 1846 and there seems to be no convincing evidence of harm resulting from it, except perhaps increased bleeding from the incision. In other parts of the world, particularly the USA, the departure from physiological normality is regarded with concern and it is usual either to assist spontaneous respiration by manual compression of the reservoir bag or, more commonly, to paralyse and ventilate artificially as a routine.

Artificial ventilation. Quite different conditions apply during anaesthesia with artificial ventilation. The minute volume can then be set at any level which seems appropriate to the anaesthetist. Values up to 17.5 l/min were recorded during unmonitored routine anaesthesia with manual ventilation (Nunn, 1958a). Hypocapnia almost invariably results from unmonitored artificial ventilation during anaesthesia, observed values for PCO_2 extending from the normal range down to about 2.4 kPa (18 mmHg). Without measurement of PCO_2, there is a natural tendency to hyperventilate the patient. Again it has proved difficult to demonstrate that hypocapnia does any significant harm during anaesthesia, but most anaesthetists now tend to avoid extreme hypocapnia because of its effects on cerebral blood flow (page 519). There is some consensus that one should aim for an arterial PCO_2 of about 4.5 kPa (34 mmHg). Hypothermia, either intentional or accidental, may result in severe hypocapnia unless the minute volume is reduced in accord with the reduced metabolic rate.

Monitoring end-expiratory PCO_2 has radically altered the control of minute volume during anaesthesia. In the case of preserved spontaneous breathing, the anaesthetist can ensure that hypoventilation does not allow the PCO_2 to exceed the limit which he considers appropriate. Artificial ventilation, on the other hand, can very easily be adjusted to maintain the target PCO_2 selected by the anaesthetist. This is more satisfactory than monitoring ventilatory volumes since the patient's metabolic rate and dead space are not usually known.

The three-compartment model of gas exchange

This model has been described on pages 167 et seq. In essence it presents the lung as though it comprised three compartments – ideally perfused and ventilated alveoli, alveolar dead space and shunt. Physiological (= anatomical + alveolar) dead space is quantified by the Bohr equation (page 171) and shunt by the shunt equation (page 179), with or without direct measurement of the mixed venous oxygen content. It is obviously not a true representation of the lung during anaesthesia but, *as a model*, it has the following very cogent advantages:

1. The model is simple to understand.
2. It is a valid model to explain changes in arterial PCO_2 and PO_2 during anaesthesia with inspired oxygen concentrations in the range 30–100%.
3. The parameters of dysfunction (dead space and shunt) can be measured with facilities available in most hospitals.
4. These parameters offer clear quantitative guidance for optimizing minute volume of ventilation and inspired oxygen concentration.

Physiological dead space
(see page 176)

The increase in physiological dead space during anaesthesia was first observed by Campbell, Nunn and Peckett in 1958 and subsequently confirmed in many studies. With allowance for the apparatus dead space of the tracheal tube and its connections, the dead space/tidal volume ratio *from carina downwards* averages 32 per cent during anaesthesia with either spontaneous or artificial ventilation (Nunn and Hill, 1960). This is approximately equal to the ratio for the normal conscious subject *including trachea, pharynx and mouth* (approximately 70 ml) (Nunn, Campbell and Peckett, 1959). Physiological dead space equals the sum of its anatomical and alveolar components, and the subcarinal anatomical dead space is not normally increased. Therefore, the increase in subcarinal physiological dead space during anaesthesia must be in the alveolar component (Nunn and Hill, 1960). There is no measurable difference between physiological and anatomical dead space in the normal conscious subject and therefore the alveolar dead space is negligible.

Anatomical dead space. In the study of Nunn and Hill (Figure 20.13), subcarinal anatomical dead space was always significantly less than physiological, reaching a maximum of about 70 ml at tidal volumes above 350 ml. This roughly accords with the expected geometric dimensions of the lower respiratory tract. At smaller tidal volumes, the anatomical dead space was less than the expected geometric volume. Values of less than 30 ml were recorded in some patients with a tidal volume less than 250 ml. This is attributed to axial streaming and the mixing effect of the heart beat (page 174), and is clearly an important and beneficial factor in patients with depressed breathing.

Alveolar dead space increases with tidal volume so that the sum of anatomical and alveolar (= physiological) dead space remains about 32% of tidal volume (Figure 20.13). The cause of the increase in alveolar dead space during anaesthesia is not

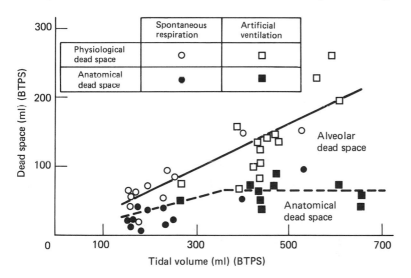

Figure 20.13 Data and regression lines for physiological and anatomical dead space (the difference indicating alveolar dead space) as a function of tidal volume. There were no significant differences between anaesthesia with and without paralysis. Note the range over which physiological dead space appeared to be a constant fraction of tidal volume. Anatomical dead space was constant above a tidal volume of 350 ml. At smaller tidal volumes it was reduced for reasons which are discussed in the text. (Modified from Nunn and Hill (1960) by permission of the Editor and publishers of the Journal of Applied Physiology)

immediately obvious. There is no evidence that it is due to pulmonary hypotension causing development of a zone 1 (page 149) and the reduced vertical height of the lung in the supine position would militate against this. The alternative explanation is maldistribution with overventilation of *relatively* underperfused alveoli. Studies of ventilation/perfusion relationships (see below) give some support to this view, but such patterns of maldistribution have not invariably been observed during anaesthesia.

Apparatus dead space. For practical purposes the apparatus dead space of the tracheal tube and its connections must be included for the purpose of calculating alveolar ventilation during anaesthesia. The total dead space then increases to a mean of 50% of tidal volume (Figure 20.14). If the trachea is not intubated, it is necessary to add the volume of the facemask and its connections to the physiological dead space, which now includes trachea, pharynx and mouth. The total dead space then amounts to about two-thirds of the tidal volume (Kain, Panday and Nunn, 1969). Thus, a seemingly adequate minute volume of 6 l/min, may be expected to result in an alveolar ventilation of only 2 l/min, which would almost inevitably result in hypercapnia.

Compensation for increased dead space may be made by increasing the minute volume to maintain the alveolar ventilation. In practice, the problem hardly exists. The artificially ventilated anaesthetized patient may have a large dead space, but the high minute volumes commonly selected usually provide more than adequate

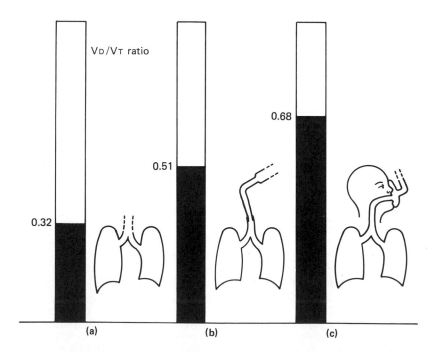

Figure 20.14 Physiological plus apparatus dead space (where applicable) as a fraction of tidal volume in anaesthetized patients: (a) from carina downwards; (b) including tracheal tube and connector; and (c) including upper airway, facemask and connector.

compensation. Thus the alveolar ventilation is almost always greater than necessary for carbon dioxide homoeostasis. With monitoring of end-expiratory PCO_2, there is very seldom any difficulty in maintaining a value in the range 4–5 kPa (30–37.5 mmHg). However, the existence of an alveolar dead space means that the arterial PCO_2 during anaesthesia is usually 0.5–1 kPa (3.8–7.5 mmHg) greater than the end-expiratory PCO_2. In the case of the hypoventilating patient who is allowed to breathe spontaneously during anaesthesia, the reduction in dead space shown in Figure 20.13 prevents some of the alveolar hypoventilation which would be expected if the *volume* of the dead space remained constant. This, together with the reduced metabolic rate, results in the hypercapnia being much less than the values for minute volume sometimes observed during anaesthesia might lead one to expect. No doubt, over the years, many patients have owed their lives to these factors.

Shunt

Magnitude of the change during anaesthesia. In the conscious healthy subject, the shunt or venous admixture amounts to only 1–2% of cardiac output (page 178) and this results in an alveolar/arterial PO_2 gradient of less than 1 kPa (7.5 mmHg) in the young healthy subject breathing air, but the gradient increases with age. During anaesthesia, the alveolar/arterial PO_2 difference is usually increased to a value which corresponds to an average shunt of about 10%. Figure 20.15 shows the mean values for shunt, taken from a large number of different studies, plotted on the iso-shunt diagram which is explained in detail on page 183. Throughout the range of inspired oxygen concentrations, the means for the studies are grouped along the 10% shunt line. Formal measurements of pulmonary venous admixture, taking into account the mixed venous oxygen content, have also been made (Table 20.5) and these concur with shunts being of the order of 10%. This provides an acceptable basis for predicting arterial PO_2 during an uncomplicated anaesthetic and it also permits calculation of the concentration of oxygen in the inspired gas which will provide an acceptable arterial PO_2. Some 30–40% inspired oxygen is usually adequate in an uncomplicated anaesthetic.

The cause of the venous admixture during anaesthesia was long debated but it is now clear that about half is true shunt through the areas of compression atelectasis described above (see Figure 20.9). There is a very strong correlation between the shunt (measured as perfusion of alveoli with a ventilation/perfusion ($\dot{V}/\dot{Q}$) ratio of less than 0.005) and the area of atelectasis (Gunnarsson et al., 1991). However, the venous admixture during anaesthesia also contains components due to dispersion of the $\dot{V}/\dot{Q}$ distribution, and to perfusion of alveoli with low $\dot{V}/\dot{Q}$ ratios (0.005–0.1). The effect of all of these changes would be enhanced by the effect of anaesthetics on the pulmonary hypoxic vasoconstrictor reflex (see below). The effect of age is complex and is considered below.

Effect of positive end-expiratory pressure (PEEP). It has long been known that, in contrast to the situation in intensive care, PEEP does little to improve the arterial PO_2 during anaesthesia (Nunn, Bergman and Coleman, 1965). The work of Colgan, Barrow and Fanning (1971) in dogs suggested that, although the shunt might be reduced, the associated decrease in the cardiac output reduced the saturation of the

Table 20.5 Values for pulmonary venous admixture measured during anaesthesia in man, by solution of the shunt equation (Figure 8.9) with sampling of mixed venous blood

Reference	Circumstances	FI_{O_2} (%)	$\dot{Q}s/\dot{Q}t$ (%)
Michenfelder, Fowler and Theye (1966)	{ Artificial ventilation { Inhalational anaesthesia	{ 40* { 100*	10.2 13.7
Price et al. (1969)	{ Conscious controls { before anaesthesia	{ 25 { 100	5.9 3.1
	{ Halothane anaesthesia { spontaneous respiration	{ 25 { 98.5	18.9 6.1
	{ Halothane anaesthesia { artificial ventilation	{ 25 { 98.5	15.1 11.1
	{ Conscious controls { before anaesthesia	{ 25 { 80	2.5 2.0
	{ Cyclopropane anaesthesia { (spont. and artif. vent.)	{ 25 { 80	11.3 7.9
	{ Halothane + N_2O anaesth. { (spont. and artif. vent.)	28	10.0
Marshall et al. (1969)	{ Conscious controls { before anaesthesia	100	4.4

	Halothane anaesthesia:
	  30 minutes after induction
	  $3\frac{1}{2}$ hours after induction
	  30 minutes after anaesthesia
	  3 hours after anaesthesia
		100*
		100*
		100
		100
			12.1
			14.8
			6.5
			5.2

Gunnarsson et al. (1991)	Conscious controls before anaesthesia Anaesthesia with paralysis	21 40	5.5 9.2

See also Bindslev et al. (1981) in Table 20.6

*These values were slightly reduced by the addition of unspecified concentrations of halothane or other inhalational anaesthetics.

blood traversing the remaining shunt and so the arterial P_{O_2} was unaltered. This was in fact demonstrated by Bindslev and his colleagues (1981) in anaesthetized man (see below). The essential difference from the patient undergoing intensive care is probably the lack of protection of intrathoracic blood vessels from raised airway pressure which is afforded by stiff lungs in most patients requiring intenssive care.

Ventilation/perfusion ($\dot{V}/\dot{Q}$) relationships

The three-compartment model of the lung provides a definition of lung function in terms of dead space and shunt, parameters which are easily measured, reproducible and provide a basis for corrective therapy. Nevertheless, it does not pretend to provide a true picture of what is going on in the lung.

A far more sophisticated approach is provided by the analysis of the distribution of pulmonary ventilation and perfusion in terms of $\dot{V}/\dot{Q}$ ratios by the multiple inert gas elimination technique, a complex and challenging technique outlined on pages 194 et seq. Studies have been undertaken in young fit subjects (Rehder et al., 1979), typical surgical patients (Bindslev et al., 1981) and elderly patients with respiratory pathology (Dueck et al., 1980). In addition, Prutow et al. (1982) have presented a study of young surgical patients in abstract. More recently Gunnarsson

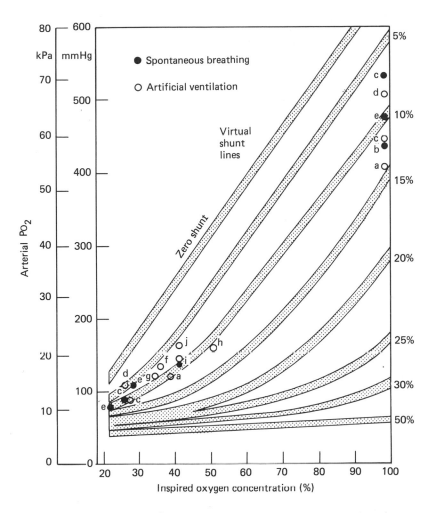

Figure 20.15 Mean values for arterial Po$_2$ are plotted against inspired oxygen concentrations for 18 published studies of anaesthetized patients, using the same co-ordinates as in Figure 8.10. (a) Michenfelder, Fowler and Theye, 1966; (b) Marshall et al., 1969; (c) Price et al., 1969; (d) Nunn, Bergman and Coleman, 1965; (e) Nunn, 1964; (f) Hewlett et al., 1974c; (g) Theye and Tuohy, 1964a; (h) Gold and Helrich, 1967; (i) Bindslev et al., 1981; (j) Gunnarsson et al., 1991.

et al. (1991) have studied a large series of patients in a systematic investigation of the influence of age.

Rehder's group studied young healthy volunteers, and both ventilation and perfusion were found to be distributed to a wider range of ventilation/perfusion ratios after induction of anaesthesia and paralysis (Figure 20.16). The true intrapulmonary shunt had a mean value of less than 1% during anaesthesia, but the alveolar/arterial Po$_2$ gradient was slightly increased and this was attributed to the increased spread of the distribution of perfusion to areas of poorer ventilation (lower V̇/Q̇ ratio). Anatomical dead space was reduced, largely because of tracheal intubation, but alveolar dead space was increased, partly due to

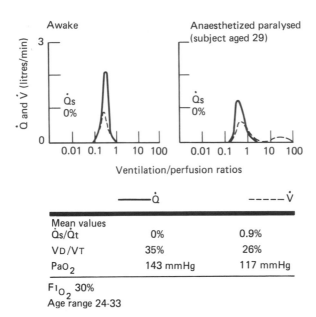

Figure 20.16 Distribution of ventilation and perfusion as a function of ventilation/perfusion ratios in the awake and anaesthetized paralysed subject. (Adapted from Rehder et al. (1979) and reproduced from Nunn (1985a) by permission of the publishers)

increased spread of distribution of ventilation to areas of poorer perfusion (higher $\dot{V}/\dot{Q}$ ratio). In a group of surgical patients of similar age range to Rehder's volunteers, Prutow et al. (1982) found an average increase in shunt of 8% during anaesthesia. Pulmonary blood flow to areas of zero and low $\dot{V}/\dot{Q}$ correlated with the reduction in FRC.

Bindslev's group studied typical surgical patients with ages ranging from 37 to 64. They were studied awake, anaesthetized and breathing spontaneously, anaesthetized paralysed and ventilated artificially and finally with PEEP (Figure 20.17 and Table 20.6). In this group of older patients, they found that the true intrapulmonary shunt was increased during anaesthesia. However, the shunt calculated from the alveolar/arterial PO_2 gradient according to the three-compartment lung model would be larger still, and the difference would be due to perfusion of areas of low $\dot{V}/\dot{Q}$ ratio. The dead space/tidal volume ratio was increased during anaesthesia in spite of the tracheal tube bypassing the upper airway, implying a large increase in subcarinal dead space (see above). Ventilation was distributed to alveoli with mean $\dot{V}/\dot{Q}$ ratio 0.81 before anaesthesia, 1.3 during anaesthesia, 2.2 with IPPV and 3.03 with PEEP. Shunt was halved by PEEP, but cardiac output was also reduced and, therefore, the mixed venous oxygen content. The decreased admixture of more desaturated blood resulted in minimal improvement in arterial PO_2. PEEP also increased ventilation of alveoli with high $\dot{V}/\dot{Q}$ ratio.

Dueck's group studied elderly patients (mean age 60) who all had some deterioration in pulmonary function. Their results can most easily be appreciated by considering the patients in three groups (Figure 20.18). In the first, there was only a small increase in the true shunt following the induction of anaesthesia but there appeared a 'shelf' of perfusion of regions of very low $\dot{V}/\dot{Q}$ ratios in the range

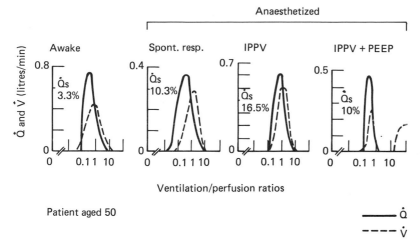

Figure 20.17 Typical changes in distribution of ventilation and perfusion as a function of ventilation/ perfusion ratios during anaesthesia in a middle-aged patient. IPPV, intermittent positive pressure ventilation; PEEP, positive end-expiratory pressure: Q̇, perfusion; V̇, ventilation; Q̇s, shunt. (Adapted from Bindslev et al. (1981) and reproduced from Nunn (1985a) by permission of publishers)

Table 20.6 Changes in factors influencing gas exchange after induction of anaesthesia

	Awake	*Anaesthesia*		
		Spont. vent.	*IPPV*	*IPPV + PEEP*
FI_{O_2}	0.21	0.4	0.4	0.4
$\dot{Q}s/\dot{Q}t$ (%)	1.6	6.2	8.6	4.1
VD/VT (%)	30	35	38	44
Cardiac output (l/min)	6.1	5.0	4.5	3.7
Pa_{O_2} (kPa)	10.5	17.6	18.8	20.5
V̇ − mean V̇/Q̇	0.81	1.30	2.20	3.03
Q̇ − mean V̇/Q̇	0.47	0.51	0.83	0.55

(Adapted from Bindslev et al. (1981) and reproduced from Nunn (1985a) by permission of the publishers)

0.01–0.1. In the second group, this 'shelf' was less prominent but there was a substantial increase in true shunt. Finally, in the third group, there was both a 'shelf' and an increase in true shunt. All of these changes are compatible with a decrease in FRC below closing capacity.

These three studies show striking differences which appear to be attributable to the different ages of the subjects or patients. However, each study was undertaken by a separate group of research workers under different conditions. In contrast, Gunnarsson et al. (1991) studied 45 patients (age range 23–69 years) as part of a single study extending over 2 years. They reached the surprising conclusion that atelectasis (as seen on computed tomography) and true intrapulmonary shunt (determined by multiple inert gas elimination technique as perfusion of alveoli with

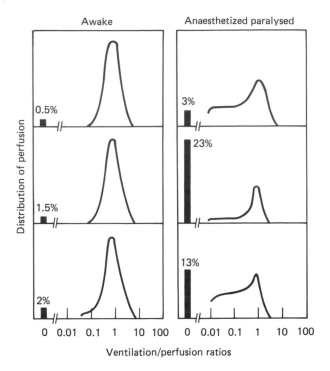

Figure 20.18 Changes in pulmonary perfusion as a function of ventilation/perfusion ratios following induction of anaesthesia in elderly patients. Numbers to the left of each block indicate the shunt. (Adapted from Dueck et al. (1980) and reproduced from Nunn (1985a) by permission of the publishers)

$\dot{V}/\dot{Q}$ ratio less than 0.005) did not relate to age. However, both were substantially increased during anaesthesia and correlated with each other. It is difficult to reconcile the lack of correlation between age and shunt with the striking differences in the studies by Rehder's group and Dueck's group. Nevertheless, Gunnarsson confirmed the enhanced decline in arterial Po_2 with increasing age during anaesthesia, and venous admixture (calculated as for the Riley three-compartment model) was increased significantly from a mean value of 5.5% of cardiac output before anaesthesia, to 9.2% during anaesthesia. Venous admixture increased steeply with age (0.17% per year), and this was attributed to an age-dependent increase in the spread of $\dot{V}/\dot{Q}$ ratios (Figure 20.19) and to greater perfusion of alveoli with low $\dot{V}/\dot{Q}$ ratios (0.005–0.1).

Summary. These studies of $\dot{V}/\dot{Q}$ relationships during anaesthesia complement one another and give us greatly increased insight into the effect of anaesthesia on gas exchange. We are now in a position to summarize the effect of anaesthesia on gas exchange as follows:

1. Uniformity of distribution of ventilation and perfusion is decreased by anaesthesia, and the magnitude of the change is age related.
2. The increase in alveolar dead space appears to be due to increased distribution of ventilation to areas of high (but not usually infinite) $\dot{V}/\dot{Q}$ ratios.

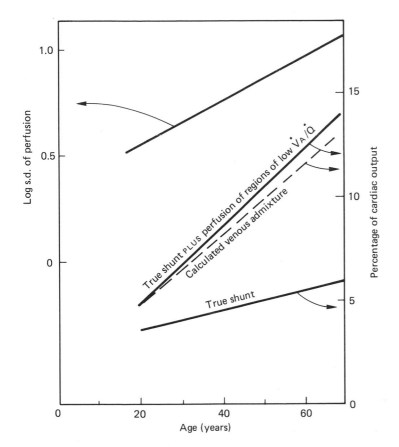

Figure 20.19 Age-dependence of various factors influencing alveolar/arterial Po_2 *difference during anaesthesia (Gunnarsson et al., 1991). The logarithm of standard deviation of distribution of perfusion is significantly greater than before anaesthesia and has a highly significant regression against age in both circumstances. True shunt is significantly increased almost tenfold compared with before anaesthesia, but the correlation with age is not significant. Perfusion of areas of poorly ventilated regions (0.005 < $\dot{V}A/ \dot{Q}$ < 0.1) was significantly increased compared with before anaesthesia and correlated with age in both circumstances. Venous admixture here refers to the value obtained from the shunt equation (see* Figure *8.9) and agrees well with the sum of shunt and perfusion of regions of low* $\dot{V}A/\dot{Q}$.

3. Venous admixture is increased in anaesthesia to a mean value of about 10%, but the change is markedly affected by age, being minimal in the young.
4. The increased venous admixture during anaesthesia is due partly to an increase in true intrapulmonary shunt (due to compression atelectasis), and partly to increased distribution of perfusion to areas of low (but not zero) V/Q ratios. The latter component increases with age.
5. The major differences are between the awake and the anaesthetized states. Paralysis and artificial ventilation do not greatly alter the parameters of gas exchange in spite of the quite different spatial distribution of ventilation.
6. PEEP reduces the shunt but the beneficial effect on arterial Po_2 is offset by the decrease in cardiac output which reduces the mixed venous oxygen content.

Effect on hypoxic pulmonary vasoconstriction

Hypoxia causes an increase in pulmonary vascular resistance (see Chapter 7, pages 145 et seq.). When confined to a single lung or localized areas of lung, hypoxic pulmonary vasoconstriction (HPV) reduces but does not eliminate perfusion through hypoxic areas and thus improves the relative distribution of ventilation and perfusion. This normally increases arterial PO_2. When HPV is abolished by vasodilators, shunting and arterial PO_2 are worsened (Marshall and Marshall, 1985).

Thilenius (1966), working with dogs, suggested that anaesthetics might interfere with HPV. Several inhalational anaesthetics were then found to inhibit HPV in the isolated lungs of both dog and cat (Sykes et al., 1972). These observations were amply confirmed in many laboratories throughout the world, but no such effect was found with intravenous anaesthetics (Bjertnaes, 1977). Further studies in the intact animal followed and were reviewed by Marshall and Marshall (1985), Sykes (1986) and Eisenkraft (1990).

Although *in vitro* studies gave clear evidence that inhalational anaesthetics depressed HPV, *in vivo* studies were inconsistent. Some studies showed that inhalational anaesthetics increased the pulmonary blood flow through hypoxic areas of lung (i.e. blocking of HPV), while others showed no change or even a slight increase. This was resolved by Marshall and Marshall (1985) who analysed a large number of studies and showed that the confusing factor was concomitant depression of cardiac output by inhalational anaesthetics. In Chapter 7 (pages 145 et seq.) it was explained how hypoxia influences pulmonary vascular resistance not only by the alveolar PO_2 but also, in part, by the mixed venous PO_2. A reduction in cardiac output must decrease the mixed venous PO_2 if oxygen consumption remains unchanged, and this would intensify pulmonary vasoconstriction. Thus an inhalational anaesthetic will inhibit HPV by direct action on the one hand while, on the other hand, it may intensify HPV by reducing mixed venous PO_2 as a result of decreasing cardiac output. Marshall and Marshall (1985) showed that most investigators' results are consistent with the view that inhalational anaesthetics depress HPV provided that allowance is made for the effect of concomitant changes of cardiac output.

Quantitative effect of inhalational anaesthetics. Suppression of HPV by inhalational anaesthetics follows a typical sigmoid dose/response curve with an ED_{50} of slightly less than twice the minimal alveolar concentration (MAC) required for anaesthesia, and an ED_{90} of 3 MAC (Marshall, 1988). Thus, during a typical anaesthetic at 1.3 MAC, HPV is attenuated by only about 30%. There are no major differences between the volatile anaesthetics. Nitrous oxide (0.3 MAC) has a slight but significant effect.

Special conditions arising during anaesthesia

Lateral position

In Chapter 8 it was explained that, in the lateral position, there is preferential distribution of inspired gas to the lower lung (see Table 8.1) and this accords approximately with the distribution of pulmonary blood flow. This favourable distribution of inspired gas is disturbed by anaesthesia whether respiration is spontaneous or artificial in the paralysed patient (Rehder et al., 1972; Rehder and Sessler, 1973). The dependent lung volume is much reduced (see Figure 6.3) and is often below its closing capacity. It is therefore liable to absorption collapse (Potgieter, 1959).

Thoracotomy
(see review by Gothard and Branthwaite, 1984)

In the early days of thoracic surgery it was commonplace to maintain spontaneous respiration. This resulted in pendulum breathing between the two lungs and routine arterial PCO_2 values were recorded in excess of 30 kPa (225 mmHg) apparently without evidence of overt harm to the patients (Ellison, Ellison and Hamilton, 1955). Spontaneous breathing with an open chest but without pendulum breathing can be achieved by collapse of the exposed lung, but at the cost of severe shunting.

It took many years to realize that the solution to the open chest was IPPV. However, when one side of the chest is opened, the exposed lung may receive a very large proportion of the total ventilation during IPPV (Nunn, 1961a). Since the patient is commonly in the lateral position, there will then be a gross mismatch between the overventilated upper and exposed lung and the overperfused lower lung. However, surgical intervention will commonly restrict the ventilation of the upper exposed lung, either by retraction of the lung or by obstruction of the bronchi. This displaces ventilation to the lower better perfused lung and is advantageous.

One-lung anaesthesia. The surgeon may find that his task is simplified by total collapse of the upper (exposed) lung. This is usually achieved by the use of a double-lumen tracheal tube, with the lumen connecting to the exposed lung left open to atmosphere. Although pulmonary blood flow through the collapsed lung is reduced, it is not zero and there is usually a substantial shunt, usually in the range 30–50% (Benumof, Augustine and Gibbons, 1987). There is seldom difficulty in maintaining a satisfactory PCO_2 but oxygenation is usually compromised. Hypoxia may be minimized by restricting the duration of one-lung anaesthesia and by increasing the inspired oxygen concentration. However, the use of even 99% oxygen does not always guarantee a normal arterial PO_2, and PEEP applied to the ventilated lung usually reduces the arterial PO_2 further (Katz et al., 1982). A better solution seems to be the application of oxygen at continuous positive pressure to the non-ventilated lung (Benumof, 1982).

It has been much debated whether it is better to avoid the inhibition of HPV by volatile anaesthetics during one-lung anaesthesia, with the hope of diverting more of the circulation to the ventilated lung. Benumof, Augustine and Gibbons (1987) were able to detect a small but significant improvement in arterial PO_2 and decrease in shunt when changing from halothane to intravenous anaesthesia during one-lung anaesthesia. The improvement was less and not significant with isoflurane. Of much greater significance is position. If one-lung anaesthesia is used in the supine position, the beneficial effect of gravity on the diversion of pulmonary blood flow to the ventilated lung is lost.

Haemorrhagic hypotension

Physiological dead space is increased in haemorrhagic hypotension (Gerst, Ratten-borg and Holaday, 1959; Freeman and Nunn, 1963) and also when hypotension is induced by ganglion blockade (Eckenhoff et al., 1963). The obvious explanation is pulmonary hypotension causing failure of perfusion of the uppermost parts of the lung fields. However, this has not yet been convincingly demonstrated. Both Gerst and colleagues and Freeman and Nunn found no evidence of increased shunting during haemorrhagic hypotension. This is one of the examples of pulmonary shunting being in direct proportion to cardiac output (page 181).

The postoperative period

Postoperative hypoxaemia is multifactorial. It may be related to the residual effects of anaesthesia, to surgery or to pulmonary complications. It may also result from certain accidents such as respiratory obstruction, tension pneumothorax and pulmonary oedema, all of which may occur in the postoperative period.

Residual effects of anaesthesia. The increased alveolar/arterial P_{O_2} gradient observed during anaesthesia usually returns to normal during the first few hours after minor operations (Nunn and Payne, 1962). The functional residual capacity rapidly returns to preoperative values, but remains decreased for several days after upper abdominal surgery (Alexander et al., 1973; Ali et al., 1974). This is associated with a persistent increase in the alveolar/arterial P_{O_2} gradient. In the first few minutes of recovery, alveolar P_{O_2} may be reduced by elimination of nitrous oxide which dilutes alveolar oxygen and carbon dioxide (page 260). However, this effect is usually transient and is easily avoided by the administration of oxygen during the early stages of wash-out of nitrous oxide. Desaturation is apparently very common during transfer to the recovery room, when monitoring is often interrupted (Moller et al., 1991). Shivering in the early postoperative period causes a large increase in oxygen consumption, which requires a corresponding increase in minute volume (Bay, Nunn and Prys-Roberts, 1968).

Intermittent obstructive apnoea during sleep was originally reported as occurring during the first postoperative night by Catley et al. (1985); it follows the general pattern of obstructive sleep apnoea described in Chapter 14. It is now clear that, after major surgery, such episodes are usually worst on the second or third postoperative night (Reeder et al., 1992). They occur predominantly during rapid eye movement (REM) sleep, which is usually absent on the first postoperative night, but exceeds the preoperative level on the second and third nights after abdominal surgery (Knill et al., 1990). Morphine abolishes REM sleep but may induce obstructive apnoea in the absence of REM sleep (Jones, Sapsford and Wheatley, 1990). Episodic hypoxaemia may be very severe and associated with signs of myocardial ischaemia (Reeder et al., 1991). Beydon et al. (1992) have identified pharyngeal hypertrophy and increased body mass index as risk factors for continuing postoperative episodic desaturation. Heavy snorers and patients known to have obstructive sleep apnoea are specially at risk.

Therapeutic implications. It is now clear that, at least after major surgery, the risk of serious hypoxaemia may extend long after discharge from the postoperative recovery room. Particularly when there are risk factors in the patient, there is a very strong case for the administration of 'sleeping oxygen' and extended monitoring by pulse oximetry. Oxygen can be very effective in preventing this type of episodic desaturation (Reeder et al., 1992), but its administration presents many practical problems, reviewed by Hanning (1992).

Chapter 21

Ventilatory failure

Definitions

Respiratory failure is defined as a failure of maintenance of normal arterial blood gas tensions. Mean of the normal arterial PCO_2 is 5.1 kPa (38.3 mmHg) with 95% limits (2 s.d.) of $\pm$ 1.0 kPa (7.5 mmHg)(page 236). The normal arterial PO_2 is more difficult to define since it decreases with age (page 268), and is strongly influenced by the concentration of oxygen in the inspired gas.

Ventilatory failure is a subdivision of respiratory failure, and is defined as a pathological reduction of the alveolar ventilation below the level required for the maintenance of normal alveolar gas tensions. Since arterial PO_2 (unlike arterial PCO_2) is so strongly influenced by shunting (page 181), the adequacy of ventilation is conveniently defined by the arterial PCO_2, although it is also reflected in end-expiratory PCO_2 and PO_2. This chapter is concerned solely with ventilatory failure.

Pattern of changes in arterial blood gas tensions

Figure 21.1 shows, on a PO_2/PCO_2 diagram, the typical patterns of deterioration of arterial blood gas tensions in respiratory failure. The shaded area indicates the normal range of tensions with increasing age corresponding to a leftward shift. Pure ventilatory failure in a young person with otherwise normal lungs would result in changes along the sloping broken line. Chronic obstructive airway disease, the commonest cause of ventilatory failure, occurs in older persons and the observed pattern of change is shown within the upper arrow in Figure 21.1 (Refsum, 1963; McNicol and Campbell, 1965). The limit of survival, while breathing air, is reached at a PO_2 of about 2.7 kPa (20 mmHg) and PCO_2 11 kPa (83 mmHg). The limiting factor is not PCO_2 but PO_2. This prevents the rise of PCO_2 to higher levels except when the patient's inspired oxygen concentration is increased. It may also be raised above 11 kPa by the inhalation of carbon dioxide. In either event, a PCO_2 in excess of 11 kPa may be considered an iatrogenic disorder. Figure 21.1 also shows the pattern of blood gas changes caused by shunting or pulmonary venous admixture (pages 261 et seq.).

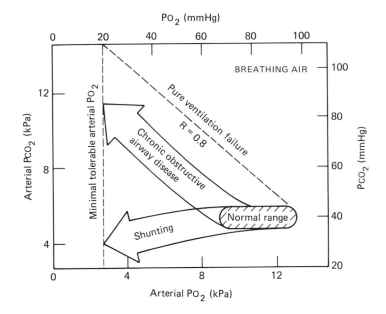

Figure 21.1 Pattern of deterioration of arterial blood gases in chronic obstructive airway disease and pulmonary shunting. The shaded area indicates the normal range of arterial blood gas tensions in which Po_2 decreases with age. The oblique broken line shows the theoretical changes in alveolar Po_2 and Pco_2 resulting from pure ventilatory failure. In chronic obstructive airway disease, the arterial Po_2 is always less than the value which would be expected in pure ventilatory failure at the same Pco_2 value. Discussion of shunting is to be found in Chapter 8.

In general the arterial Po_2 indicates the severity of respiratory failure (assuming that the patient is breathing air), while the Pco_2 indicates the differential diagnosis between ventilatory failure and shunting as shown in Figure 21.1. It is, of course, possible for ventilatory failure and shunting to coexist in the same patient.

The relationship of alveolar Pco_2 and Po_2 to alveolar ventilation (in a steady state) is governed by the alveolar air equation (page 128) and shown in Figure 6.8.

Time course of changes in blood gas tensions in acute ventilatory failure

Although the upper arrow in Figure 21.1 shows the effect of established ventilatory failure on arterial blood gas tensions, short-term deviations from this pattern occur in acute ventilatory failure. This is because the time courses of changes of Po_2 and Pco_2 in response to acute changes in ventilation are entirely different.

Body stores of oxygen are small, amounting to about 1550 ml while breathing air. Therefore, following a step change in the level of alveolar ventilation, the alveolar and arterial Po_2 rapidly reach the new value (as shown in Figure 6.8) and the half-time for the change is only 30 seconds (see page 288 and Figure 11.20). In contrast, the body stores of carbon dioxide are very large and of the order of 120 litres. Therefore, following a step change in the level of alveolar ventilation, the alveolar and arterial Pco_2 only slowly attain the value determined by the new alveolar ventilation as shown in Figure 6.8. Furthermore, the time course is slower following a reduction of ventilation than an increase (see page 238 and Figure

10.11) and the half-time of rise of P_{CO_2} following a step reduction of ventilation is of the order of 16 minutes.

The practical point is that, during the transient phase of acute hypoventilation, there may be a low P_{O_2} while the P_{CO_2} is increasing but is still within the normal range. Thus the pulse oximeter may, under certain circumstances, give an earlier warning of hypoventilation than the infrared CO_2 analyser. This breaks the rule that the P_{CO_2} is the essential index of alveolar ventilation, and it may be erroneously believed that the diagnosis is shunting rather than hypoventilation. Note that, during the acute phase of hypoventilation, the respiratory exchange ratio may fall far below its metabolic level as the carbon dioxide production is partly diverted into the body carbon dioxide stores and so does not appear in the expired air (Nunn, 1964).

Acid–base changes

An acute increase in arterial P_{CO_2} results in respiratory acidosis with the relationship between P_{CO_2} and pH defined by the whole-body CO_2 equilibration curve which approximates to that of blood with a haemoglobin concentration of 10 g/dl (see page 227 and Figure 10.5). Chronic respiratory acidosis results in partial compensation of blood pH by increase in the plasma bicarbonate level which is best quantified as the base excess.

Causes of failure of ventilation

Most of the causes of failure of ventilation have been mentioned in the first part of this book. This section reviews and classifies the causes of failure. They may be conveniently considered under the headings of the anatomical sites where they arise. These sites are indicated in Figure 21.2. Lesions or malfunctions at sites A to E result in a reduction of input to the respiratory muscles. Dyspnoea may not be apparent and the diagnosis of ventilatory failure may be overlooked on superficial inspection of the patient. Lesions or malfunctions at sites G to I result in evident dyspnoea and no one is likely to miss the diagnosis of hypoventilation. The various sites will now be considered individually.

A: The respiratory neurons of the medulla are depressed by hypoxia and also by very high levels of P_{CO_2}, probably of the order of 40 kPa (300 mmHg) in the healthy unanaesthetized subject (page 523) but at a lower P_{CO_2} in the presence of anaesthetics or narcotic drugs. Reduction of P_{CO_2} below the apnoeic threshold results in apnoea in the unconscious subject but usually not in the conscious subject (page 109). Loss of respiratory sensitivity to carbon dioxide occurs in various types of chronic ventilatory failure, particularly chronic bronchitis (the 'blue bloater'). Such patients tend to rely on their hypoxic drive to maintain ventilation. If this is abolished, as, for example, by the administration of 100% oxygen or anaesthesia, gross hypoventilation or apnoea may result (Figure 21.3).

A wide variety of drugs may cause central apnoea or respiratory depression and these include opiates, barbiturates and all anaesthetic agents. Reflex apnoea may follow noxious stimuli but the Hering–Breuer inflation reflex is weak in man and lung inflation does not normally cause apnoea (Widdicombe, 1961). The respiratory neurons may also be affected by anything which affects their blood supply, including pressure, trauma, neoplasm or vascular catastrophe.

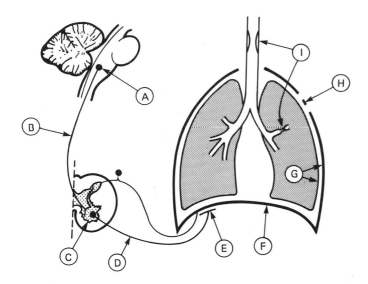

Figure 21.2 Summary of sites at which lesions, drug action or malfunction may result in ventilatory failure. (A) The 'respiratory centre'. (B) Upper motor neuron (C) Anterior horn cell. (D) Lower motor neuron. (E) The neuromuscular junction. (F) The respiratory muscles. (G) Altered elasticity of lungs or chest wall. (H) Loss of structural integrity of chest wall and pleural cavity. (I) Increased airway resistance.

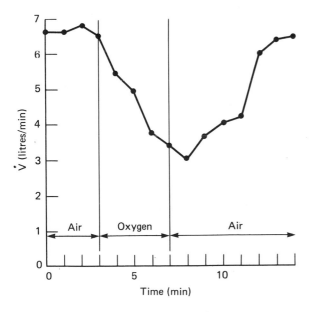

Figure 21.3 Rapid onset of hypoventilation when a patient with chronic hypercapnia and loss of chemoreceptor sensitivity to carbon dioxide breathed 100% oxygen. (Nunn, unpublished data)

B: The upper motor neurons serving the respiratory muscles are most likely to be interrupted by trauma. Only lesions above cervical 3–4 will affect the phrenic nerve and result in total apnoea. However, fracture dislocations of the lower cervical vertebrae are relatively common and result in loss of action of the intercostal and expiratory muscles while sparing the diaphragm. Upper motor neurons may be involved in various disease processes, including tumours, demyelination and, occasionally, in syringomyelia.

C: The anterior horn cell may be affected by various disease processes, of which the most important is poliomyelitis. Happily this condition is now rare in the developed world but it can produce any degree of respiratory involvement up to total paralysis of all respiratory muscles.

D: Lower motor neurons supplying the respiratory muscles are prone to normal traumatic risks and, in former times, the phrenic nerves were surgically interrupted for the treatment of pulmonary tuberculosis. Polyneuritis (e.g. Guillain–Barré syndrome) and motor neuron disease are the main conditions which may cause ventilatory failure at this level.

E: The neuromuscular junction is affected by myasthenia gravis and botulism. Drugs acting at this site include all the neuromuscular blocking agents used in anaesthesia and certain organophosphorus compounds and nerve gases. Procaine acts by preventing the synthesis of acetylcholine.

F: The respiratory muscles themselves are unlikely to be involved in any disease process which results in ventilatory failure. However, the efficiency of contraction of the diaphragm may be severely affected by 'splinting' due to abdominal distension or by flattening of the domes due, for example, to tension pneumothorax. The respiratory muscles may also become fatigued as a result of working against excessive impedance (Roussos and Macklem, 1983; Moxham, 1984). In dogs it has been shown that the administration of *Escherichia coli* endotoxin causes ventilatory failure in the presence of increased electrical activity in the respiratory muscles and unaltered respiratory impedance (Hussain, Simkus and Roussos, 1985). These authors concluded that ventilatory failure in endotoxic shock is due to enhanced fatigue in the respiratory muscles.

G: Loss of elasticity of the lungs or chest wall is a potent cause of ventilatory failure. It may arise within the lungs (e.g. pulmonary fibrosis, Hamman–Rich syndrome and respiratory distress syndrome), in the pleura (e.g. chronic empyema with fibrinous covering of the pleura), in the chest wall (e.g. kyphoscoliosis) or in the skin (e.g. contracted burn scars in children). However, it is frequently forgotten that seemingly mild pressures applied to the outside of the chest may seriously embarrass the breathing and even result in total apnoea. A sustained pressure of only 6 kPa (45 mmHg or a depth of 2 feet of water) is sufficient to prevent breathing. This is prone to occur when crowds get out of control on a staircase and people fall on top of one another. It may also occur when workers on a building site become buried under a load of sand or rubble.

H: Loss of structural integrity of the chest wall may result in ventilatory failure in the case of open pneumothorax where the reduction in overall minute volume is further complicated by pendulum breathing between the two lungs. Even if the parietal pleura is intact, ventilatory failure may result from multiple fractured ribs, a condition known as flail chest. This condition, resulting from impact on the steering wheel, was commonplace in the UK before the use of seat belts became compulsory. The condition may be successfully treated by artificial ventilation with intermittent positive pressure, although some centres prefer conservative treatment with rib fixation.

Closed pneumothorax causes interference with ventilation in proportion to the quantity of air in the chest. With a tension pneumothorax, the pressure rises above atmospheric, collapsing the ipsilateral lung, displacing the mediastinum and partially collapsing the contralateral lung. Convexity of the diaphragm is lost and ventilation may be critically impaired. The diagnosis and correction of the condition is a matter of great urgency. Gross dyspnoea with deviation of trachea and displacement of the apex beat should always alert staff to the possibility of this condition.

I: Airway resistance remains the commonest and most important cause of ventilatory failure. The causes of increased airway resistance have been described in Chapter 4 (pages 72 et seq.) and will not be discussed any further here. However, the relationship between airway resistance and ventilatory failure is a complex subject which is considered further below. In the clinical field, airway resistance is seldom measured but is most often inferred from measurement of ventilatory capacity.

Increased dead space

Very rarely, a large increase in the respiratory dead space may be the cause of ventilatory failure. Minute volume may be increased but the alveolar ventilation is reduced and the patient presents with a high PCO_2 accompanied by a high minute volume. This may be distinguished from a hypermetabolic state by measurement of either carbon dioxide output or dead space (page 238). The dead space/tidal volume ratio should be above 65% in this condition. An increase in the arterial/end-expiratory PCO_2 gradient (more than 2 kPa or 15 mmHg) indicates an increase in the alveolar dead space. This condition may be caused by ventilation of large unperfused areas of the lungs (e.g. an air cyst communicating with the bronchus), pulmonary emboli or pulmonary hypotension. External or apparatus dead space also tends to reduce alveolar ventilation and may be added either intentionally or accidentally.

Relationship between ventilatory capacity and ventilatory failure

Tests for the measurement of ventilatory capacity are described on pages 133 et seq. However, a severe reduction in ventilatory capacity does not necessarily mean that a patient will be in ventilatory failure. Figure 21.4 (Nunn et al., 1988) shows the lack of correlation between $FEV_{1.0}$ and PCO_2 in the grossly abnormal range of $FEV_{1.0}$ 0.3–1.0 litre. Most of the patients represented in Figure 21.4 had chronic obstructive airway disease and they may be classified into 'pink puffers' and 'blue bloaters'. 'Pink puffers', predominantly with emphysema, maintain a considerable degree of respiratory sensitivity to carbon dioxide and struggle to keep a normal

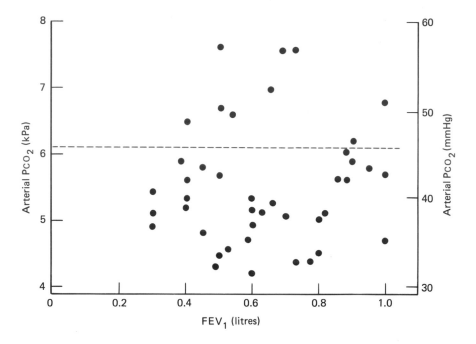

Figure 21.4 Lack of correlation between arterial Pco₂ and forced expiratory volume (1 second) in 44 patients with chronic obstructive airway disease. The broken line indicates the upper limit of normal for Pco₂. (Nunn et al., 1988)

arterial P_{CO_2} for as long as possible, although with evident dyspnoea. On the other hand, 'blue bloaters', mostly with chronic bronchitis, have lost their sensitivity to carbon dioxide and allow their P_{CO_2} to increase above the normal reference range, usually without dyspnoea. These patients rely on hypoxic drive for the maintenance of ventilation and are in a more precarious state than the 'pink puffer' in spite of the absence of dyspnoea.

Asthmatic patients tend to behave like pink puffers and, even in quite severe attacks of bronchospasm, maintain a normal or subnormal arterial P_{CO_2}. In an asthmatic, ventilatory failure, indicated by a rising P_{CO_2}, is a grave sign, indicating that the patient is no longer able to overcome the added airway resistance by increased work of breathing.

It should again be stressed that the usual tests of ventilatory capacity depend on the expiratory muscles while the work of breathing is normally achieved by the inspiratory muscles. However, expiratory resistance is usually more important than inspiratory resistance because of the factors illustrated in Figure 4.8.

The relationship between metabolic demand and ventilatory failure

In renal failure, protein intake is a major factor in the onset of uraemia. Similarly, in ventilatory failure, the onset of hypoxia and hypercapnia is directly related to the metabolic demand. Just as a patient with renal failure may benefit from a low protein diet, so a patient with a severe reduction of ventilatory capacity protects himself by limiting the exercise which he takes.

As chronic obstructive airway disease progresses, the ventilatory capacity decreases and the minute volume of breathing required for a particular level of activity increases. The increased ventilatory requirement is because both the dead space and the oxygen cost of breathing increase. The patient is thus trapped in a pincer movement of decreasing ventilatory capacity and increasing ventilatory requirement. As the jaws of the pincer close, there is first a limitation on heavy exercise, then on moderate exercise and so on until the patient is dyspnoeic at rest. At any time his work capacity is limited by the fraction of his ventilatory capacity which he is able to maintain for a given level of oxygen uptake.

The complex interaction between these factors is shown in Figure 21.5, where the upper part shows the normal state. Assuming that an untrained subject can comfortably maintain a minute volume equal to about 30% of his maximal breathing capacity (MBC) without dyspnoea, he has a reserve of ventilatory capacity which is adequate for rest and a power output of 100 watts. However, a power output of 200 watts requires a ventilation which exceeds a third of his MBC and he becomes aware of his breathing at this level of exercise.

The middle section of Figure 21.5 shows moderately severe obstructive airway disease with the following changes:

1. MBC reduced from 150 to 60 l/min.
2. Dead space/tidal volume ratio increased from 30 to 40%.
3. Oxygen cost of breathing increased by 10% for each level of activity.

Factors 2 and 3 together result in an increased minute volume for each level of activity.

Again, on the assumption that dyspnoea will not be apparent until the minute volume is 30% of MBC, the reserve of ventilation is now sufficient for rest, but 100 watts of power output will result in dyspnoea.

Finally, in Figure 21.5c, the changes have progressed to the point where resting minute volume exceeds 30% of MBC and the patient is dyspnoeic at rest.

Breathlessnesss

Breathlessness or dyspnoea has been defined by Campbell and Guz (1981) as 'undue awareness of breathing or awareness of difficulty in breathing'. This definition would apply to both the awareness of breathing during severe exercise in the healthy subject and the dyspnoea of the patient with respiratory failure or heart failure. In the first case the sensation is normal and to be expected. However, in the latter, it is pathological and should be considered as a symptom.

The origin of the sensation

Hypoxia and hypercapnia may force the patient to breathe more deeply but they are not *per se* responsible for the sensation of dyspnoea which arises from the ventilatory response rather than the stimulus itself. Dyspnoea is usually more prominent in the 'pink puffer' who keeps his blood gases relatively normal than in the 'blue bloater' who is both hypoxic and hypercapnic. Patients with respiratory paralysis caused by poliomyelitis are not usually dyspnoeic in spite of abnormal blood gas tensions.

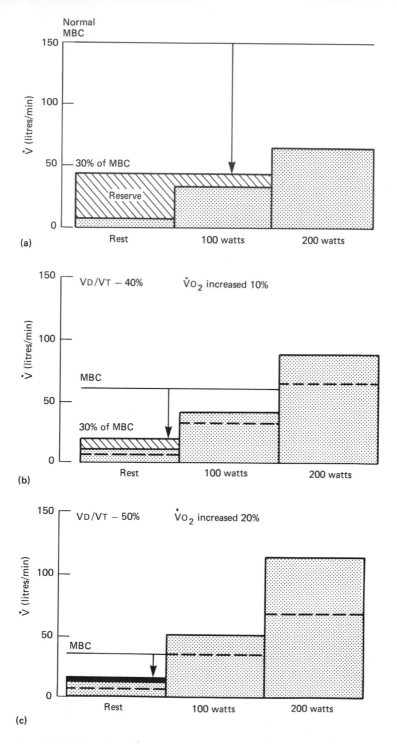

Figure 21.5 Relationship between maximal breathing capacity (MBC) and ventilatory requirements of rest and work at 100 and 200 watts. The tips of the arrows indicate 30% of MBC which can usually be maintained without dyspnoea. Ventilatory reserve is between this level and the various ventilatory requirements. (a) Normal. (b) Moderate loss of ventilatory capacity with some increase in oxygen cost of breathing. (c) Severe loss of ventilatory capacity with considerable increase in the oxygen cost of breathing.

Campbell and Guz (1981) advanced their reasons for believing that dyspnoea is not akin to pain and neither is it strictly related to the work of breathing. Some patients have dyspnoea at relatively low levels of work of breathing, while others show no dyspnoea at high levels of work. Fatigue of the respiratory muscles (page 126) may be a factor in some cases but is clearly not the only cause of dyspnoea.

Campbell and Howell (1963) suggested that a major factor in the origin of dyspnoea was an 'inappropriateness' between the tension generated in the respiratory muscles and the resultant shortening of the muscle fibres. This might arise in obstructed breathing and would tend to increase with hyperventilation when the efficiency of breathing is less.

Breath holding (pages 113 et seq.) provides some insight into the origin of the sensation of breathlessness. It has been shown that blood gas tensions are by no means the only factor limiting breath-holding time although PO_2 is more important than PCO_2. The sensation which terminates breath holding can be relieved by ventilation without change of blood gas tensions, by bilateral vagal block and by curarization. Diaphragmatic afferents appear to be more important than those from the intercostals.

It cannot be said that the problem of breathlessness is completely understood at the present time. It is, however, clear that there is no single and simple mechanism comparable to the sensations of touch, pain or temperature. The origin may well be multifactorial and the mechanisms of its generation are clearly complex.

Treatment of ventilatory failure

Many patients go about their business with arterial PCO_2 levels as high as 8 kPa (60 mmHg). Higher levels are associated with increasing disability, largely due to the accompanying hypoxaemia when the patient is breathing air (see Figure 21.1). Treatment may be divided into symptomatic relief of hypoxaemia and attempts to improve the alveolar ventilation.

Treatment of hypoxaemia due to hypoventilation by administration of oxygen

Hypoxia must be treated as the first priority, and administration of oxygen is the fastest and most effective method. However, it must be remembered that this will do nothing to improve the PCO_2 and may make it worse. It is therefore essential to ensure that palliative relief of hypoxia does not result in hypercapnia, and arterial PCO_2 should be checked if there is any doubt.

The relationship between alveolar PO_2, alveolar ventilation and inspired oxygen concentration is explained on pages 257 et seq. and illustrated in Figure 6.8. If other factors remain constant, an increase in inspired gas PO_2 will result in an equal increase in alveolar gas PO_2. Therefore only small increases in inspired oxygen concentration are required for the relief of hypoxia *due to underventilation*. Figure 21.6 shows the rectangular hyperbola relating PCO_2 and alveolar ventilation (as in Figure 6.8), but superimposed are the concentrations of inspired oxygen required to restore a normal alveolar PO_2 for different degrees of alveolar hypoventilation. It will be seen that 30% is sufficient for the degree of alveolar hypoventilation which will result in an alveolar P_{CO_2} of 13 kPa (almost 100 mmHg). Clearly this is an unacceptable P_{CO_2}, and therefore 30% can be regarded as the upper limit of inspired oxygen concentration to be used in the palliative relief of hypoxia due to ventilatory failure, without attempting to improve the alveolar ventilation. This limit is, in fact, recognized by the range of venturi masks (Campbell, 1960b). It is also the level attainable with 'walking' oxygen equipment and domiciliary oxygen.

The use of very high concentrations of inspired oxygen will prevent hypoxia even in gross alveolar hypoventilation which carries the risk of dangerous hypercapnia. Although this is itself a strong contraindication to the use of high concentrations of oxygen under these circumstances, an even graver risk exists in patients who have lost their ventilatory sensitivity to carbon dioxide and rely upon their hypoxic drive to maintain ventilation. High concentrations of oxygen will abolish the hypoxic drive and may precipitate acute-on-chronic ventilatory failure as in Figure 21.3. In 1949 Donald drew attention to the problem, but this unfortunately resulted in a tendency to withhold oxygen for fear of causing hypercapnia. The rule is that hypoxia must be treated first, because hypoxia kills quickly while hypercapnia kills slowly. However, it must always be remembered that administration of oxygen to a patient with ventilatory failure will do nothing to improve the P_{CO_2} and may make it worse. The arterial P_{CO_2} must be checked if there is any doubt.

Symptomatic relief of hypoxaemia due to shunting, in patients who have probably retained their sensitivity to carbon dioxide, requires a completely different policy for estimation of the optimal inspired oxygen concentration, and this is discussed on page 268.

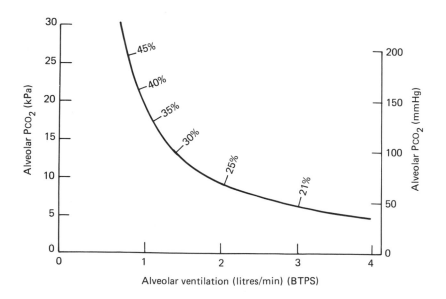

Figure 21.6 The curve indicates the alveolar P_{CO_2} as a function of alveolar ventilation at rest. The percentages indicate the inspired oxygen concentration which is then required to restore normal alveolar P_{O_2}.

Improvement of alveolar ventilation

The only way to reduce the arterial PCO_2 is to improve the alveolar ventilation. The first line of therapy is to improve ventilatory capacity by such measures as bronchodilators, control of infections and secretions, stabilization of the chest wall, closure of an open pneumothorax, relief of pain, careful control of oxygen therapy and avoidance of drugs which depress breathing. The second line is chemical stimulation of breathing. Doxapram is capable of prolonged stimulation of breathing with little tachyphylaxis. This drug stimulates breathing via the peripheral chemoreceptors (Mitchell and Herbert, 1975) and is further discussed on page 102. It may be conveniently administered by a continuous intravenous infusion at a dose of 2–8 mg/min. The third line of treatment is by tracheal intubation or tracheostomy which may improve alveolar ventilation by reducing dead space and facilitating the control of secretions.

The fourth line of therapy is the institution of artificial ventilation considered in detail in Chapter 22. It is difficult to give firm guidelines for the institution of artificial ventilation and the arterial PCO_2 should not be considered in isolation. However, a PCO_2 in excess of 10 kPa (75 mmHg) which cannot be reduced by other means in a patient who is deemed recoverable is generally considered as a firm indication. However, artificial ventilation may be required at much lower levels of PCO_2 if there is actual or impending respiratory fatigue as a result of increased work of breathing. This may be difficult to diagnose or predict. Nevertheless, it is now well recognized that intense activity by the respiratory muscles results in fatigue, as in the case of other skeletal muscles under similar conditions (see page 126). Dyscoordinated breathing with thoracic and abdominal movements out of phase is a valuable indication of fatigue. It has been mentioned above that the PCO_2 rises late in asthma, and artificial ventilation may be required before the arterial PCO_2 has risen much above the normal range.

A difficult decision may be required on whether to ventilate patients with untreatable progressive ventilatory failure. Great difficulties and much distress may arise from instituting artificial ventilation from which it proves impossible to wean the patient. However, it may be useful to ventilate a patient with chronic obstructive airway disease to tide him over a period of infection which has resulted in acute-on-chronic ventilatory failure. However, in the absence of a transient factor of this nature, it is unlikely that a period of artificial ventilation can influence the long-term progress of the disease (Nunn, Milledge and Sigaraya, 1979; Petheram and Branthwaite, 1980). Similar considerations apply to pulmonary fibrosis (Hamman–Rich syndrome).

For many years it has been accepted that artificial ventilation is the treatment of choice in severe crushed chest injury. However, there remains a school of thought which favours conservative management (Trinkle et al., 1975). Opinions differ on the management of acute epiglottitis in children. One school favours expectant treatment with antibiotics, steroids, sedation and high humidity of the inspired gas, while the other favours prophylactic intubation when the diagnosis is confirmed by lateral radiography of the larynx.

In an emergency it is frequently necessary to institute artificial ventilation to save life without consideration of the long-term aspects of the case. Under such circumstances, it may be very difficult to distinguish between acute, chronic and acute-on-chronic ventilatory failure. Resuscitation may well commit the intensive care unit to artificial ventilation of a patient who is not recoverable. It is virtually impossible to devise a system which will avoid this situation.

Artificial ventilation may be required for treatment of hypoxaemia which is not directly attributable to ventilatory failure. The benefit is often related to the increased tidal volume opening up closed airways and alveoli and so reducing shunting. This effect can be augmented by the use of positive end-expiratory pressure (page 451).

Chapter 22

Artificial ventilation

Artificial ventilation is defined as the provision of the minute volume of respiration by external forces. This is usually required when there is impaired action of the patient's respiratory muscles or a severe dysfunction of the mechanics of breathing. It may also be used to improve oxygenation of arterial blood even when P_{CO_2} is within normal limits. It is used in four main situations:

1. Resuscitation following acute apnoea.
2. Anaesthesia with paralysis.
3. Intensive care with failure of one or more vital functions.
4. Prolonged treatment of chronic ventilatory failure.

Extracorporeal gas exchange is considered separately in Chapter 23.

Artificial ventilation of the apnoeic patient during resuscitation was formerly carried out by application of direct force to the chest in an attempt to produce either inhalation or exhalation, or both. These methods have been shown to be largely ineffective and are therefore considered only briefly below. It is now universally agreed that the best method of artificial ventilation during resuscitation is inflation of the lungs with the expired air of the rescuer, and the physiology of this technique is considered below.

Much the commonest application of artificial ventilation is during anaesthesia with paralysis. It would normally be applied to some 2–5% of the population of a developed country each year. Almost without exception it is achieved by the application of intermittent positive pressure to the airway of the patient, either manually or by means of one of a large range of mechanical devices, which can be comparatively simple.

Artificial ventilation during intensive care is also undertaken almost exclusively by intermittent positive pressure ventilation (IPPV). However, in this environment, a proportion of patients present problems in ventilation and there is a requirement for more sophisticated ventilators with increased control of the manner and pattern of ventilation.

Treatment of chronic ventilatory failure has been achieved by phrenic nerve stimulation although the technique is not commonly used. The commonest methods are by the intermittent development of a positive pressure gradient between airways and the air surrounding the trunk. At the present time this is most commonly achieved by IPPV as in anaesthesia or intensive care. However, this requires tracheostomy to ensure the necessary airtight fit to the airways without the possibility of inflation of the stomach. This difficulty can be avoided by generating the intermittent pressure differential by phasic reduction of pressure in the air around the trunk, and this may be achieved by means of a tank or cuirass ventilator.

Methods used for resuscitation

Artificial ventilation by application of mechanical forces directly to the trunk

Until about 1960, the usual methods were based on the rescuer manipulating the trunk and arms of the victim. These methods, which undoubtedly saved many lives in the past, are now largely obsolete. They can be classified into those with an active expiratory phase, those with an active inspiratory phase and those with both (push–pull). None of these methods could be relied upon to provide an adequate minute volume, for reasons discussed below.

Active expiratory phase. It would appear intuitively obvious that exerting pressure on the chest wall or the abdomen would result in exhalation. This would be followed by inspiration as elastic forces restored the lung volume to functional residual capacity (FRC) when the distorting force was removed. This was the basis of the back pressure method (Schafer, 1904) and the Paul–Bragg Pneumobelt. However, neither method can be relied upon to guarantee an adequate tidal volume even if the airway is unobstructed. This is mainly because tidal exchange must take place within the expiratory reserve volume which is much reduced in the supine position (page 55). Lower limits of normal expiratory reserve volume in the supine position reported by Whitfield, Waterhouse and Arnott (1950) are of the order of 200 ml and clearly there is no possibility of obtaining a satisfactory tidal volume by this method in such a patient.

Active inspiratory phase. In an attempt to achieve tidal exchange within the inspiratory capacity, techniques have been developed which seek to expand the chest by traction on the arms or lifting of the hips. Somewhat similar is the cuirass respirator which applies an intermittent subatmospheric pressure to the epigastrium. Although these methods have the advantage of operating above FRC as in normal breathing, they cannot be relied upon to produce an adequate tidal volume in all patients.

Both active inspiratory and expiratory phases (push–pull). Of all the manual methods, these are the most efficient. The imposed tidal volume is partly above and partly below FRC. The rocking stretcher (Eve, 1932) relies on the fact that lung volume is markedly affected by posture (page 55) and phasic tilting 40 degrees on either side of horizontal can achieve a satisfactory tidal volume (Comroe and Dripps, 1946). The other push–pull methods include the arm lift/back pressure method applied to the prone victim (Holger Nielsen, 1932) and the arm lift/chest pressure method applied to the supine victim (Silvester, 1857). Safar (1959) obtained mean tidal volumes of 619 and 503 ml respectively in studies of these two methods in curarized subjects with tracheal tubes in place.

The significance of airway obstruction. Studies in curarized subjects with tracheal tubes in place do not reflect the usual circumstances of resuscitation. Virtually all unconscious patients will have some degree of airway obstruction which will be severe in many cases (page 384). Performance of the techniques described above requires the use of both hands, making it very difficult for the rescuer to protect the patency of the airway by the methods described on page 386. Recognition of the critical role of airway obstruction led to a major investigation of this factor by Safar (1959). His results (Table 22.1) clearly demonstrate that effective artificial ventilation by the manual methods can be guaranteed only if the trachea is intubated.

Even if a normal tidal volume is obtained, it does not guarantee that arterial Po_2 will be satisfactory. Considerable arterial desaturation has been found during artificial respiration using Schafer's method, which could not be entirely explained by hypoventilation. It is likely that reduction of lung volume below FRC resulted in sufficient airway closure to cause appreciable shunting.

Expired air resuscitation

Recognition of the inadequacy of the manual methods of artificial ventilation led directly to a radical new approach to artificial ventilation in the emergency situation. Around 1960 there was vigorous re-examination of the concept of the rescuer's expired air being used for inflation of the victim's lung. Elisha has been credited with use of this technique on the son of the Shunammite woman (2 Kings 4:32) but the first clear and unequivocal account of the method was by Herholdt and Rafn in 1796.

At first sight, it might appear that expired air, being 'vitiated', would not be a suitable inspired air for the victim. However, if the rescuer doubles his ventilation he is able to breathe for two. If neither party had any respiratory dead space, the simple relationship shown in Table 22.2 would apply. In fact, the rescuer's dead space improves the situation. At the start of inflation, the rescuer's dead space is filled with fresh air and this is the first gas to enter the victim's lungs. If the rescuer's dead space is artificially increased by apparatus dead space, this will improve the freshness of the air which the victim receives and it will also prevent hypocapnia in the rescuer. This concept has been exploited in certain instrumental aids (Elam, 1962).

Table 22.1 Curarized anaesthetized patients – artificial ventilation by back pressure, arm lift method (Holger Nielsen method, 1932)

Airway	Mean tidal volume (ml)	Percentage of patients with tidal volume less than dead space
Natural (head in flexion)	126	75
Oropharyngeal airway (head in flexion)	178	71
Natural (head in extension)	328	31
Oropharyngeal airway (head in extension)	351	20
Tracheal tube	619	0

Table 22.2 Alveolar gas concentrations during expired air resuscitation

	Normal spontaneous respiration	Expired air resuscitation with doubled ventilation	
		Donor	Recipient
Alveolar CO_2	6%	3%	6%
Alveolar O_2	15%	18%	15%

Doubling the donor's ventilation increases his alveolar O_2 concentration to a value midway between the normal alveolar oxygen concentration and that of room air.

Expired air resuscitation has now displaced the manual methods in all except the most unusual circumstances and its success depends on the following factors:

1. It is normally possible to achieve adequate ventilation for long periods of time without fatigue (Greene et al., 1957; Cox, Woolmer and Thomas, 1960).
2. The hands of the rescuer are free to control the patency of the victim's airway.
3. The rescuer can monitor the victim's chest expansion visually and he can also hear any airway obstruction and sense the tidal exchange from the propriocep- tive receptors in his own chest wall.
4. The method is extremely adaptable and has been used, for example, before drowning victims have been removed from the water, and on linesmen electrocuted while working on pylons. No manual method would have any hope of success in such situations.
5. The method seems to come naturally, and many rescuers have achieved success with the minimum of instruction.

Expired air resuscitation was extensively reviewed by Elam and Greene (1962) and Elam (1962). Fear of disease transmission, arising in particular from the increasing incidence of HIV infection, has prompted a number of modifications of technique reviewed by Baskett (1992). However, the essentials remain as follows:

1. The airway must be cleared, firstly by removal of any foreign matter and secondly by opening the pharynx either by extension of the head or by protrusion of the mandible (page 386).
2. The rescuer should employ a tidal volume about double normal; most people do this intuitively.
3. The first few breaths should be delivered as fast as possible; thereafter a normal respiratory rate should be employed.
4. Alternative variants of the technique should be taught as no one method is applicable to all circumstances. For example, mouth-to-nose may be preferable to mouth-to-mouth with trismus or injuries to the mouth.
5. No potential rescuer should be led to believe that success depends on the use of ancillary apparatus such as the Brooke airway. A rescue is such a rare event in the lives of all except those with professional involvement, that there is little chance of having apparatus to hand.

Intermittent positive pressure ventilation (IPPV)

Phases of the respiratory cycle

Inspiration. During IPPV, the mouth (or airway) pressure is intermittently raised above ambient pressure. The inspired gas then flows into the respiratory system in accord with the resistance and compliance of the respiratory system (Chapters 3 and 4). If inspiration is slow, the distribution is governed mainly by regional compliance. If inspiration is fast, there is preferential ventilation of parts of the lungs with short time constants (see Figure 3.6). Different temporal patterns of pressure may be applied and are discussed below. The anatomical pattern of distribution of inspired gas is different from that of spontaneous breathing, there being a relatively greater expansion of the rib cage (Vellody et al., 1978).

Expiration. During IPPV, expiration results from allowing mouth pressure to fall to ambient. Expiration is then passive and differs from expiration during spontaneous breathing in which diaphragmatic tone is gradually reduced (page 120). Expiration may be impeded by the application of positive end-expiratory pressure (PEEP) or by the addition of external resistance to gas flow (expiratory retard). Alternatively, expiration can be accelerated by the application of a subatmospheric pressure. This may be termed negative end-expiratory pressure (NEEP). Expiration to ambient pressure is also termed zero end-expiratory pressure (ZEEP).

If the inflating pressure is maintained for several seconds, the resulting tidal volume will be indicated by the following relationship:

tidal volume = sustained inflation pressure × total static compliance

Thus, for example, a sustained inflation pressure of 1 kPa (10 cmH$_2$O) with a static compliance of 0.5 l/kPa (0.05 l/cmH$_2$O) would result in a lung volume 500 ml above functional residual capacity (FRC).

Time course of inflation and deflation

Equilibration according to the above equation usually takes several seconds. When the airway pressure is raised during inspiration, it is opposed by the two forms of impedance – the elastic resistance of lungs and chest wall (Chapter 3) and resistance to air flow (Chapter 4). At any instant, the inflation pressure equals the sum of the pressures required to overcome these two forms of impedance. The pressure required to overcome elastic resistance equals the lung volume above FRC divided by the total (dynamic) compliance, while the pressure required to overcome air flow resistance equals the air flow resistance multiplied by the instantaneous flow rate.

The effect of applying a constant pressure (or square wave inflation) is shown in Figure 22.1. The two components of the inflation pressure vary during the course of inspiration while their sum remains constant. The component overcoming air flow resistance is maximal at first and declines exponentially with air flow as inflation proceeds. The component overcoming elastic resistance increases with the lung volume. With normal respiratory mechanics in the unconscious patient, the change in lung volume should be 95% complete in about 1.5 seconds, as in Figure 22.1

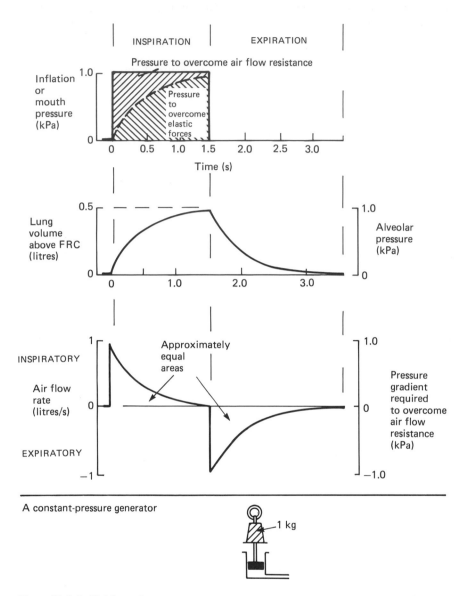

Figure 22.1 Artificial ventilation by intermittent application of a constant pressure (square wave). Passive expiration. Inspiratory and explanatory flow rates are both exponential. Assuming that air flow resistance is constant, it follows that flow rate and pressure gradient required to overcome resistance may be shown on the same graph. Lung volume and alveolar pressure may be shown on the same graph if compliance is constant. Values are typical for an anaesthetized supine paralysed patient: total dynamic compliance, 0.5 l/kPa (50 ml/cmH₂O); pulmonary resistance, 0.3 kPa l⁻¹ s) (0.3 cmH₂O/l/sec); apparatus resistance, 0.7 kPa l⁻¹ s (7 cmH₂O/l/sec); total resistance, 1 kPa l⁻¹ s (10 cmH₂O/l/sec); time constant, 0.5 s.

The approach of the lung volume to its equilibrium value is according to an exponential function of the wash-in type (see Appendix F). The time constant, which is the time required for inflation to 63% of the equilibrium value, equals the product of resistance and compliance. Normal values for an unconscious patient are as follows:

$$\text{time constant} = \text{resistance} \times \text{compliance}$$

$$0.5 \text{ second} = 1 \text{ kPa } l^{-1} \text{ s} \times 0.5 \text{ l kPa}^{-1}$$

(or, in non-SI units, $10 \text{ cmH}_2\text{O/l/s} \times 0.05 \text{ l/cmH}_2\text{O}$, which also equals 0.5 second)

The time constant is the time which would be required to reach equilibrium if the initial inspiratory flow rate were maintained. It is sometimes more convenient to use the half-time, which is 0.69 times the time constant. The inflation curve is shown in full with further mathematical detail in Appendix F.

It is normal practice for the inspiratory phase to be terminated after 1 or 2 seconds at which time the lung volume will still be increasing. Inflation pressure is not then the sole arbiter of tidal volume but must be considered in relation to the duration of the inspiratory phase.

If expiration is passive and mouth pressure remains at ambient, the driving force is the elevation of alveolar pressure above ambient, caused by elastic recoil of lungs and chest wall. This pressure is dissipated in overcoming air flow resistance during expiration. In Figure 22.1, during expiration the alveolar pressure (proportional to the lung volume above FRC) is directly proportional to expiratory flow rate, and all three quantities decline according to a wash-out exponential function with a time constant which is again equal to the product of compliance and resistance.

The effect of changes in inflation pressure, resistance and compliance

The heavy line in Figure 22.2 shows the inflation curve for the normal parameters of an unconscious paralysed patient as listed in Table 22.3. These are the same values which were considered above. The basic curve is a single exponential approaching a lung volume 0.5 litre above FRC with a time constant of 0.5 second.

Table 22.3 Parameters for inflation curves shown in Figure 22.2

	Basic curve	Pulmonary resistance doubled	Inflation pressure doubled	Compliance doubled	Compliance halved
Inflation pressure					
(kPa)	1	1	2	1	1
(cmH$_2$O)	10	10	20	10	10
Compliance					
(l/kPa)	0.5	0.5	0.5	1	0.25
(ml/cmH$_2$O)	50	50	50	100	25
Ultimate tidal volume (l)	0.5	0.5	1	1	0.25
Pulmonary resistance					
(kPa l^{-1} s)	1	2	1	1	1
(cmH$_2$O/l/sec)	10	20	10	10	10
Time constant					
(s or sec)	0.5	1	0.5	1	0.25

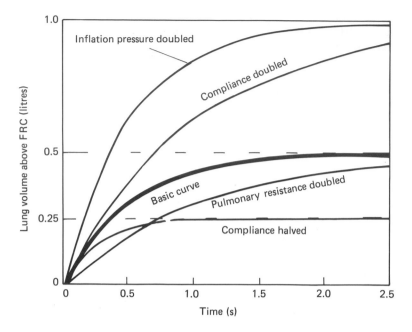

Figure 22.2 Effect of changes in various factors on inflation of the lungs. Fixed relationships: ultimate tidal volume = inflation pressure × compliance; time constant = compliance × resistance. (See also Table 22.3)

63% of inflation completed in 1 time constant   98% of inflation completed in 4 time constants
86.5% of inflation completed in 2 time constants   99% of inflation completed in 5 time constants
95% of inflation completed in 3 time constants

Changes in inflation pressure do not alter the time constant of inflation, but directly influence the amount of air introduced into the lungs in a given number of time constants. In Figure 22.2, each point on the curve labelled 'inflation pressure doubled' is twice the height of the corresponding point on the basic curve for the same time.

Effect of changes in compliance and resistance. If the compliance is doubled, the equilibrium tidal volume is also doubled. However, the time constant (product of compliance and resistance) is also doubled and therefore the equilibrium volume is approached more slowly (Figure 22.2). Conversely, if the compliance is halved, the equilibrium tidal volume is also halved and so is the time constant.

Changes in resistance have a direct effect on the time constant of inflation but do not affect the equilibrium tidal volume. Thus the effect of an increased resistance on tidal volume is through the reduction in inspiratory flow rate. Within limits, this can be counteracted by prolonging inspiration or by increasing the inflation pressure and the degree of overpressure (explained below). The effects, shown in Figure 22.2, apply not only to the whole lung but also to regions which may have different compliances, resistances and time constants (page 160).

Overpressure. Increasing the inflation pressure has a major effect on the time required to achieve a particular lung volume above FRC. In Figure 22.3, the lung characteristics are the same as for the basic curve in Figure 22.2. If the required tidal volume is 475 ml, this is achieved in 1.5 seconds with an inflation pressure of 1

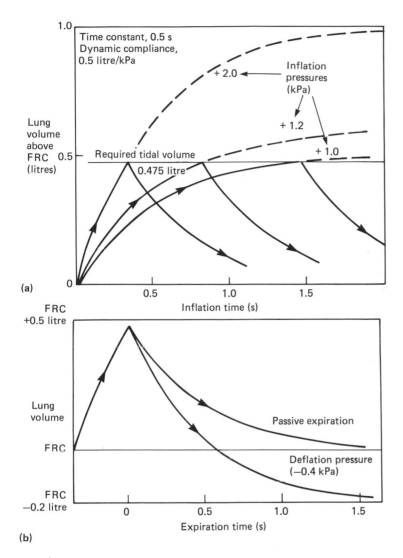

Figure 22.3 (a) How the duration of inflation may be shortened by the use of overpressure. Inflation curves are shown for +2 kPa (+20 cmH₂O) (equilibrium 1 litre), +1.2 kPa (+12 cmH₂O) (equilibrium 0.6 litre and +1 kPa (+10 cmH₂O) (equilibrium 0.5 litre). With a required tidal volume of 0.475 litre note the big reduction in duration of inflation needed when the inflation pressure is increased from 1 to 2 kPa (10 to 20 cmH₂O). (b) How expiration is influenced by the use of a subatmospheric pressure or 'negative phase'. Expiration may be terminated at the FRC after 0.6 s, or may be prolonged, in which case the lung volume will fall to 0.2 litre below the FRC.

kPa (10 cmH₂O). However, the same lung volume is achieved in only 0.3 second by doubling the inflation pressure. The application of a pressure which, if sustained, would give a tidal volume higher than that which is intended, is known as overpressure and is extensively used to increase the inspiratory flow rate and so to shorten the inspiratory phase. The use of a subatmospheric pressure to increase the rate of passive expiration is similar in principle but may be complicated by airway trapping (Figure 22.3b).

Deviations from true exponential character of expiration. It is helpful to assume that the patterns of air flow described above are exponential in character since this greatly assists our understanding of the situation. However, there are many reasons why air flow should not be strictly exponential in character. Air flow is normally partly turbulent (see Chapter 4) and therefore resistance cannot be considered as a constant. Furthermore, as expiration proceeds, the calibre of the air passages decreases and there is also a transition to more laminar flow as the instantaneous flow rate decreases. Approximation to a single exponential function is nevertheless good enough for many practical purposes.

Alternative patterns of application of inflation pressure

Constant pressure or square wave inflation has been considered above because it is the easiest for mathematical analysis. There are, however, an almost infinite number of pressure profiles which may be applied for IPPV. There is no very convincing evidence of the superiority of one over the other, except that distribution of inspired gas is improved if there is a prolongation of the period during which the applied pressure is maximal. This permits better ventilation of the 'slow' alveoli (page 45) and is not very important in patients with relatively healthy lungs.

Constant flow rate ventilators are extensively used, and Figure 22.4 shows pressure, volume and flow changes in a manner analogous to Figure 22.2. This pattern of air flow is conveniently achieved with electronically controlled ventilators such as the CPU-1 (Nunn and Lyle, 1986).

Sine wave generators were popular in the days of mechanical (as opposed to electronic) ventilators, and the pattern of inspiratory flow rate was a direct consequence of the mechanical linkage in ventilators such as the original Engstrom and Smith-Clark. Figure 22.5 shows the pattern of pressure, volume and flow rate changes with a sine wave generator.

Control of duration of inspiration

Three methods are in general use.

Time cycling terminates inspiration after a preset time. With mechanical ventilators delivering a sine pressure wave, the inspiratory time usually derives directly from the pressure generator itself. However, with constant pressure generators and constant flow generators, a separate and variable timing device is incorporated. With constant flow generators, inspiratory time has a direct effect on the tidal volume. With constant pressure generators the relationship is more complex, as described above (see Figure 22.3).

Volume cycling terminates inspiration when a preset volume has been delivered. In the absence of a leak this should guarantee the tidal volume even if the compliance or resistance of the patient changes within limits. Formerly, volume-cycled ventilators were usually based on a reciprocating pump of preset tidal volume. Nowadays they are more likely to be flow generators with an inspiratory flow sensor which terminates inspiration when the required volume (integral of flow rate) has entered the lungs.

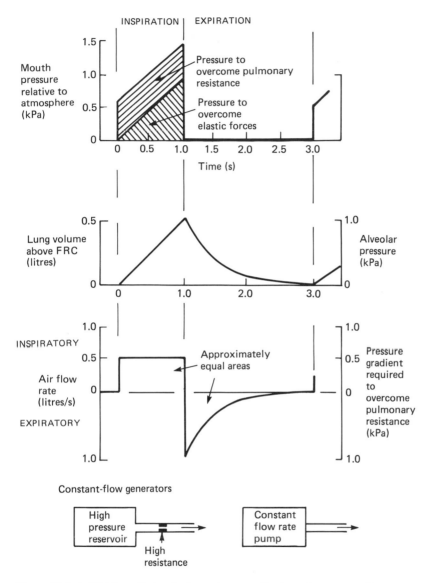

INSPIRATION | EXPIRATION

Mouth pressure relative to atmosphere (kPa)

Pressure to overcome pulmonary resistance

Pressure to overcome elastic forces

Time (s)

Lung volume above FRC (litres)

Alveolar pressure (kPa)

INSPIRATORY

Air flow rate (litres/s)

EXPIRATORY

Approximately equal areas

Pressure gradient required to overcome pulmonary resistance (kPa)

Constant-flow generators

High pressure reservoir

High resistance

Constant flow rate pump

Figure 22.4 Artificial ventilation by intermittent application of a constant-flow generator with passive expiration. Note that inspiratory flow rate is constant. Assuming that pulmonary resistance is constant, it follows that a constant amount of the inflation pressure is required to overcome flow resistance. Lung volume and alveolar pressure may be shown on the same graph if compliance is constant. Values are typical of an anaesthetized supine paralysed patient: total dynamic compliance, 0.5 l/kPa (50 ml/cmH$_2$O); pulmonary resistance, 0.3 kPa l^{-1} s (3 cmH$_2$O/l/sec); apparatus resistance, 0.7 kPa l^{-1} s (7 cmH$_2$O/l/sec); total resistance, 1 kPa l^{-1} s (10 cmH$_2$O/l/sec); time constant, 0.5 s.

Pressure cycling terminates inspiration when a particular mouth pressure is achieved. This in no way guarantees the tidal volume. Increased airway resistance, for example, would limit inspiratory flow rate and cause a more rapid increase in mouth pressure, thus terminating the inspiratory phase. Pressure-cycled ventilators are almost invariably flow generators.

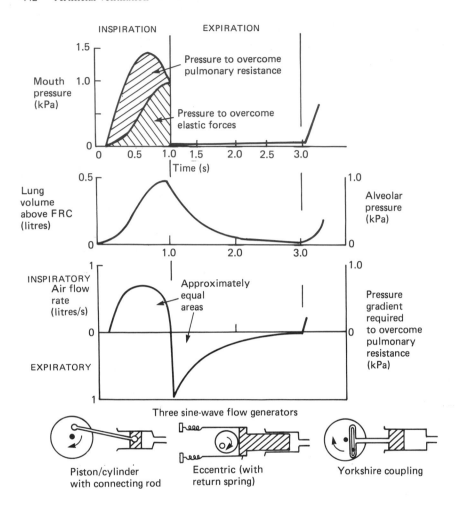

Figure 22.5 Artificial ventilation with inspiratory gas flow conforming to a sine wave. Passive expiration. Note that inspiratory gas flow rate is out of phase with the change in lung volume. (The latter conforms to a sine wave and the former to the differential of the sine which is the cosine.) Assuming that air flow resistance is constant, it follows that flow rate and pressure gradient required to overcome resistance may be shown on the same graph. Lung volume and alveolar pressure may be shown on the same graph if compliance is constant. Peak inspiratory flow rate $= \pi \times$ the minute volume $\times 1.5$. (The factor 1.5 is inserted because in this example inspiration does not last half the respiratory cycle.) Values are typical of an anaesthetized supine paralysed patient: total dynamic compliance, 0.5 l/kPa (50 ml/cmH$_2$O); pulmonary resistance, 0.3 kPa l^{-1} s (3 cmH$_2$O/l/sec); apparatus resistance, 0.7 kPa l^{-1} s (7 cmH$_2$O/l/sec; total resistance, 1 kPa^{-1} s (10 cmH$_2$O/l/sec)/ time constant, 0.5 s.

Limitations on inspiratory duration. Whatever the means of cycling, it is possible to add a limitation on inspiratory duration, usually as a safety precaution. For example, a pressure limitation can be added to a time cycled or a volume cycled ventilator. This can either function as a pressure relief valve or it can terminate the inspiratory phase.

The inspiratory/expiratory (*I/E*) ratio

For a given minute volume of ventilation, it is possible to vary within wide limits the duration of inspiration and expiration and the ratio between the two. The commonest pattern is about 1 second for inspiration, followed by 2–4 seconds for expiration (*I/E* ratio 1:2–1:4), giving respiratory frequencies in the range 12–20 breaths per minute. The problem is whether changes from this pattern confer any appreciable benefit in terms of gas exchanges. There is no guarantee that studies in animals or healthy anaesthetized patients are relevant to patients with pulmonary dysfunction in whom some benefit might be expected to accrue. Watson (1962b) demonstrated a substantial increase in dead space in patients in an intensive therapy unit when the duration of inspiration was reduced below 1 second. A similar but less marked change was found in anaesthetized patients with healthy lungs by Bergman (1967) and Fairley and Blenkarn (1966). Sykes and Lumley (1969) reported the same effect during cardiac surgery. However, the changes have mostly been too small to be of much clinical significance except in the study of Watson. The consensus view seems to be that 1 second is a reasonable minimal time for inspiration.

There seems to be no convincing evidence in any of the studies cited above that the duration of inspiration (in the range 0.5–3 seconds) has any appreciable effect on the alveolar/arterial PO_2 gradient.

Inverse I/E ratio ventilation has the effect of increasing the mean lung volume and so may be expected to achieve some of the advantages of positive end-expiratory pressure (PEEP) as considered below. It may be achieved either by slowing the inspiratory flow rate (shallow ramp) or by holding the lung volume at the end of inspiration (inspiratory pause or 'top hat' profile), the latter appearing to be more logical. *I/E* ratios as high as 4:1 have been used but 2:1 is generally preferable. A limiting factor is the time available for expiration. If this is unduly curtailed, FRC will be increased, so-called 'auto-PEEP' (see below).

Gas redistribution during an inspiratory hold reduces the dead space (page 176) and so results in a lower PCO_2 for the same minute volume (Fuleihan, Wilson and Pontoppidan, 1976). This permits the use of a lower peak inflation pressure. Shunting is also reduced (Perez-Chada et al., 1983), presumably because of the increased fraction of the respiratory cycle during which airways tend to be patent. Clinical applications were described by Cole, Weller and Sykes (1984).

Interaction of ventilator controls

The commonest controls which are provided on an artificial ventilator are drawn from the following list:

tidal volume
inspiratory flow rate
duration of inspiration
duration of expiration
I/E ratio
respiratory frequency
minute volume

It will be found that the maximum possible number of independent controls is three. A setting of any three on this list will determine the values for all the remaining variables. Opinion is divided on which of these controls the clinician likes to operate directly. However, an excellent compromise is to display computed values corresponding to the variables which are not available as controls.

Special techniques for IPPV
(see review by Slutsky, 1988)

Non-mechanical methods

Expired air resuscitation has been considered above under 'Methods used for resuscitation'.

Glossopharyngeal respiration (frog breathing) is a technique which may be helpful for short periods in patients with paresis of the respiratory muscle who retain the use of the muscles used in swallowing. Gulps of air are taken into the mouth and passed into the lungs which are thus inflated stepwise. After a number of swallows, a passive expiration takes place (Dail, Affeldt and Collier, 1955).

Venturis and jets

Venturis and jets can be used to generate a positive pressure which can be applied intermittently during bronchoscopy to maintain ventilation without any mechanical barrier to obstruct the line of vision. If oxygen is used as the driving gas, air is entrained to provide an inspired gas mixture of appropriate oxygen concentration (Sanders, 1967).

The same principle has been used in a simple, convenient and highly controllable artificial ventilator which can also provide positive pressure during expiration (Whitwam et al., 1983). Jet ventilators are essentially T-piece circuits. Fresh gas is supplied by the afferent limb while the efferent limb contains four jets. Three facing the patient can provide any required pressure during inspiration or expiration while the fourth, facing away from the patient, can provide subatmospheric pressure if required during expiration. By setting the timing and the profile of the flow rates through the various jets it is possible to provide total control of the airway pressures throughout the respiratory cycle. The system operates as a time-phased pressure generator but one which is particularly easy to control and is particularly suitable for feedback control and servo operation. Important features are that jet ventilators can operate at very high frequencies and do not require valves.

High frequency ventilation
(see reviews by Slutsky, 1988, and Smith, 1990)

Öberg and Sjöstrand (1967, unpublished) made the surprising observation that effective respiration could be maintained in dogs during artificial ventilation at a respiratory frequency of 80 b.p.m. with a tidal volume which did not appear to be sufficient to wash out the dead space (Sjöstrand, 1980). It was soon found that similar techniques could be applied to patients (Heijman et al., 1972).

High frequency ventilation may be classified into the following categories: high frequency positive pressure ventilation (HFPPV), high frequency jet ventilation (HFJV) and high frequency oscillation (HFO).

High frequency positive pressure ventilation (HFPPV) is applied in the frequency range 1–2 Hz (60–120 b.p.m.) and can be considered as an extension of conventional IPPV techniques. Although many conventional ventilators will operate in this frequency range, specially designed jet injectors have also been used. The method has enjoyed limited application for endoscopy and airway surgery but the advantages of high frequency have not been proven.

High frequency jet ventilation (HFJV) covers the frequency range 1–5 Hz. Inspiration is driven by a high velocity stream of gas from a jet, which may or may not entrain gas from a secondary supply. Usually only the latter can be humidified. The position of the jet may be proximal to the patient, in the hope of avoiding dead space, or more distal which is safer in terms of mucosal trauma and thermal injury from cooling due to the Joule–Kelvin effect (Smith, 1990). A unique advantage is the possibility of ventilating through a narrow cannula, as for example through the cricothyroid membrane.

HFJV has been extensively used both in the operating theatre and during intensive therapy. Jet systems are extremely versatile. Jets may face towards or away from the patient and may thus power inspiration, retard expiration, assist expiration or provide PEEP. It has been proposed that purely passive expiration be designated by the suffix -P and actively assisted expiration by the suffix -A (Froese and Bryan (1987).

High frequency oscillation (HFO) covers the frequency range 3–50 Hz and the flows are usually generated by an oscillating pump or diaphragm making a fourth connection to a T-piece with a low pass filter on the open limb (Figure 22.6). At these high frequencies, the respiratory waveform is usually sinusoidal. Tidal volumes are inevitably small and are difficult to measure.

Studies in dogs have shown that satisfactory gas exchange may be maintained by this technique, for periods up to at least 36 hours, with oscillator frequencies in the range 13–28 Hz. Small pleural effusions were found in dogs ventilated at high frequency but otherwise there were no important differences in respiratory or cardiovascular function when high frequency was compared with conventional artificial ventilation (Rehder, Schmid and Knopp, 1983). However, in another study by the same group it was shown that oxygenation and the uniformity of distribution of ventilation and perfusion were somewhat better at 5.8 Hz than at 15 or 29.8 Hz or with conventional artificial ventilation (Brusasco et al., 1984).

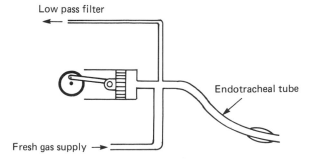

Figure 22.6 Circuit for provision of high frequency oscillation.

Satisfactory results have been obtained in anaesthetized man (Crawford and Rehder, 1985). Butler et al. (1980), using oscillator frequencies of 15 Hz (900 b.p.m.) with volume settings in the range 50–150 ml, obtained satisfactory levels of P_{CO_2} and P_{O_2} in 12 patients requiring artificial ventilation for respiratory failure. Cardiac output was much the same for both IPPV and HFO. Mean shunt was decreased with HFO in all 8 patients in whom the measurement was made, the benefit being greatest in those patients thought to have an extensive mismatch of ventilation and perfusion. However, in spite of intense research interest in this revolutionary technique, its adoption into clinical practice has been slow.

The relationship between tidal volume and dead space during high frequency ventilation is crucial to an understanding of the technique. It is useless to infer values for tidal volume and dead space from measurements made under other circumstances and yet it is very difficult to make direct measurements of these variables under the actual conditions of high frequency ventilation, especially in man. Chakrabarti, Gordon and Whitwam (1986) studied anaesthetized man during HFPPV up to frequencies of 2 Hz, holding arterial P_{CO_2} approximately constant at about 5 kPa (37.5 mmHg). As frequency increased from conventional ventilation at 15 b.p.m. to HFPPV at 2 Hz it was necessary to double the minute volume (Table 22.4). The actual volume of the physiological dead space decreased with decreasing tidal volume to reach a minimal value of about 90 ml at about 1 Hz. However, the normal proportionality between dead space and tidal volume (page 172) was not maintained. Dead space/tidal volume ratio increased from 37% at 15 b.p.m. to 75% at 2 Hz, which explains the requirement for the increased minute volume. The situation is more complex at higher frequencies. Butler et al. (1980) found that tidal volumes of at least 100 ml were still required at frequencies of 15 Hz, corresponding to an *applied* minute volume of 90 l/min which would indicate a dead space/tidal volume ratio of over 90%. There are severe technical difficulties in the measurement of the actual delivered tidal volumes which, though undoubtedly less than the pump settings, are probably much larger than the external movements of the thorax would suggest.

End-expiratory pressure is inevitably raised at high frequencies because the duration of expiration will be inadequate for passive exhalation to FRC, the time constant of the normal respiratory system being about 0.5 second (see above).

Table 22.4 Gas exchange during high frequency ventilation

		Respiratory frequency		
		15 b.p.m. *0.25 Hz*	*60 b.p.m.* *1 Hz*	*120 b.p.m.* *2 Hz*
Arterial P_{CO_2}	kPa	4.8	4.8	4.9
	mmHg	36	36	37
$\dot{V}$	l/min	6.8	10.2	14
V_T	ml	454	170	117
V_D (physiol.)	ml	165	96	88
V_D/V_T ratio	%	36	56	75

(Data from Chakrabarti, Gordon and Whitwam, 1986)

Therefore, the use of respiratory frequencies above about 2 Hz will usually result in 'auto-PEEP' (Beamer et al., 1984), and hence an increased end-expiratory lung volume which is likely to be a major factor promoting favourable gas exchange (see page 451).

Gas mixing and streaming is likely to be modified at high frequencies. The sudden reversals of flow direction are likely to set up eddies which blur the boundary between dead space and alveolar gas, thus improving the efficiency of ventilation. It has been suggested that such 'enhanced diffusion' or 'augmented dispersion' plays a major role in gas exchange during HFO (Butler et al., 1980; Rossing et al., 1981). Air passages dilated by auto-PEEP may contribute to this effect. Furthermore, cardiac mixing of gases becomes relatively more important at small tidal volumes (Nunn and Hill, 1960). It has also been suggested that high frequency ventilation causes 'accelerated diffusion', but this is difficult to demonstrate.

The clinical indications for high frequency ventilation are still not clear. HFJV seems to have a wider acceptance than HFPPV or HFO, but randomized trials have generally failed to demonstrate any clear clinical advantage over conventional methods of ventilation (Carlon, Howland and Ray, 1983; Hurst et al., 1990). There is no doubt that effective gas exchange is usually possible with high frequency ventilation but the advantages over conventional artificial ventilation are less clear. Although there are enthusiasts, others believe that it is merely a technique in search of an application. There is agreement on its special role for patients with bronchopleural fistula and the technique is particularly convenient when there is no airtight junction between ventilator and the tracheobronchial tree, at laryngoscopy, for example. Another attractive feature is the avoidance of high *peak* inspiratory pressures. However, *mean* airway pressure may still be high if exhalation is impeded, as it must be at very high frequencies. Whether high frequency ventilation is less likely to produce pulmonary barotrauma than conventional techniques of ventilation will be difficult to determine in man but animal experiments suggest this may be so (Kolton et al., 1982). It may prove valuable to combine high frequency ventilation with conventional artificial ventilation.

Perhaps the major difficulty lies in the prediction of efficiency of gas exchange in a particular patient. Tidal volume cannot easily be measured and reliance must be placed on arterial blood gas tensions.

Differential lung ventilation

There are many circumstances, such as posture, surgery and disease, which impose different requirements for optimal ventilatory patterns for the two lungs (Nunn, 1961a; Hedenstierna, 1985; Zandstra, 1989). Techniques are now available for use of selective tidal volumes and selective PEEP for the two lungs. Such techniques are complex and require double-lumen tracheal intubation. Nevertheless, there is no question that they can optimize gas exchange (Hedenstierna et al., 1984). A similar problem is considered in relation to one-lung anaesthesia' (page 415).

Application of subatmospheric pressure to the trunk

Cabinet ventilators differ from conventional IPPV in reducing the pressure surrounding the trunk rather than raising the airway pressure. However, in terms of the airway-to-ambient pressure gradient they are identical in principle (Figure 22.7). The special attraction of the technique is that it can be used for patients without tracheostomies or tracheal tubes. However, vomiting or regurgitation of gastric contents exposes the patient to the danger of aspiration during the inspiratory phase, and fatalities have occurred under particularly distressing circumstances. The method is now seldom used.

Cuirass ventilators are a simplified form of cabinet ventilators in which the application of subatmospheric pressure is confined to the anterior abdominal wall. Function depends on a good airtight seal. They are less efficient than cabinet ventilators and suffer from the same disadvantages. However, they are much more convenient to use and may be useful to supplement inadequate spontaneous breathing. High frequency ventilation by chest wall compression is possible

ARTIFICIAL VENTILATION BY INTERMITTENT POSITIVE PRESSURE

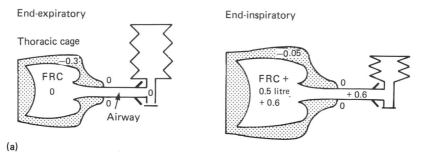

(a)

ARTIFICIAL VENTILATION BY CABINET RESPIRATOR

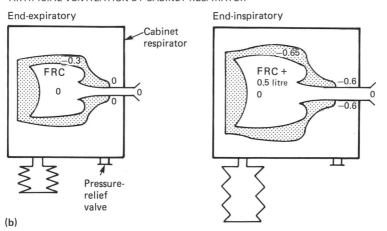

(b)

Figure 22.7 Comparison of artificial ventilation by (a) intermittent positive pressure (IPP) and (b) cabinet respirator (subatmospheric pressures only). The actual pressures differ in the two techniques, but the following pressure gradients are the same in both cases: mouth-to-ambient; alveolar-to-intrathoracic (transmural); intrathoracic-to-ambient. Ambient pressure refers to the pressure surrounding the trunk and is therefore cabinet pressure in the latter case. Static values for supine anaesthetized patient: lung compliance, 1.5 l/kPa (150 ml/cmH₂O); thoracic cage compliance, 2 l/kPa (200 ml/cmH₂O); total compliance, 0.85 l/kPa (85 ml/cmH₂O). (Intrathoracic space is shown stippled.) Figures indicate pressures relative to atmosphere in kilopascals.

(Zidulka et al., 1983) and this may be favourable for clearance of secretions. It may find a role in combination with IPPV.

Intermittent mandatory ventilation (IMV)

IMV was introduced by Downs and his colleagues in Gainsville in 1973. The essential feature is provision of a parallel inspiratory gas circuit which allows the patient to take a spontaneous breath between artificial breaths. This confers three major advantages. Firstly, a spontaneous inspiration is not obstructed by a closed inspiratory valve and this helps to prevent the patient fighting the ventilator. It is very distressing for a conscious patient to attempt to inhale against the closed valves of a mechanical ventilator and it results in a large abdominal/thoracic pressure gradient which may cause gastric regurgitation. It has been claimed that the use of IMV reduces the demand for sedatives. The second advantage is the facilitation of weaning, which is considered further below. IMV permits a gradual resumption of spontaneous breathing, during which ventilator support is only gradually reduced (Downs, Perkins and Modell, 1974). Thirdly, the patient is enabled to breathe spontaneously at any time during prolonged ventilation; this may prevent respiratory muscle atrophy and helps to reduce the mean intrathoracic pressure.

Most modern ventilators now provide IMV as a normal feature. The parallel circuit for spontaneous breathing should provide humidified inspired gas with the correct oxygen concentration. The pressure should also be appropriate to any expiratory pressure which is in use, and this is discussed below. Unfortunately, many ventilators using demand valves impose a substantial inspiratory load for spontaneous breaths. This increases the work of breathing (Gibney, Wilson and Pontoppidan, 1982).

A review by Weisman et al. (1983) challenged the concept that continuous spontaneous breathing is beneficial for a patient on IPPV. They pointed out that few of the advantages claimed for IMV have been demonstrated in controlled trials. Nevertheless, the conduct of a controlled trial in these circumstances is not easy, as it is extremely difficult to control the variables.

Airway pressure release ventilation

This technique is essentially IMV, with the reverse of intermittent positive pressure ventilation. It consists of constant positive airway pressure (CPAP), which may be intermittently released to cause the patient to *exhale* to FRC with a subsequent inspiration when CPAP is reapplied (Downs and Stock, 1987; Downs, 1992). The patient is able to breathe as he wishes during the periods when CPAP is applied, but this is from the lung volume following an inspiration after reapplication of CPAP. Artificial breaths are thus within the conventional tidal range set by his FRC, while spontaneous inspirations are within his inspiratory reserve. The CPAP release valve is controlled to provide mandatory ventilation as for IMV. The pattern of the imposed breaths is basically similar to that of reversed *I/E* ratio (see above). Dead space was found to be significantly less, but intrapulmonary shunt more, than with synchronized intermittent positive pressure ventilation (Valentine et al., 1991).

Interaction between patient and ventilator

The major weakness of all the ventilator systems mentioned above is that they lack feedback from the patient to the ventilator, which cannot, therefore, respond to any spontaneous respiratory activity by the patient. However, for many years there have been ventilators in which the inspiratory phase could be triggered with a spontaneous breath. More recently there has appeared a generation of ventilators in which the applied minute volume can be modified by the spontaneous minute volume which the patient is able to achieve.

Triggered and synchronized ventilators

The onset of the inspiratory phase of a ventilator may be brought forward by detection of inspiratory flow or the subatmospheric pressure generated by a spontaneous breath. This has three distinct applications. The original purpose was as an aid to weaning, for which it was rather disappointing (see below). Later it came to be used to assist an inadequate inspiration in a partially paralysed patient in whom it was thought desirable to preserve the spontaneous respiration rhythm. More recently it has been found to be a most effective method of synchronizing the ventilator to spontaneous respiration. In this application, it is an adjunct to IMV and is called synchronized IMV (SIMV). Figure 22.8 shows the synchronization of artificial ventilation to a spontaneous respiratory rhythm with the CPU-1 ventilator (Nunn and Lyle, 1986).

Inspiratory pressure support ventilation

In this system a spontaneous inspiration triggers a variable flow of gas that increases until airway pressure reaches a preselected level (see reviews by Wahba, 1990, and Downs, 1992). The purpose is not to provide a prescribed tidal volume,

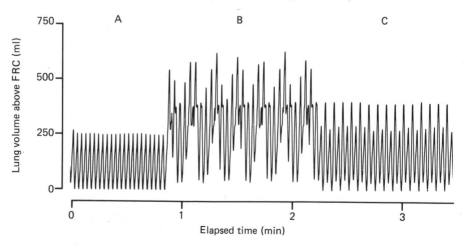

Figure 22.8 Synchronization of artificial ventilation with spontaneous breathing in a model patient using the Ohmeda CPU-1 ventilator. A: spontaneous breathing (tidal volume 250 ml at 26 b.p.m.). B: artificial ventilation superimposed (tidal volume 350 ml at 20 b.p.m.). C: synchronization mode used to obtain augmentation of alternative breaths at 13 b.p.m. (Reproduced from Nunn and Lyle (1986) by permission of the Editors of the British Journal of Anaesthesia)

but to assist the patient in making an inspiration of a pattern which lies largely within his own control, and patients usually find this very acceptable (MacIntyre, 1986). The level of support may be increased until the pressure is sufficient to provide the full tidal volume (maximal pressure support) or may be gradually reduced as the patient's ventilatory capacity improves. Design features were considered at a conference reported by MacIntyre et al. (1990). Valentine et al. (1991) found the essential parameters of gas exchange not greatly different from synchronized intermittent mandatory ventilation.

Mandatory minute volume (MMV)

Hewlett, Platt and Terry (1977) described a simple technique for controlling the volume of artificial ventilation so that the total of spontaneous and artificial ventilation did not fall below a preset value. The principle is outlined in Figure 22.9a. If the patient is able to achieve the preset level of MMV, the ventilator remains inoperative. If the patient stops breathing, the ventilator then supplies the preset level of MMV. If the patient is able to achieve a part of the MMV, his contribution is subtracted from the total and the ventilator supplies the difference (Figure 22.9b). There must be provision for the spontaneous ventilation to exceed the MMV.

This system has a number of applications. Firstly, it can be an effective technique for weaning (see below). Secondly, spontaneous breaths by a ventilated patient do not necessarily increase the minute volume as would occur with IMV. Thus hypocapnia is avoided and the patient's respiratory efforts are not discouraged. Thirdly, for a patient who is breathing spontaneously, MMV provides an excellent safeguard against any reduction in spontaneous breathing which might result from such causes as sleep, administration of opiate, respiratory muscle fatigue or the fluctuations of a myasthenic crisis.

Positive end-expiratory pressure (PEEP)

A great variety of pathological conditions, as well as general anaesthesia, result in a decrease in FRC. The deleterious effect of this on gas exchange has been considered elsewhere (page 395) and it is reasonable to consider increasing the FRC by the application of PEEP, first described by Hill and his colleagues in 1965.

Expiratory pressure can be raised during both artificial ventilation and spontaneous breathing, and both forms are best considered together. The terminology is confusing and this chapter adheres to the definitions illustrated in Figure 22.10. Note in particular sPEEP in which a patient inhales spontaneously from ambient pressure but exhales against PEEP. This involves him in a considerable amount of additional work of breathing because he must raise his entire minute volume to the level of PEEP which is applied. This is undesirable and continuous positive airway pressure (CPAP) is much to be preferred to sPEEP. Unfortunately, true CPAP is more difficult to achieve than sPEEP. Biased demand valves may be used but usually result in a pronounced dip in inspiratory pressure, increasing the total work of breathing. Loaded bellows are better but less convenient to manufacture. A high degree of constancy of airway pressure may be achieved with a weighted inspiratory bellows and balanced PEEP valve, with which the inspiratory/expiratory pressure difference was only about 0.1 kPa (1 cmH$_2$O) during spontaneous breathing

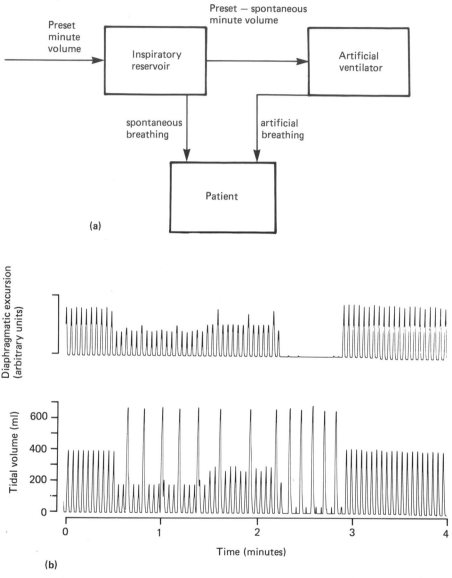

(a)

(b)

Figure 22.9 (a) The principle of mandatory minute volume (MMV). The mandatory minute volume is set on the rotameters and the patient breathes as much as he is able from the inspiratory reservoir. What is left is supplied as artificial ventilation (see text). (b) The upper trace shows the 'diaphragmatic excursion' of a model patient. The lower trace shows lung volume in the mandatory minute volume mode using the system of Hewlett, Platt and Terry (1977). For the first 30 seconds, the tidal volume of 400 ml at 18 b.p.m. (minute volume 7.2 l/min) is in excess of the mandatory minute volume setting (6.3 l/min). Thereafter, changes in spontaneous tidal volume result in intermittent breaths of artificial ventilation to preserve the required mandatory minute volume. Total apnoea supervenes at 2.3 minutes and ventilation is then totally artificial. (Reproduced from Nunn (1983) by courtesy of the Editors of the Japanese Journal of Clinical Anaesthesia*)*

(Hewlett, Platt and Terry, 1977). The simplest approach is a T-piece with a high fresh gas flow venting through a PEEP valve at the expiratory limb throughout the respiratory phase. This has been successfully used in the treatment of sleep apnoea (page 337). The problem was considered in some detail by Hillman and Finucane (1985).

PEEP may be achieved by many techniques. The simplest is to exhale through a preset depth of water but more convenient methods are spring-loaded valves or diaphragms pressed down by gas or a column of water. It is also possible to use venturis and fans opposing the direction of expiratory gas flow (see above). If a passive expiration is terminated before the lung volume has returned to FRC, there will be residual end-expiratory raised alveolar pressure variously known as intrinsic or auto-PEEP (Milic-Emili, 1992).

Respiratory effects

Lung volume. End-expiratory alveolar pressure will equal the level of applied PEEP and this will reset the FRC in accord with the pressure/volume curve of the respiratory system (see Figure 3.8). For example, PEEP of 1 kPa (10 cmH$_2$O) will increase FRC by 500 ml in a patient with a compliance of 0.5 l/kPa (50 ml/cmH$_2$O). In many patients this may be expected to raise the tidal range above the closing capacity (page 56). Opening of previously closed alveoli is probably the greatest single advantage of PEEP. It will also reduce airway resistance according to the

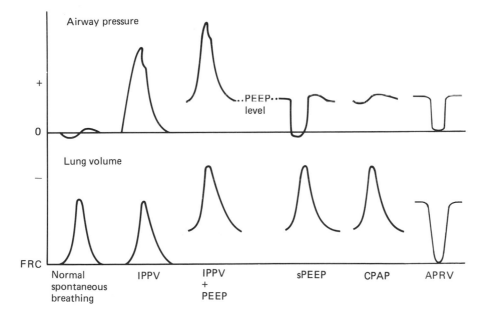

Figure 22.10 Definitions of nomenclature applied in this book to: IPPV, intermittent positive pressure ventilation; PEEP, positive end-expiratory pressure; sPEEP, true PEEP applied during spontaneous breathing; CPAP, continuous positive airway pressure applied during spontaneous breathing; and APRV, airway pressure release ventilation. Note the unsatisfactory pressure swings during sPEEP. (Reproduced from Nunn (1984) by permission of the Editors of Anesthesiology Clinics)

inverse relationship between lung volume and airway resistance (see Figure 4.11). It may also change the relative compliance of the upper and lower parts of the lung (Figure 22.11), thereby improving the ventilation of the dependent overperfused parts of the lung.

Dead space. Acute application of PEEP causes only a slight increase in dead space/tidal volume ratio (Bindslev et al., 1981; Lawler, 1987, personal communication). However, there is indirect evidence that long-term application of PEEP may cause a very large increase in the dead space, probably because of bronchiolar dilatation (see below).

Arterial P_{O_2}. It is unlikely that PEEP will improve arterial oxygenation appreciably in patients with healthy lungs, but there is no doubt of the decrease in pulmonary shunting which is obtained in a wide range of pulmonary pathology, including oedema, collapse and the adult respiratory distress syndrome. This has resulted in PEEP being widely applied in the field of intensive care, and Kirby and his colleagues (1975) extended its use to levels in excess of 1.5 kPa (15 cmH₂O). During anaesthesia, it has been repeatedly observed that PEEP does little to improve arterial oxygenation in the patient with sound lungs. Pulmonary shunting is decreased, but the accompanying decrease in cardiac output reduces the mixed venous oxygen saturation which counteracts the effect of a reduction in the shunt, resulting in minimal increase in arterial P_{O_2} (Bindslev et al., 1981). Dantzker, Lynch and Weg (1980) have suggested that shunt reduction in patients with adult respiratory distress syndrome is secondary to reduction in cardiac output (page 181).

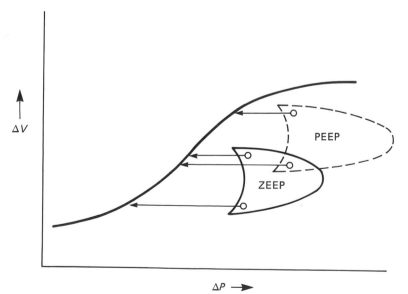

Figure 22.11 Effect of positive end-expiratory pressure (PEEP) on the relationship between regional pressure and volume in the lung (supine position). Note that compliance is greater in the upper part of the lung with zero end-expiratory pressure (ZEEP) and in the lower part of the lung with PEEP, which thus improves ventilation in the dependent zone of the lung. (Diagram kindly supplied by Professor J. Gareth Jones)

'*Best PEEP*' was originally defined as the level of PEEP at which the highest value for arterial P_{O_2} was attained. This is not necessarily the same value of PEEP which optimizes oxygen delivery (or flux) and Suter, Fairley and Isenberg (1975) suggested that the definition of 'best PEEP' be based on oxygen delivery. The definition may be further elaborated to include optimization of cardiac output in the face of PEEP by volume loading and administration of inotropes (see below).

Lung water. It was for many years believed that PEEP 'squeezed' oedema fluid out of the lung and that this was the cause of the dramatic improvement in arterial P_{O_2} which often followed the application of PEEP to patients with pulmonary oedema. However, there is good evidence that lung water is not decreased by PEEP (Miller et al., 1981; Rizk and Murray, 1982). The improvement in arterial P_{O_2} is probably due to opening up of closed alveoli, transfer of oedema fluid to the interstitial compartment (page 491) and the reduction in cardiac output which reduces shunting in a wide range of circumstances (Cheney and Colley, 1980).

Intrapleural pressure. The intrapleural pressure is protected from the level of PEEP by the transmural pressure gradient of the lungs. Patients with diseased lungs tend to have an increased transmural pressure gradient which limits the rise in intrapleural pressure (Figure 22.12). Therefore their cardiovascular systems are better protected against the adverse effects of PEEP (see below).

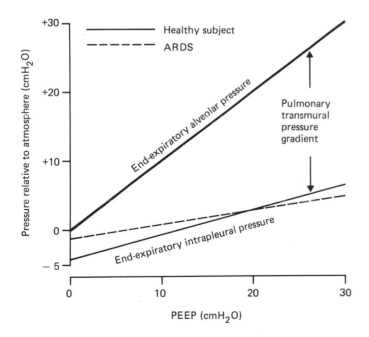

Figure 22.12 End-expiratory alveolar and intrapleural pressures as a function of positive end-expiratory pressure (PEEP). The lower continuous line shows intrapleural pressure in the relaxed healthy subject (Butler and Smith, 1957). The broken line shows values of intrapleural pressure in patients with adult respiratory distress syndrome (ARDS) taken from the work of Jardin et al. (1981). Absolute values of pressure probably reflect experimental technique and cannot be compared between the two studies. (Reproduced from Nunn (1984) by permission of the Editor of Anesthesiology Clinics)

Permeability. It has been found that PEEP increases the permeability of the lung to DTPA, a tracer molecule which does not readily cross the alveolar/capillary membrane (Rizk et al., 1984). However, it appears that this effect may be related to lung volume rather than to any damage to the membrane.

Barotrauma. A sustained increase in the transmural pressure gradient can damage the lung. The commonest forms of barotrauma attributable to artificial ventilation with or without PEEP are subcutaneous emphysema, pneumomediastinum and pneumothorax (Kumar et al., 1973). Tension lung cysts and hyperinflation of a lung or lobe have also been reported but the incidence of these complications is very variable. Pulmonary barotrauma probably starts as disruption of the alveolar membrane, with air entering the interstitial space and tracking back to the mediastinum along the bronchovascular bundles into the mediastinum from which it can reach the peritoneum, the pleural cavity or the subcutaneous tissues. Radiological demonstration of pulmonary interstitial gas may provide an early warning of barotrauma.

There is no agreement on the effect of PEEP on pulmonary barotrauma but Kumar et al. (1973) concluded that moderate levels of PEEP did not increase the level of barotrauma. However, Downs and Chapman (1976) found a very high incidence of barotrauma in patients exposed to PEEP in excess of 2 kPa (20 cmH$_2$O).

In patients who died following a prolonged period of exposure to PEEP, Slavin and his colleagues (1982) demonstrated at autopsy a gross dilatation of terminal and respiratory bronchioles which they termed bronchiolectasis (Figure 22.13). Development of the condition was found to be related to the level of PEEP and the

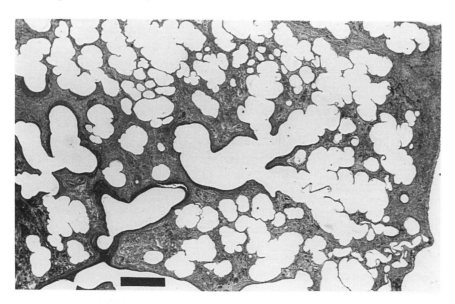

Figure 22.13 Histological appearances of bronchiolectasis in a patient who died after 16 days of artificial ventilation with positive end-capillary pressure of 0.5 kPa (5 cmH$_2$O). Terminal and respiratory bronchioles are grossly dilated and surrounding alveoli are collapsed. Diameter of a normal terminal bronchiole is 0.5 mm. Scale bar is 1 mm. (Reproduced from Nunn (1984) by permission of the Editors of Anesthesiology Clinics)

duration of its application. Indirect evidence suggested that it resulted in a large increase in dead space. Follow-up of a group of patients who had survived the use of PEEP indicated a return to normal pulmonary function with normal values for dead space (Navaratnarajah et al., 1984). The condition of bronchiolectasis appears to be analogous to bronchopulmonary dysplasia described in infants ventilated for respiratory distress syndrome (Taghizadeh and Reynolds, 1976). Pulmonary oedema has also been reported following the use of very high inflation pressures, but only with overdistension of the lungs (Dreyfuss et al., 1988).

The Valsalva effect

It has long been known that an increase in intrathoracic pressure has complex circulatory effects, characterized as the Valsalva effect, which is the circulatory response to a subject increasing his airway pressure to about 5 kPa (50 cmH$_2$O) against a closed glottis for about 30 seconds. The normal response is in four parts (Figure 22.14a). Initially the raised intrathoracic pressure alters the baseline for circulatory pressures and the arterial pressure (measured relative to atmosphere) is consequently increased (phase 1). At the same time, ventricular filling is decreased by the adverse pressure gradient from peripheral veins to the ventricle in diastole, and cardiac output therefore decreases. The consequent decline in arterial pressure in phase 2 is normally mitigated by three factors: tachycardia, increased systemic vascular resistance (afterload) and by an increase in peripheral venous pressure which tends to restore the venous return. As a result of these compensations, the arterial pressure normally settles to a value fairly close to the level before starting the Valsalva manoeuvre. When the intrathoracic pressure is restored to normal, there is an immediate decrease in arterial pressure due to the altered baseline. Simultaneously the venous return improves and therefore the cardiac output increases within a few seconds. However, the arteriolar bed remains constricted temporarily, and there is therefore a transient overshoot of arterial pressure.

Figure 22.14b shows the abnormal 'square wave' pattern which occurs with raised end-diastolic pressure or left ventricular failure or both. The initial increase in arterial pressure (phase 1) occurs normally, but the decline in pressure in phase 2 is missing because the output of the congested heart is not usually limited by end-diastolic pressure. Since the cardiac output is unchanged, there is no increase in pulse rate or systemic vascular resistance. Therefore there is no overshoot of pressure when the intrathoracic pressure is restored to normal.

Figure 22.14c shows a different abnormal pattern which may be seen with defective systemic vasoconstriction (e.g. with ganglion block or a spinal anaesthetic). Phase 1 is normal, but in phase 2 the decreased cardiac output is not accompanied by an increase in systemic vascular resistance and the arterial pressure therefore continues to decline. The normal overshoot is replaced by a slow recovery of arterial pressure as the cardiac output returns to control values.

Cardiovascular effects of PEEP

Initially there was great reluctance to use PEEP, partly because of the well known Valsalva effect, and partly because of the circulatory hazard which had been described in the classic paper of Cournand and his colleagues in 1948. Not too many papers in this field have two Nobel prize winners among their authors.

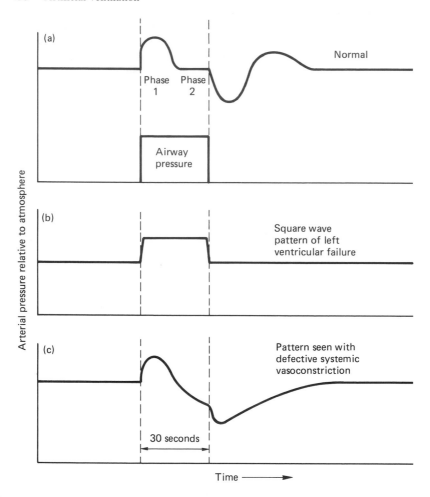

Figure 22.14 Qualitative changes in mean arterial pressure during a Valsalva manoeuvre as seen in the normal subject and for two abnormal responses. See text for explanation of the changes.

Cardiac output. Moderate levels of PEEP have relatively little effect on cardiac output. Suter, Fairley and Isenberg (1975) found in patients with acute pulmonary failure that PEEP had little effect on cardiac output up to the level of PEEP which maximized oxygen flux. However, in anaesthetized patients without pulmonary pathology, Bindslev et al. (1981) reported a 7% decrease in cardiac output with 0.9 kPa (9 cmH_2O) of PEEP. Progressive reduction in cardiac output was demonstrated for PEEP in the range 0.5–3 kPa (5–30 cmH_2O) in patients with adult respiratory distress syndrome (Jardin et al., 1981), but the effect was partially reversed by blood volume expansion (Figure 22.15).

There is general agreement that the main cause of the reduction in cardiac output is obstruction to filling of the right atrium, caused by the rise in intrathoracic pressure. The role of other factors has been hotly debated and consideration has been given to factors such as increased pulmonary capillary resistance (increased right ventricular afterload), decreased left ventricular compliance and decreased

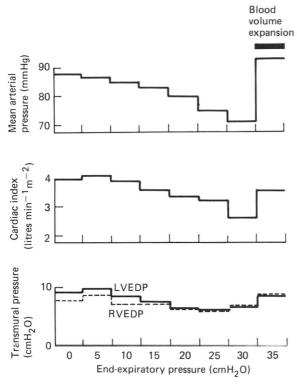

Figure 22.15 Cardiovascular responses as a function of positive end-expiratory pressure (PEEP) in patients with adult respiratory distress syndrome. Left and right ventricular end-diastolic pressure (LVEDP and RVEDP) were measured relative to intrapleural pressure. (Drawn from the data of Jardin et al. (1981) and reproduced from Nunn (1984) by permission of the Editors of Anesthesiology Clinics)

myocardial contractility. Furthermore, plasma from animals subjected to PEEP will depress contractility of isolated heart muscle preparations, suggesting the release of a negative inotrope (Grindlinger et al., 1979). Interactions of some of the factors by which PEEP may influence cardiac output and systemic arterial pressure are shown in Figure 22.16.

There are two pathological conditions in which the circulatory effects of PEEP are mitigated. With low pulmonary compliance, and therefore high transpulmonary pressure gradient, much of the raised intrapulmonary pressure is not transmitted to the great vessels in the chest. The effect on venous return and therefore cardiac output may then be minimal. The second condition is raised ventricular end-diastolic pressure with or without ventricular failure. Cardiac performance is then on the flat part of the cardiac output/filling pressure curve, and a reduction in end-diastolic pressure may not be deleterious and may even be favourable. This corresponds to the square wave pattern of Valsalva response (see Figure 22.14b) and is probably a factor in the success of continuous positive airway pressure in the treatment of cardiogenic pulmonary oedema (Räsänen et al., 1985).

Oxygen delivery. In many patients with pulmonary disease, PEEP tends to improve the arterial PO_2 while decreasing the cardiac output. As PEEP is increased the

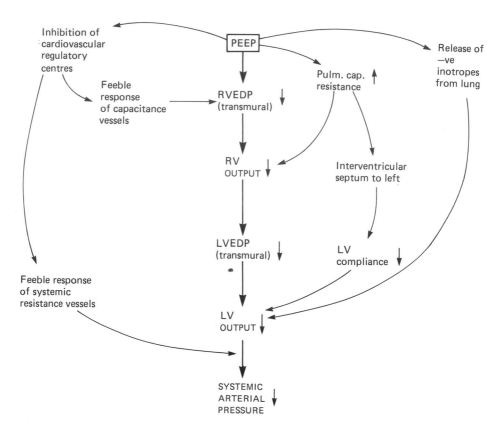

Figure 22.16 Summary of the cardiovascular effects of positive end-expiratory pressure (PEEP). See text for full explanation. RVEDP and LVEDP, right and left ventricular end-diastolic pressure; RV and LV, right and left ventricular

oxygen delivery (the product of cardiac output and arterial oxygen content, page 283) tends to rise to a maximum and then falls (Suter, Fairley and Isenberg, 1975). Suter and his colleagues described their 'best PEEP' as the level which maximized oxygen delivery. However, they did not optimize cardiac output with fluid replacement (see Figure 22.15) or with α-adrenergic stimulation or positive inotropes. It seems likely that they would have achieved better oxygen delivery at higher levels of PEEP had they done so.

Arterial blood pressure. Figure 22.15 shows the decline in arterial pressure closely following the change in cardiac output with increasing PEEP in Jardin's study. Although there was some increase in systemic vascular resistance, this was only about half that required for maintenance of the arterial pressure in the face of the declining cardiac output. It has been suggested that this is due to PEEP causing inhibition of the cardiovascular regulatory centres (Cassidy, Gaffney and Johnson, 1981).

Interpretation of vascular pressures. Atrial pressures are normally measured relative to atmospheric pressure. When PEEP is applied, atrial pressures tend to be increased relative to atmospheric. However, relative to intrathoracic pressure, they are reduced at higher levels of PEEP (Figure 22.15). It is the transmural pressure gradient and not the level relative to atmosphere which is relevant to atrial filling.

An additional problem arises if the tip of a Swan–Ganz catheter should lie in zone 1 of the lung where there is no pulmonary blood flow (page 149). It is possible that the application of PEEP increases the extent of zone 1, and an artefact may thus be introduced into the measurement of pulmonary capillary wedge pressure (Roy et al., 1977).

Renal effects

Patients undergoing IPPV tend to become oedematous. Protein depletion and inappropriate fluid loading may be factors but there is now evidence that PEEP may itself reduce glomerular filtration (Marquez et al., 1979). Arterial pressure tends to be reduced as described above, while central venous pressure is raised. Therefore, the pressure gradient between renal artery and vein is reduced and this has a direct effect on renal blood flow. In addition, PEEP causes elevated levels of vasopressin, possibly due to activation of left atrial receptors. However, the change in vasopressin level is insufficient to explain the changes in urinary flow rate.

Negative (subatmospheric) end-expiratory pressure (NEEP)

The potentially deleterious effect of PEEP on the circulation not only delayed its introduction into clinical practice, but also led to the use of NEEP, partly to facilitate expiration and partly for its supposedly beneficial effect on the circulation. NEEP was a fashionable extra on ventilators between about 1960 and 1970.

Respiratory effects

It might appear that the application of NEEP would increase the tidal volume by instituting a type of push–pull tidal exchange on either side of FRC. This, however, is unlikely to occur if FRC is close to residual volume, which tends to be the case during anaesthesia (page 393) and also in many patients who have severe respiratory problems. In such patients the inspiratory reserve remains the only practicable zone for increasing the tidal volume.

NEEP during expiration was originally seen as the counterpart of overpressure during inspiration, and Figure 22.3b shows how it might be used to obtain a reduction in the time required for expiration. However, expiration is fundamentally different from inspiration during IPPV. During inspiration there can be no question of airway collapse because the inflation pressure acts to distend the airways. During expiration, pressure gradients are acting to compress the airways as shown in Figure 4.8. Application of NEEP may then act directly to collapse the airways and so make matters worse. This is most likely to occur in patients with increased tendency to flow-related airway collapse, who are just the patients in whom some assistance to expiration might be required.

There has been no demonstration of any improvement of gas exchange with NEEP. In fact, Sykes et al. (1970) found the alveolar/arterial Po_2 gradient to be increased and Watson (1962b) found an increase in dead space.

Circulatory effects

If PEEP embarrasses the circulation, it appeared logical that NEEP would be beneficial. Unfortunately, this has not been borne out in practice. Scott, Stephen and Davie (1972), using NEEP of 0.5–0.7 kPa (5–7 cmH$_2$O), found no significant improvement in either cardiac output or arterial blood pressure in six patients undergoing artificial ventilation in an intensive care unit. Similar results were reported during anaesthesia (Prys-Roberts et al., 1967). Part of the difficulty probably lies in communicating the subatmospheric pressure to the intrathoracic space. Figure 20.12 shows that below FRC in the anaesthetized patient, the pressure/volume curve is very flat and the pulmonary transmural pressure gradient becomes very large as the lung volume decreases below FRC. It is not possible to communicate a subatmospheric pressure from the inside of a collapsed balloon to the exterior. As in the case of the respiratory effects, the supposed circulatory benefits of NEEP have not stood the test of time and the technique is now virtually obsolete.

Weaning

Weaning depends upon obtaining stable and satisfactory values for a range of respiratory variables, and typical criteria are listed in Table 22.5. The commonest technique of weaning is the abrupt cessation of artificial ventilation for periods of 2–3 minutes, with gradual prolongation of these periods depending upon the performance of the patient during the last period. Whereas this approach is satisfactory for an uncomplicated case and for healthy patients recovering from neuromuscular block, it may well be unsatisfactory for patients in whom ventilatory capacity and gas exchange function are marginal. Ventilatory capacity cannot, of course, be measured while the patient is still on a ventilator. Attempts to wean such patients often result in deterioration of minute volume and blood gases during short periods of spontaneous breathing, but there may be late deterioration caused by factors such as fatigue of the respiratory muscles (page 126).

No single variable is a reliable indicator of the success of a wean. Minute volume is probably the most useful, but it is also necessary to take into account arterial P$_{O_2}$ and P$_{CO_2}$, bearing in mind that the latter will rise only slowly (page 240). In addition to these measurements, it is necessary to observe the patient for signs of

Table 22.5 Criteria for weaning

Tests of ventilatory capacity	
VC	$\geq$ 10–15 ml/kg
FEV$_{1.0}$	$\geq$ 10 ml/kg
Peak insp. pressure	-20 to -30 cmH$_2$O
Resting minute volume	> 10 l/min (doubled with max. effort)
Tests of blood oxygenation	
(A–a) P$_{O_2}$ difference	< 40–47 kPa (300–350 mmHg)
Shunt	< 10–20%
Dead space/tidal volume	< 55–60%

(After Weisman et al., 1983)

fatigue, distress and dyscoordinated breathing. In cases of difficulty, various alternative techniques of weaning may be tried.

Triggered ventilators (page 450) have been used to encourage the patient to re-establish spontaneous respiration. However, results were generally disappointing and the technique is now seldom used. It has even been suggested that the patient might come to realize that he need not make a full respiratory effort and so be discouraged.

Respiratory stimulants may be helpful, and doxapram is the best agent since it shows minimal tachyphylaxis. An intravenous infusion in the range 1–8 mg/min may be started just before disconnecting the ventilator. This may be continued for some days, with gradual reduction of the infusion rate.

Intermittent mandatory ventilation (page 449) is a very valuable aid to weaning, which is accomplished by progressive reduction of the mandatory ventilation. This approach avoids the abrupt transition between artificial and spontaneous ventilation and supplies the patient with a fall-back level of ventilation which is progressively reduced. Clearly a dangerous situation might arise if spontaneous ventilation suddenly deteriorated in the late phase of a wean when the mandatory ventilation had been reduced to a level insufficient to maintain life. However, monitoring of the patient should avoid this eventuality and the method has gained wide acceptance. Nevertheless, differing opinions have been expressed on the value of IMV for weaning (Downs, Perkins and Modell, 1974; Weisman et al., 1983).

Mandatory minute volume (page 451) assists weaning from a completely different standpoint. The patient is left to resume spontaneous breathing if and when he is able. Artificial ventilation is reduced by whatever amount he is able to breathe, so that total minute volume and arterial P_{CO_2} should remain approximately the same. No active intervention is required by staff and the ratio of spontaneous to artificial ventilation may fluctuate widely for a considerable period before spontaneous breathing becomes fully established. Essentially the patient is allowed to wean himself in his own time, with the guarantee that his minute volume will be protected whether he breathes or not.

It should, however, be stressed that, although the minute volume is protected, there is no guarantee that the alveolar ventilation will remain constant. If the patient takes rapid and shallow breaths, this may be interpreted by the apparatus as an adequate minute volume while an increased dead space/tidal volume ratio may make the alveolar ventilation inadequate. In this connection it should be noted that the Erica ventilator in the MMV mode disregards low levels of spontaneous respiration. The efficacy of MMV for weaning has not yet been tested in a controlled trial.

Ventilation of the newborn

This subject is considered in Chapter 18.

Chapter 23

Physiological basis of extracorporeal gas exchange

Extracorporeal gas exchangers were first developed for cardiac surgery. Certain procedures were possible with stopped circulation, often prolonged by the induction of hypothermia. However, more intricate operations required an open heart for periods in excess of 20 minutes and this could not be achieved safely with simple cardiac arrest and hypothermia. Subsequently the use of extracorporeal gas exchange was extended into the treatment of respiratory failure.

Factors in design

The lungs of an adult have an interface between blood and gas of the order of 126 m^2 (page 29). It is not possible to achieve this in an artificial substitute and artificial lungs can be considered to have a very low 'diffusing capacity'. Nevertheless, they function satisfactorily within limits, for many reasons.

Factors favouring performance

1. The real lung is adapted for maximal exercise, while patients on cardiopulmonary bypass are usually close to basal metabolic rate or less if hypothermia is used.
2. Under resting conditions at sea level, there is an enormous reserve in the capacity of the lung to achieve equilibrium between pulmonary capillary blood and alveolar gas (see Figure 9.2). Therefore a subnormal diffusing capacity does not necessarily result in arterial hypoxaemia.
3. It is possible to operate an artificial lung with an 'alveolar' oxygen concentration in excess of 90%, compared with 14% for real alveolar gas under normal circumstances. This greatly increases the gas transfer for a given 'diffusing capacity' of the artificial lung (page 203).
4. There is no great difficulty in increasing the 'ventilation/perfusion ratio' of a membrane artificial lung above the value of about 0.8 in the normal lung at rest.
5. The 'capillary transit time' of an artificial lung can be increased beyond the 0.75 second in the real lung. This facilitates the approach of blood P_{O_2} to 'alveolar' P_{O_2} (see Figure 9.2).
6. It is possible to use countercurrent flow between gas and blood. This does not occur in the lungs of mammals although it is used in the gills of fishes.

Carbon dioxide exchanges much more readily than oxygen because of its greater blood and lipid solubility. Therefore, in general, elimination of carbon dioxide does not present a major problem and the limiting factor of an artificial lung is oxygenation.

Unfavourable factors

Against these favourable design considerations, there are certain advantages of the real lung, apart from its very large surface area, which are difficult to emulate in an artificial lung.

1. The pulmonary capillaries have a diameter close to that of the erythrocyte. Therefore, each erythrocyte is brought into very close contact with the alveolar gas (see Figure 2.8). Streamline flow through much wider channels in a membrane artificial lung tends to result in a stream of erythrocytes remaining at a distance from the interface. Much thought has been devoted to the creation of turbulent flow to counteract this effect. In contrast, there is a very favourable diffusion distance in a bubble oxygenator when foaming occurs.
2. The vascular endothelium is specially adapted to prevent undesirable changes in the formed elements of blood, particularly neutrophils and platelets. Most artificial surfaces cause clotting of blood, and artificial lungs therefore require the use of anticoagulants. Further adverse changes result from denaturation of protein (see below).
3. No artificial lung has the extensive non-respiratory functions of the real lung, which include uptake, synthesis and biotransformation of many constituents of the blood (see Chapter 12). This function is lost when the lungs are bypassed.
4. The lung is an extremely efficient filter with an effective pore size of about 10 μm for flow rates of blood up to about 25 l/min. This is difficult to achieve with any man-made filter.

Types of extracorporeal gas exchangers

Systems with direct blood/gas interface

Bubble oxygenators. The simplest design of extracorporeal oxygenator stems from the well-tried wash bottle of the chemist. By breaking up the gas stream into small bubbles, it is possible to achieve very large surface areas of interface. However, the smaller the bubbles, the greater the tendency for them to remain in suspension when the blood is returned to the patient. This is dangerous because of the direct access of the blood to the cerebral circulation. A compromise is to break the gas stream into bubbles ranging from 2 to 7 mm diameter, giving an effective area of interface of the order of 15 m^2. With a mean red cell transit time of 1–2 seconds, a 'ventilation/perfusion ratio' of unity or slightly more, and an oxygen concentration of more than 90%, this gives an acceptable outflow blood P_{O_2} with blood flow rates up to about 6 l/min (Finlayson and Kaplan, 1979). The P_{CO_2} of the outflowing blood must be controlled by admixture of carbon dioxide with the inflowing oxygen in the gas phase. Priming volumes range from 400 to 900 ml. Gas is passed through the blood in a reservoir of about 1 litre capacity in which foaming takes place.

Blood is then passed to a second reservoir for 'debubbling' to take place with the help of an antifoaming compound.

Disc and vertical screen oxygenators. These devices have been used to film blood over a large surface area which is directly exposed to gas. This prevents the danger of bubbles remaining in the blood and there tends to be less damage to the blood. However, it is not practicable to obtain the large surface areas of a bubble oxygenator and the apparatus is troublesome to clean and maintain.

Extracorporeal membrane oxygenation (ECMO)
(see Zapol and Kolobow, 1991)

Two types of membrane are in use. Silicone rubber can be formed into a continuous thin uniform membrane. Rubber is a lipid and is freely permeable to oxygen, carbon dioxide and anaesthetic gases. An alternative approach is the use of membranes of polypropylene, Teflon or polyacrylamide which contain small pores ranging from 0.1 to 5 μm diameter (Finlayson and Kaplan, 1979). These pores tend to fill with protein which then forms a layer over the blood side of the membrane, the whole being freely permeable to the respiratory gases. However, performance declines over several hours which is not the case with a silicone rubber membrane. Microporous membranes can weep if the apparatus is primed with a protein-free solution, but in normal use can withstand a hydrostatic pressure gradient of the order of normal arterial blood pressure. Surface areas of the order of 10 m^2 can be achieved.

A major problem has been the mixing of blood as it flows across the membrane. The blood pathway is much thicker than the normal pulmonary capillary and a slow moving boundary layer impairs gas exchange. This has been avoided by designs which encourage mixing of the blood stream.

Intravascular membrane oxygenators have been described for placement within the venae cavae (Mortensen and Berry, 1889). Prototypes have remained in dogs for up to 7 days, with the capability of transferring 100 ml of oxygen per minute.

Blood pumps

Roller pumps are now universally used to move blood to and from the extracorporeal oxygenator and they are adjusted to be not quite occlusive. This minimizes damage to the formed elements of the blood. There is no convincing evidence that performance is better with pulsatile blood flow.

Damage to blood

Damage due to non-occlusive roller pumps is almost negligible. Damage due to oxygenators is probably far less than that which results from surgical suction in removing blood from the operative site and, during cardiac surgery, this factor outweighs any differences attributable to the type of oxygenator. However, during prolonged extracorporeal oxygenation for respiratory failure, the influence of the type of oxygenator becomes important, and membrane oxygenators are then clearly superior to bubble oxygenators.

Protein denaturation

Contact between blood and either gas bubbles or plastic surfaces results in protein denaturation and plastic surfaces become coated with a layer of protein. With membrane oxygenators this tends to be self-limiting, but bubble oxygenators cause a continuous and progressive loss of protein. This is the main factor which limits their prolonged use.

Complement activation

Complement activation occurs when blood comes into contact with any artificial surface and complement C5a is known to be formed after cardiopulmonary bypass surgery (Chenoweth et al., 1981). This results in margination of neutrophils on vascular endothelium, possible consequences of which are considered on page 548.

Erythrocytes

Shear forces, resulting from turbulence or foaming may cause shortened survival or actual destruction of erythrocytes. However, surgical suction is generally more damaging than the oxygenator. Without suction, the damage to erythrocytes with membrane oxygenators remains within reasonable limits for many days. Released haemoglobin is initially bound to proteins but eventually saturates the receptors and is excreted through the kidneys. Red cell ghosts are now believed to be more damaging than free haemoglobin and they may need to be removed by filtration.

Leucocytes and platelets

Counts of these elements are usually reduced by an amount which is in excess of the changes attributable to haemodilution. Platelets are lost by adhesion and aggregation, and postoperative counts are commonly about half the preoperative value (Finlayson and Kaplan, 1979).

Coagulation

No oxygenator can function without causing coagulation of the blood. Anticoagulation is therefore a *sine qua non* of the technique and heparinization is universally employed for this purpose. This inevitably results in excess bleeding from any surgical incision.

Prolonged extracorporeal oxygenation for respiratory failure

It has long been known that extracorporeal oxygenation can be maintained for a few days in patients with respiratory failure. For reasons outlined above, membrane oxygenators are superior to bubble oxygenators for this application. It was hoped that the 'resting of the lung' might permit healing and recovery in patients with the adult respiratory distress syndrome (ARDS), considered in Chapter 29.

This hypothesis led to the multi-centre randomized prospective trial of extracorporeal membrane oxygenation (ECMO) for patients with ARDS (Zapol et al., 1979). Entry criteria were either:

1. Arterial P_{O_2} below 6.7 kPa (50 mmHg) for more than 2 hours, while breathing 100% oxygen, with positive end-expiratory pressure (PEEP) at least 0.5 kPa (5 cmH$_2$O).

or

2. Arterial P_{O_2} below 6.7 kPa (50 mmHg) for more than 12 hours, while breathing 60% oxygen, with PEEP at least 0.5 kPa (5 cmH$_2$O) and a shunt fraction greater than 30%.

Exclusion criteria included a pulmonary capillary wedge pressure of more than 3.3 kPa (25 mmHg), chronic pulmonary disease, malignancy, etc. Patients were then randomly allocated to conventional intermittent positive pressure ventilation (IPPV) or ECMO.

The study was terminated after treatment of the first 90 patients when it was found that mortality was more than 90% in both groups with no statistically significant difference between the two forms of treatment. There has been much discussion of the reasons for the failure of the ECMO trial but Zapol pointed out that the use of venoarterial bypass would have reduced pulmonary perfusion and pulmonary arterial pressure by about 30%. Possible adverse consequences of loss of pulmonary perfusion are outlined above. More recent results in adults have shown little improvement (Iatridis, 1988).

Prolonged extracorporeal oxygenation has been more successful in children. More than 800 neonates are reported to have undergone ECMO with 79% overall survival (Klein, 1988). There also appears to be a role in preserving life while waiting for transplantation.

Extracorporeal carbon dioxide removal (ECCO$_2$R)

A radically new approach to artificial gas exchange was developed by Gattinoni and his colleagues in Milan. In essence, they restricted extracorporeal gas exchange to removal of carbon dioxide, and maintained oxygenation by a modification of apnoeic mass movement oxygenation. The lungs were either kept motionless or were ventilated two to three times per minute (low-frequency positive-pressure ventilation with extracorporeal CO$_2$ removal – LFPPV–ECCO$_2$R) (Gattinoni et al., 1980; Pesenti et al., 1981; Gattinoni et al., 1986).

The technique depends on two important differences between the exchange of carbon dioxide and oxygen. Firstly, membrane oxygenators remove carbon dioxide some 10–20 times more effectively than they take up oxygen. Secondly, the normal arterial oxygen content (20 ml/100 ml) is very close to the maximum oxygen capacity, even with 100% oxygen in the gas phase (22 ml/100 ml). Therefore, there is little scope for superoxygenation of a fraction of the pulmonary circulation to compensate for a larger fraction of the pulmonary circulation in which oxygenation does not take place. In contrast, the normal mixed venous carbon dioxide content is 52 ml/100 ml compared with an arterial carbon dioxide content of 48 ml/100 ml. There is therefore ample scope for removing a larger than normal fraction of carbon dioxide from a part of the pulmonary circulation to compensate for the remaining fraction which does not undergo any removal of carbon dioxide (Figure 23.1).

It is therefore possible to maintain carbon dioxide homoeostasis by diversion of only a small fraction of the cardiac output through an extracorporeal membrane oxygenator (Gattinoni et al., 1980). This is best illustrated by means of the Fick equation for carbon dioxide:

$$\begin{array}{l}\text{carbon}\\\text{dioxide}\\\text{removal}\end{array} = \begin{array}{l}\text{pulmonary}\\\text{blood flow}\end{array} \left(\begin{array}{l}\text{mixed venous}\\\text{CO}_2 \text{ content}\end{array} - \text{arterial CO}_2 \text{ content}\right)$$

Under normal circumstances, typical values might be:

$$240 = 6000\ (52/100 - 48/100)$$
$$\text{(values in ml and ml/min)}$$

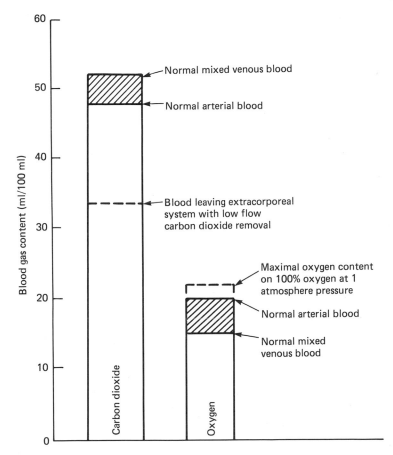

Figure 23.1 Comparison of absolute contents of carbon dioxide and oxygen in blood at 1 atmosphere pressure. Note that there is ample reserve potential for removing carbon dioxide below the level attained in normal arterial blood. In contrast, the maximal possible oxygen content of blood at 1 atmosphere is not greatly in excess of the level in normal arterial blood. This difference makes possible the extracorporeal removal of carbon dioxide (but not the supply of oxygen) by passing a small fraction of the cardiac output through an extracorporal gas exchanger.

With a flow through the membrane oxygenator of 1.3 l/min, typical values might be:

$$240 = 1300 (52/100 - 33.5/100)$$

The outflow from the membrane oxygenator would thus be 1.3 l/min with a carbon dioxide content of 33.5 ml/100 ml, corresponding to a P_{CO_2} of about 2 kPa (15 mmHg). This would account for removal of the whole of the normal metabolic production of carbon dioxide. Furthermore, there is no necessity for the bypass to be venoarterial and the far simpler venovenous bypass may be used. Therefore there need be no reduction in pulmonary blood flow, and the non-respiratory functions of the lung are preserved.

With P_{CO_2} held constant by extracorporeal removal of carbon dioxide, there is no obstacle to the continued uptake of oxygen by mass movement apnoeic oxygenation, a process which is otherwise terminated by progressive increase in P_{CO_2} (see page 241). All that is necessary is to replace the alveolar gas with oxygen and connect the trachea to a supply of oxygen, which is then drawn into the lungs at a rate equal to the metabolic consumption of oxygen, and this should continue indefinitely. Alternatively the lungs may be ventilated two to three times a minute, with long end-expiratory pauses and PEEP of about 1.5 kPa (15 cmH$_2$O). This is clearly beneficial for preservation of compliance and airway patency but imposes minimal danger of barotrauma.

The technique would seem to expose the lungs to very high concentrations of oxygen and the possibility of oxygen toxicity (Chapter 32). In practice this does not appear to have been a problem, possibly due to induction of superoxide dismutase during an earlier stage of therapy (page 550). Furthermore, the air which flows through the membrane exchanger maintains the nitrogen tension of the body and this does not appear to interfere with the uptake of oxygen. Alternatively, the oxygen concentration of the gas passing through the membrane exchanger can be increased to make a contribution to oxygenation of the arterial blood.

Gattinoni et al. (1980) described the reversal of respiratory failure in three patients who fulfilled the entry criteria of the ECMO trial and might therefore have been expected to have a 90% mortality. Subsequent reports from Milan have confirmed the original optimism (Gattinoni et al., 1983; Gattinoni et al., 1986). Use of this technique has also been reported by Hickling (1986) and Hickling et al. (1986).

Chapter 24

The transplanted lung

Transplantation of a human lung was successfully accomplished in 1983 and has now become an established form of treatment. Key developments included steps to ensure revascularization of the airway anastomosis (such as omentopexy), and the use of cyclosporin-A to prevent rejection. The function of a transplanted lung is important for the wellbeing of the recipient, but also furthers our understanding of certain fundamental issues of pulmonary physiology. Lung transplant is still in its infancy and neither indications nor techniques are yet finalized.

Types of lung transplant
(see reviews by Egan and Cooper, 1991, and Shaw, Kirk and Conacher, 1991)

Single lung transplant is the simplest procedure and is performed for isolated pulmonary disease with minimal cardiac involvement. It is particularly useful for end-stage restrictive lung disease, but the indications are widening to include emphysema and pulmonary vascular disease.

The recipient's pneumonectomy is undertaken using one-lung anaesthesia (page 415), with or without cardiopulmonary bypass. The donor lung is implanted, with anastomoses of the main bronchus, the left or right pulmonary artery and a ring of left atrium containing both pulmonary veins of one side.

Double lung transplant performed at a single operation is a more complex procedure for which total cardiopulmonary bypass is mandatory. A simpler alternative is to transplant two lungs sequentially. The main indications are severe chronic obstructive airway disease, infective lung disease and cystic fibrosis.

After establishing total cardiopulmonary bypass and removing both lungs through a sternal incision, the paired donor lungs are implanted, with anastomoses of either the trachea or both bronchi, the main pulmonary artery and the posterior part of the left atrium containing all four pulmonary veins.

Combined heart–lung transplant was originally used for patients with primary pulmonary hypertension and Eisenmenger's syndrome but the indications have widened to include right heart failure secondary to lung disease. Cardiac rejection is less common after heart–lung transplant than after isolated heart transplant.

Total cardiopulmonary bypass is, of course, essential and the anastomoses involve the right atrium, the aorta and the trachea. Omentopexy is not required, probably because of collateral circulation from pericardium and the coronary circulation.

Functional deficits

Transplantation inevitably disrupts innervation, lymphatics and the bronchial circulation. The condition of the recipient is further compromised by immuno-suppressive therapy.

The denervated lung

The transplanted lung has no afferent or efferent innervation and there is, as yet, no evidence that reinnervation occurs in patients. However, in dogs, vagal stimulation has been observed to cause bronchoconstriction 3–6 months after reimplantation (Edmunds, Graf and Nadel, 1971), and sympathetic reinnervation has been demonstrated after 45 months (Lall et al., 1973).

Respiratory rhythm. In Chapter 5, considerable attention was paid to the weakness of the Hering–Breuer reflex in man. It was therefore to be expected that denervation of the lung, with block of pulmonary baroreceptor input to the medulla, would have minimal effect on the respiratory rhythm. This is in contrast to the dog and most other laboratory animals in whom vagal block is well known to cause slow deep breathing. Bilateral vagal block in human volunteers was already known to leave the respiratory rhythm virtually unchanged (Guz et al., 1966b), and it was therefore no great surprise when it was shown that bilateral lung transplant had no significant effect on the respiratory rate and rhythm in patients, after the early postoperative period (Shaw, Kirk and Conacher, 1991). Breathing during sleep is also normal. In contrast, dogs and cats exhibit abnormal breathing patterns when both lungs are denervated.

The cough reflex, in response to afferents arising from below the level of the tracheal or bronchial anastomosis, is permanently lost after lung transplantation. It is clear that this does not preclude long term survival of the graft, but there can be no doubt that the patient is at a disadvantage in clearing secretions and must consequently have greater liability to infection.

Bronchial hypersensitivity. Enhanced sensitivity to the bronchoconstrictor effects of inhaled methacholine and histamine can be demonstrated after heart-lung transplantation (Glanville et al., 1987). This is thought to be due to hypersensitivity of receptors in airway smooth muscle (see Figure 4.7), following denervation of the predominantly constrictor autonomic supply.

Lymph drainage

The hilar lymphatics are severed at pneumonectomy and it is not feasible to anastomose with the lymphatics of the donor lung. It appears likely that restoration of pulmonary lymphatics occurs spontaneously within a few weeks. In the meantime lymph drains from the severed ends of the donor lung into the recipient's pleural cavity and chest tubes frequently drain excessively for periods of more than 2 weeks (Egan and Cooper, 1991). Nevertheless, extravascular water of the reimplanted lung is substantially increased in the dog during the early post-operative period (Cowan, Staub and Edmunds, 1976). Compliance is reduced during the same period but surfactant production appears to be unaffected (Egan and Cooper, 1991).

Mucociliary clearance

Mucociliary clearance is defective after transplantation. The actual cause appears to be defective mucus production, rather than changes in the frequency of cilial beat (Egan and Cooper, 1991). This, together with the absent cough reflex below the line of the airway anastomosis and immunosuppression, contributes to the enhanced susceptibility to infection of the transplanted lung. Expectoration from transplanted lungs should be facilitated by postural drainage, physiotherapy and 'voluntary' coughing.

Bronchial and tracheal circulation

The tracheal or bronchial circulation of the donor lung is usually compromised, and the problem of stenosis, leakage or even occasional dehiscence of the airway anastomosis remains (Egan and Cooper, 1991). The earliest approach was omento-pexy, in which omentum was brought up through the diaphragm and wrapped around the anastomosis to provide collateral circulation. More recently direct anastomosis of the internal mammary artery to the donor bronchial circulation has been advocated.

Immunosuppression

Except in the case of identical twins, survival of the transplanted lung depends on immunosuppression, and cyclosporin-A is not only currently the best drug but has, in fact, made lung transplant possible. The continued use of immunosuppression greatly reduces resistance to infection and the transplanted lung is particularly vulnerable to cytomegalovirus, herpes simplex and *Pneumocystis carinii*. Cyclosporin-A also has a wide variety of drug interactions and side effects, including nephrotoxicity and hepatotoxicity (Shaw, Kirk and Conacher, 1991). The risk of infection decreases 6 months after transplantation but persists as long as patients receive immunosuppressants and steroids.

Overall function

Ventilatory performance
(see Egan, Kaiser and Cooper, 1989)

After single lung transplant, total lung capacity and vital capacity reached 60% of predicted value within 2 months. Forced expiratory volume (1 second) showed gradual improvement over a year to attain a plateau 80% of predicted value, from only 47% of predicted before transplant. However, this measurement depends on many factors (page 133) and it would be difficult to define the precise factors involved in the slow recovery. Values in excess of 2.5 litres are often attained after double lung transplant and this can be considered very satisfactory.

Pulmonary perfusion

A single transplanted lung is often overperfused in relation to the remaining lung. The Toronto Lung Transplant Group (1988) reported mean values for perfusion of the transplanted lung of 66% of total pulmonary blood flow at 1 week, 72% at 3 weeks and a gradual increase thereafter.

Diffusing capacity

It has been explained in Chapter 9 that the diffusing capacity (or transfer factor) for carbon monoxide is a useful and sensitive test of the efficiency of gas exchange, although a decreased value does not necessarily result in significant arterial hypoxaemia. Egan, Kaiser and Cooper (1989) reported that, following single lung transplant, diffusing capacity increased from a preoperative value 37% of predicted to a plateau of 70% of predicted, attained gradually over 1 year.

Chemical control of ventilation and pulmonary vasoconstriction

Chemical control of ventilation (pages 97 et seq.) does not depend on either afferent or efferent innervation of the lung, and there is no evidence of any abnormality after lung transplant. Hypoxic pulmonary vasocontriction appears to be an entirely local mechanism and, as might be expected, has been shown to persist in the human transplanted lung (Robin et al., 1987).

Exercise performance

The attainable level of exercise depends on many factors which in addition to pulmonary function include circulation, condition of the voluntary muscles, motivation and freedom from pain on exertion (see Chapter 13). Improvement in performance increases fairly steadily for 6 months to reach walking speeds of about 100 m/min over 6 minutes (Egan and Cooper, 1991).

Rejection

Great progress has been made in overcoming the problem of rejection, but the problem still exists. In heart–lung transplant, pulmonary rejection usually precedes cardiac rejection and it is rare for cardiac rejection to occur without lung rejection. Obliterative bronchiolitis is more common after heart–lung transplant than after transplantation of lungs alone (Shaw, Kirk and Conacher, 1991).

Detection of rejection. There is a major difficulty in detecting the early stages of rejection and it is difficult to distinguish rejection from infection on clinical evidence. Both conditions feature arterial hypoxaemia, pyrexia, leucocytosis, dyspnoea and a reduced capacity for exercise. These changes are followed by a decrease in diffusing capacity and the forced expiratory volume, and later by perihilar infiltration or graft opacification on the chest X-ray. Pulmonary blood flow through the threatened lung may then be reduced from the high levels noted above.

None of the symptoms and signs described above is truly diagnostic of threatened rejection. The gold standard is the histopathology of an open-lung biopsy which shows perivascular lymphocytic infiltration. However, this procedure is unsuitable for routine screening. Transbronchial biopsy is less invasive, but unreliable in comparison with open-lung biopsy, and also not entirely free from hazard. A still less invasive alternative is bronchoalveolar lavage. When rejection is threatened the fluid recovered shows an increase in the number of T-lymphocytes, followed by an increase in B-lymphocytes and certain changes in their behaviour. These changes precede radiographic evidence of rejection. However, there is currently no test which can be applied to lavage fluid that is specific for threatened rejection, and this is an important area for research in the future.

Chapter 25

Anaemia

Anaemia is a widespread pathophysiological disorder which interferes with oxygen transport to the tissues. In developed countries it has a varied aetiology, including iron deficiency, chronic haemorrhage, loss of erythropoietin in end-stage renal failure and depletion of vitamin B_{12}. However, in the third world it is endemic with major factors including malnutrition and infestation with various parasites such as hook worm and *Schistosoma*. In many countries, haemoglobin concentrations within the range 8–10 g/dl are regarded as normal.

Anaemia *per se* has no major direct effects on pulmonary function. Arterial PO_2 and saturation should remain within the normal range in uncomplicated anaemia, and the crucial effect is on the arterial oxygen content and therefore oxygen delivery. Important compensatory changes are increases in cardiac output, greater oxygen extraction from the arterial blood and to a less extent the small rightward displacement of the oxyhaemoglobin dissociation curve. However, there are limits to these adaptations, which define the minimal tolerable haemoglobin concentration, and also the exercise limits attainable at various levels of severity of anaemia.

Pulmonary function

Gas exchange

Alveolar PO_2 is determined by dry barometric pressure, inspired oxygen concentration and the ratio of oxygen consumption to alveolar ventilation (page 257). Assuming that the first two are unchanged, and there being good evidence that the latter two factors are unaffected in the resting state by anaemia down to a haemoglobin concentration of at least 5 g/dl (see below), then there is no reason why alveolar PO_2 or PCO_2 should be affected by uncomplicated anaemia down to this degree of severity.

The increased cardiac output (see below) will cause a small reduction in pulmonary capillary transit time which, together with the reduced mass of haemoglobin in the pulmonary capillaries, causes a modest decrease in diffusing capacity or transfer factor (page 201). However, such is the reserve in the capacity of pulmonary capillary blood to reach equilibrium with the alveolar gas (Figure 9.2), that it is highly unlikely that this would have any measurable effect on the alveolar/end-pulmonary capillary P_{O_2} gradient which in the normal subject is now believed to be of the order of only 10^{-6} mmHg. Thus pulmonary end-capillary P_{O_2} should also be normal in uncomplicated anaemia.

Continuing down the cascade of oxygen partial pressures from ambient air to the site of utilization in the tissues, the next step is the gradient in P_{O_2} between pulmonary end-capillary blood and mixed arterial blood. The P_{O_2} gradient at this stage is caused by shunting and the perfusion of relatively underventilated alveoli. There is no evidence that these factors are enhanced in anaemia, and arterial P_{O_2} should therefore be normal. Because the peripheral chemoreceptors are stimulated by reduction in arterial P_{O_2} and not arterial oxygen content (page 99), there should be no stimulation of respiration unless the degree of hypoxia is sufficient to cause anaerobic metabolism and lactacidosis.

The haemoglobin dissociation curve

It is well established that intraerythrocytic 2,3-diphosphoglycerate is increased in anaemia (page 277), typical changes being from a normal value of 5 to reach 7 mmol/l at a haemoglobin concentration of 6 g/dl (Torrance et al., 1970). This results in an increase in P_{50} from 3.6 to 4 kPa (27 to 30 mmHg). This rightward shift of the dissociation curve will have a negligible effect on arterial saturation, which has indeed been reported to be normal in anaemia. The rightward shift will, however, increase the P_{O_2} at which oxygen is unloaded in the tissues, mitigating to a certain extent the effects of reduction in oxygen delivery so far as tissue P_{O_2} is concerned.

Arterial oxygen content

Although the arterial oxygen saturation usually remains normal in anaemia, the oxygen content of the arterial blood is reduced in approximate proportion to the decrease in haemoglobin concentration. Arterial oxygen content can be expressed as follows:

$$Ca_{O_2} = ([Hb] \times Sa_{O_2} \times 1.31) + 0.3 \qquad \qquad ...(1)$$

ml/dl   g/dl   %/ 100   ml/g   ml/dl

e.g.   19 $= (14.7 \times 0.97 \times 1.31) + 0.3$

where Ca_{O_2} is arterial oxygen content
                [Hb]   is haemoglobin concentration
                Sa_{O_2} is arterial oxygen saturation
                1.31   is combining power of haemoglobin with oxygen (page 271)
                0.3   is dissolved oxygen at normal arterial P_{O_2}.

Oxygen delivery

The important concept of oxygen delivery ($\dot{D}_{O_2}$) is considered in detail on page 283. It is defined as the product of cardiac output ($\dot{Q}$) and arterial oxygen content (Ca_{O_2}).

$$\dot{D}o_2 \quad = \dot{Q} \quad \times Ca_{O_2} \qquad\qquad ...(2)$$

ml/min   l/min   ml/dl

e.g. 1000 = 5.25 × 19

(the right-hand side is multiplied by a scaling factor of 10)

Combining equations (1) and (2):

$$\dot{D}o_2 \quad = \dot{Q} \quad \times \{([Hb] \times Sa_{O_2} \times 1.31) \quad + 0.3\} \qquad ...(3)$$

ml/min   l/min   g/dl   %/100   ml/g   ml/dl

e.g. 1000   = 5.25   × {(14.7 × 0.97 × 1.31)   + 0.3}

(the right-hand side is multiplied by a scaling factor of 10)

Normal values give an oxygen delivery of approximately 1000 ml/min, which is about four times the normal resting oxygen consumption of 250 ml/min. Extraction of oxygen from the arterial blood is thus 25% and this accords with an arterial saturation of 97% and mixed venous saturation of 72%.

If the small quantity of dissolved oxygen (0.3 ml/dl) is ignored, then oxygen delivery is seen to be proportional to the product of cardiac output, haemoglobin concentration and arterial oxygen saturation. There is, of course, negligible scope for any compensatory increase in saturation in a patient with uncomplicated anaemia at sea level.

Effect of anaemia on cardiac output

Equation (3) shows that, if other factors remain the same, a reduction in haemoglobin concentration will result in a proportionate reduction in oxygen delivery. Thus a haemoglobin concentration of 7.5 g/dl with unchanged cardiac output would halve delivery to give a resting value of 500 ml/min, which would be approaching the likely critical value. However, patients with quite severe anaemia usually show little evidence of hypoxia at rest and, furthermore, achieve surprisingly good levels of exercise. Since arterial saturation cannot be increased, full compensation can be achieved only by a reciprocal relationship between cardiac output and haemoglobin concentration. Thus if haemoglobin concentration is halved, then maintenance of normal delivery will require a doubling of cardiac output. Full compensation does not normally occur, but fortunately a reduction in haemoglobin concentration is usually accompanied by some increase in cardiac output. This is partly due to reduction in systemic vascular resistance in response to tissue hypoxia and partly due to reduction in blood viscosity as haematocrit is reduced.

Duke and Abelmann (1969) measured cardiac output in 15 patients before and after treatment of uncomplicated anaemia, and demonstrated that cardiac output was significantly greater before they increased their patients' haemoglobin concentration from 5.9 to 10.9 g/dl. Their results are represented by the lower curve in the upper part of Figure 25.1, for which it is assumed that the mean surface area of their patients was 1.7 m². They did, however, show a negative correlation between age and cardiac index in the anaemic state, reflecting the relative inability of the older patient to compensate. Woodson, Wills and Lenfant (1978) carried out an important study in volunteers whose haemoglobin concentration was isovolaemically reduced from a mean control value of 15.3 to 10 g/dl by replacement of blood with the same volume of albumin solution: anaemia was then maintained at the same level for 14 days. Immediately after induction of anaemia there was a marked increase in cardiac output (55.5%), but this decreased to only 14% above control levels after 14 days of sustained anaemia (Figure 25.1).

More dramatic effects have been demonstrated in dogs. The effect of haematocrit on cardiac output was studied in normovolaemic anaesthetized dogs by Richardson and Guyton (1959). They demonstrated a linear negative relationship between haematocrit and cardiac output. This extended from haematocrit values of 20%, through the normal to polycythaemic values of 70%. Circulatory measurements were made within minutes of establishing values for haematocrit. Their normal value for cardiac output was 100 ml kg^{-1} min^{-1}, increasing to 160 at a haematocrit of 20% and decreasing to 30 at a haematocrit of 70%. Cain (1977) obtained very similar results in dogs, following acute isovolaemic haemodilution with dextran. When haematocrit was reduced from 43.6 to 8.9 and then to 6.6%, cardiac output (ml kg^{-1} min^{-1}) was increased from 133 to 299 and 192 respectively. Qualitatively similar observations were made by Crowell, Ford and Lewis (1959) in acutely hypovolaemic dogs bled to a mean arterial pressure of 30 mmHg. However, their absolute values for cardiac output were very much less than those of Cain due to the decreased filling pressure of the heart.

The influence of cardiac output on oxygen delivery

The interaction of haemoglobin concentration and cardiac output on oxygen delivery (equation 3) is shown for the human studies in the lower part of Figure

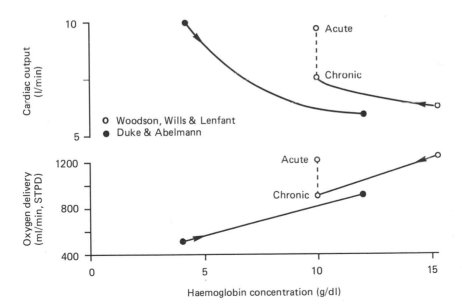

Figure 25.1 Changes in cardiac output and oxygen delivery as a function of haemoglobin concentration. The right-hand curves (open symbols) show the effect of induced anaemia in volunteers (Woodson, Wills and Lenfant, 1978). The left-hand curves (closed symbols) show the effect of treatment of anaemic patients (Duke and Abelmann, 1969).

25.1. Following the acute reduction of haemoglobin concentration to about 65% of control value in the volunteers, cardiac output increased sufficiently to maintain normal or near normal oxygen delivery. However, in sustained anaemia, the increase in cardiac output (only 14%) was insufficient to maintain oxygen delivery, which decreased to 25% below control values. Similarly in the anaemic patients studied by Duke and Abelmann (1969), delivery was reduced in proportion to the degree of anaemia. Extrapolation of the curves in the lower part of Figure 25.1 suggests that a critical oxygen delivery (probably about 500 ml/min) would be reached at a haemoglobin concentration of about 3 g/dl which is close to the minimum level compatible with life. At this point cardiac output would be about double the normal value and mixed venous saturation would be reduced from the normal value of 72% down to about 50%.

Without an increase in cardiac output, it is likely that a haemoglobin concentration of 6–8 g/dl would be the minimum level compatible with life. It is clear that the ability of the cardiovascular system to respond to anaemia with an increase in cardiac output is an essential aspect of accommodation to anaemia, and this is less effective in the elderly.

Relationship between oxygen delivery and consumption

The relationship between oxygen delivery and consumption has been considered in detail on pages 284 et seq. The basic grid is shown in Figure 11.18, where the black dot indicates the normal resting point, with extraction of about 25% and mixed venous SO_2 of about 72%. When oxygen delivery is reduced, for whatever reason, oxygen consumption is at first maintained at its normal value, but with increasing oxygen extraction and therefore decreasing mixed venous saturation. This is termed 'supply-independent oxygenation', a condition which applies provided that delivery remains above a critical value (Figure 11.19). Below the critical oxygen delivery, consumption decreases as a function of delivery. This is termed 'supply-dependent oxygenation' and is usually accompanied by evidence of hypoxia, such as increased lactate in peripheral blood. Values for critical delivery depend upon the pathophysiological state of the patient and vary from one condition to another.

It has not been clearly established what is the critical level of oxygen delivery in chronic uncomplicated anaemia in man. However, in the study by Woodson, Wills and Lenfant (1978) of volunteers maintained at a haemoglobin concentration of 10 g/dl for 14 days, oxygen delivery decreased from about 1200 to 900 ml/min while oxygen consumption remained virtually unchanged (Figure 25.2). Duke and Abelmann (1969) found no increase in oxygen consumption in a group of 15 anaemic patients when haemoglobin concentration was increased from a mean value of 5.9 to 10.9 g/dl. The corresponding change in oxygen delivery would have been from 600 to 900 ml/min. Thus these patients and subjects all remained in a state of supply-independent oxygenation down to haemoglobin values of about 6 g/dl, implying a critical delivery at some value less than 600 ml/min. This accords with animal data showing that critical oxygen delivery in uncomplicated anaemia is about half the normal value.

The optimal haemoglobin concentration

The evidence cited above and the human data summarized in Figure 25.1 suggest that oxygen delivery increases progressively with haemoglobin concentration and

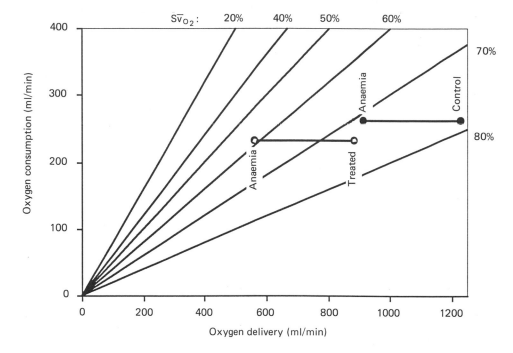

Figure 25.2 Oxygen consumption remained supply-independent in experimental isovolaemic anaemia (open symbols) (Woodson, Wills and Lenfant, 1978) and also in treated anaemic patients (closed symbols) (Duke and Abelmann, 1969).

haematocrit. However, Crowell and colleagues (Crowell, Ford and Lewis, 1959) showed that, in their acutely bled dog preparation, described above, both oxygen delivery and consumption were maximal at the normal haematocrit in their laboratory of 42%. However, the time required for irreversible shock to develop was maximal at a haematocrit of 36% rather than the normal value of 42%. The increased tissue perfusion at the lower haematocrit may thus confer advantages which outweigh the reduction in oxygen delivery.

Another aspect of this problem is the question of improving athletic performance by increasing haemoglobin concentration above the normal range. This may be achieved either by the administration of erythropoietin or by removal of blood for replacement of red cells after a few weeks when the subject has already partially restored his haemoglobin concentration, a procedure known as blood doping. Studies of trained athletes in this area are notoriously difficult, and it is easy to confuse the effects of changes in blood volume and haemoglobin concentration. Furthermore, blood doping involves the subject continuing his training after removal of blood while he is anaemic. This may well make his training more effective, as is the case when training is undertaken at altitude. In the pioneer study of Ekblom, Goldbarg and Gullbring (1972), it was reported that, following reinfusion of blood (resulting in an increase in haemoglobin concentration from 13.2 to 14.9 g/dl), maximal oxygen consumption was increased from 4.40 to 4.79 l/min, and time to exhaustion during uphill treadmill running was extended from 5.43 to 6.67 minutes. Oxygen cost of the exercise task was unaltered. These findings were challenged in subsequent studies, but confirmed in the well controlled study of highly trained runners by Buick et al. (1980), in which a mean haemoglobin concentration of 16.7 g/dl was attained with significant increases in maximal oxygen uptake from 4.85 to 5.1 l/min. Differences of this magnitude are critically important in the arena of modern athletic competition.

Anaemia and exercise

Figure 25.3 shows that, in patients with moderately severe anaemia, oxygen consumption is maintained constant in the face of reduction in delivery. This is achieved at the expense of reduction in mixed venous saturation, as a result of increased extraction of oxygen from the arterial blood. In Woodson's study of chronic isovolaemic anaemic volunteers (see above), the resting mixed venous saturation was reduced from 78% to 70%. This curtails the ability of the anaemic patient to encroach on his reserve of mixed venous oxygen saturation, which is an important adaptation to exercise. In Woodson's study, reduction of haemoglobin to 10 g/dl resulted in a curtailment of oxygen consumption attained at maximal exercise from the control values of 3.01 l/min (normalized to 70 kg body weight) down to 2.53 l/min in the acute stage, and 2.15 l/min after 14 days of sustained anaemia (Figure 25.3). The increase in cardiac output required for the same increase in oxygen consumption was greater in the anaemic state, and cardiac output at maximal oxygen consumption was slightly less than with a normal haemoglobin concentration. Maximal exercise in the anaemic state resulted in a reduction of mixed venous oxygen saturation to the exceptionally low value of 12%, compared with control values of 23% during maximal exercise with a normal haemogolobin concentration.

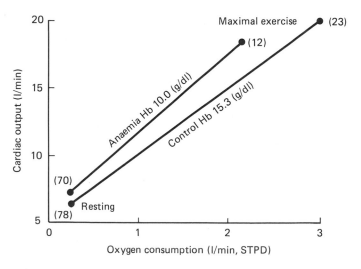

Figure 25.3 Cardiac output as a function of oxygen consumption during rest and maximal exercise under control and isovolaemic anaemic conditions. Numbers in parentheses indicate mean mixed venous saturation. (Redrawn from Woodson, Wills and Lenfant (1978) on the assumption that mean weight of the subjects was 70 kg, with permission of the authors, and the Editors and publishers of Journal of Applied Physiology)

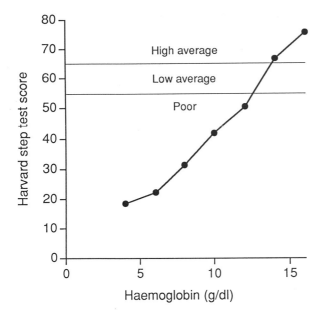

Figure 25.4 Relationship between capacity for exercise and haemoglobin concentration. (Redrawn from Viteri and Torún (1974) with permission of the authors, and the Editor and publishers of Clinics in Hematology)

Brisk walking on level gound normally requires an oxygen consumption of about 1 l/m and a cardiac output of the order of 10 l/min. At a haemoglobin level of 5 g/l, this would require a cardiac output of about 20 l/min to permit an oxygen consumption of 1 l/min with a satisfactory residual level of mixed venous oxygen saturation. It will be clear that, at this degree of anaemia, cardiac function is a critical factor determining the mobility of a patient.

Exercise tolerance may be limited by either respiratory or circulatory capacity. In uncomplicated anaemia, there is no reason to implicate respiratory limitation, and exercise tolerance is therefore, to a first approximation, governed by the remaining factors in the oxygen delivery equation (3) (above). On the assumption that the maximal sustainable cardiac output is only marginally affected by anaemia, it is to be expected that exercise tolerance will be reduced in direct proportion to the haemoglobin concentration. Available evidence supports this hypothesis (Figure 25.4).

Chapter 26
Pulmonary oedema

Pulmonary oedema is defined as an increase in pulmonary extravascular water, which occurs when transudation or exudation exceeds the capacity of the lymphatic drainage. In its more severe forms there is free fluid in the alveoli.

Anatomical factors
(see Chapter 2)

The pulmonary capillary endothelial cells abut against one another at fairly loose junctions which are of the order of 5 nm (50 Å) wide (DeFouw, 1983). These junctions permit the passage of quite large molecules and the pulmonary lymph contains albumin at about half the concentration in plasma. Epithelial cells meet at tight junctions with a gap of only about 1 nm (DeFouw, 1983). The tightness of these junctions is crucial for prevention of the escape of large molecules, such as albumin, from the interstitial fluid into the alveoli.

The lung has a well developed lymphatic system draining the interstitial tissue through a network of channels around the bronchi and pulmonary vessels towards the hilum. Lymphatic vessels cannot be identified at alveolar level but may be seen in association with bronchioles. Down to airway generation 11 (see Table 2.1), the lymphatics lie in a potential space around the air passages and vessels, separating them from the lung parenchyma.

In the hilum of the lung, the lymphatic drainage passes through several groups of tracheobronchial lymph glands, where they receive tributaries from the superficial subpleural plexus. Most of the lymph from the left lung usually enters the thoracic duct where it can be conveniently sampled in the sheep. The right side drains into the right lymphatic duct. However, the pulmonary lymphatics often cross the midline and pass independently into the junction of internal jugular and subclavian veins on the corresponding sides of the body. Studies in dogs have indicated that approximately 15% of the flow in the thoracic dust derives from the lungs (Meyer and Ottaviano, 1972).

The normal lymphatic drainage from human lungs is astonishingly small – only about 10 ml/h. However, lymphatic flow can increase greatly when transudation into the interstitial spaces is increased. This presumably occurs when pulmonary oedema is threatened but it cannot be conveniently measured in man.

Stages of pulmonary oedema

There is presumably a prodromal stage in which pulmonary lymphatic drainage is increased, but there is no increase in extravascular water. This may progress to the following stages.

Stage I. Interstitial pulmonary oedema

In its mildest form, there is an increase in interstitial fluid but without passage of oedema fluid into the alveoli. With the light microscope this is first detected as cuffs of distended lymphatics, typically '8'-shaped around the adjacent branches of the bronchi and pulmonary artery (Plate 2 and Figure 26.1). When well developed, the cuffing accounts for the butterfly shadow in the chest radiograph. Electron microscopy shows fluid accumulation in the alveolar septa but this is characteristically confined to the 'service' side of the pulmonary capillary which contains the stroma, leaving the geometry of the 'active' side unchanged (see Figure 2.10). Thus, gas exchange is better preserved than might be expected from the overall increase in lung water.

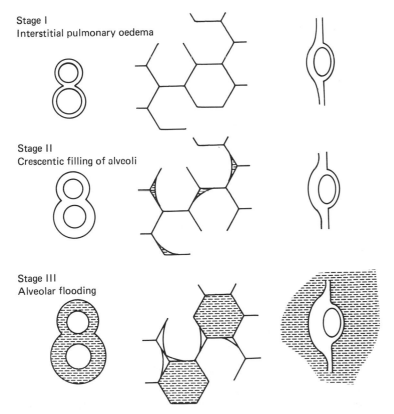

Stage I
Interstitial pulmonary oedema

Stage II
Crescentic filling of alveoli

Stage III
Alveolar flooding

Figure 26.1 Stages in the development of pulmonary oedema. On the left is shown the development of the cuff of distended lymphatics around the branches of the bronchi and pulmonary arteries. In the middle is the appearance of the alveoli by light microscopy (fixed in inflation). On the right is the appearance of the pulmonary capillaries by electron microscopy. The active side of the capillary is to the right. For an explanation of the stages, see text.

Physical signs are generally absent in stage I and the alveolar/arterial P_{O_2} gradient is normal or only slightly increased. Diagnosis rests on the chest radiograph and the demonstration of causative factors such as an increased wedge pressure.

Stage II. Crescentic filling of the alveoli

With further increase in extravascular lung water, interstitial oedema of the alveolar septa is increased and fluid begins to pass into some alveolar lumina. It first appears as crescents in the angles between adjacent septa, at least in lungs which have been fixed in inflation (Figure 26.1). The centre of the alveoli and most of the alveolar walls remain clear, and gas exchange is not grossly abnormal.

Stage III. Alveolar flooding

In the third stage, there is quantal alveolar flooding. Some alveoli are totally flooded while others, frequently adjacent, have only the crescentic filling or else no fluid at all in their lumina. It appears that fluid accumulates up to a point at which a critical radius of curvature results in surface tension sharply increasing the transudation pressure gradient. This produces flooding on an all-or-none basis for each individual alveolus.

Clearly there can be no effective gas exchange in the capillaries of an alveolar septum which is flooded on both sides, and the overall defect of gas exchange may be considered as venous admixture or shunt. It is not helpful to consider the condition as an impaired diffusing capacity. Rales can be heard during inspiration and the lung fields show an overall opacity superimposed on the butterfly shadow. Due to the effect of gravity on pulmonary vascular pressures (page 140), alveolar flooding tends to occur in the dependent parts of the lungs.

Stage IV. Froth in the air passages

When alveolar flooding is extreme, the air passages become blocked with froth which moves to and fro with breathing. This effectively stops all gas exchange and is rapidly fatal unless treated.

The mechanism of pulmonary oedema

The Starling equation and fluid exchange across the endothelium

Transudation of intravascular fluid must be considered in two stages, the first from the microcirculation into interstitial space (i.e. across the endothelium) and the second from the interstitial space into the alveoli (i.e. across the epithelium) (Figure 26.2). Passage of fluid across the endothelium is promoted by the hydrostatic pressure differential but counteracted by the osmotic pressure of the plasma proteins. The balance of pressures is normally sufficient to prevent any appreciable transudation but it may be upset in a wide variety of pathological circumstances.

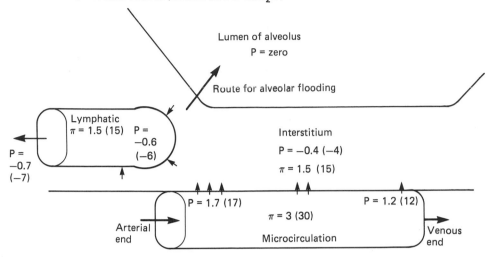

P = Hydrostatic pressure (kPa or cmH$_2$O) — relative to atmosphere
π = Protein osmotic pressure (kPa or cmH$_2$O)

Lumen of alveolus
P = zero

Route for alveolar flooding

Lymphatic
π = 1.5 (15)   P = −0.6 (−6)

Interstitium
P = −0.4 (−4)
π = 1.5 (15)

P = −0.7 (−7)

P = 1.7 (17)

P = 1.2 (12)

Arterial end

π = 3 (30)

Microcirculation

Venous end

Figure 26.2 Normal values for hydrostatic and plasma protein osmotic pressures in the pulmonary microcirculation and interstitium. Values are taken from Staub (1984).

It is customary to display the relationship between fluid flow and the balance of pressures in the form of the Starling equation. For the endothelial barrier this is as follows:

$$\dot{Q} = K[(Pmv - Ppmv) - \Sigma(\Pi mv - \Pi pmv)]$$

$\dot{Q}$ is the flow rate of transudated fluid which, in equilibrium, will be equal to the lymphatic drainage.

K is the hydraulic conductance (i.e. flow rate of fluid per unit pressure gradient across the endothelium).

Pmv is the hydrostatic pressure in the microvasculature.

Ppmv is the hydrostatic pressure in the perimicrovascular tissue (i.e. the interstitium).

Σ is the reflection coefficient, in this case applying to albumin. It is an expression of the permeability of the endothelium to the solute (albumin). A value of unity indicates total reflection corresponding to zero concentration of the solute in the interstitial fluid. A value of zero indicates free passage of the solute across the membrane and, with equal concentrations on both sides of the membrane, the solute could exert no osmotic pressure across the membrane. This normally applies to the crystalloids in plasma.

Πmv is the osmotic pressure the solute exerts within the microvasculature.

Πpmv is the osmotic pressure the solute exerts in the perimicrovascular tissue.

Under normal circumstances in man, the pulmonary lymph flow ($\dot{Q}$) is about 10 ml/hour with a protein content about half that of plasma. The pulmonary microvascular pressure (Pmv) is in the range 0–2 kPa ((0–15 mmHg), relative to atmosphere, depending on the vertical height within the lung field (see Figure 7.4). Furthermore, there is a progressive decrease in capillary pressure from its arterial to its venous end, since approximately one-half of the pulmonary vascular resistance is across the capillary bed (see Figures 7.3 and 26.2). It is meaningless to think of a single value for the mean pulmonary capillary pressure.

The hydrostatic pressure in the perimicrovascular tissue is not easy to measure. However, using implanted pressure-measuring capsules, Meyer, Meyer and Guyton (1968) found an average pressure of 1.3 kPa (10 mmHg) below atmospheric. Bhattacharya, Gropper and Staub (1984), studying the excised dog lung held at an inflation pressure of 0.5 kPa (5 cmH$_2$O), found interstitial pressures at the alveolar junctions some 0.4 kPa (4 cmH$_2$O) less than the alveolar pressure (Figure 26.2). There was a gradient in interstitial pressure from alveoli to hilum where the pressure was about 0.7 kPa (7 cmH$_2$O) less than alveolar pressure. There was no vertical gradient in interstitial pressures such as might have been expected from the effect of gravity.

With increasing pulmonary oedema, the interstitial space can accommodate large volumes of water with only small increases in pressure, the interstitial compliance being high. Some 500 ml can be accommodated in the interstitium and lymphatics of the human lungs with a rise of pressure of only about 0.2 kPa (2 cmH$_2$O) (Staub, 1984). However, above a certain critical level of pressure, fluid in the interstitial space floods into the alveoli through a high conductance pathway which has not yet been defined. Staub (1983) has compared this with an overflowing bath tub.

The capacity and compliance of the interstitium for water are increased at larger lung volumes (Gee and Williams, 1979) and this is considered to be one of the mechanisms by which positive end-expiratory pressure (PEEP) improves gas exchange although it does not decrease the total amount of lung water (page 455).

The reflection coefficient for albumin (Σ) in the healthy lung is about 0.5. The overall osmotic pressure gradient between blood and interstitial fluid is about 1.5 kPa (11.5 mmHg). Thus there is a fine balance between forces favouring and opposing transudation. There is a considerable safety margin in the upper part of the lung where the microvascular hydrostatic pressure is lowest. However, in the dependent part of the lung, where the hydrostatic pressure is highest, the safety margin is slender.

Gram-for-gram, albumin exerts about twice the osmotic pressure of the globulins which have a higher molecular weight. However, the total osmotic pressure of the plasma proteins is not simply the summation of the albumin and globulin fractions because of protein–protein interaction (Staub, 1984).

Fluid exchange across the alveolar epithelium

The permeability of this membrane is considered in Chapter 9 (page 216). It is freely permeable to gases, water and hydrophobic substances but virtually impermeable to albumin.

It is possible to construct a Starling equation for the epithelium (Staub, 1983) but there are considerable uncertainties about the osmotic pressure of the alveolar lining fluid. It has even been suggested that the alveolar lining is largely dry (Hills, 1982; Colacicco, 1985), which would make the concept meaningless. The evidence for the presence of water at the epithelial surface has been reviewed by Hills (1990). Nevertheless, it does appear that transudation across the alveolar epithelium is virtually zero unless the integrity of the barrier is compromised or the interstitial pressure increases above a critical level.

Aetiology

On the basis of the Starling equations, it is possible to make a rational approach to the aetiology of pulmonary oedema. There are four groups of aetiological factors, classified according to their effect on factors in the Starling equation.

Increased capillary pressure (haemodynamic pulmonary oedema)

This group comprises the commonest causes of pulmonary oedema. Basically the mechanism is an elevation of the hydrostatic pressure gradient across the pulmonary capillary wall, until it exceeds the osmotic pressure of the plasma proteins. Interstitial fluid accumulates until its pressure exceeds a critical value which then results in alveolar flooding. The oedema fluid has a protein content which is less than that of normal pulmonary lymph (Staub, 1984). Apart from transudation in accord with the Starling equation, severe pulmonary capillary hypertension may result in loss of structural integrity (see below).

Absolute hypervolaemia may result from overtransfusion, from excessive and rapid administration of other blood volume expanders or from accidental access of irrigation fluids through open venous channels in hollow organs, as for example during prostatectomy.

Relative pulmonary hypervolaemia may result from redistribution of the circulating blood volume into the lungs. This may result from use of the Trendelenburg position or occlusive limb tourniquets. Vasopressor mechanisms and drugs act on the systemic circulation to a greater extent than the pulmonary circulation and so redirect blood into the pulmonary circulation.

Raised pulmonary venous pressure will inevitably result in an increase in pulmonary capillary pressure. This may occur from any form of left heart failure, including left ventricular failure, dysrhythmias, mitral valve lesions and rare conditions such as atrial myxoma. There may also be vasoconstriction in the pulmonary veins and this appears to be caused by histamine (page 147) and perhaps also in Gram-negative septicaemia (Kuida et al., 1958). Annular constrictions or sphincters have recently been described in the pulmonary veins of rats, and they appear to respond to a blow on the head (Schraufnagel and Patel, 1990).

Increased pulmonary blood flow may raise the pulmonary capillary pressure sufficiently to precipitate pulmonary oedema. This may result from a left-to-right cardiac shunt, anaemia or, rarely, as a result of exercise.

Subatmospheric airway pressure was once popular in an attempt to improve cardiac output (page 461). It is uncertain whether this could increase the transmural hydrostatic pressure gradient or whether the capillary pressure would change with the alveolar pressure.

Increased permeability of the alveolar/capillary membrane (permeability oedema)

This group comprises the next commonest causes of pulmonary oedema. The mechanism is the loss of integrity of the alveolar/capillary membrane, allowing albumin and other macromolecules to enter the alveoli. The osmotic pressure gradient which opposes transudation is then lost. The oedema fluid has a protein content which approaches that of plasma (Staub, 1984).

The alveolar/capillary membrane can be damaged either directly or indirectly by many agents which are reviewed in Chapter 29. Apart from the possibility of the condition progressing to the adult respiratory distress syndrome, permeability pulmonary oedema is always potentially very dangerous. The presence of protein in the alveoli tends to make the oedema refractory and the protein may become organized into a so-called hyaline membrane.

Stress failure of the pulmonary capillaries. When the pulmonary capillary pressure is increased in the range 3–5 kPa (30–50 cmH$_2$O), discontinuities appear in the capillary endothelium and alveolar epithelium (type I cells), while the basement membrane often remains intact (Tsukimoto et al., 1991; West et al., 1991). This would appear to result in increased permeability and leakage of protein into the alveoli. The gaps tend to occur in the cell body, rather that at the junctions between the cells.

Decreased osmotic pressure of the plasma proteins

The Starling equation indicates that the osmotic pressure of the plasma proteins is a crucial factor opposing transudation. Although seldom the primary cause of pulmonary oedema, a reduced plasma albumin concentration is very common in the seriously ill patient and it must inevitably decrease the microvascular pressure threshold at which transudation commences.

Lymphatic obstruction

As in other tissues, obstruction of the pulmonary lymphatic drainage is a potential cause of pulmonary oedema. Because the pulmonary lymphatics drain into the great veins, raised systemic venous pressure has an adverse effect on pulmonary lymph flow and therefore the accumulation of lung water (Laine et al., 1986). In the first few weeks after lung transplantation, lymph drains from the cut ends of the pulmonary lymphatics into the pleural cavity (Chapter 24). Eventually the lymphatics reform and normal drainage is resumed.

Miscellaneous causes

'Neurogenic' pulmonary oedema may follow head injuries or other cerebral lesions. It has been demonstrated that it does not occur in the denervated lung. Schraufnagel and Patel (1990) suggested the pulmonary venous sphincters, which they described, as a possible mechanism for neurogenic pulmonary oedema (see above).

Sudden expansion of a collapsed lung may result in pulmonary oedema confined to the one side and probably caused by increased permeability (Pavlin, Nessly and Cheney, 1981). The problem may arise after aspiration of a pneumothorax or a pleural effusion. Lungs which have been collapsed for some time should be re-expanded slowly and by not more than 1 litre at one time. Pulmonary oedema has been reported as a form of pulmonary barotrauma (page 456).

Pulmonary oedema occurring at high altitude is well documented although the mechanism is still open to speculation. It is considered in Chapter 15 (page 343).

Also within the miscellaneous category is pulmonary oedema following diamorphine overdosage.

Pathophysiology

The most important physiological abnormality caused by pulmonary oedema is venous admixture or shunt due to blood draining flooded alveoli. This results in an increased alveolar/arterial PO_2 gradient and hypoxaemia which may be life threatening. Hypercapnia is not generally a problem. In less severe pulmonary oedema, there is usually an increased respiratory drive, due partly to hypoxaemia and partly to stimulation of J receptors (page 111). As a result the PCO_2 is usually normal or somewhat decreased. However, if a patient with severe pulmonary oedema is treated with a high concentration of inspired oxygen there may be hypercapnia due to the withdrawal of the hypoxic drive to ventilation.

Physiological principles of treatment

Immediate treatment

The highest priority is to restore the arterial PO_2. The inspired oxygen concentration should be increased, up to 100% if necessary. Sitting the patient up is a simple means of reducing the central blood volume. Morphine may exert its beneficial effect by peripheral vasodilatation.

If there is froth in the airway, this should be aspirated through a tracheal tube. Artificial ventilation is necessary if the oedema is severe, and the results are often spectacular. Artificial ventilation is often combined with positive end-expiratory pressure (PEEP). It was originally thought that this drove the fluid back into the circulation, but there is no evidence that extravascular lung water is reduced by PEEP (page 455). The success of PEEP probably depends on forcing airway liquid down the tracheobronchial tree and opening up alveoli which were previously not ventilated. By increasing the lung volume, the capacity of the interstitium to hold liquid is increased (Gee and Williams, 1979). Pare et al. (1983), studying dogs with haemodynamic pulmonary oedema, found that PEEP did not alter the total amount of lung water but a greater proportion was in the extra-alveolar interstitial space.

Treatment of the cause

Treatment of the underlying cause of pulmonary oedema follows directly from the Starling equation and an understanding of the aetiology.

Haemodynamic pulmonary oedema. The essential feature of treatment is reduction of the left atrial pressure. Depending on the precise aetiology, treatment is directed towards improvement of left ventricular function and/or reduction of blood volume. Venous occlusive cuffs on the limbs are a valuable emergency method of reduction of circulating blood volume. Diuretics act more slowly. Essentially the patient is titrated to the left along his Frank–Starling curve (Figure 26.3). In addition the curve is moved upwards and to the left, if this is possible, using positive inotropes as an adjunct to correction of left ventricular malfunction. The further

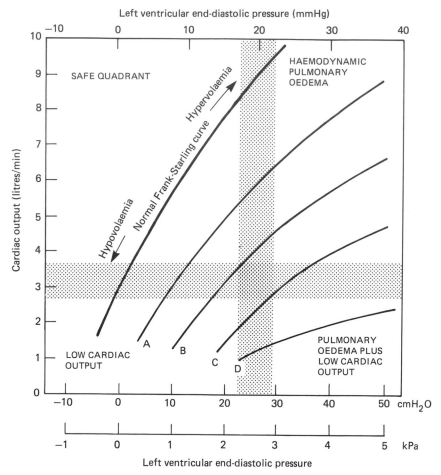

Figure 26.3 Quadrant diagram relating cardiac output to left ventricular end-diastolic pressure. The thick curve is a typical normal Frank–Starling curve. To the right are shown curves representing progressive left ventricular failure. Top left *is the safe quadrant which contains a substantial part of the normal Frank–Starling curve but progressively less of the curves representing ventricular failure.* Top right *is the quadrant representing normal cardiac output but raised left atrial pressure, attained at the upper end of relatively normal Frank–Starling curves (e.g. hypervolaemia). There is a danger of haemodynamic pulmonary oedema.* Bottom left *is the quadrant representing normal or low left atrial pressure but low cardiac output, attained at the lower end of all Frank–Starling curves (e.g. hypovolaemia). The patient is in shock.* Bottom right *is the quadrant representing both low cardiac output and raised left atrial pressure. There is simultaneous danger of pulmonary oedema and shock, and the worst Frank–Starling curves hardly leave this quadrant.*

the curve can be moved, the greater will be that part of it lying in the safe quadrant between low cardiac output on one hand and pulmonary oedema on the other.

Permeability pulmonary oedema. Treatment should be directed towards restoration of the integrity of the alveolar/capillary membrane. Unfortunately, no particularly successful measures are available towards this end (see Chapter 29). It is, however, important to minimize left atrial pressure even though this is not the primary cause of the oedema. Attempts may be made to increase the plasma albumin concentration if it is reduced.

Clinical measurement

Pulmonary venous pressure. As an indication of impending or actual haemodynamic pulmonary oedema, the most useful measurement is the pulmonary venous or wedge pressure. The Swan–Ganz catheter has revolutionized management in such patients.

Permeability of the alveolar/capillary membrane (see page 216). Laboratory methods are available for animals but the only practical approach for clinical use is measurement of the rate of loss of a gamma-emitting tracer molecule from the lung into the circulation. The most sensitive tracer is ^{99m}Tc-DTPA (metastable technetium-99-labelled diethylene triamine penta-acetate, molecular weight 492 daltons) (Jones, Royston and Minty, 1983). The half-time of clearance from the lung fields is usually in the range 40–100 minutes in the healthy non-smoker. The half-time is reduced below 40 minutes following a variety of lung insults. However, it is within the range 10–40 minutes in apparently healthy smokers (page 382) and this limits its scope for the early detection of a damaged alveolar/capillary membrane.

Lung water. This would be an extremely valuable diagnostic and prognostic aid to the management of pulmonary oedema. It is easy enough to measure lung water gravimetrically at postmortem in terms of the wet/dry difference or ratio, and there is usually sufficient protein in alveolar fluid for it to stain and be clearly visible by light microscopy.

Measurement of lung water during life has proved elusive. A great deal of effort has been devoted to the double indicator method. This uses the techniques for the measurement of pulmonary or central blood volume by dye dilution (page 151) but with two indicators. One indicator is chosen to remain within the circulation while the other (usually 'coolth' or tritiated water) diffuses into the interstitial fluid. Extravascular lung water is then derived as the difference between the volumes as measured with the two indicators. Staub (1974) discussed the limitations of these methods and there is still widespread agreement that the method is technically very difficult, since a high level of accuracy is required to demonstrate small changes in lung water. Magnetic resonance imaging appears to be as sensitive as gravimetric methods to measure lung water in rats (Cutillo et al., 1988). Thoracic electrical impedance is an alternative approach but is also beset with difficulties. Only rarely will control measurements be available before the onset of pulmonary oedema. In the event, reliance is usually placed on experienced interpretation of the chest X-ray.

Chapter 27

Pulmonary collapse and atelectasis

Pulmonary collapse may be defined as an acquired state in which the lungs or a part of the lungs become airless. Atelectasis is strictly defined as a state in which the lungs of a newborn have never been expanded, but the term is often used loosely as a synonym for collapse.

Collapse may be caused by two different mechanisms. The first of these is loss of the forces opposing the elastic recoil of the lung, which then decreases in volume to the point at which airways are closed and gas is trapped behind the closed airways. The second is obstruction of airways at normal lung volume, which may be due to many different causes. This also results in trapping of gas behind the obstructed airway. Whatever the cause of the airway closure, there is rapid absorption of the trapped gas because the total partial pressure of gases in mixed venous blood is always less than atmospheric (page 539). This generates a subatmospheric pressure more than sufficient to overcome any force tending to hold the lung expanded.

Loss of forces opposing retraction of the lung

The lungs are normally prevented from collapse by the outward elastic recoil of the rib cage and any resting tone of the diaphragm (page 48). The pleural cavity normally contains no gas but, if a small bubble of gas is introduced, its pressure is subatmospheric (see Figure 3.4). Pulmonary collapse due to loss of forces opposing lung retraction may be considered under five headings as follows.

Voluntary reduction of lung volume

It seems unlikely that voluntary reduction of lung volume below closing capacity will cause overt collapse of lung in a subject breathing air. However, in older subjects, there is an increase in the alveolar/arterial P_{O_2} gradient, suggesting trapping of alveolar gas (see Figure 20.8). If the subject has been breathing 100% oxygen, absorption collapse may follow reduction of lung volume (see below).

Excessive external pressure

Ventilatory failure is the more prominent aspect of an external environmental pressure in excess of about 6 kPa (60 cmH$_2$O) which is not communicated to the airways (page 422). However, some degree of pulmonary collapse could also occur and this is a normal consequence of the great depths attained by diving mammals while breath holding (page 360). An approximately normal lung volume is maintained during conventional diving operations when respired gas is maintained at the surrounding water pressure.

It is theoretically possible to induce collapse by the application of a subatmospheric pressure to the airways. Velasquez and Farhi (1964) demonstrated increased shunting in dogs under these circumstances.

Loss of integrity of the rib cage

Multiple rib fractures or the old operation of thoracoplasty may impair the elastic recoil of the rib cage to the point at which partial lung collapse results. This depends entirely on the extent of the injury to the rib cage, but six or more ribs fractured in two places will usually result in collapse. However, extensive trauma to the rib cage also causes interference with the mechanics of breathing, which is generally more serious than collapse.

Intrusion of abdominal contents into the chest

Extensive atelectasis results from a congenital defect of the diaphragm. Abdominal contents may completely fill one-half of the chest with total atelectasis of that lung. Paralysis of one side of the diaphragm causes the diaphragm to lie higher in the chest with a tendency to basal collapse on that side. An extensive abdominal mass (e.g. tumour or ascites) may force the diaphragm into the chest.

Space occupation of the pleural cavity

Air introduced into the pleural cavity reduces the forces opposing retraction of the lung and this is a potent cause of collapse. A *closed pneumothorax* is a fixed volume of air in the pleural cavity causing collapse in relation to the volume of air introduced. The intrapleural pressure rises in proportion to the volume of air in the cavity and is above atmospheric in a *tension pneumothorax*. The affected lung is then totally collapsed and the mediastinum is displaced towards the opposite side. This is a life-threatening condition requiring immediate relief of the pressure. An *open pneumothorax* communicates with the atmosphere and results in pendulum breathing in addition to collapse. At thoracotomy, pendulum breathing is prevented by artificial ventilation, but collapse may still occur and indeed is often induced to improve surgical access. In 'one-lung anaesthesia', a divided airway is used to ventilate the non-exposed lung while the exposed lung is allowed to collapse.

The pleural cavity may also be occupied by an effusion, empyema or a haemothorax. All of these may result in collapse. Less commonly there may be a significant intrusion in the thoracic cavity by tumour, cardiomegaly or haemopericardium.

Absorption of trapped gas

Absorption of alveolar gas trapped beyond obstructed airways may be the consequence of reduction in lung volume by the mechanisms described above.

However, it is the primary cause of collapse when there is total or partial airway obstruction at normal lung volume. Obstruction is commonly due to secretions, pus, blood or tumour but may be due to intense local bronchospasm or mucosal oedema. Bronchial blockers have been used for the deliberate production of collapse.

Gas trapped beyond the point of airway closure is absorbed by the pulmonary blood flow. The total of the partial pressures of the gases in mixed venous blood is always less than atmospheric (see Table 32.2), although pressure gradients for the individual component gases between alveolar gas and mixed venous blood may be quite different.

The effect of respired gases

If the patient has been breathing 100% oxygen prior to obstruction, the alveoli will contain only oxygen, carbon dioxide and water vapour. Since the last two together normally amount to less than 13.3 kPa (100 mmHg), the alveolar PO_2 will usually be in excess of 88 kPa (660 mmHg). However, the PO_2 of the mixed venous blood is unlikely to exceed about 6.7 kPa (50 mmHg), so the alveolar/mixed venous PO_2 gradient will be of the order of 80% of an atmosphere. Absorption collapse will thus be rapid and there will be no nitrogen in the alveolar gas to maintain inflation.

The situation is much more favourable in a patient who has been breathing air, since most of the alveolar gas is then nitrogen which is at a tension only about 0.5 kPa (4 mmHg) below that of mixed venous blood (Klocke and Rahn, 1961). Alveolar nitrogen tension rises above that of mixed venous blood as oxygen is absorbed and eventually the nitrogen will be fully absorbed. Collapse must eventually occur but the process is much slower than in the patient who has been breathing oxygen. Figure 27.1 shows a computer simulation of the time required for collapse with various gas mixtures (Webb and Nunn, 1967). Nitrous oxide/oxygen mixtures may be expected to be absorbed even more rapidly than 100% oxygen. This is partly because nitrous oxide is much more soluble in blood than nitrogen, and partly because the mixed venous tension of nitrous oxide is usually much less than the alveolar tension, except after a long period of inhalation.

When the inspired gas composition is changed *after* obstruction and trapping occur, complex patterns of absorption may ensue. The inhalation of nitrous oxide, after airway occlusion has occurred while breathing air, results in temporary expansion of the trapped volume (Figure 27.1). This is caused by large volumes of the more soluble nitrous oxide passing from blood to alveolus in exchange for smaller volumes of the less soluble nitrogen passing in the reverse direction. This phenomenon also applies to air embolus, pneumothorax, residual air from a pneumoencephalogram and, indeed, any air space in the body. It is potentially dangerous and may contraindicate the use of nitrous oxide as an anaesthetic (Munson and Merrick, 1967).

Magnitude of the pressure gradients

It needs to be stressed that the forces generated by the absorption of trapped gases are very large. The total partial pressure of gases in mixed venous blood is normally 87.4 kPa (656 mmHg). The corresponding pressure of the alveolar gases is 95.1 kPa (713 mmHg), allowing for water vapour pressure at 37°C. The difference, 7.7 kPa

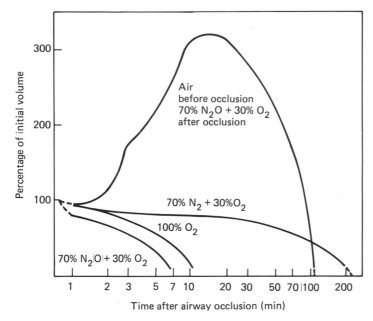

Figure 27.1 The lower curves show the rate of absorption of the contents of sections of the lung whose air passages are obstructed, resulting in sequestration of the contents. The upper curve shows the expansion of the sequestered gas when nitrous oxide is breathed by a patient who has recently suffered regional airway obstruction while breathing air. In all other cases, it is assumed that the inspired gas is not changed after obstruction has occurred. Similar considerations apply to gas sequestered in other parts of the body, and the data apply to pneumothorax, gas emboli and air introduced during pneumoencephalography. (Reproduced from Webb and Nunn (1967) by permission of the authors and the Editor of Anaesthesia)

(57 mmHg or 77 cmH$_2$O), is sufficient to overcome any forces opposing recoil of the lung. Absorption collapse after breathing air may therefore result in drawing the diaphragm up into the chest, reducing rib cage volume or displacing the mediastinum. If the patient has been breathing oxygen, the total partial pressure of gases in the mixed venous blood is barely a tenth of an atmosphere (see Table 32.2) and absorption of trapped alveolar gas generates enormous forces.

Effect of reduced ventilation/perfusion ratio

Absorption collapse may still occur in the absence of total airway obstruction provided that the ventilation/perfusion ($\dot{V}/\dot{Q}$) ratio is sufficiently reduced. It is now well established that older subjects as well as those with a pathological increase in scatter of $\dot{V}/\dot{Q}$ ratios may have substantial perfusion of areas of lung with $\dot{V}/\dot{Q}$ ratios in the range 0.01–0.1. This shows as a characteristic 'shelf' in the plot of perfusion against $\dot{V}/\dot{Q}$ (Figure 27.2). These grossly hypoventilated areas are liable to collapse if the patient breathes oxygen (Figure 27.2b). If the $\dot{V}/\dot{Q}$ ratio is less than 0.05, ventilation even with 100% oxygen cannot supply the oxygen which is removed (assuming the normal arterial/mixed venous oxygen content difference of 0.05 ml/ml). As the $\dot{V}/\dot{Q}$ ratio decreases below 0.05, so the critical inspired oxygen concentration necessary for collapse also decreases (Figure 27.2c). The flat part of the curve between $\dot{V}/\dot{Q}$ ratios of 0.001 and 0.004 means that small differences in inspired oxygen concentration in the range 20–30% may be very important in determining whether collapse occurs or not. There is no difficulty in demonstrating that pulmonary collapse may be induced in healthy middle-aged subjects breathing oxygen close to residual volume (Nunn et al., 1965b, 1978).

Perfusion through the collapsed lung

Perfusion through a collapsed lung or part of lung is one of the most important causes of intrapulmonary shunting (page 180). At least in the short term, some perfusion continues through the collapsed area and this is regulated mainly by hypoxic pulmonary vasoconstriction (page 145). In the absence of alveolar gas, the PO_2 which governs pulmonary vascular resistance is the mixed venous PO_2 (Marshall and Marshall, 1983). It has been observed that, in the presence of

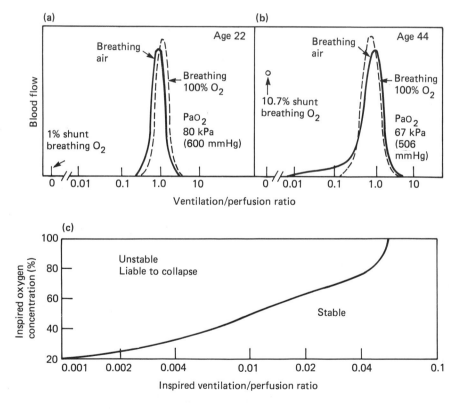

Figure 27.2 Inspiration of 100% oxygen causes collapse of alveoli with very low ventilation/perfusion ratios. (a) The minor change in the distribution of blood flow (in relation to $\dot{V}/\dot{Q}$ ratio) when a young subject breathes oxygen. Collapse is minimal and a shunt of 1% develops. (b) The changes in an older subject with a 'shelf' of blood flow distributed to alveoli with very low $\dot{V}/\dot{Q}$ ratios. Breathing oxygen causes collapse of these alveoli and this is manifested by disappearance of the shelf and appearance of an intrapulmonary shunt of 10.7%. (c) The inspired oxygen concentration relative to the inspired $\dot{V}/\dot{Q}$ ratio which is critical for absorption collapse. (Redrawn from Wagner et al. (1974) by permission of the authors and the Editor of the Journal of Clinical Investigation, and from Dantzker, Wagner and West (1975) by permission of the authors and the Editor of the Journal of Applied Physiology)

collapse, the shunt fraction of the pulmonary blood flow is directly proportional to the cardiac output (page 181), and this has been attributed to the effect of cardiac output on the mixed venous PO_2 (Marshall and Marshall, 1985). Thus, with a reduced cardiac output, the mixed venous PO_2 will be reduced (according to the Fick principle) and hypoxic pulmonary vasoconstriction in the area of the collapse will be increased. Therefore the shunt fraction will be decreased. However, the blood flowing through the shunt is more desaturated and these two effects counteract each other so that the arterial PO_2 is little changed. This complex problem is discussed further on pages 261 et seq.

Sudden re-expansion of an area of collapsed lung may result in pulmonary oedema (page 490).

Diagnosis of pulmonary collapse

The diagnosis may be made on physical signs but reliance is usually placed on chest radiography. In the upright position, collapse is commonest in the basal segments, often concealed behind the cardiac shadow unless the exposure is appropriate. Collapse in the supine position may well occur in the dorsal parts of the lung which are then dependent. This is not easy to detect radiologically since the collapsed areas may form a thin sheet parallel to the X-ray plate in an anteroposterior exposure. In the lateral view it may be obscured by the vertebral column. Computed tomography was successfully used to detect dorsal collapse during anaesthesia, after conventional means had failed (Brismar et al., 1985).

Collapse results in a reduction in pulmonary compliance, which has been suggested as a diagnostic aid (Butler and Smith, 1957; Bendixen, Hedley-Whyte and Laver, 1963; Velasquez and Farhi, 1964). Its value in diagnosis is limited by the wide scatter in normal values. However, a sudden reduction may give an indication of collapse provided, of course, that control measurements were available before collapse.

Collapse also reduces the functional residual capacity and arterial PO_2. However, in a study of absorption collapse, there was little to choose between these measurements and changes in the chest radiograph for the detection of minimal collapse (Nunn et al., 1978). When present, it was detected by all three methods. In patients undergoing intensive care, a reduction in arterial PO_2 cannot distinguish between the three very common conditions of pulmonary collapse, consolidation and oedema.

Treatment

This should be directed at the cause. Factors opposing the elastic recoil of the lung should be removed wherever possible. For example, pneumothorax, pleural effusion and ascites should be drained as necessary. In other cases, particularly impaired integrity of the chest wall, it may be preferable to treat the patient with intermittent positive pressure ventilation. It is usually possible to restore normal lung volume by appropriate control of airway pressures.

When collapse is caused by regional airway obstruction, the most useful methods in both treatment and prevention are by chest physiotherapy, combined when necessary with tracheobronchial toilet, through either a tracheal tube or a bronchoscope. Fibreoptic bronchoscopy alone will often clear an obstructed airway and permit re-expansion.

A logical approach is hyperinflation of the chest or an artificial 'sigh'. Some ventilators are equipped to provide an intermittent 'sigh' but evidence of its efficacy is elusive. It does nothing to reduce the alveolar/arterial PO_2 gradient during anaesthesia (Panday and Nunn, 1968). However, voluntary maximal inspirations have been effective in clearing areas of absorption collapse in subjects who had been breathing oxygen near residual volume (Nunn et al., 1978). The process imparted a distinctive tearing sensation in the chest, but rapidly restored to normal both chest radiograph and arterial PO_2. This process is the basis of the 'incentive spirometer' as a means of preventing postoperative collapse. Mention has been made above of the possibility of pulmonary oedema following sudden re-expansion of collapsed lung.

Chapter 28

Pulmonary embolism

The pulmonary circulation may be blocked by embolism, which may be gas, thrombus, fat, tumour or foreign body. The architecture of the microvasculature is well adapted to minimize the resultant infarct. Large numbers of pulmonary capillaries tend to arise from metarterioles at right angles and there are abundant anastomoses throughout the microcirculation (see Plate 5). This tends to preserve circulation distal to the impaction of a small embolus. Nevertheless, a large pulmonary embolus is a serious and potentially lethal complication, causing some 50 000 deaths a years in the USA (Moser, 1990).

Air embolism

An embolus may arise from pneumothorax and pulmonary barotrauma but is most commonly iatrogenic during either neurosurgery or cardiac surgery. Compressed air was formerly used to increase the speed of a blood transfusion and this was associated with some disastrous cases of embolism if the blood was exhausted before the pressure was released. Some small degree of air embolism is almost inevitable in all types of intravenous therapy.

In neurosurgery, the usual cause of air embolism is the use of the sitting position for posterior fossa surgery. This results in a subatmospheric venous pressure at the operative site and air may enter dural veins which are held open by their structure. In open cardiac surgery, it is almost impossible to remove all traces of air from the ventricles before closing the heart.

Detection of air embolism

Early diagnosis of air embolism is essential in neurosurgery, and there are three principal methods in routine use. Bubbles in circulating blood give a very characteristic sound with a precordial Doppler probe. The method is, if anything, too sensitive, since a shower of very small bubbles produces a particularly large signal. The second method is based on the appearance of nitrogen in the expired air. There should be no significant exhaled nitrogen after the first 15 minutes of an anaesthetic in which the patient breathes a mixture of oxygen and nitrous oxide. The appearance of nitrogen is easily detected with a mass spectrometer and is diagnostic of air entering the circulation. The third and simplest method is based on the end-expired carbon dioxide concentration which is easily measured with an infrared analyser. Many factors influence the end-expiratory concentration but a sudden decrease is likely to be either cardiac arrest or air embolism. More recently it has been shown that transoesophageal echocardiography is an efficient method of detecting air embolism and, furthermore, it is the only practicable method of detecting paradoxical air embolism (see below) (Cucchiara et al., 1984; Furuya and Okumura, 1984).

Effects of air embolus

Provided there is no major intracardiac right-to-left shunt, small quantities of air are filtered out by the lungs where they are gradually absorbed and no harm results. However, massive air embolism (probably in excess of 100 ml) may cause cardiac arrest either by frothing in the right ventricle or by massive occlusion of the pulmonary circulation. Treatment then requires aspiration of air through a cardiac catheter, which is difficult.

Paradoxical air embolism. Rarely, there may be passage of air emboli from the right to left heart without there being an overt right-to-left shunt. This is important because air then enters the systemic arterial circulation where there may be embolism and infarction, particularly of the brain. The cause is failure of complete closure of the foramen ovale. It is possible to pass a probe through such a foramen ovale in 20–35% of the adult population (Edward, 1960) but paradoxical embolism does not usually occur because pressure is slightly higher in the left atrium than the right. However, Perkins-Pearson, Marshall and Bedford (1982) demonstrated that in anaesthetized patients in the sitting position, right atrial pressure exceeded the pulmonary capillary wedge pressure in about half of them. Furthermore, right atrial pressure increased further in relation to wedge pressure when positive end-expiratory pressure was applied, presumably due to increased pulmonary vascular resistance (Perkins and Bedford, 1984).

Apart from intracardiac passage of an air embolus, it is possible that air bubbles may pass through the pulmonary circulation, although surface forces in the microvasculature render this unlikely. In small vessels, the radii of curvature of the air bubbles are so small that the interfaces are able to support very large pressure differences. This effect may be demonstrated *in vitro* by noting the very high pressures which can be maintained across a series of bubbles in water lying in a glass capillary tube (Jamin's tube). Nevertheless, one clinical report suggests that paradoxical pulmonary air embolism through the pulmonary circulation is possible (Marquez et al., 1981).

Pulmonary arterial pressure is increased by a large embolus due to the right ventricle working against an increased pulmonary vascular resistance.

Alveolar dead space is increased according to the proportion of the pulmonary circulation which is occluded (Severinghaus and Stupfel, 1957). The resultant increase in arterial/end-tidal PCO_2 gradient is the basis of detection of air embolism by infrared CO_2 as described above.

Thromboembolism

The commonest pulmonary embolus consists of detached venous thromboses, particularly from veins in the thigh and the pelvic venous plexuses. Smaller thrombi are filtered in the lungs without causing symptoms but larger emboli may impact in major vessels, typically at a bifurcation forming a saddle embolus. This may cause a catastrophic increase in pulmonary vascular resistance with acute right heart failure or cardiac arrest. The only effective treatment is then embolectomy. In less severe cases, dispersal of the thrombus may be accelerated with streptokinase which can be infused though a pulmonary artery catheter lying in the blocked branch.

The primary physiological lesion is an increase in alveolar dead space with an increased arterial/end-tidal P_{CO_2} gradient. However, this does not usually cause hypercapnia since hyperventilation is almost always present and arterial P_{CO_2} is usually below the normal range. Arterial P_{O_2} is also decreased and, in dogs, this has been shown to be due to increased intrapulmonary shunting (Stein et al., 1961).

Other deleterious effects result from breakdown and removal of the thrombus, a process for which the lung is well adapted. Many proteins and particularly fibrin monomers are known to counteract the effect of surfactant, so decreasing compliance (Seeger et al., 1985). Bronchospasm is a well recognized complication (Windebank, Boyd and Moran, 1973) and has been attributed to local release of serotonin (5-hydroxytryptamine) from the platelets in the clot and also to local hypocapnia in the part of the lung without effective pulmonary circulation.

Diagnosis of pulmonary thromboembolus

In massive pulmonary thromboembolus, the diagnosis is only too obvious but, in less severe cases, the diagnosis is much more difficult. The gold standard of diagnosis is pulmonary angiography although more use is made of pulmonary radioisotope perfusion or ventilation/perfusion scans (Hull et al., 1985; Bone, 1990; Morrell and Seed, 1992). Recent investigations, particularly the Prospective Investigation of Pulmonary Embolism Diagnosis (PIOPED, 1990), have demonstrated the relatively low sensitivity of high-probability scans, and Bone concluded that scans are inadequate to ascertain the presence of pulmonary embolism. Bone and also Morrell and Seed stress the value of reinforcing the diagnosis by looking for deep venous thrombi in the legs, since the great majority of pulmonary thromboemboli arise in these veins. Venous thromboembolism has been reviewed by Moser (1990).

The methods based on gas analysis described above for air embolism are not applicable to thromboembolism. Measurement of physiological dead space may help in the diagnosis, but the wide scatter of normal values reduces the discrimination of the test.

Fat embolism

Fracture of long bones may be associated with fat embolism which stains characteristically with osmic acid. It has been thought that blood lipids might coalesce and form the emboli. However, fragments of bone marrow with the normal architecture have been found embedded in the lung fields at postmortem after fat embolism.

Lipid appears to pass through the pulmonary circulation to invade the systemic circulation. Surface forces between blood and lipid are much less than between blood and air and so would not offer the same hindrance to passage through the lungs. In the systemic circulation, fat emboli cause the characteristic petechiae in the anterior axillary folds. In addition, fat may be found in the urine and there is often evidence of cerebral involvement.

There is initially an increase in physiological dead space (Greenbaum et al., 1965) but this is soon accompanied by an increase in shunt (Prys-Roberts et al., 1970) which is probably caused by the release of substances in the lung which cause spasm of the airways and open up anastomotic channels between pulmonary artery and vein. The position is often further complicated by superadded infection.

Chapter 29

Adult respiratory distress syndrome

Ashbaugh and his colleagues (1967) described a condition in adults which appeared similar to the respiratory distress syndrome in infants, and later Petty and Ashbaugh (1971) introduced the term 'adult respiratory distress syndrome' (ARDS). It is a characteristic form of severe parenchymal lung failure, often terminal, which may follow any one or more of a wide range of predisposing conditions. There are a great many synonyms for ARDS, including acute respiratory failure, acute lung injury, shock lung, respirator lung, pump lung and Da Nang lung.

Definition

There is no single diagnostic test, and much confusion has arisen from differing diagnostic criteria. This has greatly complicated comparisons of incidence, mortality, aetiology and efficacy of therapy in different centres. Many authors have stressed the importance of establishing a firm and quantitative basis for diagnosis and made specific proposals (Pepe et al., 1982; Fein et al., 1983; Fowler et al., 1983; Lloyd, Newman and Brigham, 1984; Stevens and Raffin, 1984; Murray et al., 1988). Most proposals have concentrated on the following aspects of the condition:

1. Severe hypoxaemia with a large increase in the alveolar/arterial P_{O_2} gradient. There is no agreement on the precise degree of hypoxaemia for the definition of ARDS, and proposals range from an arterial P_{O_2} of 6.7 to 10 kPa (50–75 mmHg) while breathing an inspired oxygen concentration variously cited within the range 50–100%. Alternatively, the critical level of hypoxaemia has been defined as an arterial P_{O_2} which is less than a certain fraction of the alveolar or inspired P_{O_2}.
2. Bilateral diffuse infiltration on the chest radiograph.
3. Stiff lungs with a total compliance of the respiratory system which is less than 5 ml/kPa (50 ml/cmH$_2$O). It should, however, be noted that this is within the normal range for an anaesthetized patient who has healthy lungs.
4. Pulmonary oedema should not be cardiogenic and the pulmonary wedge pressure should not be elevated. Different definitions of ARDS require the wedge pressure to be less than various values ranging from 1.6 to 2.4 kPa (12–18 mmHg). However, this would exclude the diagnosis of true ARDS where it

coexisted with a condition which caused an increased left atrial pressure (Lloyd, Newman and Brigham, 1984).

In addition to the criteria listed above, various authors suggest that one or more of the known predisposing conditions should have been present and that the clinical course has followed the recognized pattern (see below). In addition, it is noted that the histology is usually diagnostic but it is seldom indicated or advisable to take a lung biopsy. There is no reliable laboratory test to confirm the diagnosis.

In part, the diagnosis of ARDS depends on exclusion of other conditions. Sometimes it is not easy to separate it from other conditions such as pulmonary embolus, fibrosing alveolitis, bronchopneumonia and virus pneumonia, which may present many similar features. There has been much debate on whether ARDS exists as a discrete entity or whether it is more profitable to regard the conditions following the various predisposing factors as separate disorders.

Scoring systems

Various attempts have been made to derive a single numerical value to assess the severity of the condition. This greatly facilitates comparison of incidence and therapeutic trials, as well as helping in prognosis and assessment of progress in an individual patient. APACHE II (acute physiology and chronic health evaluation) is widely used (Kraus et al., 1985). Murray et al. (1988) have proposed an expanded three-part definition comprising distinction between acute and chronic phases, identification of aetiological and associated conditions and a numerical lung injury score. The lung injury score is based on all or some of the following (Table 29.1):

1. The extent of alveolar consolidation seen on chest X-ray.
2. Arterial PO_2/fractional concentration of oxygen in inspired gas.
3. The level of positive end-expiratory pressure (PEEP) in use.
4. Compliance of the respiratory system.

Predisposing conditions and risk factors

Although the clinical and histopathological picture of ARDS is remarkably consistent, it has been described as the sequel to a very large range of predisposing conditions (Table 29.2). There are, however, very important differences in the disease and its response to treatment, depending on the underlying cause and associated pathology (Murray et al., 1988). Nevertheless, recognition of the predisposing conditions is crucially important for predicting which patients are at risk and for the establishment of early diagnosis.

By no means are all the conditions in Table 29.2 equally likely to proceed to ARDS. Analysis of some of the more important risk factors has been undertaken by Pepe et al. (1982), Fein et al. (1983) and Fowler et al. (1983). Pepe's group found the highest single risk factor was the sepsis syndrome: 38% of patients in this category developed ARDS. The incidence was 30% in patients who aspirated gastric contents, 24% in patients with multiple emergency transfusions (more than 22 units in 12 hours) and 17% in patients with pulmonary contusions. Multiple minor fractures produced an incidence of only 8%, and numbers were too small to evaluate near-drowning, pancreatitis and prolonged hypotension. Over all, 25% of

Table 29.1 Lung injury score (Murray, 1988)

From chest X-ray	No alveolar consolidation		0
	Alveolar consolidation confined to 1 quadrant		1
	Alveolar consolidation confined to 2 quadrants		2
	Alveolar consolidation confined to 3 quadrants		3
	Alveolar consolidation in all 4 quadrants		4
Hypoxaemia score Pa_{O_2}/FI_{O_2}	> 40 kPa	> 30 mmHg	0
	30–39.9 kPa	225–299 mmHg	1
	23.3–29.9 kPa	175–224 mmHg	2
	13.3–23.2 kPa	100–174 mmHg	3
	< 13.3 kPa	< 100 mmHg	4
Positive end-expiratory pressure (when ventilated)	< 0.5 kPa	< 5 cmH$_2$O	0
	0.6–0.8 kPa	6–8 cmH$_2$O	1
	0.9–1.1 kPa	9–11 cmH$_2$O	2
	1.2–1.4 kPa	12–14 cmH$_2$O	3
	> 1.5 kPa	> 15 cmH$_2$O	4
Respiratory system compliance (when available)	> 0.8 l/kPa	> 80 ml/cmH$_2$O	0
	0.6–0.79 l/kPa	60–79 ml/cmH$_2$O	1
	0.4–0.59 l/kPa	40–59 ml/cmH$_2$O	2
	0.2–0.39 l/kPa	20–39 ml/cmH$_2$O	3
	< 0.19 l/kPa	< 19 ml/cmH$_2$O	4

Pa_{O_2}/FI_{O_2} is the arterial P_{O_2} divided by the fractional concentration of oxygen in the inspired gas. The final score is the mean of the individual scores for each of the components which are included in the assessment.

Score	
0	No lung injury
0.1–2.5	Mild to moderate lung injury
> 2.5	Severe lung injury (ARDS)

Table 29.2 Some predisposing conditions for ARDS

Direct injury	*Indirect injury*
Pulmonary contusion	Septicaemia
Gastric aspiration	Shock or prolonged hypotension
Near-drowning	Non-thoracic trauma
Inhalation of toxic gases and vapours	Cardiopulmonary bypass
Some infections	Head injury
Fat embolus	Pancreatitis
Amniotic fluid embolus	Diabetic coma
Radiation	Multiple blood transfusions
Bleomycin	Excessive fluid replacement

patients with a single risk factor developed ARDS but this rose to 42% with two factors and 85% with three. Sepsis was, however, seldom associated with the other factors, and in most of the patients with sepsis who developed ARDS it was the only risk factor. The number and nature of the risk factors was a better predictor than the injury severity score or measurements of initial oxygenation.

Fein's group followed 116 patients with septicaemia and found an 18% incidence of ARDS but this was greatly increased if the patient also had thrombocytopenia (46% incidence) or a period of 60 minutes with a systolic blood pressure less than 8 kPa (60 mmHg) (64% incidence). No patient without hypotension proceeded to develop ARDS. Most infections were Gram negative but some were Gram positive and a few were fungal. Age and sex did not affect the likelihood of development of ARDS. Fowler's group followed 993 patients considered to be at risk as a result of cardiopulmonary bypass surgery, burns, bacteraemia, transfusions of 10 or more units of blood, major fractures, disseminated intravascular coagulation (DIC), aspiration of gastric contents or pneumonia. As a single factor, aspiration had the highest incidence of ARDS (35.6%) followed by DIC (22.2%) and pneumonia (11.9%). Other factors, including bacteraemia, all showed an incidence of less than 6%. Patients with multiple risk factors had an incidence of 24.6% compared with 5.8% for a single risk factor.

These studies clearly show major differences in the incidence and causation of ARDS in particular patient populations. Others in this field have encountered many cases attributable to multiple trauma and also to treatment with bleomycin. Difficult though it may be to extrapolate from a particular study to one's own practice, the major predisposing conditions are now agreed to be septicaemia (particularly Gram negative), aspiration of gastric contents, DIC, multiple trauma (particularly with pulmonary contusion) and multiple transfusions. It is now rare to see the condition following evacuation and resuscitation of exsanguinated casualties from the battlefield. This was commonplace in Vietnam, where overenthusiastic replacement of circulatory volume may have been a factor. No case of ARDS occurred in the Falklands campaign (J.M. Beeley, personal communication).

It is extremely difficult, if not impossible, to separate the toxic effects of high concentrations of oxygen from the pathological condition which required their use. This problem is considered on page 553 but it seems unlikely that high concentrations of oxygen *per se* are a major aetiological factor in the causation of ARDS.

The sepsis syndrome

The sepsis syndrome is defined as a systemic response to proven or presumed infection, with hypo- (or hyper-) thermia, tachycardia, tachypnoea, and one or more organs exhibiting hypoperfusion or dysfunction (Bone et al., 1989a). There is usually altered cerebral function, arterial hypoxaemia, lactacidosis and oliguria. Plasma albumin concentration is usually decreased. Many cases of ARDS represent the pulmonary manifestation of the multi-organ dysfunction syndrome (MODS) which is a feature of this condition, and ARDS is frequently associated with circulatory failure (septic shock). Bacteraemia may or may not be present, and has little effect on outcome. In a study of 191 patients with the sepsis syndrome, 25% developed ARDS and 36% septic shock (Bone et al., 1989a).

Incidence and mortality

The much-quoted American Lung Program of 1972 estimated the incidence in the USA to be 150 000 cases a year, which would correspond to 130 per year in a typical British health district of 200 000 people. This seemed at variance with personal experience, and a 1-year survey of one regional health authority in the UK (population 3 102 500) showed an incidence of 9 per year per health district (population 200 000), or 0.045 per year per 1000 resident population. It comprised 2.5% of all admissions to intensive therapy units (Webster, Cohen and Nunn, 1988). This was barely 7% of the incidence reported by the American Lung Program.

The reasons for this discrepancy are not clear. Possibly the diagnostic criteria tend to be different and the definition cited above has considerable latitude in the precise degree of arterial hypoxaemia. Furthermore, the studies were separated by 16 years, during which there was increasing awareness of how to avoid the predisposing conditions.

There is, however, considerable agreement that the overall mortality of ARDS is of the order of 50% whatever the criteria of diagnosis. It was 38% in the survey of Webster, Cohen and Nunn. It tends to be higher in cases which follow septicaemia, in which it was 81% (Fein et al., 1983) and 78% (Fowler et al., 1983).

Clinical course

Four phases may be recognized in the development of ARDS. In the first the patient is dyspnoeic and tachypnoeic but there are no other abnormalities. The chest radiograph is normal at this stage, which lasts for about 24 hours. In the next phase there is hypoxaemia but the arterial PCO_2 remains normal or subnormal. There are minor abnormalities of the chest radiograph. This phase may last for 1 or 2 days. Diagnosis is easily missed in these prodromal stages and is very dependent on the history of one or more predisposing conditions.

It is only in phase three that the diagnostic criteria of true ARDS become established. There is severe arterial hypoxaemia due to an increased alveolar/arterial PO_2 gradient, and the PCO_2 may be slightly elevated. The lungs become stiff and the chest radiograph shows the characteristic bilateral diffuse infiltrates. Artificial ventilation is usually instituted at this stage.

The fourth phase is often terminal and comprises massive bilateral consolidation with unremitting hypoxaemia, the arterial PO_2, characteristically being less than 7 kPa (52.5 mmHg) when the inspired oxygen concentration is 100%. Dead space is substantially increased and the arterial PCO_2 is only with difficulty kept in the normal range by the use of a large minute volume (10–20 l/min).

Not every patient progresses through all these phases and the condition may resolve at any stage. It is difficult to predict whether the condition will progress and there is no useful laboratory test. Serial observations of the chest radiograph, the alveolar/arterial PO_2 gradient and function of other compromised organs are the best guides to progress. The more systems in failure, the worse is the outlook.

Histopathology

Although of diverse aetiology, the histological appearances of ARDS are remarkably consistent and this lends support for ARDS being considered a discrete clinical entity. Bachofen and Weibel (1982), after extensive study of autopsy material, have divided the histological changes into two stages: acute and subacute or chronic.

The acute stage

The acute stage is characterized by damaged integrity of the blood/gas barrier. The changes are primarily in the interalveolar septa and cannot be satisfactorily seen with light microscopy. Electron microscopy shows extensive damage to the type I alveolar epithelial cells (page 30), which may be totally destroyed (Figure 29.1). Meanwhile the basement membrane is usually preserved and the endothelial cells still tend to form a continuous layer with apparently intact cell junctions. Endothelial permeability is nevertheless increased with access of albumin to the extravascular space. Interstitial oedema is found, predominantly on the 'service' side of the capillary where endothelium and epithelium are separated by a tissue space (see Figure 2.8). Fortunately, the oedema tends to spare the 'active' side of the capillary where endothelium and epithelium are in close apposition. This differentiation between the two sides of the pulmonary capillary is also seen in cardiogenic oedema.

Protein-containing fluid leaks into the alveoli, which also contain erythrocytes and leucocytes in addition to amorphous material comprising strands of fibrin (Figure 29.1). The exudate may form into sheets which line the alveoli as the so-called hyaline membrane. Intravascular coagulation is common at this stage and, in patients with septicaemia, capillaries may be completely plugged with leucocytes, and the underlying endothelium may then be damaged.

The subacute or chronic stage

Attempted repair and proliferation predominate in the chronic stage of ARDS. Within a few days of the onset of the condition, there is a thickening of endothelium, epithelium and the interstitial space. The type I epithelial cells are destroyed and replaced by type II cells (page 30) which proliferate but do not differentiate into type I cells as usual. They remain cuboidal and about ten times the thickness of the type I cells which they have replaced. This appears to be a non-specific response to damaged type I cells, and is similar to that which results from exposure to high concentrations of oxygen (page 552). Type I cells are end-cells and cannot divide. They are derived from type II cells which appear to be much more robust.

The interstitial space is greatly expanded by oedema fluid, fibres and a variety of proliferating cells. Fibrosis commences after the first week and ultimately fibrocytes predominate: extensive fibrosis is seen in resolving cases. Within the alveoli, the protein-rich exudate may organize to produce the characteristic 'hyaline membrane' which effectively destroys the structure of the alveoli. This is clearly visible with light microscopy.

Pathophysiology

Oxygen consumption of the lung

Measurement of pulmonary oxygen consumption (as the difference between spirometry and the reversed Fick method – see page 304) has repeatedly shown very high values for infected lungs and in ARDS (Light, 1988; Takala et al., 1989; Behrendt et al., 1987; Smithies et al., 1991). It seems quite possible that some of this represents free radical formation (see Chapter 32).

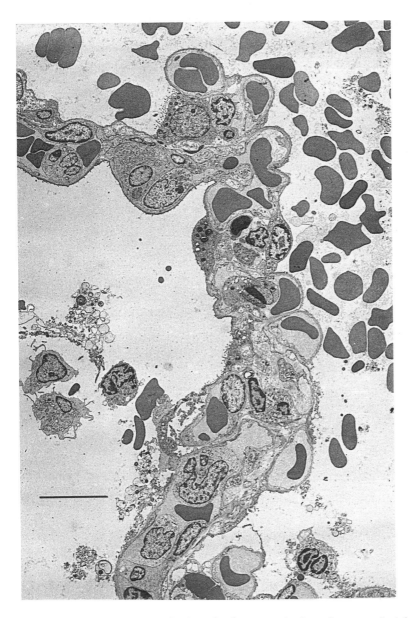

Figure 29.1 Electron micrograph of an alveolar septum in the early stages of adult respiratory distress syndrome. On the right-hand side of the septum there are many examples of damage to alveolar epithelium but the endothelium tends to remain intact. The alveolar gas spaces to left and right contain many erythrocytes, leucocytes, cell debris and fibrin strands. No hyaline membrane has yet formed. The scale bar (bottom left) is 10 μm. (Reproduced from Bachofen and Weibel (1982) by permission of the authors and the Editors of Chest Medicine*)*

Maldistribution of ventilation and perfusion.

Computed tomography (CT) of patients with ARDS shows that opacities representing collapsed areas are distributed throughout the lungs in a non-homogeneous manner but predominantly in the dependent parts (Gattinoni et al., 1988). Following a change in posture, the opacities move to the newly dependent zones within a few minutes (Gattinoni et al., 1991a, b). The most conspicuous functional disability is the shunt (Figure 29.2), which is usually so large (often more than 40%) that increasing the inspired oxygen concentration cannot produce a normal arterial PO_2 (see the iso-shunt chart, Figure 8.11). The increased dead space, which may exceed 70% of tidal volume, requires a large increase in minute volume in an attempt to preserve a normal arterial PO_2. Both shunt and dead space correlate strongly with the non-inflated lung tissue seen at CT scan (Figure 29.2). Alveolar/capillary permeability is increased in patients at risk for ARDS (Tennenberg et al., 1987), and this may be demonstrated by the enhanced transit of various tracer molecules across the alveolar/capillary membrane (page 216).

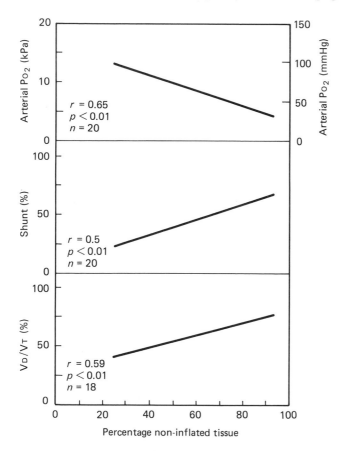

Figure 29.2 Relationship of arterial PO_2, shunt and physiological dead space (VD/VT) to the percentage of non-inflated lung tissue seen by computed tomography in patients with adult respiratory distress syndrome, artificially ventilated with positive end-expiratory pressure of 0.5 kPa (5 cmH$_2$O). (Redrawn from data of Gattinoni et al., 1988)

Dantzker and his colleagues (1979) applied the technique of multiple inert gas wash-out (page 194) to patients with ARDS to determine the pattern of distribution of ventilation and perfusion. They found a bimodal distribution of perfusion, one part to areas of normal ventilation/perfusion ($\dot{V}/\dot{Q}$) ratio and another to areas of zero or very low $\dot{V}/\dot{Q}$ ratio.

Effect of PEEP. PEEP reduces the amount of non-inflated lung tissue seen at CT scan (Gattinoni et al., 1988), and also the shunt fraction and therefore increases the arterial PO_2 (Figure 29.3). Cardiac output is better maintained than might be expected, with a reduction of the order of 20% with PEEP of 1.5 kPa (15 cm H_2O)

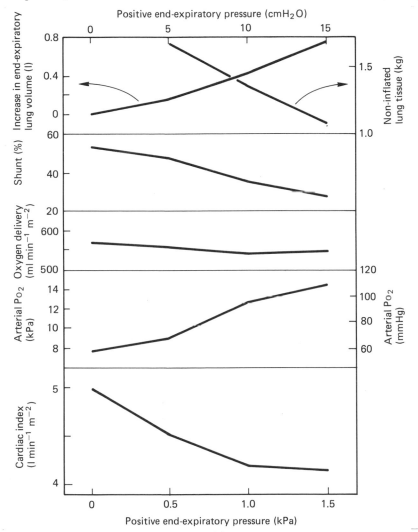

Figure 29.3 Effect of positive end-expiratory pressure on various factors influencing oxygen delivery, in patients with adult respiratory distress syndrome. Although arterial PO_2 is increased, cardiac output is decreased and there is no significant change in oxygen transport. (Data on non-inflated lung tissue are from Gattinoni et al., 1988; remaining data are from Ranieri et al., 1991)

(Figure 29.3; see also Figure 22.15). Gattinoni et al. and Ranieri et al. (1991) are agreed that the resultant reduction in oxygen delivery is insignificant. Inspiratory resistance is unaffected but, surprisingly, expiratory resistance of the respiratory system is increased, particularly by high levels of PEEP (Pesenti et al., 1991).

Lung mechanics

In established ARDS, lung compliance is greatly reduced and the static compliance of the respiratory system (lungs + chest wall) is of the order of 300 ml/kPa (30 ml/cm H_2O) (Eissa et al., 1991; Tantucci et al., 1992). This seems to be adequately explained by the histological changes described above. It is also very likely that there is impaired production and function of surfactant (Fein et al., 1982). Functional residual capacity is reduced by collapse, tissue proliferation and increased elastic recoil.

Mean total resistance to air flow was found to be 2 kPa l^{-1} s (20 cm H_2O/l/s) (Eissa et al., 1991) and 1.43 kPa l^{-1} s (14.3 cmH_2O/l/s) (Tantucci et al., 1992), values about three times those of anaesthetized patients with normal lungs, measured by the same techniques (D'Angelo et al., 1989). Using the model shown in Figure 4.6c, some two-thirds of the total resistance in patients with ARDS could be assigned to viscoelastic resistance of tissue, although the airway resistance was still about twice normal. Mean time constant was 0.16 s (Eissa et al., 1991), which is about a third of normal.

Mechanisms of causation of ARDS

The diversity of predisposing conditions suggests that there may be several possible mechanisms, at least in the early stages of development of ARDS. Nevertheless, the end-result is remarkably similar (Stevens and Raffin, 1984). In all cases initiation of the syndrome seems to be damage to the alveolar/capillary membrane with transudation often increased by pulmonary venoconstriction (Malik, Selig and Burhop, 1985). Thereafter, development of the condition is accelerated by a series of positive feedback mechanisms. The initial insult to the alveolar/capillary membrane may be direct or indirect by one of several postulated mechanisms.

Direct injury to the lung

Direct injury to the lung seems to be sufficient to explain the initiation of ARDS in certain situations. These include gastric aspiration, near-drowning, inhalation of toxic gases, pulmonary contusion and, possibly, pulmonary oxygen toxicity. Certain bacterial toxins may act directly on pulmonary endothelium.

Indirect injury to the lung

Much attention has recently been given to cellular and humoral mechanisms which may damage the alveolar/capillary membrane (Weiner-Kronish, Gropper and Matthay, 1990). The cells which appear capable of damaging the membrane include neutrophils, basophils, macrophages and also probably platelets. Damage may be inflicted by a large number of substances, including bacterial endotoxin, oxygen-derived free radicals, tumour necrosis factor (TNF), proteases, thrombin, fibrin,

fibrin degradation products, histamine, bradykinin, 5-hydroxytryptamine (serotonin), platelet-activating factor (PAF) and some arachidonic acid metabolites. Various chemotactic agents, especially complement C5a, probably play a major role in directing formed elements onto the pulmonary endothelium. It seems improbable that any one mechanism is responsible for all cases of ARDS. It is more likely that different mechanisms operate in different predisposing conditions and in different animal models of ARDS.

Malik, Selig and Burhop (1985) have drawn attention to the fact that many of the humoral mediators, including histamine and some arachidonic acid metabolites, cause pulmonary venoconstriction. This raises pulmonary capillary pressure and compounds the effect of increased permeability. It has also been noted that many proteins, including albumin but particularly fibrin monomer, can antagonize the action of surfactant (Seeger et al., 1985).

Neutrophil-mediated injury has been extensively considered as a possible mechanism (see reviews by Fantone and Ward, 1982; Rinaldo and Rogers, 1982; Tate and Repine, 1983; Brigham and Meyrick, 1984; Glauser and Fairman, 1985). The postulated sequence of events begins with activation of complement C5a which is known to cause margination of neutrophils on the vascular endothelium. Complement C5a is known to be activated in sepsis (Hammerschmidt, 1983), after cardiopulmonary bypass surgery (Chenoweth et al., 1981) and in many other conditions which may lead to ARDS. Neutrophils have been seen packed in the pulmonary capillaries of lung specimens from patients with ARDS.

Margination of very large numbers of neutrophils in the pulmonary circulation may occur without any resultant pulmonary damage (Glauser and Fairman, 1985). This occurs, for example, during the early stages of an anaphylactoid reaction and also during haemodialysis with a cellophane membrane. However, under other circumstances it seems very likely that neutrophils marginated in the pulmonary circulation may damage the endothelium. The postulated sequence of events is that the neutrophils are first primed with the bactericidal contents of their lysosomes. This may occur in response to endotoxin, which will also cause neutrophils to adhere firmly to the pulmonary capillary endothelium. In addition, complement C5a results in temporary adherence to endothelium but its most important effect is to trigger the neutrophil into inappropriate release of its lysosomal contents. Instead of being released into phagocytic vesicles, they come into direct contact with the endothelium which is thereby damaged.

Four groups of substances released from neutrophils have been considered as potentially damaging to the endothelium. Firstly, there are oxygen-derived free radicals and related compounds (see Chapter 32). These are powerful and important bactericidal agents, which also have the capacity to damage the endothelium by lipid peroxidation and other means. In addition, they inactivate α_1-antitrypsin. The second group comprises proteolytic enzymes, which not only damage the endothelium directly but also produce elastin fragments which are chemotactic for monocytes and macrophages (Senior, Griffen and Mecham, 1980). Of the proteases, elastase is particularly damaging. The third group comprises the arachidonic metabolites, prostaglandins, thromboxanes and leukotrienes, various members of which cause vasoconstriction, increase vascular permeability and are chemotactic for neutrophils. They are discussed further in Chapter 12. The fourth group comprises platelet-activating factors (PAF) resulting in intravascular coagulation. Fibrin and fibrin degradation products may themselves contribute to the tissue damage. It will be seen that numerous positive feedback loops amplify the tissue damage once it is started.

Proof of the role of neutrophils has been sought by studies of neutrophil-depleted animals, but with contradictory results. While neutrophils certainly possess the potential for endothelial damage, it seems very unlikely that they are the sole cause of ARDS. Their role in the causation of increased alveolar/capillary permeability has been critically reviewed by Glauser and Fairman (1985).

Macrophages and basophils. Macrophages are already present in the normal alveolus (page 30) but their numbers increase greatly in ARDS. They produce a wide range of bactericidal agents similar to those of the neutrophil. In addition, their antibacterial armoury includes cytokines, a group of peptides including TNF and the interleukins, known to be capable of causing tissue damage. Infusion of human recombinant TNF (but not interleukin-1) into dogs resulted in severe lung injury similar to that seen in septic shock (Eichacker et al., 1991).

Platelets are present in the pulmonary capillaries in large number in ARDS. Aggregation in that site is associated with increased capillary hydrostatic pressure, possibly due to release of arachidonic acid metabolites. They may also play a role in maintenance of the integrity of the endothelium (Malik, Selig and Burhop, 1985). Platelet function may well be implicated in the formation of the 'hyaline' membrane which lines the alveoli in ARDS (Weiner-Kronish, Gropper and Matthay, 1990).

Principles of management

Specific therapy is the goal of much research which is particularly directed towards the control of infection and the development of antagonists to the various mediators considered above (Bone, 1992). In most cases it has proved difficult to demonstrate their efficacy and the financial implications of their widespread use have caused grave concern in some cases, such as the monoclonal antibody to endotoxin. In the meantime, management is essentially supportive, with the following main objectives:

1. To maintain a safe arterial P_{O_2}.
2. To minimize pulmonary transudation.
3. To prevent complications, particularly sepsis.
4. To maintain the circulation.

Patients are always ventilated, often with positive end-expiratory pressure (PEEP) to improve arterial P_{O_2} (Figure 29.3). At one time it seemed that the early use of PEEP might prevent the development of ARDS (Schmidt et al., 1976). However, it now seems unlikely that there is any such effect (Fein et al., 1982; Pepe, Hudson and Carrico, 1984). Inspired oxygen concentration should be carefully controlled to prevent dangerous hypoxia, on the one hand, and the possibility of pulmonary oxygen toxicity on the other hand. Oxygen delivery and consumption were found to be greater in survivors of ARDS, and consumption was related to delivery (Russel et al., 1990); this is also true for septic shock (page 508). A most exciting development is the long-term use of inhaled nitric oxide (5–20 p.p.m.), which causes selective vasodilatation in the *ventilated* alveoli (page 311) and so reduces shunt as well as pulmonary hypertension (Rossaint et al., 1993).

Satisfactory gaseous exchange may be impossible by conventional means and high frequency ventilation and extracorporeal techniques have both been used (see Chapters 22 and 23). To discourage oedema formation attempts may be made to raise the serum albumin which is commonly reduced. Also the fluid balance should be adjusted to keep the wedge pressure rather low (0.7–1.3 kPa or 5–10 mmHg) (Fein et al., 1982).

Initial optimism for the use of steroids, prostaglandin E_1, naloxone and heparin has not withstood the test of randomized controlled trials in ARDS and septic shock (Bone et al., 1987, 1989b; Weiner-Kronish, Gropper and Matthay, 1990; Bone, 1992). Therapy for ARDS remains disappointing, with a very high mortality in spite of great expenditure of resources in both therapy and research. However, monoclonal antibody to endotoxin appears safe and effective for Gram-negative septic shock (Ziegler et al., 1991).

Problems of research into ARDS

Research into ARDS is notoriously difficult. Human studies are bedevilled by the diverse aetiology and the relatively small and decreasing number of cases which are seen in some research centres. When the condition has developed, the patient is clearly not in any condition to give informed consent for research and there are evident difficulties in approaching the relatives of a patient with a condition carrying a 50% mortality.

The obvious solution to these difficulties would appear to be the use of an animal model. There have, however, been great difficulties in establishing an animal model which reproduces all aspects of the disease in man. Various substances have been used to mimic ARDS, including oleic acid, paraquat, TNF, phorbol myristate acetate, α-naphthylthiourea (ANTU) and high concentrations of oxygen. Although severe lung damage can be produced in certain species, there is no certainty that the condition is a true model of ARDS. Furthermore, the evaluation of effective therapy is complicated by marked species differences in response.

Chapter 30

The effects of changes in the carbon dioxide tension

The effects of changes in P_{CO_2} were a matter of grave concern some 35 years ago, when there were no convenient techniques for monitoring or measurement of P_{CO_2} in the clinical environment. Gross departures from normality were relatively common, and hypercapnia was an appreciable cause of mortality. All of this has changed with monitoring of end-expiratory P_{CO_2} and the ease of direct measurement of arterial P_{CO_2}. It should now be possible to prevent both hypo- and hypercapnia under almost all clinical circumstances. Nevertheless, the effects of changes in P_{CO_2} involve some fundamental aspects of physiology and remain of interest.

A number of special difficulties hinder an understanding of the effects of changes in P_{CO_2}. Firstly, there is the problem of species difference, which is a formidable obstacle to the interpretation of animal studies in this as in other fields. The second difficulty arises from the fact that carbon dioxide can exert its effect either directly or in consequence of (respiratory) acidosis. The third difficulty arises from the fact that carbon dioxide acts at many different sites in the body, sometimes producing opposite effects upon a particular function, such as blood pressure (see Figure 30.3, below). The subject was reviewed by Foëx (1980), Prys-Roberts (1980) and Utting (1980).

Effects upon the nervous system

Carbon dioxide has at least five major effects upon the brain:

1. It is the major factor governing cerebral blood flow.
2. It influences the CSF pressure through changes in cerebral blood flow.
3. It is the main factor influencing the intracellular pH, which is known to have important effects upon the metabolism of the cell.
4. It may be presumed to exert the inert gas narcotic effect in accord with its physical properties which are similar to those of nitrous oxide.
5. It influences the excitability of certain neurons, particularly relevant in the case of the reticuloactivating system.

The interplay of these effects is difficult to understand, although the gross changes produced are well established.

Effects on consciousness

Carbon dioxide has long been known to cause unconsciousness in dogs entering the Grotto del Cane in Italy, where carbon dioxide issuing from a fumarole forms a layer near the ground. It was used as an anaesthetic by Henry Hill Hickman in 1824, later by Ozanam (1862), and finally by Leake and Waters (1928). Inhalation of 30% carbon dioxide is sufficient for the production of anaesthesia, and results in an isoelectric electroencephalogram (Clowes, Hopkins and Simeone, 1955). However, use of carbon dioxide as an anaesthetic in man is complicated by the frequent occurrence of convulsions at about the concentration required for anaesthesia (Leake and Waters, 1928). Higher concentrations have been shown to be tolerated in dogs, in whom the tendency to convulsions disappears when the PCO_2 rises above about 33.3 kPa (250 mmHg). Carbon dioxide has been widely used as a routine anaesthetic agent for very short procedures in small laboratory animals. In patients with ventilatory failure, carbon dioxide narcosis occurs when the PCO_2 rises above 12–16 kPa (90–120 mmHg) (Westlake, Simpson and Kaye, 1955; Refsum, 1963).

It has been claimed that hyperventilation and hypocapnia enhance the actions of agents used to produce general anaesthesia (Gray and Rees, 1952) and this is supported by the demonstration of a reduced threshold to the pain of tibial pressure (Clutton-Brock, 1957). These effects have been variously attributed to decreased excitation of the reticuloactivating system or to cerebral hypoxia resulting from the combined effects of cerebral vasconstriction and shift of the oxyhaemoglobin dissociation curve. However, Eisele, Eger and Muallem (1967) found that, in dogs, the minimal alveolar concentration (MAC) of halothane required for anaesthesia was unaltered by changes of PCO_2 within the range 2–12.7 kPa (15–95 mmHg). Above 12.7 kPa the narcotic effect of carbon dioxide was apparent and the halothane requirement was progressively reduced until, at PCO_2 32.7 kPa (245 mmHg), anaesthesia was achieved with carbon dioxide alone.

Narcosis by carbon dioxide is probably not due primarily to its inert gas narcotic effects, because its oil solubility predicts a very much weaker narcotic than it appears to be. It seems likely that the major effect on the central nervous system is by alteration of the intracellular pH with consequent derangements of metabolic processes (Woodbury and Karler, 1960). Eisele, Eger and Muallem (1967) showed that the narcotic effect correlated better with cerebrospinal fluid pH than with arterial PCO_2.

Cerebral blood flow

Cerebral blood flow (CBF) increases with PCO_2 within the range 3–13 kPa (approximately 20–100 mmHg). The effect is exerted on the cerebral vascular resistance by means of changes in the extracellular pH in the region of the arterioles. The full response curve is S-shaped (Figure 30.1). The response at very low PCO_2 is probably limited by the vasodilator effect of tissue hypoxia, and the response above 16 kPa (120 mmHg) seems to represent maximal vasodilation (Reivich, 1964). The changes shown in Figure 30.1 represent the brain as a whole and it is not possible to generalize about regional changes. It should also be remembered that sensitivity to carbon dioxide may be lost in the region of tumours, infarctions or trauma. There is commonly a fixed vasodilatation in these areas giving rise to so-called luxury perfusions (Lassen, 1966). Far from being luxurious, this may cause dangerous increases in intracranial pressure. Conversely, some

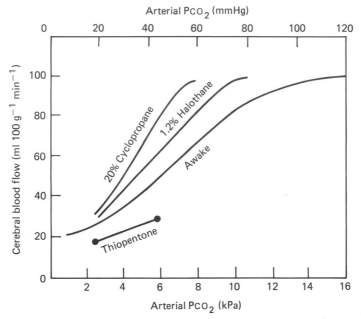

Figure 30.1 Relationship of cerebral blood flow to arterial P_{CO_2} in awake and anaesthetized patients. Lower concentrations of cyclopropane (5% and 13%) appear to reduce cerebral blood flow (Alexander et al., 1968). Data are drawn from various sources, including Reivich (1964), Lassen (1959), Pierce et al. (1962), Smith and Wollman (1972) and Alexander et al. (1968).

areas of the brain may develop focal ischaemia without the ability to respond to increased P_{CO_2}.

Areas with either luxury perfusion or focal ischaemia may respond to altered P_{CO_2} in the opposite direction to normal. Thus a high P_{CO_2} may increase blood flow through normal brain tissue and actually decrease perfusion through ischaemic areas which have lost their response to carbon dioxide. This has been termed the intracerebral steal (Hoedt-Rasmussen et al., 1967). The reverse phenomenon may occur when P_{CO_2} is lowered in patients with an area of luxury perfusion. Vasoconstriction in the surrounding normal tissue may divert blood flow towards the abnormal area of luxury perfusion which has no ability to respond to lowered P_{CO_2}. This has been termed the inverse steal or Robin Hood syndrome (Lassen and Palvalgyi, 1968).

Pierce et al. (1962) investigated the influence of anaesthesia on the effect of P_{CO_2} on CBF. Thiopentone reduced CBF at normal P_{CO_2} in accord with the reduced cerebral oxygen consumption (Table 30.1), but further vasoconstriction occurred with hyperventilation (Figure 30.1), resulting in a substantial fall in jugular venous P_{O_2}. Brain tissue P_{O_2} would undoubtedly have been reduced but there is no convincing biochemical or psychometric evidence that the practice of hyperventilation during anaesthesia results in any significant level of cerebral damage. Inhalational anaesthetics have a direct cerebral vasodilator effect and accentuate the response to P_{CO_2}.

Intracranial pressure tends to rise with increasing P_{CO_2}, probably as a result of cerebral vasodilatation. This has important implications in the management of

Table 30.1 Effects of hyperventilation and anaesthesia on cerebral blood flow and oxygenation in man

State of patient or subject	Cerebral oxygen consumption ($ml\ 100\ g^{-1}\ min^{-1}$)	Cerebral blood flow ($ml\ 100\ g^{-1}\ min^{-1}$)	Internal jugular venous P_{O_2} kPa	Internal jugular venous P_{O_2} mmHg
Conscious				
Arterial P_{CO_2}				
5.3 kPa (40 mmHg)	3.0	44.0	4.7–5.3	35–40
Arterial P_{CO_2}				
2.7 kPa (20 mmHg)	3.0	22.0	—	—
Anaesthetized:				
thiopentone				
Arterial P_{CO_2}				
5.9 kPa (44 mmHg)	1.5	27.6	4.7	35
Arterial P_{CO_2}				
2.4 kPa (18 mmHg)	1.7	16.4	2.4	18
halothane 1.0%				
Arterial P_{CO_2}				
5.5 kPa (41 mmHg)	2.2*	54.4*	5.3†	40†

Data on the conscious subject from Smith and Wollman (1972).
Data on patients anaesthetized with thiopentone from Pierce et al. (1962).
*Data on patients anaesthetized with halothane from Christensen, Hoedt-Rasmussen and Lassen (1967).
†Data on blood from superior sagittal sinus of dogs breathing 2% halothane (derived from oxygen saturation) (McDowall, 1967).

patients with head injuries and during neurosurgery. Hyperventilation has long been a standard method of reducing intracranial pressure after head injury (Shenkin and Bouzarth, 1970), but some patients react in the opposite direction and it is therefore essential to monitor intracranial pressure.

Hyperventilation is also used for controlling brain tension during neurosurgical operations (Marrubini, Rossanda and Tretola, 1964). However, halothane and other inhalational anaesthetics may cause a dangerous rise in intracranial pressure in patients with intracranial tumours (Jennett, McDowall and Barker, 1967) but this effect may be partly mitigated by prior induction of hypocapnia, as suggested by Jennett and his co-workers and later confirmed by Adams et al. (1972).

Effects upon the autonomic and endocrine systems

Survival in severe hypercapnia is, to a large extent, dependent on the autonomic response. A great many of the effects of carbon dioxide on other systems are due wholly or in part to the autonomic response to carbon dioxide.

Nahas, Ligou and Mehlman (1960) and Millar (1960) clearly showed the increase in plasma levels of both adrenaline and noradrenaline caused by an elevation of P_{CO_2} during apnoeic mass-movement oxygenation (Figure 30.2). In moderate hypercapnia there is a proportionate rise of adrenaline and noradrenaline, but in gross hypercapnia (P_{CO_2} more than 27 kPa or 200 mmHg) there is an abrupt rise of adrenaline. Similar, though very variable, changes have been obtained over a lower

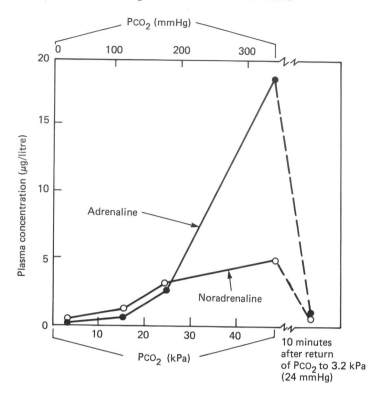

Figure 30.2 This graph shows the changes in plasma catecholamine levels in the dog during the rise of P_{CO_2} from 2.9 to 45 kPa (22 to 338 mmHg) in the course of 1 hour of apnoeic oxygenation. After 10 minutes of ventilation with oxygen, P_{CO_2} returned to 3.2 kPa (24 mmHg). Catecholamines were almost back to control values but the adrenaline remained higher than the noradrenaline. (Prepared from table 4 of Millar, 1960).

range of P_{CO_2} in human volunteers inhaling carbon dioxide mixtures (Sechzer et al., 1960).

The relationship between P_{CO_2} and plasma catecholamine levels is considerably influenced by the administration of inhalational anaesthetic agents. Higher levels of adrenaline and noradrenaline are obtained during cyclopropane anaesthesia than in the unanaesthetized subject. Price et al. (1960) reported levels of 10 μg/l with a P_{CO_2} increase to only 10.7 kPa (80 mmHg) during cyclopropane administration. However, the same group found that plasma catecholamine levels of patients under halothane anaesthesia rose in much the same way as in conscious suubjects.

The effect of an increased level of circulating catecholamines is, to a certain extent, offset by a decreased sensitivity of target organs when the pH is reduced (Tenney, 1956). This is additional to the general depressant direct effect of carbon dioxide on target organs. There is also evidence that the anterior pituitary is stimulated by carbon dioxide, resulting in increased secretion of ACTH (Tenney, 1960). Acetylcholine hydrolysis is reduced at low pH and therefore certain parasympathetic effects may be enhanced during hypercapnia.

It has been suggested that sudden reduction of P_{CO_2} after a period of hypercapnia results in a further elevation of the plasma catecholamine level (see review by

Tenney and Lamb, 1965). However, Millar (1960) showed a rapid fall of both adrenaline and noradrenaline within minutes of reduction of a gross elevation of P_{CO_2} (Figure 30.2). Some support for the theory of posthypercapnic elevation of plasma catecholamine levels has been derived from the cardiovascular response to reduction of an elevated P_{CO_2}. This is considered below.

Effects upon the respiratory system

Control of breathing

Chapter 5 discusses the role of carbon dioxide in the control of breathing. In general the maximal stimulant effect is attained within the P_{CO_2} range 13.3–20 kPa (10–150 mmHg) (Graham, Hill and Nunn, 1960). At higher levels of P_{CO_2} the stimulation is reduced, while at very high levels respiration is depressed and later ceases altogether. Graham, Hill and Nunn (1960) made the curious observation that dogs maintained at a very high tension of carbon dioxide (above 46.7 kPa or 350 mmHg) eventually started breathing again. The breathing was of a gasping character but was sufficient to maintain life for at least an hour without any artificial assistance to ventilation. The breathing in this state (termed supercarbia) is uninfluenced by changes in P_{CO_2} or by vagal section.

The P_{CO_2}/ventilation response curve is generally displaced to the right and its slope reduced by the action of anaesthetic agents and other depressant drugs (see Chapter 20). In profound anaesthesia the response curve may be flat, or even sloping downwards, and carbon dioxide then acts as a respiratory depressant.

Reduction of P_{CO_2} does not always lead to apnoea in the naive subject, who is unaware of Haldane's classic work (page 109). However, during anaesthesia reduction of P_{CO_2} below the threshold value usually results in apnoea (Fink, 1961). Therefore, to restore spontaneous respiration at the end of an operation in which artificial hyperventilation has been employed, it is necessary either to raise the P_{CO_2} above the apnoeic threshold value (Ivanov and Nunn, 1969) or to awaken the patient. References to the effects of carbon dioxide on the control of breathing are given in Chapter 5.

Pulmonary circulation. A raised P_{CO_2} causes vasoconstriction in the pulmonary circulation (page 146) but the effect is less marked than that of hypoxia (Barer, Howard and McCurrie, 1967).

Effects upon oxygenation of the blood

Quite apart from the effect of carbon dioxide upon ventilation, it exerts two other important effects which influence the oxygenation of the blood. Firstly, if the concentration of nitrogen (or other 'inert' gas) remains constant, the concentration of carbon dioxide in the alveolar gas can increase only at the expense of oxygen which must be displaced. Secondly, an increase in P_{CO_2} causes a displacement of the oxygen dissociation curve to the right (page 275). In a patient with gross hypercapnia, Prys-Roberts, Smith and Nunn (1967) reported visibly desaturated arterial blood although the P_{O_2} was 14 kPa (105 mmHg). Unfortunately, the saturation was not measured but subsequent studies suggested that a value of the order of 90% would be expected.

Effects upon the circulatory system
(see review by Foëx, 1980)

The effects of carbon dioxide upon the circulation are complicated by the alternative modes of action upon the different components of the system (Figure 30.3). Many actions are in opposition to each other and, under different circumstances, the overall effect of carbon dioxide upon certain circulatory functions can be entirely reversed.

Myocardial contractility and heart rate

Both contractility and rate are diminished by elevated P_{CO_2} in the isolated preparation (Jerusalem and Starling, 1910), probably as a result of change in pH. However, in the intact subject the direct depressant effect of carbon dioxide is overshadowed by the stimulant effect mediated through the sympathetic system. Blackburn et al. (1972) clearly showed a positive inotropic effect with increasing P_{CO_2} in the dog and demonstrated that this is prevented by β-adrenergic blockade. Cullen and Eger (1974) agreed with Prys-Roberts et al. (1967) that, in artificially ventilated man, increased P_{CO_2} raises cardiac output and slightly reduces total peripheral resistance. As a result, blood pressure tends to be increased. Cullen and Eger obtained similar results during spontaneous breathing.

At very high levels of P_{CO_2} it is likely that cardiac output falls. Study of a single dog by Severinghaus, Mitchell and Nunn (1961, unpublished) showed a progressive decline of cardiac output with increasing P_{CO_2} in supercarbia (Table 30.2). The response of cardiac output to increased P_{CO_2} is diminished by most anaesthetics and by spinal analgesia (Gregory et al., 1974; and a survey of other studies by Cullen and Eger, 1974).

Arrhythmias

Arrhythmias have been reported in unanaesthetized man during acute hypercapnia, but appear to be seldom of serious import. The position is, however, more dangerous under anaesthesia with cyclopropane (Lurie et al., 1958) and with halothane (Black et al., 1959), and possibly with other anaesthetics. With cyclopropane and halothane, it appears that arrhythmias will always occur above a 'P_{CO_2} arrhythmic threshold', which is reported to be surprisingly constant for a particular patient under particular conditions. The mean value is 9.9 kPa (74 mmHg) for cyclopropane and 12.3 kPa (92 mmHg) for halothane. Multifocal ventricular extrasystoles have been reported and the danger of ventricular fibrillation cannot be discounted. These arrhythmias occurred at catecholamine levels which were above normal, but not high enough to cause arrhythmias by themselves. It therefore seems that arrhythmias are caused, at least in part, by a direct action of carbon dioxide on the heart (Price et al., 1958).

Graham, Hill and Nunn (1960) raised the P_{CO_2} of a series of dogs to 73.3 kPa (550 mmHg) and found no arrhythmias regardless of whether the dogs were receiving cyclopropane or halothane. This is a good example of the importance of species difference and illustrates the pitfall which may result from extrapolation of animal data to man.

Brown and Miller (1952) reported that ventricular fibrillation might follow the sudden reduction of a high P_{CO_2} in dogs. Graham, Hill and Nunn (1960) were

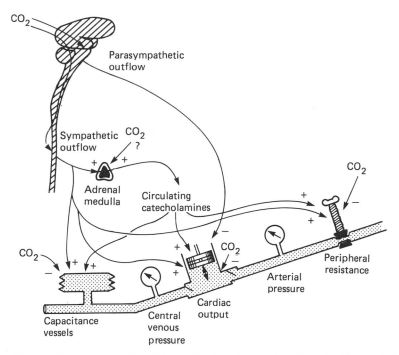

Figure 30.3 The complexity of the mechanisms by which carbon dioxide may influence the circulatory system. The overall effect in the anaesthetized patient is an increase in cardiac output which is roughly proportional to the arterial P_{CO_2}. The rise in cardiac output exceeds the rise in blood pressure and this may be described as a fall in peripheral resistance (total). In spite of the rise of cardiac output, there is an increase in central venous pressure. This implies that capacitance vessels are contracted to cause a rise in filling pressure with which the increased cardiac output does not keep pace. In the absence of sympathetic nervous system activity, the direct effect of carbon dioxide upon the myocardium causes a fall of cardiac output and a profound fall in peripheral resistance is also seen. A fall in arterial blood pressure is then inevitable.

Table 30.2 Circulatory changes at very high P_{CO_2} observed in a single dog by Severinghaus, Mitchell and Nunn (unpublished)

	Arterial blood					Cardiac output (*l/min*)	Blood pressure syst/diast	
Time	P_{CO_2}		*pH*	P_{O_2}				
	kPa	*mmHg*		*kPa*	*mmHg*		*kPa*	*mmHg*
11:51	6.8	51	7.32	39.2	294	3.14	22.0/15.3	165/115
12:35	52.4	393	6.50	27.2	204	2.34	22.0/14.7	165/110
13:00	62.4	468	6.42	20.3	152	0.98	12.0/ 8.0	90/60
13:15	72.0	540	6.41	16.0	120	0.64	11.3/ 6.0	85/45
14:33	6.4	48	7.28	39.1	293	1.29	15.3/12.7	115/95

The dog breathed spontaneously in the state of 'supercarbia' above a P_{CO_2} of 44.9 kPa (337 mmHg) which was attained at 12:25

P_{CO_2} was gradually reduced from 13:16 until 14:33

Cyclopropane anaesthesia was used when the P_{CO_2} was low.

Anaesthesia was terminated at 14:40 and the dog regained consciousness at 14:55. Recovery was uneventful.

unable to confirm these observations after precipitous falls of P_{CO_2} caused by ventilation with oxygen. They suggested that, in the study of Brown and Miller, the dogs may have suffered hypoxia caused by ventilation with air in the presence of a high P_{CO_2}.

Blood pressure

The effect of P_{CO_2} is the result of the interaction of a great many individual actions, some tending to increase and some to decrease the blood pressure. In fact, pressure is generally raised as P_{CO_2} increases in both conscious and anaesthetized patients. However, the response is variable and certainly cannot be relied upon as an infallible diagnostic sign of hypercapnia. At very high levels of P_{CO_2}, the blood pressure declines and appears to be the cause of death if the condition of supercarbia persists for much more than an hour (Graham, Hill and Nunn, 1960). Hypotension accompanies an elevation of P_{CO_2} if there is blockade of the sympathetic system by ganglioplegic drugs or spinal blockade (Payne, 1958). There is general agreement that hypotension follows a sudden fall of an elevated P_{CO_2}.

Regional blood flow
(see Tenney and Lamb, 1965)

Brain (Kety and Schmidt, 1948; Lassen, 1959), coronary and skin blood flow increases with rising P_{CO_2}, while skeletal muscle blood flow is reduced, although this effect is much diminished by general anaesthesia (McArdle and Roddie, 1958). Vance, Brown and Smith (1973) showed that hypocapnia (P_{CO_2} 3.3 kPa or 25 mmHg) in anaesthetized dogs caused a highly significant reduction in myocardial blood flow. However, oxygen extraction was increased and myocardial oxygen consumption was unchanged.

Effect upon the kidney

Renal blood flow and glomerular filtration rate are little influenced by minor changes of P_{CO_2}. However, at high levels of P_{CO_2} there is constriction of the glomerular afferent arterioles, leading to anuria. This effect is abolished in the denervated kidney (Irwin, Draper and Whitehead, 1957).

Chronic hypercapnia results in increased resorption of bicarbonate by the kidneys, further raising the plasma bicarbonate level, and constituting a secondary or compensatory metabolic alkalosis. Chronic hypocapnia decreases renal bicarbonate resorption, resulting in a further fall of plasma bicarbonate and producing a secondary or compensatory 'metabolic acidosis'. In each case the arterial pH returns towards the normal value but the bicarbonate ion concentration departs even further from normality.

Although acute changes of P_{CO_2} do not produce a true metabolic acid–base change, the interpolation technique of Siggaard-Andersen et al. (1960) indicates an apparent base deficit of about 2 mmol/l when the P_{CO_2} of a normal patient is acutely raised from 5.3 to 10.7 kPa (40 to 80 mmHg). Similarly, a base excess of about 2 mmol/l appears when the P_{CO_2} is acutely lowered to 2.7 kPa (20 mmHg) The explanation of this artefact is to be found above (page 227).

Effect upon blood electrolyte levels

Hypercapnia is accompanied by a leakage of potassium ions from the cells into the plasma (Clowes, Hopkins and Simeone, 1955). Hepatectomy has demonstrated that most of the potassium comes from the liver, probably in association with glucose which is mobilized in response to the rise in plasma catecholamine levels (Fenn and Asano, 1956). Since it takes an appreciable time for the potassium ions to be transported back into the intracellular compartment, repeated bouts of hypercapnia at short intervals result in a stepwise rise in plasma potassium.

A reduction in the ionized fraction of the total calcium has, in the past, been thought to be the cause of the tetany which accompanies severe hypocapnia. However, the changes which occur are too small to account for tetany, which only occurs in parathyroid disease when there has been a fairly gross reduction of ionized calcium (Tenney and Lamb, 1965). Hyperexcitability affects all nerves and spontaneous activity ultimately occurs. The spasms probably result from activity in proprioceptive fibres causing reflex muscle contraction.

Effect upon drug action

Changes in P_{CO_2} may affect drug action as a result of a great number of different mechanisms. Firstly, the distribution of the drug may be influenced by changes in perfusion of organs. Secondly, the ionization of drugs may be altered by the change in blood pH. Thirdly, the solubility of the drug in body fluids and the protein binding may be influenced. The effects of changes in P_{CO_2} and pH on the older neuromuscular blockers have been studied by Hughes (1970), who also reviewed the earlier literature. Dann (1971) reported no effect of P_{CO_2} on the duration of action of pancuronium.

Gross hypercapnia in clinical practice

Relatively few cases of gross hypercapnia are documented, but there are sufficient to indicate that complete recovery from gross hypercapnia without hypoxia is possible and may even be the rule. Inhaled concentrations of about 30% were formerly used in psychiatry for abreaction, apparently without ill effect. Gross hypercapnia during anaesthesia was reported (Payne, 1962; Birt and Cole, 1965; Prys-Roberts, Smith and Nunn, 1967), as well as in relation to thoracotomy without artificial ventilation (page 415). Arterial P_{CO_2} values in excess of 30 kPa (225 mm Hg) were apparently not unusual. Goldstein, Shannon and Todres (1990) reported five instances of hypercapnia without hypoxia in children with arterial P_{CO_2} in the range 21–36 kPa (155–269 mm Hg). All were comatose or stuperose but recovered. Further cases from the earlier literature were reviewed by Prys-Roberts, Smith and Nunn, but the general conclusion is that *of the reported cases* full recovery was the usual outcome. Arrhythmias did not appear to be a problem in these patients. In general, hypoxia seems to be much more dangerous than hypercapnia.

Bedside recognition of hypercapnia

Hyperventilation is the cardinal sign of hypercapnia due to an increased concentration of carbon dioxide in the inspired gas, whether it be endogenous or exogenous. However, this sign will be absent in the paralysed patient and also in those in whom hypercapnia is the result of hypoventilation. Such patients, including those with chronic obstructive airway disease, constitute the great majority of those with hypercapnia.

Dyspnoea may or may not be present. In patients with central failure of respiratory drive (including 'blue bloaters'), dyspnoea may be entirely absent. On the other hand, when hypoventilation results from mechanical failure in the respiratory system (airway obstruction, pneumothorax, pulmonary fibrosis, etc.), dyspnoea is usually obvious. This problem is discussed further on page 420 in relation to Figure 21.2.

In patients with chronic bronchitis, hypercapnia is usually associated with a flushed skin and a full and bounding pulse with occasional extrasystoles. The blood pressure is often raised but this is not a reliable sign. Muscle twitchings and a characteristic flap of the hands may be observed when coma is imminent. Convulsions may occur. The patient will become comatose when the P_{CO_2} is in the range 12–16 kPa (90–120 mmHg) (see above). Hypercapnia should always be considered in cases of unexplained coma.

Hypercapnia cannot be reliably diagnosed on clinical examination. This is particularly true when there is a neurological basis for hypoventilation. Now that it has become so simple to measure the arterial P_{CO_2}, an arterial sample should be taken in all cases of doubt.

Chapter 31

Hypoxia

Biochemical changes in hypoxia

Chapter 1 explained how all but the simplest forms of life have evolved to exploit the immense advantages of oxidative metabolism. The price they have paid is to become dependent on oxygen for their survival. The essential feature of hypoxia is the cessation of oxidative phosphorylation (page 248) when the mitochondrial PO_2 falls below the critical level. Anaerobic pathways, in particular the glycolytic pathway (see Figure 11.3), then come into play. Glycolysis is initiated under hypoxic conditions by the accumulation of adenosine diphosphate (ADP) which acts on rate-limiting steps in the metabolic pathway.

Depletion of high energy compounds

Anaerobic metabolism produces only one-nineteenth of the yield of the high energy phosphate compound adenosine triphosphate (ATP) per mole of glucose, when compared with aerobic metabolism (page 249). In organs with a high metabolic rate such as the brain, it is impossible to increase glucose transport sufficiently to maintain the normal level of ATP production. Therefore, during hypoxia, the ATP/ADP ratio falls and there is a rapid decline in the level of all high energy compounds, including phosphocreatine (Figure 31.1). Very similar changes occur in response to arterial hypotension. These changes will rapidly block cerebral function but organs with a lower energy requirement will continue to function for a longer time, and are thus more resistant to hypoxia (see below).

Under hypoxic conditions, two molecules of ADP combine to form one of ATP and one of AMP (the adenylate kinase reaction). This reaction is driven forward by the removal of AMP (adenosine monophosphate) which is converted to adenosine (a potent vasodilator) and thence to inosine, hypoxanthine, xanthine and uric acid, with irreversible loss of adenine nucleotides (Gutierrez, 1991). The implications for production of free radicals are discussed on page 546.

The role of calcium in hypoxia

Hypoxia inhibits the ATP-driven calcium pumps, and the consequent increase in intracellular calcium is generally harmful (Cheung et al., 1986). ATPases are activated just when ATP may be critically low, and proteases may be activated to

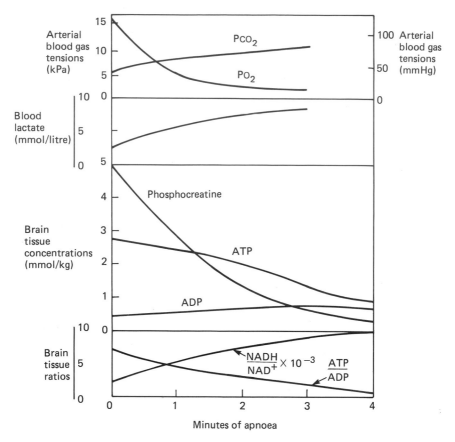

Figure 31.1 Time course of changes during 4 minutes of respiratory arrest in anaesthetized and curarized rats previously breathing 30% oxygen. Recovery of all values, except blood lactate, was complete within 5 minutes of restarting pulmonary ventilation after 3 minutes' apnoea. Effects of sustained levels of hypoxaemia were reported by Siesjö and Nilsson (1971). (Drawn from the data of Kaasik, Nilsson and Siesjö, 1970a)

damage sarcolemma and the cytoskeleton. Phospholipases are also activated and may result in damage to phospholipids

End-products of metabolism

The end-products of aerobic metabolism are carbon dioxide and water, both of which are easily diffusible and lost from the body. The main anaerobic pathway produces hydrogen and lactate ions which, from most of the body, escape into the circulation, where they may be conveniently quantified in terms of the base deficit, excess lactate or lactate/pyruvate ratio. However, the blood/brain barrier is relatively impermeable to charged ions, and therefore hydrogen and lactate ions are retained within the neurons of the hypoxic brain. Lactacidosis can occur only when circulation is maintained to provide the large quantities of glucose required for conversion to lactic acid.

In severe cerebral hypoxia, there is some evidence that a major part of the dysfunction and damage is due to intracellular acidosis rather than depletion of high energy compounds. Gross hypoperfusion is more damaging than total ischaemia, because the latter limits glucose supply and therefore the formation of lactic acid (Gutierrez, 1991). Similarly, when anoxia follows chronic hypoxia, there is less evidence of cell damage than in acute anoxia. It has been suggested that this is due to the reduction in lactic acid formation, because of glucose depletion during the period of chronic hypoxaemia (Lindenberg, 1963; Geddes, 1967). Hypoxia may cause pH to fall below the optimum for certain enzymes and intracellular acidosis may be the main cause of the development of postanoxic cerebral oedema.

Fructose-1,6-diphosphate as substrate

Acidosis inhibits the rate-limiting enzyme 6-phosphofructokinase (see Figure 11.3). This limits the production of ATP and may even result in hyperglycaemia. Fructose-1,6-diphosphate enters the glycolytic pathway below the stage which is rate-limited by lactacidosis, and also avoids the expenditure of two molecules of ATP in its derivation from glucose. Therefore four molecules of ATP are produced from one of fructose-1,6-diphosphate in comparison with two from one molecule of glucose. There is no subsequent stage in the glycolytic pathway which is significantly rate-limited by acidosis. Initial results suggested that it might have a promising role in the treatment of various types of hypoxia (Webb, 1984).

PO$_2$ levels and hypoxia

Cellular PO$_2$

Oxidative phosphorylation to form ATP in the mitochondria will continue down to a PO$_2$ of about 0.13 kPa, or 1 mmHg (the Pasteur point, page 253). PO$_2$ gradients within the cell are considered on page 287, and neurons will no longer function when the PO$_2$ at their surface is reduced below about 2.7 kPa (20 mmHg). PO$_2$ varies from one cell to another and is also different in different parts of the same cell. There are therefore insuperable difficulties in defining or measuring 'the tissue PO$_2$'.

Venous PO$_2$

Venous PO$_2$ approximates to the mean PO$_2$ at the surface of the cells in the most unfavourable location near the venous end of the capillaries (see Figure 9.4). A familiar example is the centrilobular zone of the liver. The venous PO$_2$ may thus be a useful and practicable measure of the state of oxygenation of an organ, and consciousness is usually lost when the internal jugular venous PO$_2$ falls below about 2.7 kPa (20 mmHg) whatever the cause. The significance of the venous PO$_2$ is lost when there are shunts which permit arterial blood to mix with blood draining the tissue, but significant shunts do not occur in the organs which are most vulnerable to hypoxia.

Critical arterial P_{O_2} for cerebral function

The minimum safe level of arterial P_{O_2} is that which will maintain a safe tissue (and therefore venous) P_{O_2}. This will depend on many factors besides arterial P_{O_2}, including haemoglobin concentration, tissue perfusion and tissue oxygen consumption. These factors accord with Barcroft's classification of 'anoxia' into anoxic, anaemic and stagnant (page 284). This has been shown as a Venn diagram (see Figure 11.17) and also considered in relation to oxygen delivery (page 282).

This argument may be extended to consider in which circumstances the *venous* P_{O_2} may fall below its critical level corresponding, in normal blood, to 32% saturation and 6.4 ml/100 ml oxygen content. If the brain has a mean oxygen consumption of 46 ml/min and a blood flow of 620 ml/min, the arterial/venous oxygen content difference will be 7.4 ml/100 ml. Therefore, *with normal cerebral perfusion, haemoglobin concentration, pH, etc.*, this would correspond to a critical arterial oxygen content of 13.8 ml/100 ml, saturation 68% and P_{O_2} 4.8 kPa (36 mmHg). This calculation and others under various different conditions are set out in Table 31.1.

However, the other factors in italics above will probably not be normal. They may be unfavourable as a result of multiple disability in the patient (e.g. anaemia or a decreased cerebral blood flow). Alternatively, there may be favourable factors, including compensatory mechanisms such as polycythaemia with chronic arterial hypoxaemia and increased blood flow in anaemia and hypoxia. Cerebral vascular resistance is diminished by reduced arterial blood pressure and arterial hypoxaemia. Cerebral oxygen requirements are reduced by hypothermia and anaesthesia (see Table 30.1). The possible combinations of circumstances are so great that it is not feasible to consider every possible situation. Instead, certain important examples have been selected which illustrate the fundamentals of the problem, and these are set out in Table 31.1.

A twofold increase of cerebral blood flow would allow the arterial P_{O_2} to decrease further from 4.8 to 3.6 kPa (36 to 27 mmHg) before the cerebral venous P_{O_2} reached 2.7 kPa (20 mmHg). This is important, as an increase in cerebral blood flow may be expected to follow severe hypoxia. Polycythaemia (e.g. a haemoglobin concentration of 18 g/dl) does not confer the same degree of benefit and the critical arterial P_{O_2} would then be 4.3 kPa (32 mmHg). Alkalosis, which may be expected to result from the hypoxic drive to respiration, confers no advantage at all. Considerable advantage derives from hypothermia, due to the reduction in cerebral metabolism but not the shift of the dissociation curve.

Uncompensated ischaemia is dangerous and, with a 45% reduction in cerebral blood flow, any reduction of arterial P_{O_2} exposes the brain to risk of hypoxia. Uncompensated anaemia is almost equally dangerous, although an increase in cerebral blood flow restores a satisfactory safety margin. In the example in Table 31.1, a 40% reduction of blood oxygen capacity and a 40% increase of cerebral blood flow permits the arterial P_{O_2} to fall to 5.3 kPa (40 mmHg) without the cerebral venous P_{O_2} falling below 2.7 kPa (20 mmHg). The last line in Table 31.1 shows the very dangerous combination of anaemia (haemoglobin concentration 11 g/dl) and cerebral blood flow three-quarters of normal. Neither abnormality is very serious considered separately, but in combination the arterial P_{O_2} cannot be reduced below its normal value without the risk of cerebral hypoxia.

Table 31.1 is not be taken too literally, since there are many minor factors which have not been considered. However, it is a general rule that maximal cerebral vasodilatation may be expected to occur in any condition (other than cerebral

Table 31.1 Lowest arterial oxygen levels compatible with a cerebral venous Po_2 of 2.7 kPa (20 mmHg) under various conditions

	Blood O_2 capacity (ml/100 ml)	Brain O_2 consump. (ml/min)	Cerebral blood flow (ml/min)	Cerebral venous blood Po_2 (kPa)	(mmHg)	Sat (%)	O_2 content (ml/100 ml)	Art./ven. O_2 content difference (ml/100 ml)	Arterial blood O_2 content (ml/100 ml)	Sat. (%)	Po_2 (kPa)	(mmHg)
Normal values	20	46	620	4.4	33	63	12.6	7.4	20.0	97.5	13.3	100
Uncompensated arterial hypoxaemia	20	46	620	2.7	20	32	6.4	7.4	13.8	68	4.8	36
Arterial hypoxaemia with increased cerebral blood flow	20	46	1240	2.7	20	32	6.4	3.7	10.1	50	3.6	27
Arterial hypoxaemia with polycythaemia	25	46	620	2.7	20	32	8.0	7.4	15.4	61	4.3	32
Arterial hypoxaemia with alkalosis*	20	46	620	2.7	20	46	9.2	7.4	16.6	82	4.9	37
Arterial hypoxaemia with hypothermia†	20	23	620	2.7	20	57	11.4	3.7	15.1	75	3.6	27
Uncompensated cerebral ischaemia	20	46	340	2.7	20	32	6.4	13.5	19.9	98	14.9	112
Uncompensated anaemia	12	46	620	2.7	20	32	3.8	7.4	11.2	93	8.9	67
Anaemia with increased cerebral blood flow	12	46	870	2.7	20	32	3.8	5.3	9.1	75	5.3	40
Combined anaemia and iscnaemia	15	46	460	2.7	20	32	4.8	10.0	14.8	97	12.3	92

*pH 7.6   †temp. 30°C; cerebral O_2 consumption reduced to half normal

ischaemia) which threatens cerebral oxygenation. Also there are circumstances in which the critical organ is not the brain but the heart, liver or kidney.

The most important message of this discussion is that there is no simple answer to the question 'What is the safe lower limit of arterial P_{O_2}?' Acclimatized mountaineers have remained conscious during exercise at high altitude with arterial P_{O_2} values as low as 2.7 kPa (20 mmHg) (page 351). Patients presenting with severe respiratory disease tend to remain conscious down to the same level of arterial P_{O_2} (Refsum, 1963; McNicol and Campbell, 1965). However, both acclimatized mountaineers and patients with chronic respiratory disease have compensatory polycythaemia and maximal cerebral vasodilatation. Uncompensated subjects who are acutely exposed to hypoxia are unlikely to remain conscious with an arterial P_{O_2} of less than about 3.6 kPa (27 mmHg) but considerable individual variation must be expected.

The question of fitness for surgery and anaesthesia in the presence of a factor which limits oxygen delivery should not be decided in isolation, but can be answered only after considering the other relevant factors and the patient as a whole. It is particularly important to consider the additional disturbances which may be expected to result from the proposed intervention.

Relationship between oxygen delivery and consumption

Much research has been devoted to relating oxygen consumption to delivery (see Figures 11.18, 11.19 and 25.2). Above a critical value for delivery, oxygen consumption is constant and independent of supply; below the critical value for delivery, oxygen consumption declines as a linear function of delivery and there is evidence of lactacidosis (page 286). The critical value for delivery in healthy subjects is probably of the order of 400 ml/min. However, in patients with septic shock, it has been repeatedly found that oxygen consumption increases with supply up to very high values of both delivery and consumption (Astiz et al., 1987; Wolf et al., 1987; Skootsky and Abraham, 1988; Edwards et al., 1989). There is also evidence that optimized oxygen delivery and consumption is associated with a favourable outcome in septic shock (Shoemaker, Bland and Appel, 1985) and also in the adult respiratory distress syndrome (Russell et al., 1990). The implication is that these patients have a very high oxygen demand. Multiple pathology limits their oxygen delivery below the critical level and they are therefore in a state of relative hypoxia.

Compensatory mechanisms in hypoxia

Hypoxia presents a serious threat to the body, and compensatory mechanisms usually take priority over other changes. Thus, for example, in hypoxia with concomitant hypocapnia, hyperventilation and increase in cerebral blood flow occur in spite of the decreased P_{CO_2} (Turner et al., 1957). Certain compensatory mechanisms will come into play whatever the reason for the hypoxia, although their effectiveness will depend on the cause. For example, hyperventilation will be relatively ineffective in stagnant or anaemic hypoxia since hyperventilation while breathing air can do little to increase the oxygen content of arterial blood, and usually nothing to increase perfusion.

Hyperventilation results from a decreased arterial P_{O_2} but the response is non-linear (Figure 5.6). There is little effect until arterial P_{O_2} is reduced to about 7 kPa (52.5 mmHg); maximal response is at 4 kPa (30 mmHg). The interrelationship between hypoxia and other factors in the control of breathing is discussed in Chapter 5.

Pulmonary distribution of blood flow is improved by hypoxia as a result of increase in pulmonary arterial pressure (page 145).

Cardiac output is increased by hypoxia, together with the regional blood flow to almost every major organ, particularly the brain.

Haemoglobin concentration is not increased in acute hypoxia in man (unlike the seal, page 360), but it is increased in chronic hypoxia due to residence at altitude or chronic respiratory disease.

The dissociation curve is displaced to the right by an increase in 2,3-DPG and by acidosis which may also be present. This tends to increase tissue P_{O_2} (see Figure 11.14).

The sympathetic system is concerned in many of the responses to hypoxia, particularly the increase in organ perfusion. The immediate response is reflex and is initiated by chemoreceptor stimulation: it occurs before there is any measurable increase in circulating catecholamines although this does occur in due course. Reduction of cerebral and probably myocardial vascular resistance is not dependent on the autonomic system but depends on local responses in the vicinity of the vessels themselves.

Anaerobic metabolism is increased in severe hypoxia in an attempt to maintain the level of ATP (see above).

Organ survival times

Lack of oxygen stops the machine and then wrecks the machinery. The time of circulatory arrest up to the first event (survival time) must be distinguished from the duration of anoxia which results in the second event (revival time), the latter being defined as the time beyond which no recovery of function is possible. Incomplete recovery of function may follow anoxia lasting more than the survival time but less than the revival time.

Survival times depend on many factors. There is a very large difference between different organs, ranging from less than 1 minute for the cerebral cortex to about 2 hours for skeletal muscle. Heart is intermediate with a survival time of about 5 minutes, liver and kidney probably being about 10 minutes. Revival times tend to be about four times as long as survival times.

Apart from the inherent differences in sensitivity of organs, survival time is influenced by oxygen consumption and oxygen stores in the tissue. An inactive organ (such as a heart in asystole or the brain in hypothermia) has increased resistance to hypoxia, and there is a small but definite increase in survival time when tissue P_{O_2} has been increased by hyperbaric oxygenation. Hypothermia both decreases oxygen demand and increases the solubility of oxygen in the tissue.

Survival of an organ after anoxia depends on many secondary factors which influence oxygen transport during the recovery phase. If the heart has been severely affected by generalized hypoxaemia, there may be a reduced perfusion of other organs during recovery. Tissue oedema, particularly of the brain, may decrease the local perfusion and oxygen transport for a considerable time during recovery.

Quantification of cerebral hypoxia

This presents considerable difficulty since the usual indicators (hydrogen and lactate ions) are not released into the jugular venous blood. It is possible to detect rapid changes of CSF pH and lactate during arterial hypotension (Kaasik, Nilsson and Siesjö, 1970a) since the CSF is on the same side of the blood/brain barrier as the neurons. However, an index of hypoxia available from the jugular venous blood is more elusive. Venous P_{O_2} is perhaps the best of the simple measurements. Arterial/venous differences offer further possibilities but, again, lactate and base deficit are not helpful. A better index is the ratio of arterial/venous differences of oxygen and glucose. With full aerobic metabolism the theoretical ratio is 6:1 (moles). A decrease indicates anaerobic consumption of glucose (usually in increased quantity) and the validity of this index is not affected by the blood/brain barrier. The redox state of the neuronal cytochromes may be determined in infants by near-infrared spectroscopy with transmission through the skull.

Chapter 32

Hyperoxia and oxygen toxicity

Hyperoxia

Hyperventilation, while breathing air, can raise the arterial P_{O_2} to about 16 kPa (120 mmHg). Higher levels can be obtained only by oxygen enrichment of the inspired gas or by elevation of the ambient pressure. Although the arterial P_{O_2} can be raised to very high levels, the increase in arterial oxygen content is usually relatively small (Table 32.1). The arterial oxygen saturation is normally close to 95% and, apart from raising saturation to 100%, additional oxygen can be carried only in physical solution. Provided that the arterial/mixed venous oxygen content difference remains constant, it follows that venous oxygen content will rise by the same value as the arterial oxygen content. The consequences in terms of venous P_{O_2} (Table 32.1) are important because tissue P_{O_2} approximates more closely to venous P_{O_2} than to arterial P_{O_2}. The rise in venous P_{O_2} is trivial when breathing 100% oxygen at normal barometric pressure, and it is necessary to breathe oxygen at 3 atmospheres absolute (ATA) pressure before there is a large increase in venous and therefore tissue P_{O_2}. This is because most of the body requirement can then be met by dissolved oxygen, and the saturation of capillary and venous blood remains close to 100%.

It is convenient to consider two degrees of hyperoxia. The first applies to the inhalation of oxygen-enriched gas at normal pressure, while the second involves inhaling oxygen at raised pressure and is termed hyperbaric oxygenation. The inhalation of air at raised pressures results in hyperoxia and an air-breathing diver at a depth of 50 metres of sea water (6 ATA) would have an arterial P_{O_2} comparable to that of a man breathing oxygen at sea level.

Hyperoxia resulting from breathing oxygen-enriched gas at normal pressure

The commonest indications for oxygen enrichment of the inspired gas are the prevention of arterial hypoxaemia ('anoxic anoxia') caused either by hypoventilation (page 128) or by venous admixture (page 178). Oxygen enrichment of the

Table 32.1 Oxygen levels attained in the normal subject by changes in the oxygen tension of the inspired gas

	At normal barometric pressure		At 2 ATA	At 3 ATA
Inspired gas	Air	Oxygen	Oxygen	Oxygen
Inspired gas P_{O_2} (humidified)				
(kPa)	20	95	190	285
(mmHg)	150	713	1425	2138
Arterial P_{O_2}*				
(kPa)	13	80	175	270
(mmHg)	98	600	1313	2025
Arterial oxygen content†				
(ml/100 ml)	19.3	21.3	23.4	25.5
Arterial/venous oxygen content				
difference (ml/100 ml)	5.0	5.0	5.0	5.0
Venous oxygen content				
(ml/100 ml)	14.3	16.3	18.4	20.5
Venous P_{O_2}				
(kPa)	5.2	6.4	9.1	48.0
(mmHg)	39	48	68	360

Tissue perfusion may be reduced by elevation of P_{O_2}. This tends to increase the arterial/venous oxygen content difference which will limit the rise in venous P_{O_2}. The increases in venous P_{O_2} shown in this Table will therefore be too great in certain circumstances.

*Reasonable values have been assumed for P_{CO_2} and alveolar/arterial P_{O_2} difference.

†Normal values are assumed for Hb, pH, etc.

inspired gas may also be used to mitigate the effects of hypoperfusion ('stagnant hypoxia'). The data in Table 32.1 show that there will be only marginal improvement oxygen delivery (page 282), but it may be critical in certain situations. Freeman (1962) demonstrated reduction in mortality in critically bled dogs following the administration of oxygen, but improvement of perfusion is generally more important than raising a normal arterial P_{O_2}.

'Anaemic anoxia' will be only partially relieved by oxygen therapy but, since the combined oxygen is less than in a subject with normal haemoglobin concentration, the effect of additional oxygen carried in solution will be relatively more important.

Clearance of gas loculi in the body may be greatly accelerated by the inhalation of oxygen, which greatly reduces the *total* tension of the dissolved gases in the venous blood (Table 32.2). This results in the capillary blood having additional capacity to carry away gas dissolved from the loculi. Total gas tensions in venous blood are always slightly less than atmospheric, and this is of critical importance in prevention of the accumulation of air in potential spaces such as the pleural cavity, where the pressure is subatmospheric (page 42). Oxygen is useful in the treatment of air embolus and pneumothorax, and has also been used to relieve intestinal distension (Down and Castleden, 1975).

Carbon monoxide poisoning has long been recognized as an indication for oxygen therapy. Not only is the oxygen content of the arterial blood improved, but also the rate of dissociation of carboxyhaemoglobin is increased (Sharp, Ledingham and Norman, 1962).

Table 32.2 Normal arterial and mixed venous blood gas tensions

	kPa		*mmHg*	
	Arterial blood	*Venous blood*	*Arterial blood*	*Venous blood*
Breathing air				
P_{O_2}	13.3	5.3	100	40
P_{CO_2}	5.3	6.1	40	46
P_{N_2}	76.0	76.0	570	570
Total gas tensions	94.6	87.4	710	656
Breathing oxygen				
P_{O_2}	80.0	6.7	600	50*
P_{CO_2}	5.3	6.1	40	46
P_{N_2}	0	0	0	0
Total gas tensions	85.3	12.8	640	96

*See Table 32.1

Hyperbaric oxygenation

Mechanisms of benefit

Effect on P_{O_2}. Hyperbaric oxygenation is the only means by which arterial P_{O_2} values in excess of 90 kPa (675 mmHg) may be obtained. However, it is easy to be deluded into thinking that the tissues will be exposed to much the same P_{O_2} as applies in the chamber. Terms such as 'drenching the tissues with oxygen' have been used but are really meaningless. In fact, the simple calculations shown in Table 32.1, supported by experimental observations, show that large increases in venous and presumably tissue P_{O_2} do not occur until the P_{O_2} of the arterial blood is of the order of 270 kPa (2025 mmHg), when the whole of the tissue oxygen requirements can be met from the dissolved oxygen. However, the relationship between arterial and tissue P_{O_2} varies from one tissue to another, and oxygen-induced vasoconstriction in the brain and other tissues limits the rise in venous and tissue P_{O_2}. Direct access of ambient oxygen may increase P_{O_2} in superficial tissues.

Effect on P_{CO_2}. An increased haemoglobin saturation of venous blood reduces its buffering power and carbamino carriage of carbon dioxide. It was suggested that carbon dioxide retention might result (Gessel, 1923) but, in fact, the increase in tissue P_{CO_2} from this cause is unlikely to exceed 1 kPa (7.5 mmHg). However, in the brain this might result in a significant increase in cerebral blood flow, causing a secondary rise in tissue P_{O_2}.

Vasoconstriction, due to increase in P_{O_2}, may be valuable for reduction of oedema in the reperfusion of ischaemic limbs and in burns (Thom, 1989).

Antibacterial effect. Oxygen plays a major role in bacterial killing by the formation of free radicals and derived species, particularly in polymorphs and macrophages (see below). Apart from its direct effect, relief of hypoxia improves the performance of polymorphs (Mandell, 1974).

Wound healing is improved by hyperbaric oxygenation, even when used intermittently. In particular, angiogenesis is improved when oxygen is increased above 1 ATA (Thom, 1989).

Boyle's law effect. The volume of gas spaces within the body is reduced inversely to the absolute pressure according to Boyle's law (page 562). This effect is additional to that resulting from reduction of the total tension of gases in venous blood (see above).

Clinical applications of hyperbaric oxygenation

Around 1960 it appeared that hyperbaric oxygenation would become a most important and widespread form of therapy. Since then, enthusiasm has waxed and waned, but its use is still confined to relatively few centres. Clear answers to its value have been slow to emerge from controlled trials, which are admittedly very difficult to conduct in the conditions for which benefit is claimed. There is a natural temptation to overemphasize the potential applications for such an expensive facility.

Infection is the most enduring field of application of hyperbaric oxygenation, following good results obtained with anaerobic infections by Brummelkamp (1965). High partial pressures of oxygen increase the production of oxygen-derived free radicals which are cidal not only to anaerobes but also to aerobes (page 548). The strongest indications are for clostridial myonecrosis, chronic refractory osteomyelitis and necrotizing soft tissue infections, including cutaneous ulcers (Thom, 1989).

Carbon monoxide poisoning has been a strong indication for hyperbaric oxygenation since the pioneer work of Sharp, Ledingham and Norman (1962). However, its clinical value is maximal at the very early stages when hyperbaric facilities are least likely to be available. This consideration led to interest in the possibility of mounting small pressure chambers in ambulances (Williams and Hopkinson, 1965). In spite of the exploitation of natural gas, there remains a high incidence of carbon monoxide poisoning from automobile exhausts and fires. The rationale of therapy is considered above under orthobaric oxygenation.

Gas embolus and decompression sickness are unequivocal indications for hyperbaric therapy, and the rationale of treatment is considered above.

Hypoxia due to hypoperfusion can be relieved by hyperbaric oxygenation when the perfusion is only marginally inadequate. The small increase in oxygen content of the arterial blood clearly cannot compensate for a gross failure of perfusion. Satisfactory results have been obtained in experimental ligation of the left circumflex coronary artery in dogs (Smith and Lawson, 1958). However, evidence of satisfactory results in clinical myocardial infarction has remained elusive (Cameron et al., 1965). There have been isolated case reports of patients with severe cerebral ischaemia who have regained consciousness during hyperbaric oxygenation (Ingvar, 1965). Better results have been obtained with partially severed limbs and compromised skin flaps (Smith et al., 1961; Thom, 1989). It has also been claimed that mortality from haemorrhagic shock has been reduced by hyperbaric oxygenation (Attar, Scanlan and Cowley, 1966). There were reports of a beneficial effect in patients with cerebral infarction secondary to occlusion of a carotid or middle cerebral artery (Kapp, 1981).

Burns. There is experimental and clinical evidence (including controlled trials) that hyperbaric oxygen reduces fluid requirements, improves the microcirculation, reduces oedema, encourages earlier epithelialization and reduces the need for grafting (Thom, 1989).

Prolongation of the safe period of circulatory arrest would seem at first sight to be an obvious application. However, the realities in terms of venous and therefore tissue PO_2 (see Table 32.1) show why it was less promising than was hoped. Results have proved to be disappointing at normal temperatures, although somewhat better during hypothermia (Ledingham and Norman, 1965), when oxygen consumption is reduced and the solubility of oxygen in tissue fluids is increased.

Intrapulmonary shunting Hyperbaric oxygen has a minor and largely theoretical role in the management of severe pulmonary shunting. The iso-shunt diagram (page 184) shows that even 100% oxygen can do little to improve arterial PO_2 when the shunt is greater than about 40%. However, hyperbaric oxygenation will restore a normal arterial PO_2 in the presence of a shunt up to 50% (Table 32.3).

Radiotherapy has been employed under conditions of hyperbaric oxygenation since 1955, the rationale being based on the synergistic effect of radiation and oxygen which tends to spare hypoxic areas of tumours. The subject was reviewed by Foster (1965) but results have been disappointing and the technique is seldom used today.

Table 32.3 Oxygen levels with 50% shunt

	Pulmonary end-capillary blood			Arterial blood			Mixed venous blood		
	PO_2		O_2 content	PO_2		O_2 content	PO_2		O_2 content
Oxygen at:	*(kPa)*	*(mmHg)*	*(ml/100 ml)*	*(kPa)*	*(mmHg)*	*(ml/100 ml)*	*(kPa)*	*(mmHg)*	*(ml/100 ml)*
1 ATA*	80	600	21	6.3	47	16	4.0	30	11
2 ATA*	173	1 300	23	8.3	62	18	4.7	35	13
3 ATA*	267	2 000	25	26.7	200	20	5.6	42	15

*The pressure in atmospheres absolute (ATA) is equal to the sum of the barometric pressure and the gauge pressure (which shows the difference between the chamber pressure and the atmosphere). It is very important to distinguish clearly between absolute and gauge pressure because both scales are in routine use in different laboratories.

Multiple sclerosis. At the time of the previous edition, there was great interest in the therapeutic value of hyperbaric oxygenation in multiple sclerosis. Fischer, Marks and Reich (1983) had reported a favourable response after 12 months in a double-blind controlled clinical trial of 40 patients, in which the treated group received 2 ATA oxygen, while the placebo group inhaled 10% oxygen in nitrogen, also at 2 atmospheres. However, these findings were not confirmed in larger studies by Wiles et al. (1986) and Barnes et al. (1987).

Techniques for the administration of oxygen under orthobaric and hyperbaric conditions are described on pages 290 et seq. Toxicity of hyperbaric oxygen is considered below.

Oxygen toxicity

The oxygen molecule and derived species

Although ground state oxygen (dioxygen) is a powerful oxidizing agent, the molecule is stable and with an indefinite half-life. However, the oxygen molecule can be transformed into a range of free radicals and other highly toxic substances, most of which are far more reactive than oxygen itself (see reviews by Halliwell and Gutteridge, 1985; Royston, 1988; Webster and Nunn, 1988).

The dioxygen molecule (Figure 32.1) is unusual in having two unpaired electrons in the outer (2P) shell. Thus dioxygen itself qualifies as a 'double' free radical, but stability is conferred by the fact that the orbits of the two unpaired electrons are parallel. The two unpaired electrons also confer the property of paramagnetism which has been exploited as a method of gas analysis that is almost specific for oxygen.

Singlet oxygen. Internal rearrangements of the unpaired electrons of dioxygen result in the formation of two highly reactive species, both known as singlet oxygen ($1O_2$). In $1\Delta gO_2$ one unpaired electron is transferred to the orbit of the other (Figure 32.1), imparting an energy level 22.4 kcal/mol above the ground state. There being no remaining unpaired electron, $1\Delta gO_2$ is not a free radical. In $1\Sigma g^+$, the rotation of one unpaired electron is reversed, which imparts an energy level 37.5 kcal/mol above the ground state and this species is still a free radical. $1\Sigma g^+$ is extremely reactive, and rapidly decays to the $1\Delta gO_2$ form, which is particularly relevant in biological systems and especially to lipid peroxidation (see below).

Superoxide anion. Under a wide range of circumstances, considered below, the oxygen molecule may be partially reduced by receiving a single electron, which pairs with one of the unpaired electrons forming the superoxide anion ($O_2^{\cdot-}$ in Figure 32.1), which is both an anion and a free radical. It is the first and crucial stage in the production of a series of toxic oxygen-derived free radicals and other compounds. The superoxide anion is relatively stable in aqueous solution at body pH, but has a rapid biological decay due to the ubiquitous presence of superoxide dismutase (see below). Being charged, superoxide anion does not readily cross cell membranes.

Hydroperoxyl radical. Superoxide anion may acquire a hydrogen ion to form the hydroperoxyl radical thus:

$$O_2^{\cdot-} + H^+ = HO_2^{\cdot}$$

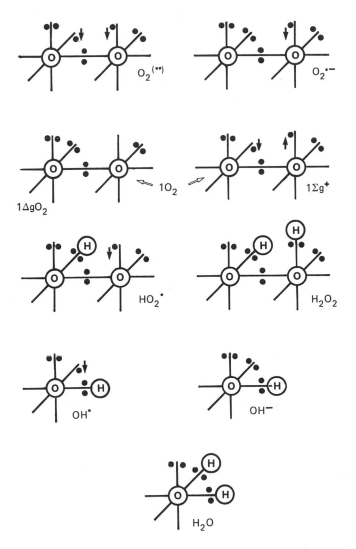

Figure 32.1 Outer orbital ring of electrons in (from the top left): ground state oxygen or dioxygen (O_2); superoxide anion (O_2^{-}); two forms of singlet oxygen ($1O_2$); peroxy free radical (HO_2^{-}); hydrogen peroxide (H_2O_2); hydroxyl free radical ($HO^{\cdot}$); hydroxyl ion (OH^{-}); and water H_2O. The arrows indicate the direction of rotation of unpaired electrons. See text for properties and interrelationships.

The reaction is pH dependent with a pK of 4.8 so the equilibrium is far to the left in biological systems.

Hydrogen peroxide. Superoxide dismutase (SOD) catalyses the transfer of an electron from one molecule of the superoxide anion to another. The donor molecule becomes dioxygen while the recipient rapidly combines with two hydrogen ions to form hydrogen peroxide (Figure 32.1). Although hydrogen peroxide is not a free radical, it is a powerful and toxic oxidizing agent, that plays an important role in oxygen toxicity. Superoxide dismutase is widely distributed in different organs and different species but is deficient in most obligatory anaerobic bacteria. The overall reaction is as follows:

$$2O_2^{\cdot-} + 2H^+ \rightarrow H_2O_2 + O_2$$

Reduction of hydrogen peroxide to water. Hydrogen peroxide is continuously generated by the dismutation and other reactions in the body. Two enzymes ensure its rapid removal. Catalase is a highly specific enzyme active against only hydrogen, methyl and ethyl peroxides. Hydrogen peroxide is reduced to water thus:

$$2H_2O_2 \rightarrow 2H_2O + O_2$$

Glutathione peroxidase acts against a much wider range of peroxides (R—OOH) which react with glutathione (G—SH) thus:

$$R—OOH + 2G—SH \rightarrow R—OH + G—S—S—G + H_2O$$

Deficiency of catalase or glutathione peroxidase has been reported in man, and obligatory anaerobes are normally without catalase.

Three-stage reduction of oxygen. Figure 32.2 summarizes the three-stage reduction of oxygen to water, which is the fully reduced and stable state. This contrasts with the more familiar single-stage reduction of oxygen to water which occurs in the

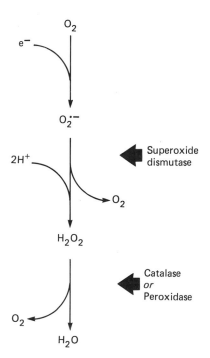

Figure 32.2 Three-stage reduction of oxygen to water. The first reaction is a single electron reduction to form the superoxide anion free radical. In the second reaction the first products of the dismutation reaction are dioxygen and a short-lived intermediate which then receives two protons to form hydrogen peroxide. The final stage forms water, the fully reduced form of oxygen.

terminal cytochrome (page 250). Unlike the single-stage reduction of oxygen, the three-stage reaction shown in Figure 32.2 is not inhibited by cyanide.

Secondary derivatives of the products of dioxygen reduction

The Fenton reaction. Although both the superoxide anion and hydrogen peroxide have direct toxic effects, they interact to produce even more dangerous species. To the right of Figure 32.3 is shown the Fenton or Haber–Weiss reaction which results in the formation of the harmless hydroxyl ion together with two extremely reactive species, the hydroxyl free radical ($OH^{\bullet}$) and singlet oxygen ($1O_2$).

$$O_2^{\bullet-} + H_2O_2 \rightarrow OH^- + OH^{\bullet} + 1O_2$$

The hydroxyl free radical is much the most dangerous species derived from oxygen. The Fenton reaction is more likely than the Haber–Weiss reaction to take place under biological circumstances and it is catalysed by metals, particularly ferrous iron.

The myeloperoxidase reaction. To the left of Figure 32.3 is shown the reaction of hydrogen peroxide with chloride ion to form hypochlorous acid. This occurs in the phagocytic vesicle of the neutrophil and plays a major role in bacterial killing. The reaction is accelerated by the enzyme myeloperoxidase which comprises some 7%

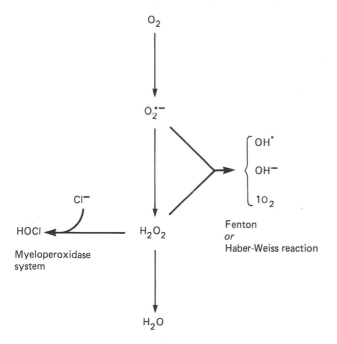

Figure 32.3 Interaction of superoxide anion and hydrogen peroxide in the Fenton or Haber–Weiss reaction to form hydroxyl free radical, hydroxyl ion and singlet oxygen. Hypochlorous acid is formed from hydrogen peroxide by the myeloperoxidase system. (Reproduced from Nunn (1985b) by courtesy of the Editor of the Journal of the Royal Society of Medicine)

of the dried weight of a neutrophil. The clinical significance of the myeloperoxidase reaction was reviewed by Del Maestro (1980) and Fantone and Ward (1982). Hypochlorite has long been known as an effective antibacterial agent and was used in the First World War as Dakin's solution. The myeloperoxidase reaction also occurs immediately after fertilization of the ovum, and hypochlorous acid so formed causes polymerization of proteins to form the membrane which prevents the further entry of sperms.

Relationship to ionizing radiation. The changes described above have many features in common with those caused by ionizing radiation, the hydroxyl free radical (OH·) being the most dangerous product in both cases. Gerschman and her colleagues (1954) were the first to draw the comparison, and to suggest that oxygen-derived free radicals were responsible for the pathophysiology of oxygen poisoning. It is hardly surprising that the effect of radiation is increased by high partial pressures of oxygen, to which reference was made above. As tissue PO_2 is reduced below about 2 kPa (15 mmHg), there is progressively increased resistance to radiation damage until, at zero PO_2, resistance is increased threefold (Gray et al., 1953). This unfortunate effect favours survival of malignant cells in hypoxic areas of tumours.

Sources of electrons for the reduction of oxygen to superoxide anion

Figure 32.3 shows the superoxide anion as the starting point for the production of more toxic free radicals and related species. The first stage reduction of dioxygen to the superoxide anion is therefore critically important in oxygen toxicity.

Xanthine and reperfusion injury. The existence of the superoxide anion was first deduced by McCord and Fridovich in 1968 from a reaction in which the electron was donated by the conversion of xanthine to uric acid by the enzyme xanthine oxidase (Figure 32.4). This long remained a laboratory technique for the production of oxygen-derived free radicals in cell cultures and organ perfusion techniques. However, hypoxanthine may be formed from ATP under hypoxic or ischaemic conditions (page 529), and, especially during reperfusion, reaction with oxygen and xanthine oxidase may result in liberation of oxygen-derived free radicals. Xanthine oxidase catalyses the conversion of both hypoxanthine to xanthine, and xanthine to uric acid. It seems probable that, under certain circumstances, this mechanism may play a role in reperfusion tissue damage or postischaemic shock (McCord and Roy, 1982; Parks, Bulkley and Granger, 1983; Traystman, Kirsch and Koehler, 1991). It has also been implicated in Dupuytren's contracture (Murrell, Francis and Bromley, 1987; Murrell, 1992). Xanthine oxidase occurs naturally as xanthine dehydrogenase (type D) which does not produce superoxide anion unless it has been converted to xanthine oxidase itself (type O).

Xanthine and tumour necrosis factor. Xanthine is also involved in the cytotoxic effects of tumour necrosis factor (TNF) (Larrick and Wright, 1990). Binding to receptors on the cell wall initiates many intracellular biochemical pathways, which include the conversion of xanthine dehydrogenase to xanthine oxidase, and thereby the formation of superoxide anion (Figure 32.5).

Ferrous iron loses an electron during conversion to the ferric state. This is an important aspect of the toxicity of ferrous iron and has been proposed as a

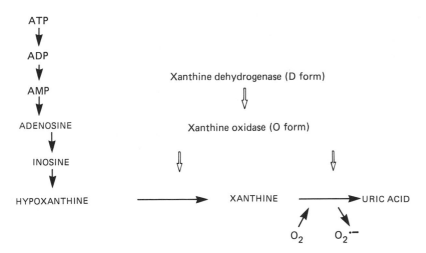

Figure 32.4 Generation of superoxide anion from oxygen by the reaction of xanthine and xanthine oxidase. Also shown are the pathways from ATP to hypoxanthine and the conversion of xanthine dehydrogenase to xanthine oxidase, both of which changes occur in hypoxia.

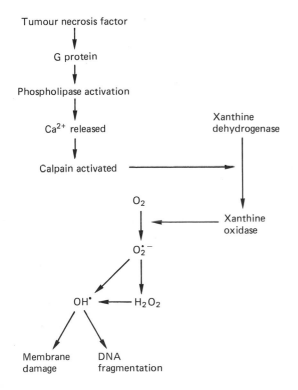

Figure 32.5 Sequence of events in the cytotoxic effects of tumour necrosis factor (TFN). Conversion of xanthine dehydrogenase (D form) to xanthine oxidase (O form) results in the formation of superoxide anion (see Figure 32.4), which then proceeds to the formation of hydroxyl free radical by the Fenton reaction (see Figure 32.3).

mechanism of rheumatoid arthritis (Blake et al., 1981). A similar reaction also occurs during the spontaneous oxidation of haemoglobin to methaemoglobin (page 279). It is for this reason that large quantities of SOD, catalase and other protective agents are present in the young erythrocyte. Their depletion may well determine the life of the cell. Apart from ferrous iron acting as an electron donor, it is a catalyst in the Fenton reaction (see above).

The NADPH oxidase system is the major electron donor in neutrophils and macrophages (Babior, Kipnes and Curnutte, 1973). The electron is donated from NADPH by the enzyme NADPH oxidase which is located within the membrane of the phagocytic vesicle (Figure 32.6), NADPH being generated by the hexose monophosphate shunt. This mechanism is activated by phagocytosis and is accompanied by an enormous increase in the oxygen consumption of the cells. This is the so-called respiratory burst, which is probably responsible for most of the oxygen consumption by shed blood (page 298), a process which is known to be cyanide resistant. Superoxide anion is released into the phagocytic vesicle, where it is reduced to hydrogen peroxide which then reacts with chloride ions to form hypochlorous acid in the myeloperoxidase reaction (see Figure 32.3). NADPH oxidase is absent in chronic granulomatous disease which results in a serious disability to contend with infection. Absence of myeloperoxidase is less serious. Oxygen-derived free radicals are also involved in the killing of malarial parasites (Clark and Hunt, 1983).

Although the NADPH oxidase system has extremely important biological advantages, there seems little doubt that its inappropriate activation in marginated neutrophils can damage the endothelium of the lung, and it may well play a part in the production of the adult respiratory distress syndrome (ARDS) (Chapter 29). Bronchoalveolar lavage fluid from patients with ARDS has been found to contain myeloperoxidase (Weiland et al., 1986). The endothelium is damaged by lipid peroxidation and other mechanisms (see below), causing increased permeability to macromolecules which causes further damage (Fantone and Ward, 1982; Rinaldo and Rogers, 1982; Tate and Repine, 1983).

Exogenous compounds, including various drugs and toxic substances, can act as an analogue of NADPH oxidase and transfer an electron from NADPH to molecular oxygen. The best example of this is paraquat which can, in effect, insert itself into an electron transport chain, alternating between its singly and doubly ionized form (Figure 32.7). This process is accelerated at high levels of Po_2 and so there is a

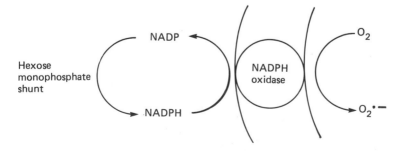

Figure 32.6 Single-stage reduction of oxygen by NADPH oxidase located in the membrane of the phagocytic vesicle of a neutrophil.

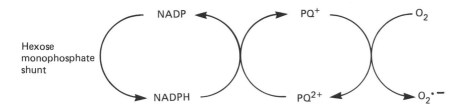

Figure 32.7 Role of paraquat (PQ) in the reduction of oxygen to superoxide anion. Compare with Figure 32.6.

synergistic effect between paraquat and oxygen. Paraquat is concentrated in the alveolar epithelial type II cell where the PO_2 is as high as anywhere in the body. Due to the very short half-life of the oxygen-derived free radicals, damage is confined to the lung. Bleomycin and various antibiotics can act in a similar manner but usually at high dose levels.

High PO_2. Whatever other factors may apply, the production of oxygen-derived free radicals is increased at high levels of PO_2 by the law of mass action (Freeman and Crapo, 1981; Freeman, Topolsky and Crapo, 1982). It would appear that the normal tissue defences against free radicals (discussed below) are usually effective only up to a tissue PO_2 of about 60 kPa (450 mmHg). This accords with the development of clinical oxygen toxicity as discussed below. There is also evidence that generation of oxygen-derived free radicals is increased when normal oxygen usage is increased. Thus during severe exercise, lipid peroxidation occurs which can be reversed by pretreatment with vitamin E (Clark, Cowden and Hunt, 1985).

Additional factors promoting the formation of superoxide anion include complement activation, interaction with nitric oxide (see page 311) and glucose oxidase.

Biochemical targets of oxygen-derived free radicals

The three main targets are deoxyribonucleic acid (DNA), lipids and sulphydryl-containing proteins. All three are also sensitive to ionizing radiation. The mechanisms of both forms of damage have much in common and synergism occurs.

Breakage of chromosomes in cultures of Chinese hamster lung fibroblasts by high concentrations of oxygen was demonstrated by Sturrock and Nunn (1978) (Figure 32.8). The same authors showed that 48 hours' exposure to 95% oxygen increased the rate of mutations by a factor of 25. It is not yet clear to what extent damage to DNA is responsible for pulmonary oxygen toxicity.

There is little doubt that lipid peroxidation is a major mechanism of tissue damage by oxygen-derived free radicals. The interaction of a free radical with an unsaturated fatty acid not only disrupts that particular lipid molecule but also generates another free radical so that a chain reaction ensues until stopped by a free radical scavenger (Webster and Nunn, 1988). Lipid peroxidation disrupts cell membranes and accounts for the loss of integrity of the alveolar/capillary barrier in pulmonary oxygen toxicity.

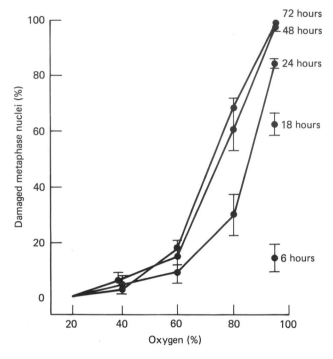

Figure 32.8 Breakage of chromosomes in a culture of Chinese hamster lung fibroblasts by oxygen at various concentrations and for varying durations of exposure. (Reproduced from Sturrock and Nunn (1978) by courtesy of the Editors of Mutation Research)

Damage to sulphydryl-containing proteins is caused primarily by formation of disulphide bridges, which inactivate a range of enzymes including some which may be involved in oxygen convulsions (see below).

Defences against oxygen-derived free radicals

Life in an oxidizing environment is possible only because of powerful antioxidant defences, which all aerobes have developed (see Chapter 1, page 8). The defensive systems are freely duplicated and operate in depth.

Enzymes. Actions of the enzymes superoxide dismutase (SOD) and catalase (CAT) are described above. These are widely distributed in all aerobic organisms and can be induced, particularly in the young. Thus, 7 days' exposure of rats to 85% oxygen increased tissue levels of SOD and also increased tolerance to subsequent exposure to 100% oxygen (Crapo and Tierney, 1974). SOD may also be induced by injection of endotoxin (Frank, Summerville and Massaro, 1980). There are difficulties in the therapeutic use of SOD and CAT because they are intracellular enzymes with very short half-lives in plasma. There is therefore little scope for their use by direct intravenous injection. In certain circumstances, induction may be feasible as a prophylactic measure and this must often have occurred during the early stages of treatment of ARDS, when the inspired oxygen concentration has been gradually increased to counter progressive failure of gas exchange. It is possible for these enzymes to enter cells if they are administered in liposomes and their plasma half-life may also be extended by conjugation with polyethylene glycol. Experimental use of SOD and CAT in these forms has been described by Turrens, Crapo and Freeman (1984), Padmanabhan et al. (1985) and McDonald et al. (1985).

Antienzymes. Because xanthine oxidase plays a pivotal role in the reactions shown in Figures 32.4 and 32.5, it seemed logical to explore the use of allopurinol which inhibits a range of enzymes including xanthine oxidase.

Free-radical scavengers. The glutathione/glutathione peroxidase system scavenges not only the oxygen-derived free radicals themselves but also free radicals formed during lipid peroxidation as described above. Two molecules of the tripeptide (glycine–cysteine–glutamic acid) glutathione (GSH) are oxidized to one molecule of reduced glutathione (GSSG) by the formation of a disulphide bridge linking the cysteine residue (see above). GSH is re-formed from GSSG by the enzyme glutathione reductase, hydrogen being supplied by NADPH and hydrogen ions. NADPH is formed by the pentose phosphate pathway which can be rate-limiting in the maintenance of the GSH/GSSG ratio. Other scavengers include ascorbic acid (important for the hydroxyl free radical), vitamin E (α-tocopherol), dimethylthiourea, *n*-acetyl cysteine and dimethylsulphoxide. Their therapeutic role in oxygen toxicity is still not fully clarified.

Iron-chelating agents. Since ferrous iron is both a potent source of electrons for conversion of oxygen to the superoxide anion and a catalyst in the Fenton reaction, desferrioxamine may well prove to have a therapeutic role which is likely to extend beyond the haemachromatoses and acute iron poisoning (Gutteridge et al., 1985).

Steroids. The role of steroids is not yet clarified. Sturrock and Hulands (1980) have shown that maximal doses of methylprednisolone give considerable protection from the chromosome-breaking effect of oxygen described above (Sturrock and Nunn, 1978). Dexamethasone in high dosage has been found to have therapeutic value in the late stage of pulmonary oxygen toxicity in rats but to decrease survival when used in the early stages of exposure (Koizumi, Frank and Massaro, 1985). It will be difficult if not impossible to confirm the value of steroids in the treatment of pulmonary oxygen toxicity in man.

Extracellular antioxidant defences can be studied in bronchoalveolar lavage (BAL) fluid, which represents the alveolar lining fluid. BAL normally contains SOD, CAT, glutathione and vitamins E and C, in addition to a number of proteins (Davis and Pacht, 1991).

Clinical oxygen toxicity

The most important clinical conditions in which oxygen has been identified as the sole precipitating cause are oxygen convulsions, pulmonary oxygen toxicity and retrolental fibroplasia.

Oxygen convulsions (the Paul Bert effect)

It is well established that exposure to oxygen at a partial pressure in excess of 2 atmospheres absolute (2 ATA) may result in convulsions, which are usually lethal to divers. This limits the depth to which closed circuit oxygen apparatus can be used. It is interesting that the threshold for oxygen convulsions is close to that at which brain tissue P_{O_2} is likely to be sharply increased (Table 32.1). The relationship to cerebral tissue P_{O_2} is supported by the observation that an elevation of P_{CO_2} lowers the threshold for convulsions (Lambertsen, 1965). High P_{CO_2} increases cerebral blood flow and therefore raises the tissue P_{O_2} relative to the arterial P_{O_2}. Hyperventilation and anaesthesia each provide limited protection.

Concentrations of gamma-aminobutyric acid (GABA) decrease in the brain prior to convulsion, and the change correlates with the severity of the convulsion (Wood and Watson, 1963). Furthermore, the threshold for change in GABA levels is similar to the threshold for convulsions (Wood, Watson and Murray, 1969). Association of two phenomena does not necessarily prove that the relationship is causal, but GABA is an inhibitory neurotransmitter and it is not unreasonable to suggest that a reduced level might result in convulsions. The change in GABA levels may be due to inactivation of sulphydryl-containing enzymes which are one of the targets for free radical attack. Both convulsions and depression of GABA levels occur when the brain tissue P_{O_2} level is sufficiently high for the increased production of free radicals to overwhelm the natural defences.

Pulmonary oxygen toxicity

Pulmonary tissue P_{O_2} is the highest in the body and the lung is therefore the organ most vulnerable to oxygen toxicity. Pulmonary oxygen toxicity is unequivocal and lethal in laboratory animals such as the rat. Man appears to be far less sensitive, but there are formidable obstacles to investigation of both human volunteers and patients. Study of oxygen toxicity in the clinical environment is complicated by the presence of the pulmonary pathology which necessitated the use of oxygen.

Cellular changes. Weibel reviewed the classic studies of his group in 1971. Electron microscopy has shown that, in rats exposed to 1 atmosphere of oxygen, the primary change is in the capillary endothelium, which becomes vacuolated and thin. Permeability is increased and fluid accumulates in the interstitial space. At a later stage, in monkeys, the epithelial lining is lost over large areas of the alveoli. This process affects the type I cell (page 30) and is accompanied by proliferation of the type II cell which is relatively resistant to oxygen. Massaro and Massaro (1978) suggested that this was an essential defence mechanism to re-establish the integrity of the blood/gas interface. Weibel postulated that the cytological differentiation of the type I cell decreases its resistance to oxygen-induced damage. Over all, the alveolar/capillary membrane is greatly thickened, partly because of the substitution of type II cells for type I and partly because of interstitial accumulation of fluid.

Limits of survival. Pulmonary effects of oxygen vary greatly between different species, probably because of different levels of provision of defences against free radicals. Most strains of rats will not survive for much more than 3 days in 1 atmosphere of oxygen. Monkeys generally survive oxygen breathing for about 2 weeks, and man is probably even more resistant. Pulmonary oxygen tolerance curves for normal man have been prepared by Clark and Lambertsen (1971), but these are based on reduction in vital capacity which is a very early stage of oxygen toxicity. There is an approximately inverse relationship between P_{O_2} and duration of tolerable exposure. Thus 20 hours of 1 atmosphere had a similar effect to 10 hours of 2 atmospheres or 5 hours of 4 atmospheres. There is also general agreement that man can withstand 10 hours' exposure to 1 atmosphere of oxygen, with nothing more than substernal distress and a measurable reduction in vital capacity.

American astronauts breathed 100% oxygen at a pressure of about one-third of an atmosphere until the Apollo fire of 1967 (see below). There is abundant evidence that prolonged exposure to this environment does not result in demonstrable pulmonary oxygen toxicity, thus establishing a P_{O_2} of 34 kPa (255 mmHg) as a safe level. It also shows that the significant factor is partial pressure and not concentration. In contrast, the concentration of oxygen rather than its partial pressure is the important factor in absorption collapse of the lung (page 496).

Clinical studies. Some limited information on human pulmonary oxygen toxicity has been obtained from patients in the course of therapeutic administration of oxygen.

Nash, Blennerhassett and Pontoppidan (1967) reviewed 70 patients who died after prolonged artificial ventilation. Pulmonary abnormalities (particularly fibrin membranes, oedema and fibrosis) were greater in those patients who had received more than 90% oxygen. However, the higher concentrations of oxygen would probably have been used in those patients with the more severe defects in gas exchange and it is, therefore, difficult to distinguish between the effects of oxygen itself and the conditions which required its use. The same problem was tackled by Gilbe, Salt and Branthwaite (1980) who, in an extensive review of patients ventilated for long periods with high concentrations of oxygen, concluded that adverse effects of oxygen on the alveolar epithelium were rarely of practical importance in hypoxaemic patients.

An elegant attempt to avoid the complicating factor of pre-existing pulmonary disease was made by Singer and his colleagues (1970), who ventilated a group of patients with 100% oxygen for 24 hours after cardiac surgery. Two further patients received oxygen for 5 and 7 days respectively. Various indices of pulmonary function (V_D/V_T ratio, shunt and compliance) were not significantly different from a control group receiving less than 42% oxygen.

Barber, Lee and Hamilton (1970) studied patients with irreversible head injuries and compared a group receiving 100% oxygen for 31−72 hours with a control group ventilated with air. There were no differences in lung histology between the two groups.

In contrast to these essentially negative studies, Register et al. (1987) obtained positive findings in a randomized study of patients ventilated after coronary bypass grafting. Venous admixture was significantly greater and arterial P_{O_2} less in patients receiving 50% oxygen compared with the group receiving less than 30%. There are many possible causes for these changes but the authors concluded that unnecessary elevation of inspired oxygen concentration should be avoided, a view from which few would dissent in the present state of knowledge.

Pulmonary absorption collapse. Whatever the uncertainties about the susceptibility of man to pulmonary oxygen toxicity, there is no doubt that high concentrations of oxygen in zones of the lung with low ventilation/perfusion ratios will result in collapse (page 498). This may be demonstrated in the healthy but middle-aged volunteer. A few minutes of breathing oxygen at residual lung volume results in radiological evidence of collapse, a reduced arterial PO_2 and substernal pain on attempting a maximal inspiration (Nunn et al., 1965b, 1978).

Ventilatory depression. Perhaps the greatest danger of oxygen therapy is the production of ventilatory depression in patients who have lost their sensitivity to carbon dioxide and rely upon the hypoxic drive to breathing (page 421). This is particularly dangerous in the patient with chronic bronchitis (the 'blue bloater'). Figure 21.3 shows the alarmingly rapid onset of respiratory depression when oxygen is breathed by a patient dependent on his peripheral chemoreceptors, a danger to which Donald first drew attention in 1949.

Balancing the risks. Prevention of dangerous hypoxia is always the first priority; if it occurs, it must be treated in spite of the various hazards associated with the use of oxygen. This point was firmly stressed by Gilbe, Salt and Branthwaite (1980). A reasonably safe arterial PO_2 is 10 kPa (75 mmHg), normally giving a saturation of 95%, but, if this cannot be maintained without resorting to dangerous levels of inspired oxygen concentrations (in excess of 60%), it may be necessary to settle for a lower arterial PO_2 and 6.7 kPa (50 mmHg), giving a saturation of 85%, was suggested by Hutchison, Flenley and Donald (1964). In fact, the safe lower level of arterial PO_2 for an individual patient depends on many factors (page 532) and no general rule can be formulated. Levels of the order of 3 kPa (23 mmHg) have been tolerated by Himalayan mountaineers.

The cornerstone of avoiding the potentially harmful effects of oxygen in the clinical environment is prevention (Fracica, Piantadosi and Crapo, 1991). Although brief periods of exposure to 100% oxygen appear to be safe, inspired oxygen concentrations should be titrated against arterial PO_2, particularly in patients exposed to paraquat or bleomycin. Pharmacological protection currently remains in the experimental stage, in spite of the interesting possibilities outlined above (see Heffner and Repine, 1991).

Retrolental fibroplasia (RLF)

Shortly after RLF was first described in 1942, it became established that hyperoxia was the major aetiological factor. This led to the use of oxygen being strictly curtailed in the management of neonates. This resulted in an increase in morbidity and mortality attributable to hypoxia and thereafter oxygen was carefully monitored and titrated in the hope of steering the narrow course between the Scylla of hypoxia and the Charybdis of RLF (see review by Lucey and Dangman, 1984). This policy has not eradicated the condition and there is now overwhelming evidence that RLF may occur in infants who have never received additional oxygen. Vitamin E has been used in the attempt to prevent RLF but it is currently believed that hyperoxia is but one of a variety of factors which may cause RLF by changes in the retinal oxygen supply. There is a well established inverse relationship between birth weight and the incidence of RLF. Flynn (1984) presented the case against major surgery (with administration of anaesthetic gases and oxygen) being a significant risk factor.

The fire hazard

Fire risk is enormously increased by the use of high concentrations of oxygen, even at reduced barometric pressure. The problem had been reviewed by Denison, Ernsting and Cresswell (1966) but was tragically highlighted by the death of the three American astronauts breathing 100% oxygen at one-third of an atmosphere, in 1967. Cabin atmospheres for the American space programme are now normal air at sea level pressure (West, 1991). This substantially reduces the fire hazard.

Techniques for orthobaric and hyperbaric oxygen therapy are considered on pages 290 et seq.

Appendix A

Physical quantities and units of measurement

SI units

The author now despairs of living to see a clean transition from the old to the new metric units. The old system was based on the centimetre–gram–second (CGS) and was supplemented with many non-coherent derived units such as the millimetre of mercury for pressure and the calorie for work, which could not be related to the basic units by factors which were powers of ten. The new system, the Système Internationale or SI, is based on the metre–kilogram–second (MKS) and comprises base and derived units which are obtained simply by multiplication or division without the introduction of numbers, not even powers of ten.

Base units are metre (length), kilogram (mass), second (time), ampere (electric current), kelvin (thermodynamic temperature), mole (amount of substance) and candela (luminous intensity).

Derived units include newton (force: kilograms metre second^{-2}), pascal (pressure: newton metre^{-2}), joule (work: newton metre) and hertz (periodic frequency: second^{-1}).

Special non-SI units are recognized as having sufficient practical importance to warrant retention for general or specialized use. These include litre, day, hour, minute and the standard atmosphere.

Non-recommended units include the dyne, bar, calorie and gravity-dependent units such as the kilogram-force, centimetre of water and millimetre of mercury, the demise of which has been expected for many years.

The introduction of SI units into anaesthesia and respiratory physiology was reviewed by Padmore and Nunn (1974). The kilopascal is replacing the millimetre of mercury for blood gas tensions, the transition being almost complete in many European countries but barely started in the USA, where mmHg had been replaced by the almost identical torr. The introduction of the kilopascal for fluid pressures in the medical field is being delayed for, what appears to the author, an entirely specious attachment to the mercury or water manometer. We appear to be condemned to a further period during which we record arterial pressure in mmHg, venous pressure in cmH_2O, cerebrospinal fluid pressure in mmH_2O and some suction pumps are still calibrated in cmHg. This absurd situation would be less dangerous if all staff knew the relationship between a millimetre of mercury and a centimetre of water.

The replacement of the calorie by the joule should end the confusion between the calorie and the Calorie (kilocalorie). It is not yet clear whether the 'amount of substance' (mol) will replace the gas volume in expressions of, for example, oxygen consumption. This transition would be fairly inconvenient. The litre is steadily replacing the '100 ml' as the reference quantity of a liquid.

As in previous editions of this book, it has proved necessary to make text and figures bilingual, with both SI and CGS units for the benefit of readers who are unfamiliar with one or other of the systems. Some useful conversion factors are listed in Table A.1. Physical quantities relevant to respiratory physiology are defined below, together with their mass/length/time (MLT) units. These units provide a most useful check of the validity of equations and other expressions which are derived in the course of studies of respiratory function. Only quantities with identical MLT units can be added or subtracted and the units must be the same on both sides of an equation.

Volume (dimensions: L^3)

In this book we are concerned with volumes of blood and gas. Strict SI units would be cubic metres and submultiples. However, the litre (l) and millilitre (ml) are recognized as special non-SI units and will remain in use. For practical purposes, we may ignore changes in the volume of liquids which are caused by changes of temperature. However, the changes in volume of gases caused by changes of temperature or pressure are by no means negligible and constitute an important source of error if they are ignored. Gas volumes are usually measured at ambient (or environmental) temperature and pressure, either dry (as from a cylinder passing through a rotameter) or saturated with water vapour at ambient temperature (e.g. an expired gas sample). Customary abbreviations are ATPD (ambient temperature and pressure, dry) and ATPS (ambient temperature and pressure, saturated).

It is not good practice to report gas volumes under the conditions prevailing during their measurement. In the case of oxygen uptake, carbon dioxide output and the exchange of 'inert' gases, we need to know the actual quantity (i.e. number of molecules) of gas exchanged and this is most conveniently expressed by stating the gas volume as it would be under standard conditions; i.e. 0°C, 101.3 kPa (760 mmHg) pressure and dry (STPD). Conversion from ATPS to STPD is by application of Charles' and Boyle's laws (see Appendix B). A table of conversion factors is given in Appendix C.

In the case of volumes which relate to anatomical measurements (e.g. vital capacity, tidal volume and dead space) gas volumes should be expressed as they would be at body temperature and pressure, saturated with water vapour (BTPS). Conversion from ATPS to BTPS is also based on Charles' and Boyle's laws, and conversion factors are listed in Appendix C.

Table A.1 Conversion factors for units of measurement

Force
   1 N (newton) $= 10^5$ dyn

Pressure
   1 kPa (kilopascal) $= 7.50$ mmHg
                                                                         $= 10.2$ cmH$_2$O
                                                                         $= 0.009\ 87$ standard atmospheres
                                                                         $= 10\ 000$ dyn/cm^2 (microbars)
   1 standard atmosphere $= 101.3$ kPa
                                                                         $= 760$ mmHg
                                                                         $= 1033$ cmH$_2$O
                                                                         $= 10$ m of sea water (specific
                                                                           gravity 1.033)
   1 mm Hg(almost equal to the torr) $= 1.36$ cmH$_2$O

Compliance
   1 l kPa^{-1} $= 0.098$ l/cmH$_2$O

Flow resistance
   1 kPa l^{-1} s $= 10.2$ cmH$_2$O/l/sec

Work
   1 J (joule) $= 0.102$ kilopond metres
                                                                         $= 0.239$ calories

Power
   1 W (watt) $= 1$ J s^{-1}
                                                                         $= 6.12$ kp m min^{-1}

Surface tension
   1 N m^{-1} (newton/metre or pascal metre) $= 1000$ dyn/cm
   Note: 1mN m^{-1} $= 1$ dyn/cm

Amount of substance
   1 mmol of oxygen $= 22.39$ ml (STPD)
   1 mmol of carbon dioxide $= 22.26$ ml (STPD)

In the figures and text of this book 1 kPa has been taken to equal 7.5 mmHg or 10 cmH$_2$O

Amount of substance (dimensionless)

In clinical chemistry there is a progressive move towards reporting concentrations in terms of 'amount of substance' concentration (mmol l^{-1}) in place of mass concentration (mg/dl). In the respiratory field this may be extended to gases and vapours. For an ideal gas, 1 mmol corresponds to 22.4 ml, and this figure applies to oxygen and nitrogen. For non-ideal gases such as nitrous oxide and carbon dioxide the figure is reduced to 22.25.

   Gas concentrations may be expressed as mmol/l, and for a mixture of ideal gases the sum of the concentrations of the components would be 44.6 mmol/l at standard temperature and pressure (dry). The advantages and disadvantages of expressing gas concentrations in terms of millimoles were reviewed by Piiper et al. (1971). If haemoglobin is expressed as millimoles of the monomer, then 1 mmol of haemoglobin combines with 1 mmol of oxygen.

Fluid flow rate (dimensions: L^3/T, or L^3T^{-1})

In the case of liquids, flow rate is the physical quantity of cardiac output, regional blood flow, etc. The strict SI units would be metre^3 second^{-1}, but litres per minute (l/min) and millilitres per minute (ml/min) are special non-SI units which may be retained. For gases, the dimension is applied to minute volume of respiration, alveolar ventilation, peak expiratory flow rate, oxygen consumption, delivery rate of fresh gases in anaesthetic gas circuits, etc. The units are the same as those for liquids except that litres per second are used for the high instantaneous flow rates which occur during the course of inspiration and expiration.

In the case of gas flow rates, just as much attention should be paid to the matter of temperature and pressure as when volumes are being measured. Measurement is usually made at ambient temperature, but gas exchange rates are reported after correction to STPD, while ventilatory gas flow rates should be corrected to BTPS. As a very rough rule, gas volumes at STPD are about 10% less than at ATPS, while volumes at BTPS are about 10% more.

Force (dimensions: MLT^{-2}) (LT^{-2} or L/T^2 are the units of acceleration)

In respiratory physiology we are chiefly concerned with force in relation to pressure, which is force per unit area. An understanding of the units of force is essential to an understanding of the units of pressure. Force, when applied to a free body, causes it to change either the magnitude or the direction of its velocity.

The units of force are of two types. The first is the force resulting from the action of gravity on a mass and is synonymous with weight. It includes the kilogram-force and the pound-force (as in the pound per square inch). All such units are non-recommended under the SI and are expected to disappear. The second type of unit of force is absolute and does not depend on the magnitude of the gravitational field. In the CGS system, the absolute unit of force was the dyne and this has been replaced under the MKS system and the SI by the newton (N) which is defined as the force which will give a mass of 1 kilogram an acceleration 1 metre per second per second.

$$1 N = 1 kg\ m\ s^{-2}$$

Pressure (dimensions: MLT^{-2}/L^2, or $ML^{-1}T^{-2}$)

Pressure is defined as force per unit area. The SI unit is the pascal (Pa) which is 1 newton per square metre.

$$1 Pa = 1 N\ m^{-2}$$

The pascal is inconveniently small (one hundred-thousandth of an atmosphere) and the kilopascal (kPa) has been adopted for general use in the medical field. Its introduction is simplified by the fact that the kPa is very close to 1% of an atmosphere. Thus a standard atmosphere is 101.3 kPa and the PO_2 of dry air is very close to 21 kPa: 1 kPa is also approximately equal to 10 cmH_2O. The kilopascal will replace the millimetre of mercury and the centimetre of water, both of which are gravity based. The centimetre of water can be considered as the pressure at the bottom of a centimetre cube of water which would be one gram-force acting on a square centimetre.

The standard atmosphere may continue to be used under SI. It is defined as $1.013\ 25 \times 10^5$ pascals.

The torr came into use only shortly before the move towards SI units. This is unfortunate for the memory of Torricelli, as the torr will disappear from use. The torr is defined as exactly equal to 1/760 of a standard atmosphere and it is therefore very close to the millimetre of mercury, the two units being considered identical for practical purposes. The only distinction is that the torr is absolute, while the millimetre of mercury is gravity based.

The bar is the absolute unit of pressure in the old CGS system and is defined as 10^6 dyn/cm². The unit was convenient because the bar is close to 1 atmosphere (1.013 bars) and a millibar is close to 1 centimetre of water (0.9806 millibars).

Compliance (dimensions: $M^{-1}L^4T^2$)

The term 'compliance' is used in respiratory physiology to denote the volume change of the lungs in response to a change of pressure. The dimensions are therefore volume divided by pressure, and the commonest units have been litres (or millilitres) per centimetre of water. It is likely that this will change to litres per kilopascal (l/kPa). Elastance is the reciprocal of compliance.

Resistance to fluid flow (dimensions: $ML^{-4}T^{-1}$)

Under conditions of laminar flow (see Figure 4.2) it is possible to express resistance to gas flow as the ratio of pressure difference to gas flow rate. This is analogous to electrical resistance which is expressed as the ratio of potential difference to current flow. The dimensions of resistance to gas flow are pressure difference divided by gas flow rate, and typical units in the respiratory field have been cmH₂O/litre/ second or dynes sec cm^{-5} in absolute units. Appropriate SI units will probably be kilopascals litre^{-1} second (kPa l^{-1} s).

Work (dimensions: ML^2T^{-2}, derived from $MLT^{-2} \times L$ or $ML^{-1}T^{-2} \times L^3$)

Work is done when a force moves its point of application or gas is moved in response to a pressure gradient. The dimensions are therefore either force times distance or pressure times volume, in each case simplifying to ML^2T^{-2}. The multiplicity of units of work has caused confusion in the past. Under SI, the erg, calorie and kilopond-metre will disappear in favour of the joule, which is defined as the work done when a force of 1 newton moves its point of application 1 metre. It is also the work done when 1 litre of gas moves in response to a pressure gradient of 1 kilopascal. This represents a welcome simplification.

$$1 \text{ joule} = 1 \text{ newton metre} = 1 \text{ litre kilopascal}$$
$$1 \text{ J} = 1 \text{ N m} \qquad = 1 \text{ l kPa}$$

The kilojoule will replace the kilocalorie in metabolism.

Power (dimensions: ML^2T^{-2}/T or ML^2T^{-3})

Power is the rate at which work is done and so has the dimensions of work divided by time. The SI unit is the watt, which equals 1 joule per second. Power is the correct dimension for the rate of continuous expenditure of biological energy, although one talks loosely about the 'work of breathing' (page 124, for example). This is incorrect and 'power of breathing' is the correct term.

Surface tension (dimensions: MLT^{-2}/L or MT^{-2})

Surface tension has become important to the respiratory physiologist since the realization of the part it plays in the 'elastic' recoil of the lungs (page 36). The CGS units of surface tension are dynes per centimetre (of interface). The appropriate SI unit would be the newton per metre. This has the following rather curious relationships:

$$1 \text{ N/m} = 1 \text{ Pa m} = 1 \text{ kg/s}^2$$

The unit for surface tension is likely to be called the pascal metre (Pa m) which is identical to the newton per metre. As an unexpected bonus, a millinewton per metre (or a millipascal metre) is identical in value to the old and familiar CGS unit, the dyn/cm.

General notes

The symbol for second is now changed from sec to s. In the case of temperature, the symbol °C now represents degrees Celsius and not degrees Centigrade. The values are identical.

Division may be indicated by a solidus (/) provided that only one is used. For example, m/s and m s^{-1} are equally correct for metres per second. In expressions with more than two terms, confusion may be avoided by the exclusive use of negative indices (see Padmore and Nunn, 1974).

Appendix B

The gas laws

A knowledge of physics is more important to the understanding of the respiratory system than of any other system of the body. Not only gas transfer but also ventilation and perfusion of the lungs occur largely in response to physical forces, with vital processes playing a less conspicuous role than is the case, for example, in brain, heart or kidney. Much of this book is concerned with physics, and it may be helpful to review those aspects which are most relevant to the behaviour of gases in the respiratory system.

Physical quantities and units of measurement are perennial sources of confusion in respiratory physiology. Apart from any inherent difficulty, we suffer from an unnecessary duplication of units, particularly those of pressure. Appendices A and B are intended to resolve some of these difficulties but need not be read by those who already understand the subject.

Certain physical attributes of gases are customarily presented under the general heading of the gas laws. These are of fundamental importance in respiratory physiology.

Boyle's law describes the inverse relationship between the volume and absolute pressure of a perfect gas at constant temperature:

$$PV = K \qquad \qquad ...(1)$$

where P represents pressure and V represents volume. At temperatures near their boiling point, gases deviate from Boyle's law. At room temperature, the deviation is negligible for oxygen and nitrogen and is of little practical importance for carbon dioxide or nitrous oxide. Anaesthetic vapours show substantial deviations.

Charles' law describes the direct relationship between the volume and absolute temperature of a perfect gas at constant pressure:

$$V = KT \qquad \qquad ...(2)$$

where T represents the absolute temperature. There are appreciable deviations at temperatures immediately above the boiling point of gases. Equations (1) and (2) may be combined as follows:

$$PV = RT \qquad \qquad ...(3)$$

where R is the universal gas constant, which is the same for all perfect gases and has the value of 8.1314 joules degrees kelvin^{-1} moles^{-1}. From this it may be derived that the mole volume of all perfect gases is 22.4 litres at STPD. Carbon dioxide and nitrous oxide deviate from the behaviour of perfect gases to the extent of having mole volumes of about 22.2 litres at STPD.

Van der Waals' equation is an attempt to improve the accuracy of equation (3) in the case of non-perfect gases. It makes allowance for the finite space occupied by gas molecules and the forces which exist between them. The Van der Waals equation includes two additional constants:

$$(P + a/V^2)\,(V - b) = RT \qquad\qquad ...(4)$$

where a corrects for the attraction between molecules, and b corrects for the volume occupied by molecules. Surprisingly the constants for anaesthetic gases are related to their anaesthetic potency (Wulf and Featherstone, 1957).

An alternative method of correction for non-ideality is to express equation (3) in the following form:

$$PV/RT = Z \qquad\qquad ...(5)$$

For a perfect gas, Z equals unity. For a particular gas at a particular temperature and pressure, the non-ideality may be expressed as the special value for Z (usually less than unity) which may be obtained from tables.

Since Z has a special value for each gas at each temperature and pressure, useful tables of Z values are necessarily very cumbersome. It is therefore much more convenient to replace Z with a power series as follows:

$$PV/RT = 1 + B/V + C/V^2 +... \qquad\qquad ...(6)$$

The constants B, C, etc., are known as virial coefficients and vary only with temperature for a particular gas. Compilations are therefore simplified and the serious student is referred to Dymond and Smith (1980) or to Kaye and Laby (1986) which is more generally available but less complete. Values for B may be positive or negative and it is seldom necessary to use more than the one coefficient.

Adiabatic heating. A great deal of respiratory physiology can fortunately be understood without much knowledge of thermodynamics. However, a recurrent problem is the heating which occurs when a gas is compressed. This effect is sufficiently large to be a readily detectable source of error in such techniques as the body plethysmograph (page 60), and the use of a large rigid container as a simulator for the paralysed thorax.

Henry's law describes the solution of gases in liquids with which they do not react. It does not apply to vapours which, in the liquid state, are infinitely miscible with the solvent (e.g. ether in olive oil) (Nunn, 1960b). The general principle of Henry's law is simple enough. The number of molecules of gas dissolving in the solvent is directly proportional to the partial pressure of the gas at the surface of the liquid, and the constant of proportionality is an expression of the solubility of the gas in the liquid. This is a constant for a particular gas and a particular liquid at a particular temperature but usually falls with rising temperature.

Unfortunately, confusion often arises from the multiplicity of units which are used. For example, when considering oxygen dissolved in blood, it has been customary to consider the amount of gas dissolved in units of vols % (ml of gas (STPD) per 100 ml blood) and the pressure in mmHg. Solubility is then expressed as vols %/mmHg, the value for oxygen in blood at 37°C being about 0.003. However, for carbon dioxide in blood, we tend to use units of mmol/l of carbon dioxide per mmHg. The units are then $mmol\ l^{-1}\ mmHg^{-1}$, the value for carbon dioxide in blood at 37°C being 0.03. Both vols % and mmol/l are valid measurements of the quantity (mass or number of molecules) of the gas in solution and are interchangeable with the appropriate conversion factor.

Physicists are more inclined to express solubility in terms of the *Bunsen coefficient*. For this, the amount of gas in solution is expressed in terms of volume of gas (STPD) per unit volume of solvent (i.e. one-hundredth of the amount expressed as vols %) and the pressure is expressed in atmospheres.

Biologists, on the other hand, prefer to use the *Ostwald coefficient*. This is the volume of gas dissolved, expressed as its volume under the conditions of temperature and pressure at which solution took place. It might be thought that this would vary with the pressure in the gas phase, but this is not so. If the pressure is doubled, according to Henry's law, twice as many molecules of gas dissolve. However, according to Boyle's law, they would occupy half the volume at double the pressure. Therefore, if Henry's and Boyle's laws are obeyed, the Ostwald coefficient will be independent of changes in pressure at which solution occurs. It will differ from the Bunsen coefficient only because the gas volume is expressed as the volume it would occupy at the temperature of the experiment rather than at 0°C. Conversion is thus in accord with Charles' law and the two coefficients will be identical at 0°C. This should not be confused with the fact that, like the Bunsen coefficient, the Ostwald coefficient falls with rising temperature.

The partition coefficient is the ratio of the number of molecules of gas in one phase to the number of molecules of gas in another phase when equilibrium between the two has been attained. If one phase is gas and the other liquid, the liquid/gas partition coefficient will be identical to the Ostwald coefficient. Partition coefficients are also used to describe partitioning between two media (e.g. oil/water, brain/blood, etc.). It is still too early to say when SI units will come into general use for expression of solubility (see Appendix A). The coherent unit is millimole litre^{-1} kilopascal^{-1}.

Graham's law of diffusion governs the influence of molecular weight on the diffusion of a gas through a gas mixture. Diffusion rates through orifices or through porous plates are inversely proportional to the square root of the molecular weight. This factor is only of importance in the gaseous part of the pathway between ambient air and the tissues, and is, in general, only of importance when the molecular weight is greater than that of oxygen or carbon dioxide. Graham's law is not relevant to the process of 'diffusion' through the alveolar/capillary membrane (page 202).

Dalton's law of partial pressure states that, in a mixture of gases, each gas exerts the pressure which it would exert if it occupied the volume alone. This pressure is known as the partial pressure (or tension) and the sum of the partial pressures equals the total pressure of the mixture. Thus, in a mixture of 5% carbon dioxide in oxygen at a total pressure of 101 kPa (760 mmHg), the carbon dioxide exerts a partial pressure of $5/100 \times 101 = 5.05$ kPa (38 mmHg). In general terms:

$$P_{CO_2} = F_{CO_2} \times P_B$$

(Note that fractional concentration is expressed as a fraction and not as a percentage: per cent concentration $= F \times 100$.)

In the alveolar gas at sea level there is about 6.2% water vapour, which exerts a partial pressure of 6.3 kPa (47 mmHg). The available pressure for other gases is therefore (P_B − 6.3) kPa or (P_B − 47) mmHg. Gas concentrations are usually measured in the dry gas phase and therefore it is necessary to apply this correction for water vapour in the lungs.

Tension is synonymous with partial pressure and is applied particularly to gases dissolved in a liquid such as blood. Molecules of gases dissolved in liquids have a tendency to escape, but net loss may be prevented by exposing the liquid to a gas mixture in which the partial pressure of the gas exactly balances the escape tendency. The two phases are then said to be in equilibrium, and *the tension of a gas in a liquid is defined as the tension of the gas in a gas mixture with which the liquid is in equilibrium*. Thus a blood P_{CO_2} of 5.3 kPa (40 mmHg) means that there would be no net exchange of carbon dioxide if the blood were exposed to a gas mixture which had a P_{CO_2} of 5.3 kPa (40 mmHg).

Appendix C

Conversion factors for gas volumes

Conversion factors for gas volume – ATPS to BTPS

Gas volumes measured by spirometry and other methods usually indicate the volume at ambient temperature and pressure, saturated (ATPS). Tidal volume, minute volume, dead space, lung volumes, etc., should be converted to the volumes they would occupy in the lungs of the patient at body temperature and pressure, saturated (BTPS).

Derivation of conversion factors:

$$\text{volume}_{(BTPS)} = \text{volume}_{(ATPS)} \left(\frac{273 + 37}{273 + t} \right) \left(\frac{PB - PH_2O}{PB - 6.3} \right)$$

Table C.1 Factors for conversion of gas volumes measured under conditions of ambient temperature and pressure, saturated (ATPS) to the volumes which would be occupied under conditions of body temperature and pressure, saturated (BTPS)

Ambient temperature (°C)	Conversion factor	Saturated water vapour pressure	
		kPa	*mmHg*
15	1.129	1.71	12.8
16	1.124	1.81	13.6
17	1.119	1.93	14.5
18	1.113	2.07	15.5
19	1.108	2.20	16.5
20	1.103	2.33	17.5
21	1.097	2.48	18.6
22	1.092	2.64	19.8
23	1.086	2.80	21.0
24	1.081	2.99	22.4
25	1.075	3.16	23.7
26	1.069	3.66	25.2

PB   is barometric pressure (kPa) and the Table has been prepared for a barometric pressure of 100 kPa (750 mmHg); variations within the range 99–101 kPa (740–760 mmHg) have a negligible effect upon the factors.

t is ambient temperature (°C). The Table has been prepared for a body temperature of 37°C; variations within the range 35–39°C are of little importance.

PH$_2$O is the water vapour pressure of the sample (kPa) at ambient temperature (see Table C.1).

Conversion factors for gas volume – ATPS to STPD

Measurement of absolute amounts of gases (e.g. oxygen consumption) requires conversion of measured gas volumes to standard conditions (0°C, 101.3 kPa (760 mmHg), dry). Under these conditions, 1 mole of an ideal gas occupies 22.4 litres.

Derivation of conversion factors:

$$\text{volume}_{(STPD)} = \text{volume}_{(ATPS)} \left(\frac{273}{273 + t} \right) \left(\frac{PB - PH_2O}{101} \right)$$

PB   is barometric pressure (kPa).

t is ambient temperature (°C).

PH$_2$O is the saturated water vapour pressure of the sample (kPa) at ambient temperature (see Table C.1).

Table C.2 Factors for conversion of gas volumes measured under conditions of ambient temperature and pressure, saturated (ATPS) to the volumes which would be occupied under conditions of standard temperature and pressure, dry (STPD)−0°C, 101.3 kPa (760 mmHg)

Ambient temperature (°C)	Barometric pressure, kPa (mmHg)			
	97.3 (730)	98.7 (740)	100 (750)	101.3 (760)
15	0.895	0.907	0.919	0.932
16	0.890	0.903	0.915	0.928
17	0.886	0.899	0.911	0.923
18	0.882	0.894	0.907	0.919
19	0.878	0.890	0.902	0.915
20	0.873	0.886	0.898	0.910
21	0.869	0.881	0.893	0.906
22	0.865	0.877	0.889	0.901
23	0.860	0.872	0.885	0.897
24	0.856	0.868	0.880	0.892
25	0.851	0.863	0.875	0.887
26	0.847	0.859	0.871	0.883

Appendix D

Symbols, abbreviations and definitions

Symbols

Symbols used in this book are in accord with the recommendations of the committee for standardization of definitions and symbols in respiratory physiology (Pappenheimer et al., 1950). The use of these symbols is very helpful for an understanding of the quantitative relationships which are so important in respiratory physiology.

Primary symbols (large capitals) denoting physical quantities.

- F fractional concentration of gas
- P pressure, tension or partial pressure of a gas
- V volume of a gas
- Q volume of blood
- C content of a gas in blood
- S saturation of haemoglobin with oxygen
- R respiratory exchange ratio (RQ)
- D diffusing capacity

· denotes a time derivative; e.g. $\dot{V}$ ventilation
$\dot{Q}$ blood flow
$\dot{D}$ is now used to mean delivery (page 283)

Secondary symbols denoting location of quantity.

in gas phase (small capitals)	in blood (lower case)
I inspired gas	a arterial blood
E expired gas	v venous blood
A alveolar gas	c capillary
D dead space	t total
T tidal	s shunt
B barometric (usually pressure)	

− denotes mixed or mean; e.g. $\bar{v}$ mixed venous blood
$\bar{E}$ mixed expired gas
denotes end; e.g. E' end-expiratory gas
c' end-capillary blood

Tertiary symbols indicating particular gases.

O_2 oxygen
CO_2 carbon dioxide
N_2O nitrous oxide
etc.

f denotes the respiratory frequency

BTPS, ATPS and STPD: see Appendix C

Examples of respiratory symbols

P_{AO_2} alveolar oxygen tension
$C\bar{v}_{O_2}$ oxygen content of mixed venous blood
$\dot{V}_{O_2}$ oxygen consumption

The system is well adapted to the expression of quantitative relationships.

$$\dot{Q}\,(Ca_{O_2} - C\bar{v}_{O_2}) = \dot{V}_{O_2} \qquad \text{(Fick equation)}$$

$$V_D = V_E \left(\frac{Pa_{CO_2} - P\bar{E}_{CO_2}}{Pa_{CO_2}} \right) \text{(Bohr equation)}$$

$$R = \frac{\dot{V}_{CO_2}}{\dot{V}_{CO_2}}$$

Definitions of words used in a special sense or which have little general use

Ambient: surrounding or environmental (e.g. room air).

Parameter: a quantity which is a constant in a particular relationship, but which varies from one relationship to another; e.g. a and b in the equation $y = a + bx$ (x and y are variables).

Variable: any quantity of which the value is likely to change; e.g. haemoglobin concentration might be considered as a variable over a number of days but as a parameter when a series of blood samples are drawn in rapid succession without there being a change of haemoglobin concentration. P_{O_2} would probably be a variable in both situations.

Phase: a continuous fluid medium. The lungs contain a gas phase and a blood phase, separated by the alveolar/capillary membrane.

Appendix E

Nomograms and correction charts

Blood gas correction nomograms for time

This nomogram (Figure E.1) is designed for the application of corrections for metabolism of blood occurring between sampling and analysis. The effect of temperature is based on the cooling curve when blood is drawn at 37°C into a 5 ml glass or 2 ml plastic syringe at room temperature, followed by storage at room temperature. Elapsed time between sampling and analysis is shown on the ordinate. Line charts indicate the change in P_{CO_2} (which rises), pH (which falls) and base excess (which falls). A graph is required for the change in P_{O_2} (which falls) because the rate of fall depends upon the P_{O_2}. For details, see Kelman and Nunn (1966b).

Blood gas correction nomogram for temperature (Figure E.2)

Enter with the patient's temperature on the abscissa. *Multiply* the measured gas tension by the factor shown on the ordinate, using the appropriate curve for P_{O_2} based on the saturation of the sample. The broken line should be used for P_{CO_2}, whatever the level of P_{CO_2}. The line chart at the top of the graph may be used for the pH correction which should be *added*. For details, see Kelman and Nunn (1966b).

Nomogram for haemoglobin dissociation curve

The right-hand line charts of Figure E.3 give corresponding values for P_{O_2} and saturation under standard conditions (temperature 37°C; pH 7.40; base excess zero). The remaining lines indicate the factors by which the actual measured P_{O_2} should be multiplied to give the 'virtual P_{O_2}' with which to enter the standard dissociation curve for determination of saturation. When more than one factor is required, they should be multiplied together (page 275).

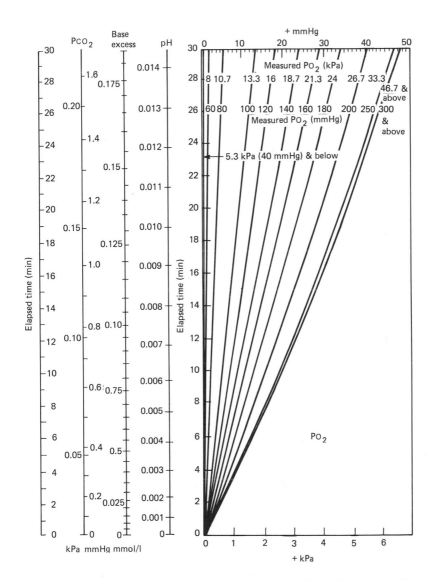

Figure E.1 Nomogram for correcting blood Pco₂, Po₂, pH and base excess for metabolic changes occurring between sampling and analysis. (Reproduced from Kelman and Nunn (1966b) by permission of the Editors of the Journal of Applied Physiology*)*

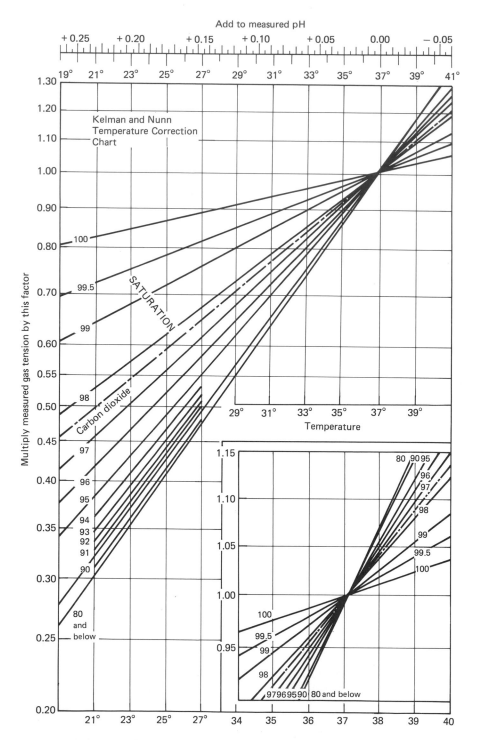

Figure E.2 Nomogram for correction of blood P_{CO_2}, P_{O_2} and pH for differences between temperature of patient and electrode system (assumed to be 37°C). (Reproduced from Kelman and Nunn (1966b) by permission of the Editors of the Journal of Applied Physiology*)*

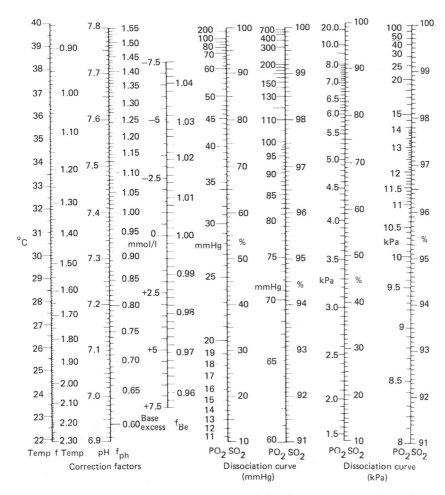

Figure E.3 Line charts representing the oxyhaemoglobin dissociation curve. (Reproduced after Kelman and Nunn (1966b) by permission of the Editors of the Journal of Applied Physiology)

The Siggaard-Andersen curve nomogram

The *in vitro* relationship between pH and P_{CO_2} of oxygenated blood is indicated either by a line joining two points obtained after *in vitro* equilibration, or by a line passing through the actual arterial values and with a slope dependent on the haemoglobin concentration. The slope is that of a line joining the normal arterial point (indicated by a small circle in the diagram) and the appropriate point on the haemoglobin scale (i.e. 14 g/dl in the example). Intersections of the buffer line indicate three indices of metabolic acid–base state: buffer base, standard bicarbonate and base excess which is currently in vogue. Interpolation of P_{CO_2} indicates corresponding (*in vitro*) pH values and *vice versa*.

The example in Figure E.4 is normal arterial blood (*in vitro* changes); other equilibration curves are shown in Figure 10.5.

Nomogram for RQ and oxygen consumption

The respiratory exchange ratio of a patient breathing air may be determined from the concentrations of oxygen and carbon dioxide in the expired gas by using the left-hand section of Figure E.5. Oxygen consumption may be determined from the mixed expired oxygen concentration and the volume of gas expired in 2 or 3 minutes, by using the right-hand section of Figure E.5. The nomogram for

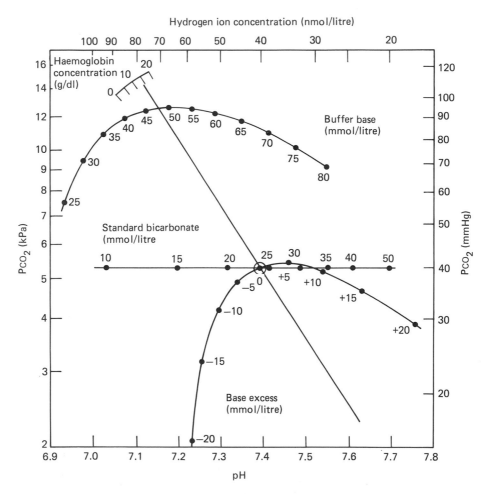

Figure E.4 The Siggaard-Andersen curve nomogram relating pH and P_{CO_2} for oxygenated blood in vitro. (Adapted from Siggaard-Andersen (1962) with permission of the author and the Editors of the Scandinavian Journal of Clinical and Laboratory Investigation)

calculation of the respiratory exchange ratio has only a very small error. The nomogram for calculating the oxygen consumption has an error of less than 10 ml/min if the respiratory exchange ratio is within the limits 0.7–0.9. For details, see Nunn (1972).

The iso-shunt chart

Figure E.6 is a diagram of the theoretical relationship between arterial PO_2 and inspired oxygen concentration for different values of virtual shunt. It is based on assumed values as follows:

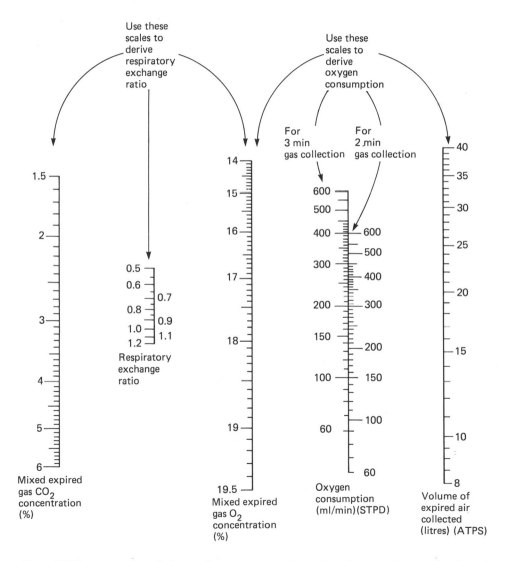

Figure E.5 Nomograms for calculation of oxygen consumption and respiratory exchange ratio of a patient breathing air. (Reproduced from Nunn (1972) by permission of the Editor of the British Medical Journal*)*

Arterial P_{CO_2} 5.3 kPa (40 mmHg).
Arterial/mixed venous oxygen content difference 5 ml/dl.
Haemoglobin concentration 14 g/dl.

Virtual shunt is defined as the shunt which gives the relationships depicted when the arterial/mixed venous oxygen content difference is 5 ml/dl. For further details, see page 183 and Benatar, Hewlett and Nunn (1973).

These curves include a small component for moderate non-uniformity of ventilation/perfusion ratios of the ventilated alveoli. This is explained on page 187, but see also Petros, Doré and Nunn (1993).

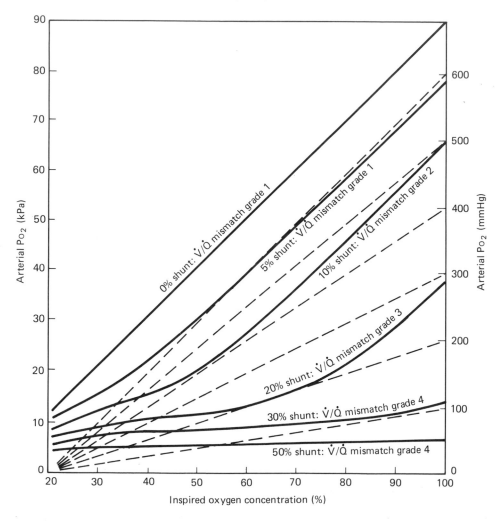

Figure E.6 Arterial P_{O_2} as a function of inspired oxygen concentration on a modified iso-shunt diagram (Figure 8.10), incorporating a factor for ventilation/perfusion mismatch (Table 8.3, Figure 8.13). Normal values are assumed for P_{CO_2}, haemoglobin concentration and arterial/mixed venous oxygen content difference. Note the reverse curves below an inspired oxygen concentration of 40% with mismatch grades of 2–4. The broken lines indicate arterial P_{O_2} expressed as a ratio of inspired oxygen concentration, as used for example in the calculation of lung injury score (Table 29.1)

Air–oxygen mixing chart

The chart shown in Figure E.7 is used for determining air and oxygen flow rates required to give various total gas flow rates at various oxygen concentrations. (Chart prepared by Dr A.M. Hewlett.)

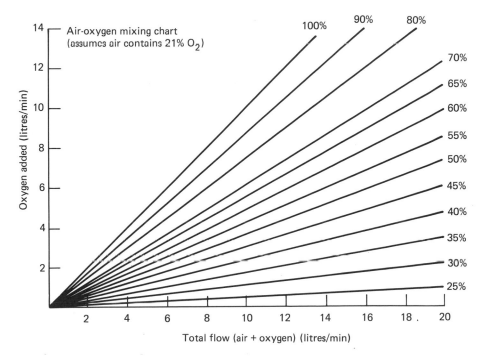

Figure E.7 Air–oxygen mixing chart for oxygen therapy. (Reproduced from Richardson, Chinn and Nunn (1976) by permission of the Editor of the British Journal of Anaesthesia)

Appendix F

Mathematical functions relevant to respiratory physiology

This book contains many examples of mathematical statements, which relate respiratory variables under specified conditions. Appendix F is intended to refresh the memory of those readers whose knowledge of mathematics has been attenuated under the relentless pressure of new information acquired in the course of study of the biological sciences.

The most basic study of respiratory physiology requires familiarity with at least four types of mathematical relationship. These are:

1. The linear function.
2. The rectangular hyperbola or inverse function.
3. The parabola or squared function.
4. Exponential functions.

These four types of function will now be considered separately with reference to examples drawn from this book.

The linear function

Examples

1. Pressure gradient against flow rate with laminar flow (page 61). There is no constant factor and the pressure gradient is zero when flow rate is zero.
2. Respiratory minute volume against PCO_2 (page 108). In this case there is a constant factor corresponding to a 'negative' respiratory minute volume when PCO_2 is zero.
3. Over a limited range, lung volume is proportional to inflating pressure (page 41). The slope of the line is then the compliance.

Mathematical statement

A linear function describes a change in one variable (dependent or y variable) which is directly proportional to another variable (independent or x variable).

There may or may not be a constant factor which is equal to y when x is zero. Thus:

$$y = ax + b$$

where a is the slope of the line and b is the constant factor. In any one particular relationship a and b are assumed to be constant but both may have different values under other circumstances. These are not therefore true constants (like π for example) and are more precisely termed parameters.

Graphical representation

Figure F.1 shows a plot of a linear function following the convention that the independent variable (x) is plotted on the abscissa and the dependent variable (y) on the ordinate. Note that the relationship is a straight line and simple regression analysis is based on the assumption that the relationship is of this type. If the slope (a) is positive, the line goes upwards and to the right. If the slope is negative, the line goes upwards and to the left.

Linear scales would normally be used, although log scales might be required to encompass a very wide range of values. A linear function would give a straight line only on logarithmic coordinates if there is no constant factor (i.e. b = zero).

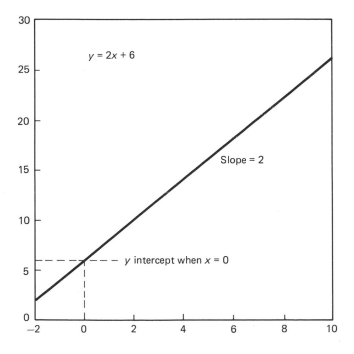

Figure F.1 A linear function plotted on linear coordinates. Examples include pressure/flow rate relationships with laminar flow (see Figure 4.2) and P_{CO_2}/ventilation response curves (see Figure 5.8).

The rectangular hyperbola or inverse function

Examples

1. The ventilatory response to hypoxia (expressed in terms of PO_2) approximates to a rectangular hyperbola (page 391), asymptotic on the horizontal axis to the respiratory minute volume at high PO_2 and, on the vertical axis, to the PO_2 at which it is assumed ventilation increases towards infinity.
2. The relationships of alveolar gas tensions to alveolar ventilation are conveniently described by rectangular hyperbolas. For carbon dioxide see page 235 and for oxygen see page 259. The curves are concave upwards for gases which are eliminated (e.g. carbon dioxide) and concave downwards for gases which are taken up from the lungs (e.g. oxygen). Curvature is governed by gas output (or uptake) and the asymptotes in each case are zero ventilation and partial pressure of the gas under consideration in the inspired gas. The relationship is extremely helpful for understanding the quantitative relationship between ventilation and alveolar gas tensions.
3. Airway resistance approximates to an inverse function of lung volume (page 82).

Mathematical statement

A rectangular hyperbola describes a relationship when the dependent variable y is inversely proportional to the independent variable x thus:

$$y = a/x + b$$

where a and b are parameters. The asymptote of x is its value when y is infinity and the asymptote of y is its value when x is infinity. If b is zero, then the relationship may be simply represented as follows:

$$xy = a$$

Graphical representation

Figure F.2a shows rectangular hyperbolas with and without constant factors. Changes in the value of a alter the curvature but not the asymptotes. Figure F.2b shows the same relationships plotted on logarithmic coordinates. The relationship is now linear but with a negative slope of unity because, if:

$$xy = a$$

then:

$$\log y = -\log x + \log a$$

The parabola or squared function

Example

With fully turbulent gas flow, pressure gradient changes according to the square of gas flow and the plot is a typical parabola (see 65).

(a)

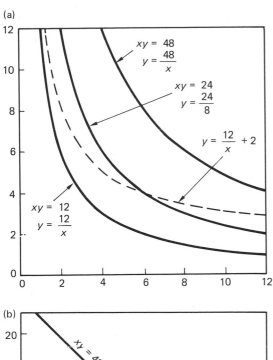

(b)

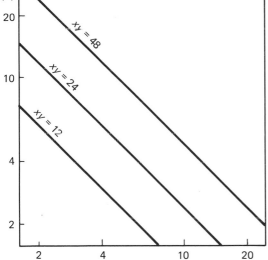

Figure F.2 Rectangular hyperbolas plotted on (a) linear coordinates and (b) logarithmic coordinates. Examples include the relationships between alveolar gas tensions and alveolar ventilation (see Figures 6.8, 10.9 and 11.6), PO₂/ventilation response curves (see Figure 5.6) and the relationship between airway resistance and lung volume (see Figures 4.11 and 20.10).

Mathematical statement

A parabola is described when the dependent variable (y) changes in proportion to the square of the independent variable (x), thus:

$$y = ax^2$$

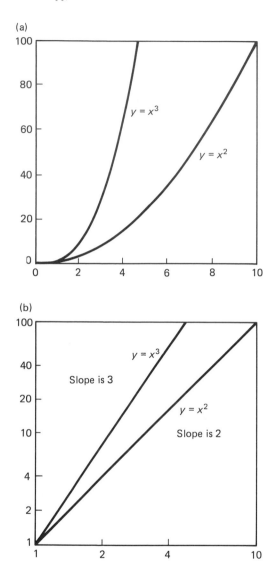

Figure F.3 Parabolas plotted on (a) linear coordinates and (b) logarithmic coordinates. An example is the pressure/volume relationship with turbulent flow (see Figure 4.3).

Graphical representation

On linear coordinates, a parabola, with positive values of the abscissa, shows a steeply rising curve (Figure F.3a), which may be confused with an exponential function (see below) although it is fundamentally different. On logarithmic coordinates for both abscissa and ordinate, a parabola becomes a straight line with a slope of two (Figure F.3b) since $\log y = \log a + 2 \log x$ (a and $\log a$ are parameters).

Exponential functions

General statement

An exponential function describes a change in which the rate of change of the dependent variable is proportional to the magnitude of the independent variable at that time. Thus, the rate of change of y with respect to x (i.e. dy/dx)* varies in proportion to the value of y at that instant. That is to say:

$$dy/dx = ky$$

where k is a constant or a parameter.

   This general equation appears with minor modifications in three main forms. To the biological worker they may be conveniently described as the tear-away, the wash-out and the wash-in.

The tear-away exponential function

This must be described first, as it is the simplest form of the exponential function. It is, however, the least important of the three in relation to respiratory function.

Simple statement

In a tear-away exponential function, the quantity under consideration increases at a rate which is in direct proportion to its actual value – the richer one is, the faster one makes money.

Examples

Classic examples are compound interest, and the mythical water-lily which doubles its diameter every day (Figure F.4). A typical biological example is the free spread of a bacterial colony in which (for example) each bacterium divides every 20 minutes. The doubling time of this example would be 20 minutes.

Mathematical statement

In the case of exponential functions relevant to respiratory function, the independent variable x almost invariably represents time, and so we shall take the liberty of replacing x with t throughout. The tear-away function may thus be represented as follows:

$$\frac{dy}{dt} = ky$$

---

*dy/dx is the mathematical shorthand for rate of change of y with respect to x. The 'd' means 'a very small bit of'. Therefore dy/dx means a very small bit of y divided by the corresponding very small bit of x. This is equal to the slope of the graph of y against x at that point. In the case of a curve, it is the slope of a tangent drawn to the curve at that point.

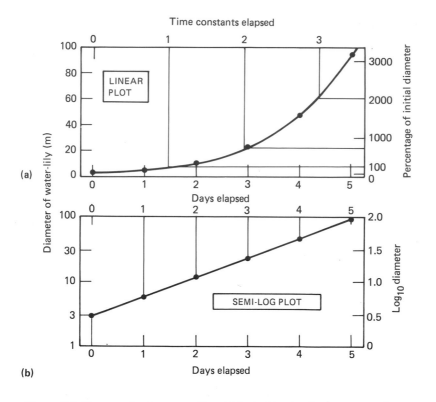

Figure F.4 The growth of a water-lily which doubles its diameter every day – a typical tear-away exponential function. Initial diameter, 3 metres; size doubled every day (i.e. doubling time = 1 day). Compare the figures in the table below with those in Table F.1.

	Elapsed time (days)	Diameter of water-lily	
		metres	percentage of initial diameter
Diameter of water-lily = $3e^{t/1.44}$	0	3	100
(t is measured in days, diameter in metres)	1	6	200
	1.44	8.2	272
	2	12	400
	2.88	22.2	739
	3	24	800
	4	48	1 600
	4.32	60.3	2 009
	5	96	3 200

A little mathematical processing will convert this equation into a more useful form, which will indicate the instantaneous value of y at any time, t.

First multiply both sides by dt/y:

$$\frac{1}{y} dy = k \, dt$$

Next integrate both sides with respect to t:

$$\log_e y + C_1 = kt + C_2$$

(C_1 and C_2 are constants of integration and may be collected on the right-hand side.)

$$\log_e y = (C_2 - C_1) + kt$$

Finally, take antilogs of each side to the base e:

$$y = e^{(C_2 - C_1)} \times e^{kt}$$

At zero time, $t = 0$ and $e^{kt} = 1$. Therefore the constant $e^{(C_2 - C_1)}$ equals the initial value of y which we may call y_0. Our final equation is thus:

$$y = y_0 \, e^{kt}$$

y_0 is the initial value of the variable y at zero time.

e is the base of natural or Naperian logarithms (discovered in 1619 before the circulation of the blood was known). This constant (2.71828...) possesses many remarkable properties which are lucidly expounded for the non-specialist by Hogben (1951).

k is a constant which defines the speed of the particular function. For example, it will differ by a factor of two if our mythical water-lily doubles its size every 12 hours instead of every day. In the case of the wash-out and wash-in, we shall see that k is directly related to certain important physiological quantities, from which we may predict the speed of certain biological changes.

Instead of using e, it is possible to take logs to the more familiar base 10, thus:

$$y = y_0 10^{k_1 t}$$

This is a perfectly valid way of expressing a tear-away exponential function, but you will notice that the constant k has changed to k_1. This new constant does not have the simple relationships of physiological variables mentioned above. It does, however, bear a constant relationship to k, as follows:

$$k_1 = 0.4343k \text{ (approx.)}$$

When an exponential function is considered to proceed by steps of whole numbers, it is known as a geometrical progression.

Graphical representation

On linear graph paper, a tear-away exponential functional rapidly disappears off the top of the paper (Figure F.4). If plotted on semi-logarithmic paper (time on a linear axis and y on a logarithmic axis), the plot becomes a straight line and this is a most convenient method of presenting such a function. The logarithmic plots in Figures F.4–F.6 are all plotted on semi-log paper.

The wash-out or die-away exponential function

The account of the tear-away exponential function has really been an essential introduction to the wash-out or die-away exponential function, which is of great importance to the biologist in general, and the respiratory physiologist in particular.

Simple statement

In a wash-out exponential function, the quantity under consideration falls at a rate which decreases progressively in proportion to the distance it still has to fall. It approaches but, in theory, never reaches zero.

Examples

Familiar examples are cooling curves, radioactive decay and water running out of the bath. In the last example the rate of flow of bath water to waste is proportional to the pressure of water, which is proportional to the depth of water in the bath, which in turn is proportional to the quantity of water in the bath (assuming that the sides are vertical). Therefore, the flow rate of water to waste is proportional to the amount of water left in the bath, and decreases as the bath empties. The last molecule of bath water takes an infinitely long time to drain away. A similar example is the mountaineer who each day ate half of the food which he carried. In this way he made his food last indefinitely.

In the field of respiratory physiology, examples include:

1. Passive expiration (Figure F.5).
2. The elimination of inhalational anaesthetics.
3. The fall of arterial P_{CO_2} to its new level after a step increase in ventilation.
4. The fall of arterial P_{O_2} to its new level after a step decrease in ventilation.
5. The fall of blood P_{CO_2} towards the alveolar level as it progresses along the pulmonary capillary.
6. The fall of blood P_{O_2} towards the tissue level as blood progresses through the tissue capillaries.

Mathematical statement

When a quantity *decreases* with time, the rate of change is *negative*. Therefore, the wash-out exponential function is written thus:

$$\frac{dy}{dt} = -ky$$

from which we may derive the following equations, which give the value of y at any time t:

$$y = y_0 e^{-kt}$$

which is simply another way of saying:

$$y = \frac{y_0}{e^{kt}}$$

y_0 is again the initial value of y at zero time. In Figure F.5, y_0 is the initial value of
(lung volume − FRC) at the start of expiration; that is to say, the tidal volume
inspired.

e is again the base of natural logarithms (2.718 28...).

k is the constant which defines the rate of decay, and is the reciprocal of a most
important quantity known as the *time constant* represented by the Greek letter
tau (τ). There are three things which should be known about the time constant:

1. Figure F.5 shows a tangent drawn to the first part of the curve. This shows the
   course events would take if the initial rate were maintained instead of slowing
   down in the manner characteristic of the wash-out curve. The time which would
   then be required for completion would be the time constant, or $1/k$, and
   designated by the Greek letter tau (τ). The wash-out exponential function may
   thus be written:

$$y = y_0 e^{-t/\tau}$$

2. After 1 time constant, y will have fallen to $1/e$ of its initial value, or
   approximately 37% of its initial value.
   After 2 time constants, y will have fallen to $1/e^2$ of its initial value, or
   approximately 13.5% of its initial value.
   After 3 time constants, y will have fallen to $1/e^3$ of its initial value, or
   approximately 5% of its initial value.
   After 5 time constants, y will have fallen to $1/e^5$ of its initial value, or
   approximately 1% of its initial value.
   (More precise values are indicated in Table F.1).

3. The time constant is often determined by physiological factors. When air
   escapes passively from a distended lung, the time constant is governed by two
   variables, compliance and resistance (see Chapters 3, 4 and 22).

We may now consider the example of passive expiration. Let V represent the
lung volume (above FRC), then $-dV/dt$ is the instantaneous expiratory gas flow
rate. Assuming Poiseuille's law is obeyed (page 63):

$$-\frac{dV}{dt} = \frac{P}{R}$$

when P is the instantaneous alveolar-to-mouth pressure gradient and R is the
airway resistance. However, compliance $C = V/P$. Therefore:

$$-\frac{dV}{dt} = \frac{1}{CR} V$$

or

$$\frac{dV}{dt} = -\frac{1}{CR} V$$

Then by integration and taking antilogs as described above:

$$V = V_0 e^{-(t/CR)}$$

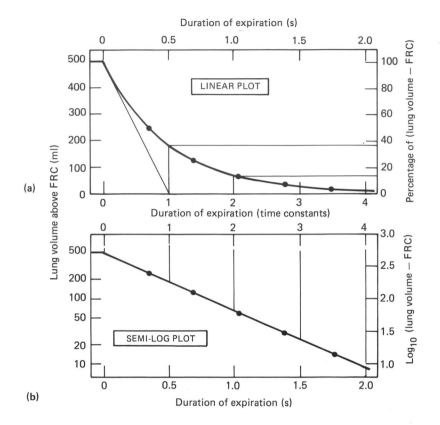

Figure F.5 Passive expiration – a typical wash-out exponential function. Tidal volume, 500 ml; compliance, 0.5 l/kPa (50 ml/cmH₂O); airway resistance 1 kPa l⁻¹ s (10 cmH₂O/1000 ml/sec); time constant, 0.5 s; half-life, 0.35 s. The points on the curves indicate the passage of successive half-lives.

		Lung volume remaining above FRC	
Lung volume above FRC $= 500e^{-(t/0.5)}$	Elapsed time (constants)	ml	percentage of tidal volume
	0	500	100
	0.69	250	50
	1	184	36.8
	2	67.5	13.5
	3	25	5.0
	4	9	1.8

Note that the logarithmic co-ordinate has no zero. This accords with the lung volume approaching, but never actually equalling, the FRC.

By analogy with the general equation of the wash-out exponential function, it is clear that $CR = 1/k = \tau$ (the time constant). Thus the *time constant equals the product of compliance and resistance.** This is analogous to the discharge of an electrical capacitor through a resistance, when the time constant of discharge equals the product of the capacitance and the resistance. Analysis of the passive expiration has been considered in greater detail on page 57 and by Bergman (1969).

Rather similar is the wash-out of anaesthetic from a body or organ. Here the 'capacitance' equals the product of the mass of the body or organ and the solubility in it of the anaesthetic. The anaesthetic's 'resistance' to escape is inversely related to ventilation, diffusion, blood flow, renal function, etc. In the more complex situations, wash-out curves remain exponential in form but are compounded of a number of individual wash-out curves. Each has its own time constant which equals the product of capacitance (for the anaesthetic) and resistance (to wash-out) for each part. An example of the technique for separation of individual components from an overall wash-out curve is the analysis of nitrogen clearance curves (Comroe et al., 1962).

Wash-out of a substance from an organ by perfusion with blood which is free of the substance is another example of a wash-out exponential function where the time constant may be stated in terms of certain physiological factors.

Let Q represent the volume of an organ and C be the concentration in the organ of a substance whose solubility in the organ equals its solubility in blood.

Imagine a small quantity of blood (dQ) to enter the organ. The concentration is then reduced by dC:

$$\frac{C - dC}{C} = \frac{Q + dQ}{Q}$$

Subtracting 1 from each side:

$$-\frac{dC}{C} = \frac{dQ}{Q}$$

If blood enters the organ at a constant rate, dQ/dt may be represented by $\dot{Q}$ (the usual symbol for blood flow rate). It then follows that:

$$-\frac{dC}{C} = \frac{\dot{Q}.dt}{Q}$$

and so:

$$-\frac{dC}{dt} = \frac{\dot{Q}}{Q} Q$$

from which if follows that:

$$C = C = C_0 e^{e-(\dot{Q}/Qt)}$$

Again, by analogy, it is clear that $Q/\dot{Q} = 1/k = \tau$ (the time constant). Thus the *time constant equals the tissue volume divided by its blood flow rate.*

---

*It is strange at first sight that two quantities as complex as compliance and resistance should have a product as simple as time. In fact, the mass/length/time units check perfectly well (see Appendix A).

$$\text{compliance} \times \text{resistance} = \text{time}$$
$$M^{-1}L^4T^2 \times ML^{-4}T^{-1} = T$$

This is also the basis of the Lassen and Ingvar (1961) technique for measurement of organ blood flow. The theory is delightfully simple. The time constant is determined for the wash-out of a freely diffusible radioactive substance from the organ. Since the reciprocal of the time constant equals the organ blood flow divided by the organ volume, the answer is immediately available in blood flow per unit volume of tissue (usually expressed as ml/min per 100 ml of tissue). This makes the assumption that the solubility of the substance is the same for blood and tissue. If it is not, a correction factor can easily be applied.

Similar principles apply to the time constant of wash-out of a substance from the alveolar gas, which equals the FRC divided by the alveolar ventilation (assuming that none of the substance crosses the alveolar/capillary membrane during the process, as is nearly true with helium, for example). This important relationship is used in the nitrogen wash-out test of uniformity of intrapulmonary gas mixing, in which gas is considered as being washed out of two compartments, one fast and one slow (page 46). A compuond wash-out curve is obtained and is subsequently analysed for different components (Comroe et al., 1962).

Half-life. It is often convenient to use the half-life instead of the time constant. This is the time required for *y* to change to half of its previous value. The special attraction of the half-life is its ease of measurement. The half-life of a radioactive element may be determined quite simply. First of all the degree of activity is measured and the time noted. Its activity is then followed and the time noted at which its activity is exactly half the initial value. The difference between the two times is the half-life and is constant at all levels of activity. Half-lives are shown in Figures F.4–F.6 as dots on the curves. For a particular exponential function there is a constant relationship between the time constant and the half-life.

$$Half\text{-}life = 0.69 \text{ times the } time\ constant$$
$$Time\ constant = 1.44 \text{ times the } half\text{-}life$$

(For practical purposes, the time constant is approximately 1.5 times the half-life.)

Graphical representation

Plotting a wash-out exponential function is similar to the tear-away function (Figure F.5). A semi-log plot is particularly convenient as the curve (being straight) may then be defined by far fewer observations. It is also easy to extrapolate backwards to zero time if the initial value is required but could not be measured directly for some reason. It is, for example, an essential step in the measurement of cardiac output with a dye which is rapidly lost from the circulation (page 152).

The wash-in exponential function

The wash-in function is also of special importance to the respiratory physiologist and is the mirror image of the wash-out function.

Simple statement

In a wash-in exponential function, the quantity under consideration rises towards a limiting value, at a rate which decreases progressively in proportion to the distance it still has to rise.

Examples

A typical example would be a mountaineer who each day manages to climb half the remaining distance between his overnight camp and the summit of the mountain. His rate of ascent declines exponentially and he will never reach the summit. A graph of his altitude plotted against time would resemble a 'wash-in' curve.

   Biological examples include the reverse of those listed for the wash-out function:

1. Inflation of the lungs of a paralysed patient by a sustained increase of mouth pressure (Figure F.6).
2. The uptake of inhalational anaesthetics.
3. The rise of arterial PCO_2 to its new level after a step decrease of ventilation.
4. The rise of arterial PO_2 to its new level after a step increase of ventilation.
5. The rise of blood PO_2 to the alveolar level as it progresses along the pulmonary capillary.
6. The rise of blood PCO_2 to the venous level as blood progresses through the tissue capillaries.

Mathematical statement

With a wash-in exponential function, y increases with time and therefore the rate of change is positive. As time advances, the rate of change falls towards zero. The initial value of y is often zero and y approaches a final limiting value which we may designate y_∞, that is the value of y when time is infinity (∞). A change of this type is indicated thus:

$$\frac{dy}{dt} = k(y_\infty - y)$$

As y approaches y_∞ so the quantity within the parentheses approaches zero, and the rate of change slows down. The corresponding equation which indicates the instantaneous value of y is:

$$y = y_\infty(1 - e^{-kt})$$

y_∞ is the limiting value of y (attained only at infinite time).
e is again the base of natural logarithms.
k is a constant defining the rate of build-up and, as is the case of the wash-out function, it is the reciprocal of the *time constant* the significance of which is described above. It is the time which would be required to reach completion, if the initial rate of change were maintained without slowing down.
   After 1 time constant, y will have risen to approximately $100 - 37 = 63\%$ of its final value.
   After 2 time constants, y will have risen to approximately $100 - 13.5 = .86.5\%$ of its final value.

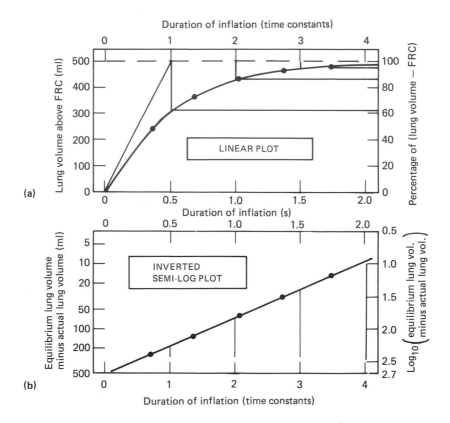

Figure F.6 Passive inflation of the lungs with a sustained mouth pressure – a typical wash-in exponential function. Eventual tidal volume, 500 ml; compliance, 0.5 l/kPa (50 ml/cmH₂O); airway resistance, 1 kPa l⁻¹ s (10 cm H₂O/1000 ml/sec); time constant, 0.5 s; half-life, 0.35 s. The points on the curves indicate the passage of successive half-lives.

	Elapsed time (constants)	Lung volume attained above FRC	
		ml	*percentage of tidal volume*
Lung volume above FRC $= 500\ (1 - e^{-(t/0.5)})$	0	0	0
	0.69	250	50
	1	316	63.2
	2	433	86.5
	3	475	95.0
	4	491	98.2

Note that, for the semi-log plot, the log scale (ordinate) is from above downwards and indicates the difference between the equilibrium lung volume (inflation pressure maintained indefinitely) and the actual lung volume. Use log graph paper upside down.

Table F.1 Percentage change of y after lapse of different numbers of time constants

Time elapsed in time constants	Tear-away function $y = y_0 e^{kt}$ (expressed as % of y_0)	Wash-out function $y = y_0 e^{-kt}$ (expressed as % of y_0)	Wash-in function $y = y_\infty(1 - e^{-kt})$ (expressed as % of y_∞)
0	100	100	0
0.693*	200	50	50
1	272	36.8	63.2
2	739	13.5	86.5
3	2 009	4.98	95.02
4	5 460	1.83	98.17
5	14 841	0.67	99.33
10	2 202 650	0.004 5	99.995 5
∞	∞	0	100

*Half-life or doubling time. *Note.* $272 = 100 \times e$
$739 = 100 \times e^2$
$2\ 009 = 100 \times e^3$
etc.

After 3 time constants, y will have risen to approximately $100 - 5 = 95\%$ of its
   final value.
After 5 time constants, y will have risen to approximately $100 - 1 = 95\%$ of its
   final value.
(More precise values are indicated in Table F.1.)

   As in the wash-out function representing passive exhalation, the time constant
for the corresponding wash-in exponential function (passive inflation of the lungs)
equals the product of compliance and resistance. For the wash-in of a substance
into an organ, the time constant equals tissue volume divided by blood flow, or
FRC divided by alveolar ventilation as the case may be. As above, the time
constant is approximately 1.5 times the half-life.
   There are many situations in which the same parameters apply to both wash-in
and a wash-out functions of the same system. The time constant for each function
will then be the same. A classic example is the charging of an electrical capacitor
through a resistance, and then allowing it to discharge to earth through the same
resistor. The time constant is the same for each process and equals the product of
capacitance and resistance. This is approximately true for passive deflation and
inflation of the lungs (Figures F.5 and F.6), on the assumption that compliance and
airway resistance remain the same.

Graphical representation

The wash-in function may be represented on linear paper as for the other types of
exponential function. However, for the semi-log plot, the paper must be turned
upside down and the plot made as indicated in Figure F.6. The curve will then be a
straight line.

References and further reading

Abraham, A.S., Cole, R.B. and Bishop, J.M. (1968) Reversal of pulmonary hypertension by prolonged oxygen administration to patients with chronic bronchitis. *Circulation Res.* **23**, 147

Abraham, A.S., Cole, R.B., Green, I.D., Hedworth-Whitty, R.B., Clarke, S.W. and Bishop, J.M. (1969) Factors contributing to the reversible pulmonary hypertension of patients with acute respiratory failure studied by serial observations during recovery. *Circulation Res.* **24**, 51

Abreu e Silva, F.A., MacFadyen, U.M., Williams, A. and Simpson, H. (1985) Sleep apnoea in infancy. *Jl R. Soc. Med* **78**, 1005

Adair, G.S. (1925) The hemoglobin system. VI. The oxygen dissociation curve of hemoglobin. *J. biol. Chem.* **63**, 529

Adams, R.W., Gronert, G.A., Sundt, T.M. and Michenfelder, J.D. (1972) Halothane, hypocania, and cerebrospinal fluid pressure in neurosurgery. *Anesthesiology* **37**, 510

Agostoni, E. (1962) Diaphragm activity and thoraco-abdominal mechanics during positive pressure breathing, *J. appl. Physiol.* **17**, 215

Agostoni, E. (1963) Diaphragm activity during breath-holding: factors related to its onset. *J. appl. Physiol.* **18**, 30

Agostoni, E., Sant'Ambrogio, G. and Carrasco, H.D.P. (1960) Electromyography of the diaphragm in man and transdiaphragmatic pressure. *J. appl. Physiol.* **15**, 1093

Aitken, R.S. and Clarke-Kennedy, A.E. (1928) On the fluctuations in the composition of the alveolar air during the respiratory cycle in muscular exercise. *J. Physiol.* **65**, 389

Alabaster, V.A. (1980) Inactivation of endogenous amines in the lungs. In: *Metabolic Activities of the Lung*, Ciba Foundation Symposium no. 78. Amsterdam: Excerpta Medica

Alexander, J.I., Spence, A.A., Parikh, R.K. and Stuart, B. (1973) The role of airway closure in postoperative hypoxaemia. *Br. J. Anaesth.* **45**, 34

Alexander, S.C., James, F.M., Colton, E.T., Gleaton, H.R. and Wollman, H. (1968) Effects of cyclopropane on cerebral blood flow and carbohydrate metabolism in man. *Anesthesiology* **29**, 170

Ali, J., Weisel, R.D., Layug, A.B., Kripke, B.J. and Hechtman, H.B. (1974) Consequences of postoperative alterations in respiratory mechanics. *Am. J. Surg.* **128**, 376

Anderson, D.O. and Ferris, B.G. (1962) Role of tobacco smoking in the causation of chronic respiratory disease. *New Engl. J. Med.* **267**, 787

Angus, G.E. and Thurlbeck, W.M. (1972) Number of alveoli in the human lung. *J. appl. Physiol.* **32**, 483

Antezana, G., Leguia, G., Guzmann, A.M., Coudert, J. and Spielvogel, H. (1982) Haemodynamic study of high altitude pulmonary edema (12 200 ft). In: *High Altitude Physiology and Medicine*, p. 232, edited by W. Brendel and R.A. Zink. New York: Springer-Verlag

Anthonisen, N.R., Danson, J., Robertson, P.C. and Ross, W.R.D. (1969) Airway closure as a function of age. *Resp. Physiol.* **8**, 58

Archie, J.P. (1981) Mathematical coupling of data. *Ann. Surg.* **193**, 296

Armitage, G.H. and Taylor, A.B. (1956) Non-bronchospirometric measurement of differential lung function. *Thorax* **11**, 281

Arndt, H., King, T.K.C. and Briscoe, W.A. (1970) Diffusing capacities and ventilation:perfusion ratios in patients with the clinical syndrome of alveolar capillary block. *J. clin. Invest.* **49,** 408

Arnone, A. (1972) X-ray diffraction study of binding of 2,3-diphosphoglycerate to human deoxyhaemoglobin. *Nature* **237,** 146

Ashbaugh, D.G., Bigelow, D.B., Petty, T.L. and Levine, B.E. (1967) Acute respiratory distress in adults. *Lancet* **2,** 319

Ashton, H., Stepney, R. and Thompson, P.W. (1979) Self-titration by cigarette smokers. *Br. med. J.* **2,** 357

Asmussen, E. (1965) Muscular exercise. *Handbk Physiol., section 3,* **2,** 939

Asmussen, E. and Neilsen, M. (1946) Studies on the regulation of respiration in heavy work. *Acta physiol. scand.* **12,** 171

Asmussen, E. and Nielsen, M. (1960) Aveolar–arterial gas exchange at rest and during work at different oxygen tensions. *Acta physiol. scand.* **50,** 153

Astiz, M.E., Rackow, E.C., Falk, J.L., Kaufman, B.S. and Weil, M.H. (1987) Oxygen delivery and consumption in patients with hyperdynamic septic shock. *Crit. Care Med.* **15,** 25

Åstrand P.-O. and Rodahl, K. (1986) *Textbook of Work Physiology*, 3rd edn. New York: McGraw-Hill

Astrup, P. and Severinghaus, J.W. (1986) *The History of Blood Gases, Acids and Bases.* Copenhagen: Munksgaard

Attar, S., Scanlan, E. and Cowley, R.A. (1966) Further evaluation of hyperbaric oxygen in haemorrhagic shock. In *Proceedings of the Third International Conference on Hyperbaric Medicine*, edited by I.W. Brown and B.G. Cox. Washington DC: National Academy of Sciences

Aub, J.C. and DuBois, E.F. (1917) The basal metabolism of old men. *Archs intern. Med.* **19,** 823

Austrian, R., McClement, J.H., Renzetti, A.D., Donald, K.W., Riley, R.L. and Cournand, A. (1951) Clinical and physiological features of some types of pulmonary diseases with impairment of alveolar–capillary diffusion. *Am. J. Med.* **11,** 667

Avery, M.E. and Mead, J. (1959) Surface properties in relation to atelectasis and hyaline membrane disease. *Archs Dis. Childh.* **97,** 517

Babior, B.M., Kipnes, R.S. and Curnutte, J.T. (1973) The production by leukocytes of superoxide, a potential bactericidal agent. *J. clin. Invest.* **52,** 741

Bachofen, M. and Weibel, E.R. (1982) Structural alterations and lung parenchyma in the adult respiratory distress syndrome. *Clins chest Med.* **3,** 35

Bachrach, A.J. (1982) A short history of man in the sea. In: *The Physiology and Medicine of Diving*, edited by P.B. Bennett and D.H. Elliott. London: Baillière Tindall

Bainton, C.R. and Mitchell, R.A. (1965) Posthyperventilation apnea in awake man. *Fedn Proc.* **24,** 273

Bake, B., Wood, L., Murphy, B., Macklem, P.T. and Milic-Emili, J. (1974) Effect of inspiratory flow rate on regional distribution of inspired gas. *J. appl. Physiol.* **37,** 8

Bakhle, Y.S. (1968) Conversion of angiotensin I to angiotensin II by cell-free extracts of dog lung. *Nature* **220,** 919

Bakhle, Y.S. (1980) Pulmonary angiotensin-converting enzyme and its inhibition. In: *Metabolic Activities of the Lung*, Ciba Foundation Symposium no. 78. Amsterdam: Excerpta Medica

Bakhle, Y.S. (1990) Pharmacokinetic and metabolic properties of the lung. *Br. J. Anaesth.* **65,** 79

Bakhle, Y.S. and Block, A.J. (1976) Effects of halothane on pulmonary inactivation of noradrenalin and prostaglandin E_2 in anaesthetized dogs. *Clin. Sci.* **50,** 87

Bakhle, Y.S. and Ferreira, S.H. (1985) Lung metabolism of eicosanoids: prostaglandins, prostacyclin, thromboxane and leukotrienes. *Handbk Physiol., section 3,* **1,** 365

Bakhle, Y.S. and Vane, J.R. (1977) (eds) *Metabolic Functions of the Lung.* New York: Marcel Dekker

Banner, N.R. and Govan, J.R. (1986) Long term transtracheal oxygen delivery through microcatheter in patients with hypoxaemia due to chronic obstructive airway disease. *Br. med. J.* **293,** 111

Bannister, R.G., Cunningham, D.J.C. and Douglas, C.G. (1954) The carbon dioxide stimulus to breathing in severe exercise. *J. Physiol.* **125,** 90

Barber, R.E., Lee, J. and Hamilton, W.K. (1970) Oxygen toxicity in man. A prospective study in patients with irreversible brain damage. *New Engl. J. Med.* **283,** 1478

Barcroft, J. (1920) Physiological effects of insufficient oxygen supply. *Nature* **106,** 125

Barer, G.R., Howard, P. and McCurrie, J.R. (1967) The effect of carbon dioxide and changes in blood pH on pulmonary vascular resistance in cats. *Clin. Sci.* **32,** 361

Barer, G.R., Howard, P., McCurrie, J.R. and Shaw, J.W. (1969) Changes in the pulmonary circulation after bronchial occlusion in anaesthetized dogs and cats. *Circulation Res.* **25**, 747

Barker, R.W., Brown, F.F., Drake, R., Halsey, M.J. and Richards, R.E. (1975) Nuclear magnetic resonance studies of anaesthetic interactions with haemoglobin. *Br. J. Anaesth.* **47**, 25

Barnes, M.P., Bates, D., Cartlidge, N.E.F., French, J.M. and Shaw, D.A. (1987) Hyperbaric oxygen and multiple sclerosis: final results of a placebo-controlled, double-blind study. *J. Neurol. Neurosurg. Psychiat.* **50**, 1402

Barnes, P.J. (1984) The third nervous system in the lung: physiology and clinical perspectives. *Thorax* **39**, 561

Barnes, P.J. (1991a) Neural control of airway smooth muscle. In: *The Lung: scientific foundations*, p. 903, edited by R.G. Crystal and J.B. West. New York: Raven Press

Barnes, P.J. (1991b) Pharmacology of airway smooth muscle. In: *The Lung: scientific foundations*, p. 977, edited by R.G. Crystal and J.B. West. New York: Raven Press

Barth, L. (1954) Untersuchungen über die Diffusionsatmung des Menschen. In *Anaesthesieprobleme. Abh. dt. Akad. Wiss. Berl., Klasse für med.*

Bartlett, D. (1989) Respiratory functions of the larynx. *Physiol. Rev.* **69**, 33

Baskett, P.J.F. (1992) Advances in cardiopulmonary resuscitation. *Br. J. Anaesth.* **69**, 182

Bates, D.V., Macklem, P.T. and Christie, R.V. (1971) *Respiratory Function in Disease*, 2nd edn. Philadelphia, Pa. and London: W.B. Saunders

Bay, J., Nunn, J.F. and Prys-Roberts, C. (1968) Factors influencing arterial Po_2 during recovery from anaesthesia. *Br. J. Anaesth.* **40**, 398

Beamer, W.C., Prough, D.S., Royster, R.L., Johnston, W.E. and Johnson, J.C. (1984) High frequency ventilation produces auto-PEEP. *Crit. Care Med.* **12**, 734

Behrendt, W., Weiland, C., Kalff, J. and Giani, G. (1987) Continuous measurement of oxygen uptake. *Acta anaesth. scand.* **31**, 10

Bellville, J.W. and Seed, J.C. (1960) The effect of drugs on the respiratory response to carbon dioxide. *Anesthesiology* **21**, 727

Benatar, S.R., Hewlett, A.M. and Nunn, J.F. (1973) The use of iso-shunt lines for control of oxygen therapy. *Br. J. Anaesth.* **45**, 711

Bend, J.R., Serabjit-Singh, C.J. and Philpot, R.M. (1985) The pulmonary uptake, accumulation and metabolism of xenobiotics. *A. Rev. Pharmacol. Toxicol.* **25**, 97

Bendixen, H.H. and Bunker, J.P. (1962) Measurement of inspiratory force in anesthetized dogs. *Anesthesiology* **23**, 315

Bendixen, H.H., Hedley-Whyte, J. and Laver, M.B. (1963) Impaired oxygenation in surgical patients during general anesthesia with controlled ventilation. *New Engl. J. Med.* **269**, 991

Bendixen, H.H., Smith, G.M. and Mead, J. (1964) Pattern of ventilation in young adults. *J. appl. Physiol.* **19**, 195

Benesch, R. and Benesch, R.E. (1967) Effects of organic phosphates from human erythrocytes on the allosteric properties of haemoglobin. *Biochem. Biophys. Res. Commun.* **26**, 162

Bennett, E.D., Jayson, M.I.V., Rubinstein, D. and Campbell, E.J.M. (1962) The ability of man to detect added non-elastic loads to breathing. *Clin. Sci.* **23**, 155

Bennett, P.B. (1982a) Inert gas narcosis. In: *The Physiology and Medicine of Diving*, edited by P.G. Bennett and D.H. Elliott. London: Baillière Tindall

Bennett, P.B. (1982b) The high pressure nervous syndrome in man. In: *The Physiology and Medicine of Diving*, edited by P.B. Bennett and D.H. Elliott. London: Baillière Tindall.

Benumof, J.L. (1982) One-lung ventilation: which lung should be PEEPed? *Anesthesiology* **56**, 161

Benumof, J.L. (1991) Management of the difficult airway. *Anesthesiology* **75**, 1087

Benumof, J.L., Augustine, S.D. and Gibbons, J.A. (1987) Halothane and isoflurane only slightly impair arterial oxygenation during one lung ventilation in patients undergoing thoracotomy. *Anesthesiology* **67**, 910

Benzinger, T. (1937) Untersuchungen über die Atmung und den Gasstoffwechsel insbesondere bei Sauerstoffmangel und Unterdruck, mit fortlaufend unmittelbar aufzeichnenden Methoden. *Ergebn. Physiol.* **40**, 1

Berger, A.J. and Hornbein, T.F. (1987) Control of respiration. In: *Physiology and Biophysics*, vol. 2, 21st edn, edited by H.D. Patton, A.F. Fuchs, B. Hille and A.M. Scher. Philadelphia, Pa: W.B.

Saunders

Bergman, N.A. (1963) Distribution of inspired gas during anesthesia and artificial ventilation. *J. appl. Physiol.* **18**, 1085

Bergman, N.A. (1966) Measurement of respiratory resistance in anesthetized subjects. *J. appl. Physiol.* **21**, 1913

Bergman, N.A. (1967) Effects of varying waveforms on gas exchange. *Anesthesiology* **28**, 390

Bergman, N.A. (1969) Properties of passive exhalations in anesthetized subjects. *Anesthesiology* **30**, 379

Bergman, N.A. and Tien, Y.K. (1983) Contribution of the closure of pulmonary units to impaired oxygenation during anesthesia. *Anesthesiology* **59**, 395

Bergman, N.A. and Waltemath, C.L. (1974) A comparison of some methods for measuring total respiratory resistance. *J. appl. Physiol.* **36**, 131

Bernstein, L. and Mendel, D. (1951) Accuracy of spirographic tracings at high rates. *Thorax* **6**, 297

Bernstein, L., D'Silva, J.L. and Mendel, D. (1952) The effect of rate on MBC determination with a new spirometer. *Thorax* **7**, 225

Bertrand, F., Hugelin, A. and Vibert, J.F. (1974) A stereologic model of pneumotaxic oscillator based on spatial and temporal distributions of neuronal bursts. *J. Neurophysiol.* **37**, 91

Beydon, L., Hassapopoulos, J., Quera, M.-A., Rauss, A., Becquemin, J.-P., Bonnet, F., Harf, A. and Goldenberg, F. (1992) Risk factors for oxgyen desaturation during sleep, after abdominal surgery. *Br. J. Anaesth.* **69**, 137

Bhattacharya, J., Gropper, M.A. and Staub, N.A. (1984) Interstitial fluid pressure gradient measured by micropuncture in excised dog lung. *J. appl. Physiol.* **56**, 271

Bickler, P.E., Dueck, R. and Prutow, R.J. (1987) Effects of barbiturate anesthesia on functional residual capacity and ribcage/diaphragm contributions to ventilation. *Anesthesiology* **66**, 147

Bindslev, L.G., Hedenstierna, G., Santesson, J., Gottlieb, I. and Carvallhas, A. (1981) Ventilation–perfusion distribution during inhalation anaesthesia. *Acta anaesth. scand.* **25**, 360

Birt, C. and Cole, P.V. (1965) Some physiological effects of closed circuit halothane anaesthesia. *Anaesthesia* **30**, 258

Biscoe, T.J. (1971) Carotid body structure and function. *Physiol. Rev.* **5**, 437

Biscoe, T.J. and Millar, R.A. (1964) The effect of halothane on carotid sinus baroreceptor activity *J. Physiol.* **173**, 24

Biscoe, T.J. and Willshaw, P. (1981) Stimulus–response relationships of the peripheral arterial chemoreceptors. In: *Regulation of Breathing*, part I, edited by T.F. Hornbein. New York: Marcel Dekker

Bitter, H.S. and Rahn, H. (1956) Redistribution of alveolar blood flow with passive lung distension. *Wright Air Dev. Ctr. Tech. Rep.* 56–466, 1

Bjertnaes, L.J. (1977) Hypoxia induced vasoconstriction in isolated perfused lungs exposed to injectable or inhalation anaesthetics. *Acta anaesth. scand.* **21**, 133

Black, A.M.S. and Torrance, R.W. (1971) Respiratory oscillations in chemoreceptor discharge in the control of breathing. *Resp. Physiol.* **13**, 221

Black, G.W., Linde, H.W., Dripps, R.D. and Price, H.L. (1959) Circulatory changes accompanying respiratory acidosis during halothane (Fluothane) anaesthesia in man. *Br. J. Anaesth.* **31**, 238

Blackburn, J.P., Conway, C.M., Leigh, J.M., Lindop, M.J. and Reitan, J.A. (1972) PaCO$_2$ and the pre-ejection period. *Anesthesiology* **37**, 268

Blake, D.R., Hall, N.D., Bacon, P.A., Dieppe, P.A., Halliwell, B. and Gutteridge, J.M.C. (1981) The importance of iron in rheumatoid disease. *Lancet* **2**, 1142

Bland, R.D. (1991) Fetal lung liquid and its removal near birth. In: *The Lung: scientific foundations*, p. 1677, edited by R.G. Crystal and J.B. West. New York: Raven Press

Bledsoe, S.W. and Hornbein, T.F. (1981) Central chemosensors and the regulation of their chemical environment. In: *Regulation of Breathing*, part I, edited by T.F. Hornbein. New York: Marcel Dekker

Blitt, C.D., Brown, B.R., Wright, B.J., Gandolfi, A.J. and Sipes, G. (1979) Pulmonary biotransformation of methoxyflurane. *Anesthesiology* **51**, 528

Bodman, R.I. (1963) Clinical applications of pulmonary function tests. *Anaesthesia* **18**, 355

Bohr, C. (1891) Über die Lungenathmung. *Skand. Arch. Physiol.* **2**, 236

Bohr, C. (1909) Über die spezifische Tätigkeit der Lungen bei der respiratorischen Gasaufnahme.

Skand. Arch. Physiol. **22,** 221

Boidin, M.P. (1985) Airway patency in the unconscious patient. *Br. J. Anaesth.* **57,** 306

Bone, R.C. (1990) Ventilation/perfusion scan in pulmonary embolism. *J. Am. med. Ass.* **263,** 2794

Bone, R.C. (1992) Adult respiratory distress syndrome. In: *Anaesthesia and the Lung*, p. 253, edited by T.H. Stanley and R.J. Sperry. Dordrecht: Kluwer.

Bone, R.C., Fisher, C.J., Clemmer, T.P., Slotman, G.J., Metz, C.A. and Balk, R.A. (1987) A controlled trial of high-dose methylprednisolone in the treatment of severe sepsis and septic shock. *New Engl. J. Med.* **317,** 653

Bone, R.C., Fisher, C.J., Clemmer, T.P., Slotman, G.J., Metz, C.A. and Balk, R.A. (1989a) Sepsis syndrome: a valid clinical entity. *Crit. Care Med.* **17,** 389

Bone, R.C., Slotman, G., Maunder, R., Silverman, H., Hyers, T.M., Kerstein, M.D. and Ursprung, J.J. (1989b) Randomized double-blind, multicentre study of prostaglandin E_1 in patients with the adult respiratory distress syndrome. *Chest* **96,** 114

Bonora, M., Shields, G.I., Knuth, S.L., Bartlett, D. and St John, W.M. (1984) Selective depression by ethanol of upper airway respiratory motor activity in cats. *Am. Rev. resp. Dis.* **130,** 156

Bookallil, M. and Smith, W.D.A. (1964) A proportional respiratory sampling apparatus. *Br. J. Anaesth.* **36,** 527

Boothby, W.M. and Sandiford, I. (1924) Basal metabolism. *Physiol. Rev.* **18,** 1085

Borland, C., Chamberlain, A., Higenbottam, T., Shipley, M. and Rose, G. (1983) Carbon monoxide yield of cigarettes and its relation to cardiorespiratory disease. *Br. med. J.* **287,** 1583

Boushey, H.A., Holtzman, M.J., Sheller, J.R. and Nadel, J.A. (1980) Bronchial hyperreactivity. *Am. Rev. resp. Dis.* **121,** 389

Bowes, G. and Phillipson, E.A. (1984) Arousal responses to respiratory stimuli during sleep. In: *Sleep and Breathing*, edited by N.A. Saunders and C.E. Sullivan. New York: Marcel Dekker

Brady, J.P., Cotton, E.C. and Tooley, W.H. (1964) Chemoreflexes in the newborn infant: effects of 100% oxygen on heart rate and ventilation. *J. Physiol.* **172,** 332

Brain, A.I.J. (1983) The laryngeal mask: a new concept in airway management. *Br. J. Anaesth.* **55,** 801

Brancatisano, T.P., Dodd, D.S. and Engel, L.A. (1984) Respiratory activity of posterior cricoarytenoid muscle and vocal cords in humans. *J. appl. Physiol.* **57,** 1143

Brashers, V.L., Peach, M.J. and Rose, E. (1988) Augmentation of hypoxic pulmonary vasoconstriction in the isolated perfused rat lung by in vitro antagonists of endothelium-dependent relaxation. *J. clin. Invest.* **82,** 1495

Braun, U., Zundel, J., Freiboth, K., Weyland, W., Turner, E., Heidelmeyer, C.F. and Hellige, G. (1989) Evaluation of methods for indirect calorimetry with a ventilated lung model. *Int. Care Med.* **15,** 196

Braunitzer, G. (1963) Molekulare struktur der Hämoglobine. *Nova Acta Acad. Caesar. Leop. Carol.* **26,** 471

Breuer, J. (1868) Die Selbsteurung der Athmung durch den Nervus Vagus. *Sber. Akad. Wiss. Wien* **58,** 909

Brigham, K.L. and Meyrick, B. (1984) Interactions of granulocytes with the lungs. *Circulation Res.* **54,** 623

Briscoe, W.A., Forster, R.E. and Comroe, J.H. (1954) Alveolar ventilation at very low tidal volumes. *J. appl. Physiol.* **7,** 27

Brismar, B., Hedenstierna, G., Lundquist, H., Strandberg, A., Svensson, L. and Tokics, L. (1985) Pulmonary densities during anesthesia with muscular relaxation – a proposal of atelectasis. *Anesthesiology* **62,** 422

Broderick, P.M., Webster, R.N. and Nunn, J.F. (1989) The laryngeal mask airway. *Anaesthesia* **44,** 238

Brown, E.B. and Miller, F. (1952) Ventricular fibrillation following a rapid fall in alveolar carbon dioxide concentration. *Am. J. Physiol.* **169,** 56

Brown, E.S., Johnson, R.P. and Clements, J.A. (1959) Pulmonary surface tension. *J. appl. Physiol.* **14,** 717

Brummelkamp, W.H. (1965) Reflections on hyperbaric oxygen therapy at 2 atmospheres absolute for *Clostridium welchii* infections. In: *Hyperbaric Oxygenation*, edited by I. Ledingham. Edinburgh and London: Churchill Livingstone

Brusasco, V., Knopp, T.J., Schmid, E.R. and Rehder, K. (1984) Ventilation–perfusion relationship during high-frequency ventilation. *J. appl. Physiol.* **56**, 454

Buick, F.J., Gledhill, N., Froese, A.B., Spriet, L. and Meyers, E.C. (1980) Effect of induced erythrocythemia on aerobic work capacity. *J. appl. Physiol.* **48**, 636

Burke-Wolin, T. and Wolin, M.S. (1990) Inhibition of cGMP-associated pulmonary arterial relaxation to H_2O_2 and O_2 by ethanol. *Am. J. Physiol.* **258**, 1267

Burton, A.C. (1951) On the physical equilibrium of small blood vessels. *Am. J. Physiol.* **164**, 319

Butler, J. (1960) The work of breathing through the nose. *Clin. Sci.* **19**, 55

Butler, J. and Smith, B.H. (1957) Pressure–volume relationships of the chest in the completely relaxed anaesthetised patient. *Clin. Sci.* **16**, 125

Butler, J., White, H.C. and Arnott, W.M. (1957) The pulmonary compliance in normal subjects. *Clin. Sci.* **16**, 709

Butler, W.J., Bohn, D.J., Bryan, A.C. and Froese, A.B. (1980) Ventilation by high frequency oscillation in humans. *Anesth. Analg.* **59**, 577

Butt, M.P., Jalowayski, A., Modell, J.H. and Giammona, S.T. (1970) Pulmonary function after resuscitation from near drowning. *Anesthesiology* **32**, 275

Bye, P.T.P., Farkas, G.A. and Roussos, C. (1983) Respiratory factors limiting exercise. *A. Rev. Physiol.* **45**, 439

Cain, C.C. and Otis, A.B. (1949) Some physiological effects resulting from added resistance to respiration. *J. Aviat. Med.* **20**, 149

Cain, S.M. (1977) Oxygen delivery and uptake in dogs during anemic and hypoxic hypoxia. *J. appl. Physiol.* **42**, 228

Cain, S.M. and Otis, A.B. (1961) Carbon dioxide transport in anesthetized dogs during inhibition of carbonic anhydrase. *J. appl. Physiol.* **16**, 1023

Cameron, A.J.V., Gibb, B.H., Ledingham, I. McA. and McGuinness, J.B. (1965) A controlled clinical trial of hyperbaric oxygen in the treatment of acute myocardial infarction. In: *Hyperbaric Oxygenation*, edited by I. Ledingham. Edinburgh and London: Churchill Livingstone

Campbell, E.J.M. (1952) An electromyographic study of the role of the abdominal muscles in breathing, *J. Physiol.* **177**, 222

Campbell, E.J.M. (1955) An electromyographic examination of the role of the intercostal muscles in breathing in man. *J. Physiol.* **129**, 12

Campbell, E.J.M. (1957) The effects of increased resistance to expiration on the respiratory behaviour of the abdominal muscles and intra-abdominal pressure. *J. Physiol.* **136**, 556

Campbell, E.J.M. (1958) *The Respiratory Muscles and the Mechanics of Breathing*. London: Lloyd-Luke.

Campbell, E.J.M. (1960a) Simplification of Haldane's apparatus for measuring CO_2 concentration in respired gases in clinical practice. *Br. med. J.* **1**, 457

Campbell, E.J.M. (1960b) A method of controlled oxygen administration which reduces the risk of carbon-dioxide retention. *Lancet* **2**, 12

Campbell, E.J.M. (1962) RIpH. *Lancet* **1**, 681

Campbell, E.J.M. and Guz, A. (1981) Breathlessness. In: *Regulation of Breathing*, part II, edited by T.F. Hornbein. New York: Marcel Dekker

Campbell, E.J.M. and Howell, J.B.L. (1960) Simple rapid methods of estimating arterial and mixed venous P_{CO_2}. *Br. med. J.* **1**, 458

Campbell, E.J.M. and Howell, J.B.L. (1962) Proprioceptive control of breathing. In: Ciba Foundation Symposium on *Pulmonary Structure and Function*, edited by A.V.S. de Rueck and M. O'Connor. Edinburgh and London: Churchill Livingstone

Campbell, E.J.M. and Howell, J.B.L. (1963) The sensation of breathlessness. *Br. med. Bull.* **19**, 36

Campbell, E.J.M., Howell, J.B.L. and Peckett, B.W. (1957) The pressure–volume relationships of the thorax of anaesthetized human subjects. *J. Physiol.* **136**, 563

Campbell, E.J.M., Nunn, J.F. and Peckett, B.W. (1958) A comparison of artificial ventilation and spontaneous respiration with particular reference to ventilation–blood-flow relationships. *Br. J. Anaesth.* **30**, 166

Campbell, E.J.M., Westlake, E.K. and Cherniack, R.M. (1957) Simple methods of estimating oxygen consumption and efficiency of the muscles of breathing. *J. appl. Physiol.* **11**, 303

Campbell, E.J.M., Freedman, S., Smith, P.S. and Taylor, M.E. (1961) The ability of man to detect added elastic loads to breathing. *Clin. Sci.* **20**, 223

Campbell, E.J.M., Freedman, S., Clark, T.J.H., Robson, J.G. and Norman, J. (1967) The effect of muscular paralysis induced by tubocurarine on the duration and sensation of breath-holding. *Clin. Sci.* **32**, 425

Campbell, E.J.M., Godfrey, S., Clark, T.J.H., Freedman, S. and Norman, J. (1969) The effect of muscular paralysis induced by tubocurarine on the duration and sensation of breath holding during hypercapnia. *Clin. Sci.* **36**, 323

Carlens, E., Hanson, H.E. and Nordenström, B. (1951) Temporary occlusion of the pulmonary artery. *J. thorac. Surg.* **22**, 527

Carlon, G.C., Howland, W.S. and Ray, C. (1983) High frequency jet ventilation. A prospective randomised evaluation. *Chest* **84**, 551

Caro, C.G., Butler, J. and DuBois, A.B. (1960) Some effects of restriction of chest cage expansion on pulmonary function in man. *J. clin. Invest.* **39**, 573

Cascorbi, H.F. and Singh-Amaranath, A.V. (1972) Fluroxene toxicity in mice. *Anesthesiology* **37**, 480

Cassidy, S.S., Gaffney, F.A. and Johnson, R.L. (1981) A perspective in PEEP. *New Engl. J. Med.* **304**, 421

Castleden, C.M. and Cole, P.V. (1974) Variations in carboxyhaemoglobin levels in smokers. *Br. med. J.* **4**, 736

de Castro, F. (1926) Sur la structure et l'innervation de la glande intercarotidienne. *Trab. Lab. Invest. biol. Univ. Madrid* **24**, 365

Cater, D.B., Garatini, S., Marina, F. and Silver, I.A. (1961) Changes of oxgyen tension in brain and somatic tissues induced by vasodilator and vasoconstrictor drugs. *Proc. R. Soc. B* **155**, 136

Cater, D.B., Hill, D.W., Lindop, P.J., Nunn, J.F. and Silver, I.A. (1963) Oxygen washout studies in the anesthetized dog. *J. appl. Physiol.* **18**, 888

Catley, D.M., Thornton, C., Jordan, C., Lehane, J.R., Royston, D. and Jones, J.G. (1985) Pronounced, episodic oxygen desaturation in the postoperative period. *Anesthesiology* **63**, 20

Cerretelli, P. (1980) Gas exchange at high altitude. In: *Pulmonary Gas Exchange*, vol II, edited by J.B. West. New York: Academic Press

Cerretelli, P., Cruz, J.C., Farhi, L.E. and Rahn, H. (1966) Determination of mixed venous O_2 and CO_2 tensions and cardiac output by a rebreathing method. *Resp. Physiol.* **1**, 258

Ceruti, E. (1966) Chemoreceptor reflexes in the newborn infant: effect of cooling on the response to hypoxia. *Pediatrics* **37**, 556

Chakrabarti, M.K., Gordon, G. and Whitwam, J.G. (1986) Relationship between tidal volume and deadspace during high frequency ventilation. *Br. J. Anaesth.* **58**, 11

Channin, E. and Tyler, J. (1962) Effect of increased breathing frequency on inspiratory resistance in emphysema. *J. appl. Physiol.* **17**, 605

Chanutin, A. and Curnish, R. (1967) Effect of organic and inorganic phosphates on the oxygen equilibrium of human erythrocytes. *Archs Biochem. Biophys.* **121**, 96

Chapman, C.R. and Morrison, D. (1989) *Cosmic Catastrophes*, p.97. London: Plenum Press

Cheney, F.W. and Colley, P.S. (1980) The effect of cardiac output on arterial blood oxygenation. *Anesthesiology* **52**, 496

Chenoweth, D.E., Cooper, S.W., Hugli, T.E., Stewart, R.W., Blackstone, E.H. and Kirlin, J.W. (1981) Complement activation during cardiopulmonary bypass. *New Engl. J. Med.* **304**, 497

Chernick, V. (1981) The fetus and the newborn. In: *Regulation of Breathing*, part II, edited by T.F. Hornbein. New York: Marcel Dekker

Cherry, P.D., Furchgott, R.F., Zawadzki, J.V. and Jothianandan, D. (1982) Role of endothelial cells in relaxation of isolated arteries by bradykinin. *Proc. Natl Acad. Sci. USA.* **72**, 2106

Cheung, J.Y., Bonventre, J.V., Malis, C.D. and Leaf, A. (1986) Calcium and ischemic injury. *New Engl. J. Med.* **314**, 1670

Christensen, M.S. (1974) Acid–base changes in cerebrospinal fluid and blood, and blood volume changes following prolonged hyperventilation in man. *Br. J. Anaesth.* **46**, 348

Christensen, M.S., Hoedt-Rasmussen, K. and Lassen, N.A. (1967) Cerebral vasodilatation by halothane anaesthesia in man and its potentiation by hypotension and hypercapnia. *Br. J. Anaesth.* **39**, 927

Christiansen, J., Douglas, C.G. and Haldane, J.S. (1914) The adsorption and dissociation of carbon dioxide by human blood. *J. Physiol.* **48,** 244

Church, D.F. and Pryor, W.A. (1991) The oxidative stress placed on the lung by cigarette smoke. In: *The Lung: scientific foundations*, p. 1975, edited by R.G. Crystal and J.B. West. New York: Raven Press

Clark, I.A. and Hunt, N.H. (1983) Evidence for reactive oxygen intermediates causing hemolysis and parasite death in malaria. *Infec. Immun.* **39,** 1

Clark, I.A., Cowden, W.B. and Hunt, N.H. (1985) Free radical-induced pathology. *Med. Res. Rev.* **5,** 297

Clark, J.M. and Lambertsen, C.J. (1971) Pulmonary toxicity – a review. *Pharmac. Rev.* **23,** 37

Clark, J.M., Hagerman, F.C. and Gelfand, R. (1983) Breathing patterns during submaximal and maximal exercise in elite oarsmen, *J. appl. Physiol.* **55,** 440

Clark, T.J.H. (1968) The ventilatory response to CO_2 in chronic airways obstruction measured by a rebreathing method. *Clin. Sci.* **34,** 559

Clark, T.J.H., Clarke, B.G. and Hughes, J.M.B. (1966) A simple technique for measuring changes in ventilatory response to carbon dioxide. *Lancet* **2,** 368

Clark, S.W., Jones, J.G. and Oliver, D.R. (1970) Resistance to two-phase gas–liquid flow in airways. *J. appl. Physiol.* **29,** 464

Clements, J.A. (1970) Pulmonary surfactant. *Am. Rev. resp. Dis.* **101,** 984

Clergue, F., Ecoffey, C., Derenne, J.P. and Viars, P. (1984) Oxygen drive to breathing during halothane anesthesia: effects of almitrine bismesilate. *Anesthesiology* **60,** 125

Cloud, P. (1988) *Oasis in Space*, p. 132. London: W. W. Norton

Clowes, G.H.A., Hopkins, A.L. and Simeone, F.A. (1955) A comparison of physiological effects of hypercapnia and hypoxia in the production of cardiac arrest. *Ann. Surg.* **142,** 446

Clutton-Brock, J. (1957) The cerebral effects of overventilation. *Br. J. Anaesth.* **29,** 111

Cobley, M. and Vaughan, R.S. (1992) Recognition and management of difficult airway problems. *Br. J. Anaesth.* **68,** 90

Cockett, F.B. and Vass, C.C.N. (1951) A comparison of the role of the bronchial arteries in the bronchiectasis. *Thorax* **6,** 268

Cohen, G., Xu, C. and Henderson-Smart, D. (1991) Ventilatory response of the sleeping newborn to CO_2 during normoxic rebreathing. *J. appl. Physiol.* **71,** 168

Cohen, J.J., Brackett, N.C. and Schwartz, W.B. (1964) The nature of the carbon dioxide titration curve in the normal dog. *J. clin. Invest.* **43,** 777

Cohen, P.J. and Behar, M.G. (1970) The *in vitro* effect of anesthesia on the oxyhemoglobin dissociation curve. *Fedn Proc.* **29,** 329

Colacicco, G. (1985) Arguments against and alternatives for an extracellular surfactant layer in the alveoli of mammalian lung. *J. theor. Biol.* **114,** 641

Cole, A.G.H., Weller, S.F. and Sykes, M.K. (1984) Inverse ratio ventilation compared with PEEP in adult respiratory failure. *Intens. Care Med.* **10,** 227

Cole, R.B. and Bishop, J.M. (1963) Effects of varying inspired oxygen tension on alveolar–arterial O_2 tension difference in man. *J. appl. Physiol.* **18,** 1043

Coleridge, J.C.G. and Coleridge, H.M. (1984) Afferent vagal C fibre innervation of the lungs and airways and its functional significance. *Rev. Physiol. Biochem. Pharmac.* **99,** 1

Colgan, F.J., Barrow, R.E. and Fanning, G. (1971) Constant positive-pressure breathing and cardiorespiratory function. *Anesthesiology* **34,** 145

Comroe, J.H. (1939) The location and function of the chemoreceptors of the aorta. *Am. J. Physiol.* **127,** 176

Comroe, J.H. and Botelho, S. (1947) The unreliability of cyanosis in the recognition of arterial anoxemia. *Am. J. med. Sci.* **214,** 1

Comroe, J.H. and Dripps, R.D. (1946) Artificial respiration *J. Am. med. Ass.* **130,** 381

Comroe, J.H. and Schmidt, C.F. (1938) The part played by reflexes from the carotid body in the chemical regulation of respiration in the dog. *Am. J. Physiol.* **121,** 75

Comroe, J.H., Nisell, O.I. and Nims, R.G. (1954) A simple method of concurrent measurement of compliance and resistance to breathing in anesthetized animals and man. *J. appl. Physiol.* **7,** 225

Comroe, J.H., Forster, R.E., DuBois, A.B., Briscoe, W.A. and Carlsen, E. (1962) *The Lung*, 2nd edn. Chicago: Year Book Medical; London: Lloyd-Luke

Conn, A.W. and Barker, G.A. (1984) Fresh water drowning and near drowning. *Can. Anaesth. Soc. J.* **31**, S38

Conn, A.W., Edmonds, J.F. and Barker, G.A. (1978) Near-drowning in cold fresh water: current treatment regimen. *Can. Anaesth. Soc. J.* **25**, 259

Connaughton, J.J., Douglas, N.J., Morgan, A.D., Shapiro, C.M., Critchley, J.A.J.H., Pauly, N. and Flenley, D.C. (1985) Almitrine improves oxygenation when both awake and asleep in patients with hypoxia and carbon dioxide retention caused by chronic bronchitis and emphysema. *Am. Rev. resp. Dis.* **132**, 206

Cooper, E.A. (1957) Infra-red analysis for the estimation of carbon dioxide in the presence of nitrous oxide. *Br. J. Anaesth* **30**, 486

Cooper, E.A. (1959) The estimation of minute volume. *Anaesthesia* **14**, 373

Cooper, E.A. (1961) Behaviour of respiratory apparatus. *Med. Res. Memo. Natn. Coal Bd med. Serv.* **2**

Cooper, E.A. and Smith, H. (1961) Indirect estimation of arterial pCO₂. *Anaesthesia* **16**, 445

Corda, M., von Euler, C. and Lennerstrand, G. (1965) Proprioceptive innervation of the diaphragm. *J. Physiol.* **178**, 161

Cormack, R.S. (1972) Eliminating two sources of error in the Lloyd–Haldane apparatus. *Resp. Physiol.* **14**, 382

Cormack, R.S. and Powell, J.N. (1972) Improving the performance of the infra-red carbon dioxide meter. *Br. J. Anaesth.* **44**, 131

Cormack, R.S., Cunningham, D.J.C. and Gee, J.B.L. (1957) The effect of carbon dioxide on the respiratory response to want of oxygen in man. *Q. Jl exp. Physiol.* **42**, 303

Cotes, J.E. (1975) *Lung Function*, 3rd edn. Oxford: Blackwell Scientific

Cotes, J.E. (1979) *Lung Function,* 4th edn. Oxford: Blackwell Scientific

Cotev, S., Lee, J. and Severinghaus, J.W. (1968) The effects of acetazolamide on cerebral blood flow and cerebral tissue Po₂. *Anesthesiology* **29**, 471

Cournand, A., Motley, H.L., Werko, L. and Richards, D.W. (1948) Physiological studies of the effects of intermittent positive pressure breathing on cardiac output in man. *Am. J. Physiol.* **152**, 162

Cowan, G.S., Staub, N.C. and Edmunds, L.H. (1976) Changes in the fluid compartments and dry weights of reimplanted dog lungs. *J. appl. Physiol.* **40**, 962

Cox, J., Woolmer, R.W. and Thomas, V. (1960) Expired air resuscitation. *Lancet* **1**, 727

Craig, A.B. (1961) Causes of loss of consciousness during underwater swimming. *J. appl. Physiol.* **16**, 583

Craig, A.B. (1968) Depth limits of breath hold diving. *Resp. Physiol.* **5**, 14

Craig, D.B., Wahba, W.M., Don, H.F., Couture, J.G. and Becklake, M.R. (1971) 'Closing volume' and its relationship to gas exchange in seated and supine positions. *J. appl. Physiol.* **31**, 717

Crandall, E.D., Bidani, A. and Forster, R.E. (1977) Postcapillary changes in blood pH *in vivo* during carbonic anhydrase inhibition. *J. appl. Physiol.* **43**, 582

Crapo, J.D. and Tierney, D.F. (1974) Superoxide dismutase and pulmonary oxygen toxicity. *Am. J. Physiol.* **226**, 1401

Crawford, M. and Rehder, K. (1985) High-frequency small-volume ventilation in anesthetized humans. *Anesthesiology* **62**, 298

Cross, K.W., Klaus, M., Tooley, W.H. and Weisser, K. (1960) The response of the new-born baby to inflation of the lungs. *J. Physiol.* **151**, 551

Crouch, E.C., Martin, G.R. and Brody, J.S. (1991) Basement membranes. In: *The Lung: scientific foundations*, p. 421, edited by R.G. Crystal and J.B. West. New York: Raven Press

Crowell, J.W., Ford, R.G. and Lewis, V.M. (1959) Oxygen transport in hemorrhagic shock as a function of the hematocrit ratio. *Am. J. Physiol.* **196**, 1033

Cucchiara, R.F., Nugent, M., Seward, J.B. and Messick, J.M. (1984) Air embolism in upright neurosurgical patients; detection and localization by two-dimensional transesophageal echocardiography. *Anesthesiology* **60**, 353

Cullen, D.J. and Eger, E.I. (1974) Cardiovascular effects of carbon dioxide in man. *Anesthesiology* **41**, 345

Cunningham, D.J.C. (1974) The control system regulating breathing in man. *Q. Rev. Biophys.* **6**, 433

Cunningham, D.J.C. and Ward, S.A. (1975a) The form of respiratory interaction between an alternate-breath oscillation of Paco₂ and hypoxia in man. *J. Physiol.* **251**, 37P

Cunningham, D.J.C. and Ward, S.A. (1975b) The separate effects of alternate-breath oscillations of P_{ACO_2} during hypoxia on inspiration and expiration. *J. Physiol.* **252**, 33P

Cunningham, D.J.C., Howson, M.G. and Pearson, S.B. (1973) The respiratory effects in man of altering the time profile of alveolar CO_2 and O_2 within each respiratory cycle. *J. Physiol.* **234**, 1

Cunningham, D.J.C., Kay, R.H. and Young, J.M. (1965) A fast response paramagnetic oxygen analyser. *J. Physiol.* **181**, 15P

Cunningham, D.J.C., Hey, E.N., Patrick, J.M. and Lloyd, B.B. (1963) The effect of noradrenalin infusion on the relation between pulmonary ventilation and the alveolar P_{O_2} and P_{CO_2} in man. *Ann. N.Y. Acad. Sci.* **109**, 756

Cushley, M.J., Tattersfield, A.E. and Holgate, S.T. (1984) Adenosine-induced bronchoconstriction in asthma. *Am. Rev. resp. Dis.* **129**, 380

Cutillo, A.G., Morris, A.H., Ailon, D.C., Case, T.A., Durney, C.H., Ganesan, K., Watanabe, F. and Akhtari, M. (1988) Assessment of lung water distribution by nuclear magnetic resonance. *Am. Rev. resp. Dis.* **137**, 1371

Cymerman, A., Reeves, J.T., Sutton, J.T., Rock, P.B., Groves, B.M., Malconian, M.K. et al. (1989) Operation Everest II: maximal oxygen uptake at extreme altitude. *J. appl. Physiol* **66**, 2446

Dail, C.W.., Affeldt, J.E. and Collier, C.R. (1955) Clinical aspects of glossopharyngeal breathing. *J. Am. med. Ass.* **158**, 445

Dalhamn, T. and Rylander, R. (1965) Ciliastatic action of cigarette smoke. *Archs Otolaryngol.* **81**, 379

Daly, I. de B. and Daly, M. de B. (1959) The effects of stimulation of the carotid body chemoreceptors on the pulmonary vascular bed in the dog. *J. Physiol.* **148**, 201

Daly, N.J., Ross, J.C. and Behnke, R.H. (1963) The effect of changes in the pulmonary vascular bed produced by atropine, pulmonary engorgement and positive pressure breathing on diffusing and mechanical capacity of the lung. *J. clin. Invest.* **42**, 1083

D'Angelo, E., Calderini, E., Torri, G., Robatto, F.M., Bonon, D. and Milic-Emili, J. (1989) Respiratory mechanics in anesthetized paralyzed humans: effects of flow, volume and time. *J. appl. Physiol.* **67**, 2556

D'Angelo, E., Robatto, F.M., Calderini, E., Tavola, M., Bono, D., Torri, G. and Milic-Emili, J. (1991) Pulmonary and chest wall mechanics in anesthetized paralyzed humans. *J. appl. Physiol.* **70**, 2602

Dann, W.L. (1971) The effects of different levels of ventilation in the action of pancuronium in man. *Br. J. Anaesth.* **43**, 959

Dantzker, D.R., Lynch, J.P. and Weg, J.G. (1980) Depression of cardiac output is a mechanism of shunt reduction in the therapy of acute respiratory failure. *Chest* **77**, 636

Dantzker, D.R., Wagner, P.D. and West, J.G. (1975) Instability of lung units with low $\dot{V}_A/\dot{Q}$ ratios during O_2 breathing. *J. appl. Physiol.* **38**, 886

Dantzker, D.R., Brock, C.J., Dehart, P., Lynch, J.P. and Weg. J.G. (1979) Ventilation–perfusion distributions in adult respiratory distress syndrome. *Am. Rev. resp. Dis.* **120**, 1039

Datta, H., Stubbs, W.A. and Alberti, K.G.M.M. (1980) Substrate utilization by the lung. In: *Metabolic Activities of the Lung*, Ciba Foundation Symposium no. 78. Amsterdam: Excerpta Medica

Davenport, H.T. and Valman, H.B. (1980) Resuscitation of the newborn. In: *General Anaesthesia*, 4th edn, vol. 2, edited by T.C. Gray, J.F. Nunn and J.E. Utting. London: Butterworths

Davidson, J.M. (1990) Biochemistry and turnover of lung interstitium. *Eur. Resp. J.* **3**, 1048

Davidson, J.T., Whipp, B.J., Wasserman, K., Koyal, S.N. and Lugliani, R. (1974) Role of carotid bodies in breath-holding. *New Engl. J. Med.* **290**, 819

Davies, P.R.F., Tighe, S.Q.M, Greenslade, G.L. and Evans, G.H. (1990) Laryngeal mask airway and tracheal tube: insertion by unskilled personnel. *Lancet* **336**, 977

Davies, R.J.O. and Hopkin, J.M. (1989) Nasal oxygen in exacerbations of ventilatory failure; an underappreciated risk. *Br. med. J.* **299**, 43

Davies, R.J.O. and Stradling, J.R. (1990) The relationship between neck circumference, radiographic pharyngeal anatomy, and the obstructive sleep apnoea syndrome. *Eur. Resp. J.* **3**, 509

Davies, R.O., Edwards, M.W. and Lahiri, S. (1982) Halothane depresses the response of carotid body chemoreceptors to hypoxia and hypercapnia in the cat. *Anesthesiology* **57**, 153

Davis, W.B. and Pacht, E.R. (1991) Extracellular antioxidant defenses. In: *The Lung: scientific foundations*, p. 1821, edited by R.G. Crystal and J.B. West. New York: Raven Press

Dawes, G.S. (1968) *Fetal and Neonatal Physiology*. Chicago: Year Book Publishers

Dawes, G.S., Fox, H.E., Leduc, B.M., Liggins, G.C. and Richards, R.T. (1972) Respiratory movements and rapid eye movement sleep in the foetal lamb. *J. Physiol.* **220,** 119

Defares, J.G., Lundin, G., Arborelius, M., Stromblad, R. and Svanberg, L. (1960) Effect of 'unilateral hypoxia' on pulmonary blood flow distribution in normal subjects. *J. appl. Physiol.* **15,** 169

DeFouw, D.O. (1983) Ultrastructural features of alveolar epithelial transport. *Am. Rev. resp. Dis.* **127,** S9

Dejours, P. (1962) Chemoreflexes in breathing. *Physiol. Rev.* **42,** 335

Dejours, P. (1964) Control of respiration in muscular exercise. *Handbk Physiol., section 3*, **1,** 631

Del Maestro, R.F. (1980) An approach to free radicals in medicine and biology. *Acta physiol. scand.* suppl. **492,** 153

Delivoria-Papadopoulos, M., Roncevic, N.P. and Oski, F.A. (1971) Postnatal changes in oxygen transport of term, premature, and sick infants. *Pediat. Res.* **5,** 235

DeMaria, E.J., Reichman, W., Kenney, P.R., Armitage, J.M. and Gann, D.S. (1985) Septic complications of corticosteroid administration after central nervous system trauma. *Ann. Surg.* **202,** 248

Dempsey, J.A., Forster, H.V. and doPico, G.A. (1974) Ventilatory acclimatization to moderate hypoxemia in man. *J. clin. Invest.* **53,** 1091

Dempsey, J.A., Skatrud, J.B., Badr, S. and Henke, K.G. (1991) Effects of sleep on the regulation of breathing and respiratory muscle function. In: *The Lung: scientific foundations*, p. 1615, edited by R.G. Crystal and J.B. West. New York: Raven Press

Denison, D.M. (1984) Geometric estimates of lung and chest wall function. In: *Techniques in Respiratory Physiology*, part II, edited by A.B. Otis. Amsterdam: Elsevier

Denison, D.M., Ernsting, J. and Cresswell, A.W. (1966) Fire and hyperbaric oxygen. *Lancet* **2,** 1404

Denison, D., Edwards, R.H.T., Jones, G. and Pope, H. (1971) Estimates of the CO_2 pressures in systemic arterial blood during rebreathing on exercise. *Resp. Physiol.* **11,** 186

Derion, T., Guy, H.J.B., Tsukimoto, K., Schaffartzik, W., Prediletto, R., Poole, D.C., Knight, D.R. and Wagner, P.D. (1992) Ventilation–perfusion relationships in the lung during head-out water immersion. *J. appl. Physiol.* **72,** 64

De Troyer, A. (1991) Respiratory muscles. In: *The Lung: scientific foundations*, p. 869, edited by R.G. Crystal and J.B. West. New York: Raven Press

De Troyer, A. and Estenne, M. (1984) Coordination between rib cage muscles and diaphragm during quiet breathing in humans. *J. appl. Physiol.* **57,** 899

Dev, N.B. and Loeschcke, H.H. (1979) Topography of the respiratory and circulatory responses to acetylcholine and nicotine of the ventral surface of the medulla oblongata. *Pflüger's Archiv.* **379,** 19

Dickinson, J.G. (1985) Terminology and classification of acute mountain sickness. *Br. med. J.* **285,** 720

Dickinson, J., Heath, D., Gosney, J. and Williams, D. (1983) Altitude-related deaths in seven trekkers in the Himalayas. *Thorax* **38,** 646

Doll, R. and Hill, A.B. (1950) Smoking and carcinoma of the lung. *Br. med. J.* **2,** 739

Doll, R. and Peto, M. (1976) Mortality in relation to smoking: 20 years' observations on male British doctors. *Br. med. J.* **2,** 1525

Dollfuss, R.E., Milic-Emili, J. and Bates, D.V. (1967) Regional ventilation of the lung studied with boluses of [133]xenon. *Resp. Physiol.* **2,** 234

Don, H.F. and Robson, J.G. (1965) The mechanics of the respiratory system during anesthesia. *Anesthesiology* **26,** 168

Don, H.F., Wahba, W.M. and Craig, D.B. (1972) Airway closure, gas trapping, and the functional residual capacity during anesthesia. *Anesthesiology* **36,** 533

Don, H.F., Wahba, M., Cuadrado, L. and Kelkar, K. (1970) The effects of anesthesia and 100 per cent oxygen on the functional residual capacity of the lungs. *Anesthesiology* **32,** 521

Donald, K.W. (1947) Oxygen poisoning in man. *Br. med. J.* **1,** 667 and 712

Donald, K.W. (1949) Neurological effects of oxygen. *Lancet* 1056

Donald, K.W. and Christie, R.V. (1949) A new method of clinical spirometry. *Clin. Sci.* **8,** 21

Donald, K.W., Renzetti, A., Riley, R.L. and Cournand, A. (1952) Analysis of factors affecting the concentrations of oxygen and carbon dioxide in gas and blood of lungs: results. *J. appl. Physiol.* **4,** 497

Donald, K.W., Bishop, J.M., Cumming, G. and Wade, O.L. (1953) Effect of nursing positions on cardiac output in man. *Clin. Sci.* **12,** 199

Dorbin, H.L., Lutchen, K.R. and Jackson, A.C. (1988) Human respiratory input impedance from 4 to 200 Hz: physiologic and modelling considerations. *J. appl. Physiol.* **64**, 823

Dorinsky, P.M. and Gadek, J.E. (1989) Mechanisms of multiple nonpulmonary organ failure in ARDS. *Chest* **96**, 885

Douglas, C.G. and Haldane, J.S. (1909) The causes of periodic or Cheyne–Stokes breathing. *J. Physiol.* **38**, 401

Douglas, N.J. and Flenley, D.C. (1990) Breathing during sleep in patients with obstructive lung disease. *Am. Rev. resp. Dis.* **141**, 1055

Douglas, N.J., White, D.P., Pickett, C.K., Weil, J.V. and Zwillich, C.W. (1982) Respiration during sleep in normal man. *Thorax* **37**, 840

Dowman, C.E. (1927) Relief of diaphragmatic tic, following encephalitis, by section of phrenic nerves. *J. Am. med. Ass.* **88**, 95

Down, R.H.L. and Castleden, W.M. (1975) Oxygen therapy for pneumatosis coli. *Br. med. J.* **1**, 493

Downs, J. (1992) New modes of ventilatory support. In: *Anesthesia and the Lung*, p. 297, edited by T.H. Stanley and R.J. Sperry. Dordrecht: Kluwer.

Downs, J. and Stock, M.C. (1987) Airway pressure release ventilation: a new concept in ventilatory support. *Crit. Care Med.* **15**, 459

Downs, J.B. and Chapman, R.L. (1976) Treatment of bronchopleural fistula during continuous positive pressure ventilation. *Chest* **69**, 363

Downs, J.B., Perkins, H.M. and Modell, J.H. (1974) IMV – an evaluation. *Archs Surg.* **109**, 519

Draper, W.B. and Whitehead, R.W. (1944) Diffusion respiration in the dog anesthetized by pentothal sodium. *Anesthesiology* **5**, 262

Dreyfuss, D., Soler, P., Basset, G. and Saumon, G. (1988) High inflation pressure pulmonary edema. *Am. Rev. resp. Dis.* **137**, 1159

Drummond, G.B. (1989a) Influence of thiopentone on upper airway muscles. *Br. J. Anaesth.* **63**, 12

Drummond, G.B. (1989b) Chest wall movements in anaesthesia. *Eur. J. Anaesthesiol.* **6**, 161

Drummond, G.B. and Wright, D.J. (1977) Oxygen therapy after abdominal surgery. *Br. J. Anaesth.* **49**, 789

Drummond, G.B., Allan, P.L. and Logan M.R. (1986) Changes in diaphragmatic position in association with induction of anaesthesia. *Br. J. Anaesth.* **58**, 1246

Drummond, G.B., Pye, D.W., Annan, F.J. and Tothill, P. (1988) Changes in blood volume distribution associated with general anaesthesia. *Br. J. Anaesth.* **60**, 331P

Drummond, G.B., Jan, M.A., Warren, P.M., Yildrim, N. and Douglas, N.J. (1991) Effect of posture on genioglossal EMG activity in normal subjects and in patients with the sleep apnea/hypopnea syndrome. *Thorax* **46**, 744P

DuBois, A.B., Botelho, S.Y. and Comroe, J.H. (1956) A new method of measuring airway resistance in man using a body plethysmograph *J. clin. Invest.* **35**, 327

DuBois, A.B., Botelho, S.Y., Bedell, G.N., Marshall, R. and Comroe, J.H. (1956) A rapid plethysmographic method for measuring thoracic gas volume. *J. clin. Invest.* **35**, 322

Dueck, R., Young, I., Clausen, J. and Wagner, P.D. (1980) Altered distribution of pulmonary ventilation and blood flow following induction of inhalational anesthesia. *Anesthesiology* **52**, 113

Duffin, J., Triscott, A. and Whitwam, J.G. (1976) The effect of halothane and thiopentone on ventilatory responses mediated by the peripheral chemoreceptors in man. *Br. J. Anaesth.* **48**, 975

Duke, H.N. (1954) The site of action of anoxia on the pulmonary blood vessels of the cat. *J. Physiol.* **125**, 373

Duke, M. and Abelmann, W.H. (1969) The hemodynamic response to chronic anemia. *Circulation* **39**, 503

Dunbar, B.S., Ovassapian, A. and Smith, T.C. (1967) The effects of methoxyflurane on ventilation in man. *Anesthesiology* **28**, 1020

Dutton, R.E., Fitzgerald, R.S. and Gross, N. (1968) Ventilatory response to square-wave forcing of carbon dioxide at the carotid bodies. *Resp. Physiol.* **4**, 101

Dymond, J.H. and Smith, E.B. (1980) *The Viral Coefficients of Pure Gases and Mixtures: a critical compilation.* Oxford: Clarendon Press

Eckenhoff, J.E., Enderby, G.E.H., Larson, A., Edridge, A. and Judevine, D.E. (1963) Pulmonary gas exchange during deliberate hypotension. *Br. J. Anaesth.* **35**, 750

Edelman, N.H. and Neubauer, J.A. (1991) Hypoxic depression of breathing. In: *The Lung: scientific foundations*, p. 1341, edited by R.G. Crystal and J.B. West. New York: Raven Press

Edlund, A., Bonfim, W., Kaijser, L., Olin, C., Patrono, C., Pinca, E. and Wennmalm, W. (1981) Pulmonary formation of prostacyclin in man. *Prostaglandins* **22**, 323

Edmunds, L.H., Graf, P.D. and Nadel, J.A. (1971) Reinnervation of reimplanted canine lung. *J. appl. Physiol.* **31**, 722

Edward, J.F. (1960) Inter-atrial communication. In: *Pathology of the Heart*, edited by J.E. Gould Springfield, Ill: Charles C Thomas

Edwards, J.D., Brown, G.C.S., Nightingale, P., Slater, R.M. and Faragher, E.B. (1989) Use of survivors' cardiorespiratory values as therapeutic goals in septic shock. *Crit. Care Med.* **17**, 1098

Effros, R.M. and Mason, G.R. (1983) Measurements of pulmonary epithelial permeability in vivo. *Am. Rev. resp. Dis.* **127**, S59

Effros, R.M., Mason, G. and Silverman, P. (1981) Asymmetric distribution of carbonic anhydrase in the alveolar–capillary barrier. *J. appl. Physiol.* **51**, 190

Egan, T.M. and Cooper, J.D. (1991) The lung following transplantation. In: *The Lung: scientific foundations*, p. 2205, edited by R.G. Crystal and J.B. West. New York: Raven Press

Egan, T.M., Kaiser, L.R. and Cooper, J.D. (1989) Lung transplantation. *Curr. Prob. Surg.* **26**, 675

Eger, E.I. (1981) Isoflurane: a review. *Anesthesiology* **55**, 559

Eger, E.I., Dolan, W.M., Stevens, W.C., Miller, R.D. and Way, W.L. (1972) Surgical stimulation antagonizes the respiratory depression produced by forane. *Anesthesiology* **36**, 544

Eichacker, P.Q., Hoffman, W.D., Farese, A., Banks, S.M., Kuo, G.C., MacVittie, T.J. and Natanson, C. (1991) TNF but not IL-1 in dogs causes lethal lung injury and multiple organ dysfunction similar to human sepsis. *J. appl. Physiol.* **71**, 1979

Eisele, J.H., Eger, E.I. and Muallem, M. (1967) Narcotic properties of carbon dioxide in the dog. *Anesthesiology* **28**, 856

Eisele, J.H., Trenchard, D., Burki, N. and Guz, A. (1968) The effect of chest wall block on respiratory sensation and control in man. *Clin. Sci.* **35**, 23

Eisele, J.H., Noble, M.I.M., Katz, J., Fung, D.L. and Hickey, R.F. (1972) Bilateral phrenic-nerve block in man. *Anesthesiology* **37**, 64

Eisenkraft, J.B. (1990) Effects of anaesthetics on the pulmonary circulation. *Br. J. Anaesth.* **65**, 63

Eissa, N.T., Ranieri, V.M., Corbeil, C., Chassé, M., Robatto, F.M., Braidy, J. and Milic-Emili, J. (1991) Analysis of behavior of the respiratory system in ARDS patients: effects of flow, volume and time. *J. appl. Physiol.* **70**, 2719

Ekblom, B., Goldbarg, A.N. and Gullbring, B. (1972) Response to exercise after blood loss and reinfusion. *J. appl. Physiol.* **33**, 175

Elam, J.O. (1962) In: *Artificial Respiration*, edited by J.L. Whittenberger. New York and London: Harper and Row

Elam, J.O. and Greene, D.G. (1962) In: *Artificial Respiration*, edited by J.L. Whittenberger. New York and London: Harper and Row

Elliott, S.E., Segger, F.J. and Osborn, J.J. (1966) A modified oxygen gauge for the rapid measurement of Po_2 in respiratory gases. *J. appl. Physiol.* **21**, 1672

Ellis, F.R. and Nunn, J.F. (1968) The measurement of gaseous oxygen tension utilising paramagnetism: an evaluation of the Servomex OA 150 analyser. *Br. J. Anaesth.* **40**, 569

Ellis, H. and Feldman, S. (1983) *Anatomy for Anaesthetists*, 4th edn. Oxford: Blackwell Scientific

Ellison, R.G., Ellison, L.T. and Hamilton, W.F. (1955) Analysis of respiratory acidosis during anaesthesia. *Ann. Surg.* **141**, 375

Enghoff, H. (1931) Zur Frage des schädlichen Raumes bei der Atmung. *Skand. Arch. Physiol.* **63**, 15

Enghoff, H. (1938) Volumen inefficax. Bemerkungen zur Frage des schädlichen Raumes. *Uppsala Läk För Förh.* **44**, 191

Enghoff, H., Holmdahl, M. H:son and Risholm, L. (1951) Diffusion respiration in man. *Nature* **168**, 830

Ernsting, J. (1963) The effect of brief profound hypoxia upon the arterial and venous oxygen tensions in man. *J. Physiol.* **169**, 292

Ernsting, J. and McHardy, G.J.R. (1960) Brief anoxia following rapid decompression from 560 to 150 mmHg. *J. Physiol.* **153**, 73P

von Euler, C. (1991) Neural organization and rhythm generation. In: *The Lung: scientific foundations*,

p. 1307, edited by R.G. Crystal and J.B. West. New York: Raven Press

Eve, F.C. (1932) Actuation of the inert diaphragm by a gravity method. *Lancet* **2,** 995

Ezi-Ashi, T.I., Papworth, D.P. and Nunn, J.F. (1983) Inhalational anaesthesia in developing countries. *Anaesthesia* **38,** 736

Fairley, H.B. and Blenkarn, G.D. (1966) Effect on pulmonary gas exchange of variations in inspiratory flow rate during intermittent positive pressure ventilation. *Br. J. Anaesth.* **38,** 320

Fairweather, L.J., Walker, J. and Flenley, D.C. (1974) 2,3-Diphosphoglycerate concentrations and the dissociation of oxyhaemoglobin in ventilatory failure. *Clin. Sci.* **47,** 577

Faithfull, N.S. (1987) Fluorocarbons – current status and future applications. *Anaesthesia* **42,** 234

Falke, K.J., Hill, R.D., Qvist, J., Schneider, R.C., Guppy, M., Liggins, G.C. et al. (1985) Seal lungs collapse during free diving: evidence from arterial nitrogen tensions. *Science* **229,** 556

Fanta, C.H. and Drazen, J.M. (1983) Calcium blockers and bronchoconstriction. *Am. Rev. resp. Dis.* **127,** 673

Fantone, J.C. and Ward, P.A. (1982) Role of oxygen-derived free radicals and metabolites in leukocyte-dependent inflammatory reactions. *Am. J. Pathol.* **107,** 397

Farhi, L.I. (1964) Gas stores of the body. *Handbk Physiol., section 3,* **1,** 873

Featherstone, R.M., Muehlbaecher, C.A., DeBon, F.L. and Forsaith, J.A. (1961) Interactions of inert gases with proteins. *Anesthesiology* **22,** 6

Fein, A.M., Goldberg, S.K., Lippmann, M.L., Fischer, R. and Morgan, L. (1982) Adult respiratory distress syndrome. *Br. J. Anaesth.* **54,** 723

Fein, A.M., Lippmann, M., Holtzman, H., Eliraz, A. and Goldberg, S.K. (1983) The risk factors, incidence, and prognosis of ARDS following septicemia. *Chest* **83,** 40

Femi-Pearse, D., Afonja, A.O., Elegbeleye, O.O. and Odusote, K.A. (1976) Value of determination of oxygen consumption in tetanus. *Br. med. J.* **1,** 74

Fencl, V., Miller, T.B. and Pappenheimer, J.R. (1966) Studies of the respiratory response to disturbances of acid–base balance, with deductions concerning the ionic composition of cerebral interstitial fluid. *Am. J. Physiol.* **210,** 459

Fenn, W.O. and Asano, T. (1956) Effects of carbon dioxide inhalation on potassium liberation from the liver. *Am. J. Physiol.* **185,** 567

Fenn, W.O., Otis, A.B., Rahn, H., Chadwick, L.E. and Hegnauer, A.H. (1947) Displacement of blood from the lungs by pressure breathing. *Am. J. Physiol.* **151,** 258

Ferguson, J.K.W. (1936) Carbamino compounds of CO_2 with human haemoglobin and their role in the transport of CO_2. *J. Physiol.* **88,** 40

Ferguson, J.K.W. and Roughton, F.J.W. (1934) The direct chemical estimation of carbamino compounds of CO_2 with haemoglobin. *J. Physiol.* **83,** 68

Ferris, B.G., Mead, J., Whittenberger, J.L. and Saxton, G.A. (1952) Pulmonary function in convalescent poliomyelitis patients. 3. Compliance of the lungs and thorax. *New Engl. J. Med.* **40,** 664

Ferris, E.B., Engel, G.L., Stevens, C.D. and Webb, J. (1946) Voluntary breath holding. *J. clin. Invest.* **25,** 734

Fidone, S.J., Gonzalez, C., Dinger, B., Gomez-Nino, A., Obeso, A. and Yoshizaki, K. (1991) Cellular aspects of peripheral chemoreceptor function. In: *The Lung: scientific foundations,* p. 1319, edited by R.G. Crystal and J.B. West. New York: Raven Press

Filley, G.F., MacIntosh, D.J. and Wright, G.W. (1954) Carbon monoxide uptake and pulmonary diffusing capacity in normal subject at rest and during exercise. *J. clin. Invest.* **33,** 530

Fink, B.R. (1961) Influence of cerebral activity in wakefulness on regulation of breathing. *J. appl. Physiol.* **16,** 15

Fink, B.R. and Demarest, R.J. (1978) *Laryngeal Mechanics.* Cambridge, Mass: Harvard University Press

Fink, B.R., Ngai, S.H. and Holaday, D.A. (1958) Effect of air resistance on ventilation and respiratory muscle activity. *J. Am. med. Ass.* **168,** 2245

Finlayson, D.C. and Kaplan, J.A. (1979) Cardiopulmonary bypass. In: *Cardiac Anesthesia,* edited by J.A. Kaplan. London: Grune & Stratton

Finley, T.N., Swenson, E.W. and Comroe, J.H. (1962) The cause of arterial hypoxemia at rest in patients with 'alveolar–capillary block syndrome'. *J. clin. Invest.* **41,** 618

Finucane, K.E. and Colebatch, H.J.H. (1969) Elastic behavior of the lung in patients with airway obstruction. *J. appl. Physiol.* **26,** 330

Fischer, B.H., Marks, M. and Reich, T. (1983) Hyperbaric-oxygen treatment of multiple sclerosis. A randomized, placebo-controlled, double-blind study. *New Engl. J. Med.* **308,** 181

Fisher, A.B. and Forman, H.J. (1985) Oxygen utilization and toxicity in the lungs. *Handbook Physiol. section 3,* **1,** 231

Fishman, A.P. (1972) Pulmonary oedema. The water exchanging function of the lung. *Circulation* **46,** 390

Fishman, A.P. (1980) Vasomotor regulation of the pulmonary circulation. *A Rev. Physiol.* **42,** 211

Fishman, A.P. (1985) Pulmonary circulation. *Handbk Physiol., section 3,* **1,** 93

Fleming, P.J. and Ponte, J. (1983) Control of respiration in the fetus and newborn. In: *Control of Respiration,* edited by D.J. Pallot. London: Croom Helm

Flenley, D.C. (1985a) Long-term home oxygen therapy. *Chest* **87,** 99

Flenley, D.C. (1985b) Disordered breathing during sleep. *Jl R. Soc. Med.* **78,** 1031

Flenley, D.C. (1985c). In: *Asthma and Bronchial Hyper-reactivity. Progress in Respiration Research 19,* edited by H. Herzog and A. Perruchoud. Basel: Karger

Flenley, D.C., Fairweather, L.J., Cooke, N.J. and Kirby, B.J. (1975) Changes in haemoglobin binding curve and oxygen transport in chronic hypoxic lung disease. *Br. med. J.* **1,** 602

Fletcher, R. (1984) Airway dead space, end-tidal CO_2 and Christian Bohr. *Acta anaesth. scand.* **28,** 408

Flynn, J.T. (1984) Oxygen and retrolental fibroplasia: update and challenge. *Anesthesiology* **60,** 397

Foëx, P. (1980) Effects of carbon dioxide on the systemic circulation. In: *The Circulation in Anaesthesia,* edited by C. Prys-Roberts. Oxford: Blackwell Scientific

Folkow, B. and Pappenheimer, J.R. (1955) Components of the respiratory dead space and their variation with pressure breathing and with broncho-active drugs. *J. appl. Physiol.* **8,** 102

Forrest, J.B. (1972) The effect of hyperventilation on pulmonary surface activity. *Br. J. Anaesth.* **44,** 313

Forster, H.V. and Pan, L.G. (1991) Exercise hyperpnea. In: *The Lung: scientific foundations,* p. 1553, edited by R.G. Crystal and J.B. West. New York: Raven Press

Forster, H.V., Dempsey, J.A. and Chosy, L.W. (1975) Incomplete compensation of $CSF[H^+]$ in man during acclimatization to high altitude (4,300 m). *J. appl. Physiol.* **38,** 1067

Forster, H.V., Dempsey, J.A., Thomson, J., Vidruk, E. and doPico, G.A. (1972) Estimation of arterial Po_2, Pco_2, pH and lactate from arterialized venous blood. *J. appl. Physiol.* **32,** 134

Forster, R.E. (1964a) Rate of gas uptake by red cells. *Handbk Physiol., section 3,* **1,** 827

Forster, R.E. (1964b) Diffusion of gases. *Handbk Physiol., section 3,* **1,** 839

Forster, R.E. (1987) Diffusion of gases across the alveolar membrane. *Handbk Physiol., section 3,* **4,** 71

Foster, C.A. (1965) Hyperbaric oxygen and radiotherapy. In: *Hyperbaric Oxygenation,* edited by I. Ledingham. Edinburgh and London: Churchill Livingstone

Fourcade, H.E., Larson, C.P., Hickey, R.F., Bahlman, S.H. and Eger, E.I. (1972) Effects of time on ventilation during halothane and cyclopropane anesthesia. *Anesthesiology* **36,** 83

Fowler, A.A., Hamman, R.F., Good, J.T. et al (1983) Adult respiratory distress syndrome: risk with common predispositions. *Ann. intern. Med.* **98,** 593

Fowler, K.T. and Hugh-Jones, P. (1957) Mass spectrometry applied to clinical practice and research. *Br. med. J.* **1,** 1205

Fowler, W.S. (1948) Lung function studies. II. The respiratory dead space. *Am. J. Physiol.* **154,** 405

Fowler, W.S. (1950a) Lung function studies. IV. Postural changes in respiratory dead space and functional residual capacity. *J. clin. Invest.* **29,** 1437

Fowler, W.S. (1950b) Lung function studies. V. Respiratory dead space in old age and in pulmonary emphysema. *J. clin. Invest.* **29,** 1439

Fowler, W.S. (1954) Breaking point of breath-holding. *J. appl. Physiol* **6,** 539

Fowler, W.S. and Blakemore, W.S. (1951) Lung function studies. VII. The effect of pneumonectomy on respiratory dead space. *J. thorac. Surg.* **21,** 433

Fracica, P.J., Piantadosi, C.A. and Crapo, J.D. (1991) Oxygen toxicity. In: *The Lung: scientific foundations,* p. 2155, edited by R.G. Crystal and J.B. West. New York: Raven Press

Frank, L., Summerville, J. and Massaro, D. (1980) Protection from oxygen toxicity with endotoxin: role of the endogenous antioxidant enzymes of the lung. *J. clin. Invest.* **65,** 1104

Frayser, R., Rennie, I.D., Gray, G.W. and Houston, C.S. (1975) Hormonal and electrolyte response to exposure to 17,500 ft. *J. appl. Physiol.* **38,** 636

Freeman, B.A. and Crapo, J.D. (1981) Hyperoxia increases oxygen radical production in rat lungs and lung mitochondria. *J. biol. Chem.* **256,** 10986

Freeman, B.A., Topolsky, M.K. and Crapo, J.D. (1982) Hyperoxia increases oxygen radical production in rat lung homogenates. *Archs Biochem. Biophys.* **216,** 477

Freeman, J. (1962) Survival of bled dogs after halothane and ether anaesthesia. *Br. J. Anaesth.* **34,** 832

Freeman, J. and Nunn, J.F. (1963) Ventilation–perfusion relationships after haemorrhage. *Clin. Sci.* **24,** 135

Freund, F., Roos, A. and Dodd, R.B. (1964) Expiratory activity of the abdominal muscles in man during general anesthesia. *J. appl. Physiol.* **19,** 693

Froese, A.B. (1985) Effects of anesthesia and paralysis on the chest wall. In: *Effects of Anesthesia,* edited by B.G. Covino, H.A. Fozzard, K. Rehder and G. Strichartz. Bethesda, Md: American Physiological Society

Froese, A.B. and Bryan, A.C. (1974) Effects of anesthesia and paralysis on diaphragmatic mechanics in man. *Anesthesiology* **41,** 242

Froese, A.B. and Bryan, A.C. (1987) High frequency ventilation. *Am. Rev. resp. Dis.* **135,** 1363

Froman, C. (1966) Correction of cerebrospinal fluid metabolic acidosis by intrathecal injection of bicarbonate. *Br. J. Anaesth.* **39,** 90

Froman, C. and Crampton-Smith, A. (1966) Hyperventilation associated with low pH of cerebrospinal fluid after intracranial haemorrhage. *Lancet* **1,** 780

Frostell, C., Fratacci, M.-D., Wain, J.C., Jones, R. and Zapol, W.M. (1991) Inhaled nitric oxide: a selective pulmonary vasodilator reversing hypoxic pulmonary vasoconstriction. *Circulation* **83,** 2038

Frumin, M.J., Epstein, R.M. and Cohen, G. (1959) Apneic oxygenation in man. *Anesthesiology* **20,** 789

Fujita, S., Zorick, F., Conway, W., Roth, T., Hartse, K.M. and Piccone, P. (1980) Uvulo-palato-pharyngoplasty: a new surgical treatment for upper airway sleep apnea. *Sleep Res.* **9,** 197

Fuleihan, S., Wilson, R.S. and Pontoppidan, H. (1976) Effect of mechanical ventilation with end-inspiratory pause on blood-gas exchange. *Anesth. Analg.* **55,** 122

Furchgott, R.F. and Zawadzki, J.V. (1980) The obligatory role of endothelial cells in the relaxation of arterial smooth muscle by acetylcholine. *Nature* **288,** 373

Furuya, H. and Okumura, F. (1984) Detection of paradoxical air embolism by transesophageal echocardiography. *Anesthesiology* **60,** 374

Gail, D.B. and Lenfant, C.J.M. (1983) Cells of the lung: biology and clinical implications. *Am. Rev. resp. Dis.* **127,** 366

Garthwaite, J. (1991) Glutamate, nitric oxide and cell–cell signalling in the nervous system. *Trends neurol. Sci.* **14,** 60

Gattinoni, L., Pesenti, A., Rossi, G.P. et al. (1980) Treatment of acute respiratory failure with low-frequency positive-pressure ventilation and extracorporeal removal of CO_2. *Lancet* **2,** 292

Gattinoni, L., Pesenti, A., Kolobow, T. and Damia, G. (1983) A new look at therapy of the adult respiratory distress syndrome: motionless lungs. *Int. Anesth. Clins* **21,** 97

Gattinoni, L., Pesenti, A., Mascheroni, D., Marcolin, R., Funagalli, R. and Rossi, F. (1986) Low frequency positive-pressure ventilation with extracorporeal CO_2 removal in severe acute respiratory failure. *J. Am. med. Ass.* **256,** 881

Gattinoni, L., Pesenti, A., Bombino, M., Baglioni, S., Rivolta, M., Rossi, F. et al. (1988) Relationships between lung computed tomographic density, gas exchange, and PEEP in acute respiratory failure. *Anesthesiology* **69,** 824

Gattinoni, L., Pelosi, P., Pesenti, A., Brazzi, L., Vitale, G., Moretto, A., Crespi, A. and Tagliabue, M. (1991a) CT scan in ARDS: clinical and physiopathological insights. *Acta anaesth. scand.* **35,** suppl. 95, 87

Gattinoni, L., Pelosi, P., Vitale, G., Pesenti, A., D'Andrea, L. and Mascheroni, D. (1991b) Body position changes redistribute lung computed-tomographic density in patients with acute respiratory failure. *Anesthesiology* **74,** 15

Gautier, H. and Bertrand, F. (1975) Respiratory effects of pneumotaxic center lesions and subsequent vagotomy in chronic cats. *Resp. Physiol.* **23,** 71

Gautier, H., Bonora, M. and Gaudy, J.H. (1981) Breuer–Hering inflation reflex and breathing pattern in anesthetized humans and cats. *J. appl. Physiol.* **51,** 1162

Geddes, I.C. (1967) Recent studies in metabolic aspects of anaesthesia. In: *Modern Trends in*

Anesthesia – 3, edited by F.T. Evans and T.C. Gray. London: Butterworths

Geddes, D.M., Nesbitt, K., Traill, T. and Blackburn, J.P. (1979) First pass uptake of ^{14}C-propranolol by the lung. *Thorax* **34**, 810

Gee, M.H. and Williams, D.O. (1979) Effect of lung inflation on perivascular cuff fluid volume in isolated dog lung lobes. *Microvasc. Res.* **17**, 192

Gehr, P., Bachofen, M. and Weibel, E.R. (1978) The normal lung: ultrastructure and morphometric estimation of diffusion capacity. *Resp. Physiol.* **32**, 121

Georg, G., Lassen, N.A., Mellemgaard, K. and Vinther, A. (1965) Diffusion in the gas phase of the lungs in normal and emphysematous subjects. *Clin. Sci.* **29**, 525

Gerbershagan, H.U. and Bergman, N.A. (1967) The effect of *d*-tubocurarine on respiratory resistance in anesthetized man. *Anesthesiology* **28**, 981

Gerrard, J.W., Cockcroft, D.W., Mink, J.T., Cotton, D.J., Poonawala, R. and Dosman, J.A. (1980) Increased nonspecific bronchial reactivity in cigarette smokers with normal lung function. *Am. Rev. resp. Dis.* **122**, 577

Gerschman, R., Gilbert, D.L., Nye, S.W., Dwyer, P. and Fenn, W.O. (1954) Oxygen poisoning and X-irradiation: a mechanism in common. *Science* **119**, 623

Gersh, B.J. (1980) Measurement of intravascular pressures. In: *The Circulation in Anesthesia*, edited by C. Prys-Roberts. Oxford: Blackwell Scientific

Gerst, P.H., Rattenborg, C. and Holaday, D.A. (1959) The effects of hemorrhage on pulmonary circulation and respiratory gas exchange. *J. clin. Invest.* **38**, 524

Gessell, R. (1923) On the chemical regulation of respiration. *Am. J. Physiol.* **66**, 5

Giammona, S.T. and Modell, J.H. (1967) Drowning by total immersion. Effects on pulmonary surfactant of distilled water, isotonic saline and sea water. *Am. J. Dis. Child.* **114**, 612

Gibney, R.T., Wilson, R.S. and Pontoppidan, H. (1982) Comparison of work of breathing on high gas flow and demand valve continuous positive airway pressure systems. *Chest* **82**, 692

Gil, J., Bachofen, H., Gehr, P. and Weibel, E.R. (1979) Alveolar volume-surface area relation in air- and saline-filled lungs fixed by vascular perfusion. *J. appl. Physiol.* **47**, 990

Gilbe, C.E., Salt, J.C. and Branthwaite, M.A. (1980) Pulmonary function after prolonged mechanical ventilation with high concentrations of oxygen. *Thorax* **35**, 907

Gillis, C.N. (1973) Metabolism of vasoactive hormones by lung. *Anesthesiology* **39**, 626

Gillis, C.N. and Pitt, B.R. (1982) The fate of circulating amines with the pulmonary circulation. *A. Rev. Physiol.* **44**, 269

Ginn, R. and Vane, J.R. (1968) Disappearance of catecholamines from the circulation. *Nature* **219**, 740

Glanville, A.R., Burke, C.M., Theodore, J., Baldwin, J.C., Harvey, J., Vankessel, A. and Robin, E.D. (1987) Bronchial hyper-responsiveness after human cardiopulmonary transplantation. *Clin. Sci.* **73**, 299

Glauser, F.L. and Fairman, R.P. (1985) The uncertain role of the neutrophil in increased permeability pulmonary edema. *Chest* **88**, 601

Glazier, J.B., Hughes, J.M.B., Maloney, J.E. and West, J.B. (1967) Vertical gradient of alveolar size in lungs of dogs frozen intact. *J. appl. Physiol.* **23**, 694

Glazier, J.B., Hughes, J.M.B., Maloney, J.E. and West, J.B. (1969) Measurements of capillary dimensions and blood volume in rapidly frozen lungs. *J. appl. Physiol.* **26**, 65

Glossop, M.W. (1963) A simple method for the estimation of carbon dioxide concentration in the presence of nitrous oxide. *Br. J. Anaesth.* **35**, 17

Gluck, L. (1971) Biochemical development of the lung. *Clin. Obstet. Gynec.* **14**, 710

Gluck, L., Kulovich, M.V., Borer, R.C., Brenner, P.H., Anderson, G.G. and Spellacy, W.N. (1971) Diagnosis of the respiratory distress syndrome by amniocentesis. *Am. J. Obstet. Gynec.* **109**, 440

Godfrey, S. and Wolf, E. (1972) An evaluation of rebreathing methods for measuring mixed venous Pco2 during exercise. *Clin. Sci.* **42**, 345

Gold, M.I. and Helrich, M. (1967) Ventilation and blood gases in anaesthetized patients. *Can. Anaesth. Soc. J.* **14**, 424

van Gold, L.M.G., Batenburg, J.J. and Robertson, B. (1988) The pulmonary surfactant system: biochemical aspects and functional significance. *Physiol. Rev.* **68**, 374

Goldman, M., Knudson, R.J., Mead, J., Paterson, N., Schwaber, J.R. and Wohl, M.E. (1970) A simplified measurement of respiratory resistance by forced oscillation. *J. appl. Physiol.* **28**, 113

Goldstein, B., Shannon, D.C. and Todres, I.D. (1990) Supercarbia in children: clinical course and outcome. *Crit. Care Med.* **18**, 166

Gooden, B.A. (1982) The diving response in clinical medicine. *Aviat. Space Environ. Med.* **53**, 273

Gordh, T. (1945) Postural circulatory and respiratory changes during ether and intravenous anesthesia. *Acta chir. scand.* **92**, suppl. 102, 26

Gothard, J.W.W. and Branthwaite, M.A. (1984) The effects of thoracic surgery. In: *Effects of anesthesia and surgery on pulmonary mechanisms and gas exchange. International Anesthesiology Clinics*, vol. 22, no. 4, edited by J.G. Jones. Boston, Mass: Little, Brown.

Gracey, D.R., Divertie, M.B. and Brown, A.L. (1968) Alveolar–capillary membrane in idiopathic interstitial pulmonary fibrosis. *Am. Rev. resp. Dis.* **98**, 16

Graham, G.R., Hill, D.W. and Nunn, J.F. (1960) Die Wirkung hoher CO_2-Konzentrationen auf Kreislauf und Atmung. *Anaesthesist* **9**, 70

Granit, R. (1955) *Receptors and Sensory Perception*. New Haven, Ct, and London: Yale University Press

Gray, L.H., Conger, A.D., Ebert, M., Hornsey, S. and Scott, O.C.A. (1953) The concentration of oxygen dissolved in tissues at the time of irradiation as a factor in radiotherapy. *Br. J. Radiol.* **26**, 638

Gray, T.C. and Rees, G.J. (1952) The role of apnoea in anaesthesia for major surgery. *Br. med. J.* **2**, 891

Greenbaum, R., Nunn, J.F., Prys-Roberts, C., Kelman, G.R. and Silk, F.F. (1965) Cardio-pulmonary function after fat embolism. *Br. J. Anaesth.* **37**, 554

Greenbaum, R., Bay, J., Hargreaves, M.D., Kain, M.L., Kelman, G.R., Nunn, J.F., Prys-Roberts, C. and Siebold, K. (1967a) Effects of higher oxides of nitrogen on the anaesthetized dog. *Br. J. Anaesth.* **39**, 393

Greenbaum, R., Nunn, J.F., Prys-Roberts, C. and Kelman, G.R. (1967b) Metabolic changes in whole human blood (*in vitro*) at 37°C. *Resp. Physiol.* **2**, 274

Greene, D.G., Bauer, R.O., Janney, C.D. and Elam, J.O. (1957) Oxygen and carbon dioxide exchange and energy cost of expired air resuscitation. *J. Am. med. Ass.* **167**, 328

Gregory, G.A. (1981) Resuscitation of the newborn. In: *Anesthesia*, vol. 2, edited by R.D. Miller. London: Churchill Livingstone

Gregory, G.A., Kitterman, J.A., Phibbs, P.H., Tooley, W.H. and Hamilton, W.K. (1971) Treatment of the idiopathic respiratory-distress syndrome with continuous positive airway pressure. *New Engl. J. Med.* **284**, 1333

Gregory, G.A., Eger, E.I., Smith, N.T. and Cullen, B.F. (1974) The cardiovascular effects of carbon dioxide in man awake and during diethyl ether anesthesia. *Anesthesiology* **40**, 301

Gregory, I.C. (1973) Assessment of Van Slyke manometric measurements of oxygen content. *J. appl. Physiol.* **34**, 715

Gregory, I.C. (1974) The oxygen and carbon monoxide capacities of foetal and adult blood. *J. Physiol.* **236**, 625

Grindlinger, G.A., Manny, J., Justice, R., Dunham, B., Shepro, D. and Hechtman, H.B. (1979) Presence of negative inotropic agents in canine plasma during positive end-expiratory pressure. *Circulation Res.* **45**, 460

Grollman, A. (1929) The determination of the cardiac output of man by the use of acetylene. *Am. J. Physiol.* **88**, 285

Groves, B.M., Reeves, J.T., Sutton, J.T., Wagner, P.D., Cymerman, A., Malconian, M.K. et al. (1987) Operation Everest II: elevated high-altitude pulmonary resistance unresponsive to oxygen. *J. appl. Physiol.* **63**, 521

Guilleminault, C., van den Hoed, J. and Mitler, M.M. (1978) Clinical overview of the sleep apnea syndromes. In: *Sleep Apnea Syndromes*, edited by C. Guilleminault and W.C. Dement. New York: Alan R. Liss

Gunnarsson, L., Tokics, L., Gustavsson, H. and Hedenstierna, G. (1991) Influence of age on atelectasis formation and gas exchange impairment during general anaesthesia. *Br. J. Anaesth.* **66**, 423

Gurtner, G. and Burns, B. (1975) Physiological evidence consistent with the presence of a specific O_2 carrier in the placenta. *J. appl. Physiol.* **39**, 728

Gurtner, G.H. and Fowler, W.S. (1971) Interrelationships of factors affecting the pulmonary diffusing capacity. *J. appl. Physiol.* **30**, 619

Gutierrez, G. (1991) Cellular effects of hypoxaemia and ischaemia. In: *The Lung: scientific foundations*, p. 1525, edited by R.G. Crystal and J.B. West. New York: Raven Press

Gutteridge, J.M.C., Rowley, D.A., Griffiths, E. and Halliwell, B. (1985) Low molecular weight iron complexes and oxygen radical reactions in idiopathic haemochromatosis. *Clin. Sci.* **68**, 463

Guy, H.J.B., Prisk, G.K., Elliott, A.R. and West, J.B. (1992) Uneven ventilation and blood flow in the lung during sustained microgravity on Spacelab SLS-1. *FASEB J.* **6**, A1772

Guz, A., Noble, M.I.M., Trenchard, D., Cochrane, H.L. and Makey, A.R. (1964) Studies on the vagus nerves in man: their role in respiratory and circulatory control. *Clin. Sci.* **27**, 293

Guz, A., Noble, M.I.M., Widdicombe, J.G., Trenchard, D. and Mushin, W.W. (1966a) Peripheral chemoreceptor block in man. *Resp. Physiol.* **1**, 38

Guz, A., Noble, M.I.M., Widdicombe, J.G., Trenchard, D., Mushin, W.W. and Makey, A.R. (1966b) The role of the vagal and glossopharyngeal afferent nerves in respiratory sensation, control of breathing and arterial pressure regulation in conscious man. *Clin. Sci.* **30**, 161

Guz, A., Noble, M.I.M., Eisele, J.H. and Trenchard, D. (1971) The effect of lung deflation on breathing in man. *Clin. Sci.* **40**, 451

Hagberg, J.M., Mullin, J.P. and Nagle, F.J. (1978) Oxygen consumption during constant-load exercise. *J. appl. Physiol.* **45**, 381

Hairston, L.E. and Sauerland, E.K. (1981) Electromyography of the human palate: discharge patterns of the levator and tensor veli palatini. *Electromyogr. clin. Neurophysiol.* **21**, 287

Haldane, J.S. (1920) A new apparatus for accurate blood-gas analysis. *J. Path. Bact.* **23**, 443

Haldane, J.S. and Priestley, J.G. (1905) The regulation of the lung ventilation. *J. Physiol.* **32**, 225

Hales, S. (1731) *Vegetable Staticks: analysis of the air*, p. 240. London

Halliwell, B. and Gutteridge, J.M.C. (1985) *Free Radicals in Biology and Medicine*. Oxford: Clarendon Press

Halsey, M.J. (1982) The effects of high pressure on the central nervous system. *Physiol. Rev.* **62**, 1341

Halsey, M.J., Wardley-Smith, B. and Green, C.J. (1978) Pressure reversal of general anaesthesia – a multi-site expansion hypothesis. *Br. J. Anaesth.* **50**, 1091

Hamberger, G.E. (1749) *De Respirationis Mechanismo et usu genuino*, Jena

Hamburger, H.J. (1918) Anionenwanderungen in serum und Blut unter dem Einfluss von CO_2. Säure und Alkali. *Biochem. Z.* **86**, 309

Hammerschmidt, D.E. (1983) Activation of the complement system and of granulocytes in lung injury: the adult respiratory distress syndrome. *Adv. Inflamm. Res.* **5**, 147

Hanks, E.C., Ngai, S.H. and Fink, B.R. (1961) The respiratory threshold for carbon dioxide in anesthetized man. *Anesthesiology* **22**, 393

Hanning, C.D. (1992) Prolongs postoperative oxygen therapy. *Br. J. Anaesth.* **69**, 115

Haponik, E.F., Smith, P.L., Bohlman, M.E., Allen, R.P., Goldman, S.M. and Bleecker, E.R. (1983) Computerized tomography in obstructive sleep apnea. *Am. Rev. resp. Dis.* **127**, 221

Harding, R. (1991) Fetal breathing movements. In: *The Lung: scientific foundations*, p. 1655, edited by R.G. Crystal and J.B. West. New York: Raven Press

Hardy, C., Robinson, C., Lewis, R.A., Tattersfield, A.E. and Holgate, S.T. (1985) Airway and cardiovascular responses to inhaled prostacyclin in normal and asthmatic subjects. *Am. Rev. resp. Dis.* **131**, 18

Harlan, W.R. and Said, S.I. (1969) Selected aspects of lung metabolism. Chapter 12 in: *The Biological Basis of Medicine*, edited by E.E. Bittar and N. Bittar. New York and London: Academic Press

Harper, R.M. and Sauerland, E.K. (1978) The role of the tongue in sleep apnea. In: *Sleep Apnea Syndromes*, edited by C. Guilleminault and W.C. Dement. New York: Alan R. Liss

Harries, M.G. (1981) Drowning in man. *Crit. Care Med.* **9**, 407

Harris, E.A., Hunter, M.E., Seelye, E.R., Vedder, M. and Whitlock, R.M.L. (1973) Prediction of the physiological dead-space in resting normal subjects. *Clin. Sci.* **45**, 375

Harris, P. and Heath, D. (1962) *The Human Pulmonary Circulation*. Edinburgh and London: Churchill Livingstone

Hasselbalch, K.A. (1916) Berechnung der Wasserstoffzahl des Blutes usw. *Biochem Z.* **78**, 112

von Hayek, H. (1960) *The Human Lung*. Translated from *Die Menschliche Lunge* by V.E. Krahl. New York and London: Hafner

Head, H. (1889) On the regulation of respiration. *J. Physiol.* **10**, 1

Heaton, R.W., Henderson, A.F. and Costello, J.F. (1984) Cold air as a bronchial provocation technique. *Chest* **86,** 810

Hedenstierna, G. (1985) Differential ventilation in bilateral lung disease. *Eur. J. Anaesthesiol.* **2,** 1

Hedenstierna, G. (1990) Gas exchange during anaesthesia. *Br. J. Anaesth.* **64,** 507

Hedenstierna, G. and McCarthy, G. (1975) Mechanics of breathing, gas distribution and functional residual capacity at different frequencies of respiration during spontaneous and artificial ventilations. *Br. J. Anaesth.* **47,** 706

Hedenstierna, G., McCarthy, G. and Bergström, X. (1976) Airway closure during mechanical ventilation. *Anesthesiology* **44,** 114

Hedenstierna, G., Baehrendtz S., Klingstedt, C., Santesson, J., Soderborg, B., Dhalborn, M. and Bindslev, L. (1984) Ventilation and perfusion of each lung during differential ventilation with selective PEEP. *Anesthesiology* **61,** 369

Hedenstierna, G., Strandberg, A., Brismar, B., Lundquist, H., Svensson, L. and Tokics, L. (1985) Functional residual capacity, thoraco-abdominal dimensions and central blood volume during general anesthesia with muscle paralysis and mechanical ventilation. *Anesthesiology* **62,** 247

Hedenstierna, G., Tokics, L., Strandberg, A., Lundquist, H. and Brismar, B. (1986) Correlation of gas exchange impairment to development of atelectasis during anaesthesia and muscle paralysis. *Acta anaesth. scand.* **30,** 183

Hedenstierna, G., Lundquist, H., Lundh, B., Tokics, L. Strandberg, A., Brismar, B. and Frostell, C. (1989) Pulmonary densities during anaesthesia. *Eur. Resp. J.* **2,** 528

Heffner, J.E. and Repine, J.E. (1991) Antioxidants and the lung. In: *The Lung: scientific foundations,* p. 1811, edited by R.G. Crystal and J.B. West. New York: Raven Press

Heiberg, J. (1874) A new expedient in administering chloroform. *Medical Times and Gazette* **10 Jan,** 36

Heijman, K., Heijman, L., Jonzon, A., Sedin, G., Sjostrand, U. and Widman, B. (1972) High frequency positive pressure ventilation during anesthesia and routine surgery in man. *Acta anaesth. scand.* **16,** 176

Heller, M.L. and Watson, T.R. (1961) Polarographic study of arterial oxygenation during apnea in man. *New Engl. J. Med.* **264,** 326

Hemmingsen, A. and Scholander, P.E. (1960) Specific transport of oxygen through hemoglobin solutions. *Science* **132,** 1379

Hempleman, H.V. and Lockwood, A.P.M. (1978) *The Physiology of Diving in Man and Other Animals.* London: Edward Arnold

Henderson, L.J. (1909) Das Gleichgewicht zwischen Basen und Säuren im tierischen Organismus. *Ergebn. Physiol.* **8,** 254

Henderson, Y., Chillingworth, F.P. and Whitney, J.L. (1915) The respiratory dead space. *Am. J. Physiol.* **38,** 1

Heneghan, C.P.H., Bergman, N.A. and Jones, J.G. (1984) Changes in lung volume and $(P_{A_{O_2}} - P_{a_{O_2}})$ during anaesthesia. *Br. J. Anaesth.* **56,** 437

Heneghan, C.P.H., Bergman, N.A., Jordan, C., Lehane, J.R. and Catley, D.M. (1986) Effect of isoflurane on bronchomotor tone in man. *Br. J. Anaesth.* **58,** 24

Herholdt, J.D. and Rafn, C.G. (1796) *Life-saving Methods for Drowning Persons.* Copenhagen: T. Tikiob. Reprinted in 1960; Aarhuus, Denmark:Stiftsbogtrykkerie

Hering, E. (1868) Die Selbststeuerung der Athmung durch den Nervus Vagus. *Sber. Akad. Wiss. Wien* **57,** 672

Hewlett, A.M., Platt, A.S. and Terry, V.G. (1977) Mandatory minute volume. *Anaesthesia* **32,** 163

Hewlett, A.M., Hulands, G.H., Nunn, J.F. and Minty, K.B. (1974a) Functional residual capacity during anaesthesia. I: Methodology. *Br. J. Anaesth.* **46,** 479

Hewlett, A.M., Hulands, G.H., Nunn, J.F. and Heath, J.R. (1974b) Functional residual capacity. II: Spontaneous respiration. *Br. J. Anaesth.* **46,** 486

Hewlett, A.M., Hulands, G.H., Nunn, J.F. and Milledge, J.S. (1974c) Functional residual capacity during anaesthesia. III: Artificial ventilation. *Br. J. Anaesth.* **46,** 495

Heymans, C. and Neil, E. (1958) *Reflexogenic Areas of the Cardiovascular System.* Boston, Mass: Little Brown; London: Churchill

Heymans, C., Bouckaert, J.J. and Dautrebande, L. (1930) Sinus carotidien et réflexes respiratoire. *Archs int. Pharmacodyn Thér.* **39,** 400

Heymans, J.F. and Heymans, C. (1927) Sur les modifications directes et sur la régulation reflexe de l'activité du centre respiratoire de la tête isolée du chien. *Archs int. Pharmacodyn. Thér.* **33**, 272

Hickey, R.F., Visick, W., Fairley, H.B. and Fourcade, H.E. (1973) Effects of halothane anesthesia on functional residual capacity and alveolar–arterial oxygen tension difference. *Anesthesiology* **38**, 20

Hickling, K.G. (1986) Extracorporeal CO_2 removal in severe adult respiratory distress syndrome. *Anaesth. intens. Care* **14**, 46

Hickling, K.G., Downward, G., Davis, F.M. and A'Court, G. (1986) Management of severe ARDS with low frequency positive pressure ventilation and extracorporeal CO_2 removal. *Anaesth. intens. Care* **14**, 79

Hickman, H.H. (1824). A letter on suspended animation. Ironbridge, W. Smith (addressed to T.A. Knight of Downton Castle)

Higgins, H.L. and Means, J.H. (1915) The effect of certain drugs on the respiration and gaseous metabolism in normal human subjects. *J. Pharmac. exp. Ther.* **7**, 1

Hill, J.D., Main, F.B., Osborn, J.J. and Gerbode, F. (1965) Correct use of respirator on cardiac patient after operation. *Archs Surg.* **91**, 775

Hillman, D.R. and Finucane, K.E. (1985) Continuous positive airway presure: a breathing system to minimize work. *Crit. Care Med.* **13**, 38

Hillman, D.R. and Finucane, K.E. (1987) A model of the respiratory pump. *J. appl. Physiol.* **63**, 951

Hills, B.A. (1982) What forces keep the air spaces of the lung dry? *Thorax* **37**, 713

Hills, B.A. (1990) The role of lung surfactant. *Br. J. Anaesth.* **65**, 13

Hirshman, C.A. and Bergman, N.A. (1990) Factors influencing intrapulmonary airway calibre during anaesthesia. *Br. J. Anaesth.* **65**, 30

Hirshman, C.A., Downes, H., Farbood, A. and Bergman, N.A. (1979) Ketamine block of bronchospasm in experimental canine asthma. *Br. J. Anaesth.* **51**, 713

Hodson, W.A. (1991) The first breath. In: *The Lung, scientific foundations*, p. 1665, edited by R.G. Crystal and J.B. West. New York: Raven Press

Hoedt-Rasmussen, K., Skinhoj, E., Paulson, O., Ewald, J., Bjerrum, J.K., Fahrenkrug, A. and Lassen, N.A. (1967) Regional cerebral blood flow in acute apoplexy. The 'luxury perfusion syndrome' of brain tissue. *Archs Neurol.* **17**, 271

Hoff, H.E. and Breckenridge, C.G. (1949) The medullary origin of respiratory periodicity in the dog. *Am. J. Physiol.* **158**, 157

Hoffman, S.J., Looker, D.L., Roehrich, J.M., Cozart, P.E., Durfee, S.L., Tedesco, J.L. and Stetler, G.L. (1990) Expression of fully functional tetrameric human haemoglobin in *Escherichia coli*. *Proc. Natl Acad. Sci. USA* **87**, 8521

Hoffstein, V. and Fredberg, J.J. (1991) The acoustic reflection technique for non-invasive assessment of upper airway area. *Eur. Resp. J.* **4**, 602

Hogben, L. (1951). *Mathematics for the Million*, 3rd edn. London: Allen and Unwin

Holmdahl, M. H:son. (1953) Apnoeic diffusion oxygenation in electroconvulsion therapy. *Acta Soc. Med. uppsal.* **58**, 269

Holmdahl, M. H:son (1956) Pulmonary uptake of oxygen acid–base metabolism and circulation during prolonged apnoea. *Acta chir. scand.* suppl. 212

Hornbein, T.F. and Pavlin, E.G. (1975) Distribution of H^+ and HCO_3^- between CSF and blood during respiratory alkalosis in dogs. *J. Physiol.* **228**, 1149

Horbein, T.F. and Roos, A. (1963) Specificity of H ion concentration as a carotid chemoreceptor stimulus. *J. appl. Physiol.* **18**, 580

Hornbein, T.F., Griffo, Z.J. and Roos, A. (1961) Quantitation of chemoreceptor activity: interrelation of hypoxia and hypercapnia. *J. Neurophysiol.* **24**, 561

Hornbein, T.H. (1992) The hypoxic brain. In: *Anesthesia and the Lung*, p. 91, edited by T.H. Stanley and R.J. Sperry. Dordrecht: Kluwer

Hornbein, T.H., Townes, B.D., Schoene, R.B., Sutton, J.R. and Houston, C.S. (1989) The cost to the central nervous system of climbing to extremely high altitude. *New Engl. J. Med.* **321**, 1714

Horner, R.L. and Guz, A. (1991) Some factors affecting the maintenance of upper airway patency in man. *Resp. Med.* **85**, suppl. A, 27

Horner, R.L., Innes, J.A., Holden, H.B. and Guz, A. (1991) Afferent pathway(s) for pharyngeal dilator reflex to negative airway pressure in man; a study using upper airway anaesthesia. *J. Physiol.*

436, 31

Horner, R.L., Mohiaddin, R.H., Lowell, D.G., Shea, S.A., Burman, E.D., Longmore, D.B. and Guz, A. (1989a) Sites and sizes of fat deposits around the pharynx in obese patients with obstructive sleep apnoea and weight matched controls. *Eur. Resp. J.* **2**, 613

Horner, R.L., Shea, S.A., McIvor, J. and Guz, A. (1989b) Pharyngeal size and shape during wakefulness and sleep in patients with obstructive sleep apnoea. *Q. Jl Med.* **268**, 719

Houston, C.S., Sutton, J.R., Cymerman, A. and Reeves, J.T. (1987) Operation Everest II: man at extreme altitude. *J. appl. Physiol* **63**, 877

Howell, J.B.L., Permutt, S., Proctor, D.F. and Riley, R.L. (1961) Effect of inflation of the lung on different parts of pulmonary vascular bed. *J. appl. Physiol.* **16**, 71

Hudgel, D.W. and Hendricks, C. (1988) Palate and hypopharynx – sites of inspiratory narrowing of the upper airway during sleep. *Am. Rev. resp. Dis.* **138**, 1547

Hughes, J.M.B., Glazier, J.B., Maloney, J.E. and West, J.B. (1968) Effect of lung volume on the distribution of pulmonary blood flow in man. *Resp. Physiol.* **4**, 58

Hughes, J.M.B., Grant, B.J.B., Greene, R.E., Iliff, L.D. and Milic-Emili, J. (1972) Inspiratory flow rate and ventilation distribution in normal subjects and in patients with simple chronic bronchitis. *Clin. Sci.* **43**, 583

Hughes, R. (1970) The influence of changes in acid–base balance on neuromuscular blockade in cats. *Br. J. Anaesth.* **42**, 658

Hugh-Jones, P. and West, J.B. (1960) Detection of bronchial and arterial obstruction by continuous gas analysis from individual lobes and segments of the lung. *Thorax* **15**, 154

Hulands, G.H., Green, R., Iliff, L.D. and Nunn, J.F. (1970) Influence of anaesthesia on the regional distribution of perfusion and ventilation in the lung. *Clin. Sci.* **38**, 451

Hull, R.D., Hirsh, J., Carter, C.J., Raskob, G.E., Gill, G.J., Jay, R.M. et al. (1985) Diagnostic value of ventilation–perfusion lung scanning in patients with suspected pulmonary embolism. *Chest* **88**, 819

Hultgren, H.N. (1978) High altitude pulmonary edema. In: *Lung Water and Solute Exchange*, edited by N. Staub. New York: Marcel Dekker

Hunninghake, G.W. and Crystal, R.G. (1983) Cigarette smoking and lung destruction. Accumulation of neutrophils in the lungs of cigarette smokers. *Am. Rev. resp. Dis.* **128**, 833

Hurst, J.M., Branson, R.D., Davis K., Barrette, R.R. and Adams, K.S. (1990) Comparison of conventional mechanical ventilation and high-frequency ventilation. *Ann. Surg.* **211**, 486

Hussain, S.N.A., Simkus, G. and Roussos, C. (1985) Respiratory muscle fatigue: a cause of ventilatory failure in septic shock. *J. appl. Physiol.* **58**, 2033

Hutchison, D.C.S., Flenley, D.C. and Donald, K.W. (1964) Controlled oxygen therapy in respiratory failure. *Br. med. J.* **2**, 1159

Hutchison, D.C.S., Cook, P.J.L., Barter, C.E., Harris, H. and Hugh-Jones, P. (1971) Pulmonary emphysema and α_1-antitrypsin deficiency. *Br. med. J.* **1**, 689

Hyatt, R.E., Zimmerman, I.R., Peters, G.M. and Sullivan, W.J. (1970) Direct write out of total respiratory resistance. *J. appl. Physiol.* **28**, 675

Iatridis, A. (1988) Review of ECMO in adults – North American experience. *Perfusion* **3**, 37

Ignarro, L.J. (1990) Biosynthesis and metabolism of endothelium-derived nitric oxide. *A. Rev. Pharmacol. Toxicol.* **30**, 535

Ignarro, L.J., Buga, G.M., Wood, K.S. and Chaudhuri, G. (1987) Endothelium-derived relaxing factor produced and released from artery and vein is nitric oxide. *Proc. Natl Acad. Sci. USA* **84**, 9265

Ingvar, D.H. (1965) In: *Hyperbaric Oxygenation*, discussion page 199, edited by I. Ledingham. Edinburgh and London: Churchill Livingstone

Irwin, R.L., Draper, W.B. and Whitehead, R.W. (1957) Urine secretion during diffusion respiration after apnea from neuromuscular block. *Anesthesiology* **18**, 594

Ivanov, S.D. and Nunn, J.F. (1968) Influence of duration of hyperventilation on rise time of P_{CO_2} after step reduction of ventilation. *Resp. Physiol.* **4**, 243

Ivanov, S.D. and Nunn, J.F. (1969) Methods of elevation of P_{CO_2} for restoration of spontaneous breathing after artificial ventilation of anaesthetised patients. *Br. J. Anaesth.* **41**, 28

Jain, S.K., Trenchard, D., Reynolds, F., Noble, M.I.M. and Guz, A. (1973) The effect of local anaesthesia of the airway on respiratory reflexes in the rabbit. *Clin. Sci.* **44**, 519

Jarasch, E.-D., Grund, C., Bruder, G., Heid, H.W., Keenan, T.W. and Franke, W.W. (1981)

Localization of xanthine oxidase in mammary-gland epithelium and capillary endothelium. *Cell* **25**, 67

Jardin, F., Farcot, J.-C., Boisante, L., Curien, N., Margairaz, A. and Bourdarias, J.-P. (1981) Influence of positive end-expiratory pressure on left ventricular performance. *New Engl. J. Med.* **304**, 387

Jennett, S. (1984) Snoring and its treatment. *Br. med. J.* **289**, 335

Jennett, W.B., McDowall, D.G. and Barker, J. (1967) The effect of halothane on intracranial pressure in cerebral tumours: report of two cases. *J. Neurosurg.* **26**, 270

Jerusalem, E. and Starling, E.H. (1910) On the significance of carbon dioxide for the heart beat. *J. Physiol.* **40**, 279

Jobe, A. and Ikegami, M. (1987) Surfactant for the treatment of respiratory distress syndrome. *Am. Rev. resp. Dis.* **136**, 1256

Johns, R.A., Linden, J.M. and Peach, M.J. (1989) Endothelium-dependent relaxation and cyclic GMP accumulation in rabbit pulmonary artery are selectively impaired by moderate hypoxia. *Circ. Res.* **65**, 1508

Johnson, S.R. (1951) The effect of some anesthetic agents on the circulation in man. *Acta chir. scand.* **102**, suppl. 158

Jones, J.G., Royston, D. and Minty, B.D. (1983) Changes in alveolar–capillary barrier function in animals and humans. *Am. Rev. resp. Dis.* **127**, S51

Jones, J.G., Sapsford, D.J. and Wheatley, R.G. (1990) Postoperative hypoxaemia: mechanisms and time course. *Anaesthesia* **45**, 566

Jones, J.G., Faithfull, D., Jordan, C. and Minty, B. (1979) Rib cage movement during halothane anaesthesia in man. *Br. J. Anaesth.* **51**, 399

Jones, J.G., Minty, B.D., Lawler, P., Hulands, G., Crawley, J.C.W. and Veall, N. (1980) Increased alveolar epithelial permeability in cigarette smokers. *Lancet* **1**, 66

Jones, J.G., Minty, B.D., Royston, D. and Royston, J.P. (1983) Carboxyhaemoglobin and pulmonary epithelial permeability in man. *Thorax* **38**, 129

Jones, R.D., Commins, B.T. and Cernik, A.A. (1972) Blood lead and carboxyhaemoglobin levels in London taxi drivers. *Lancet* **2**, 302

Jorfeldt, L., Lewis, D.H., Löfström, J.B. and Post, C. (1979) Lung uptake of lidocaine in healthy volunteers. *Acta anaesth. scand.* **23**, 567

Joyner, M.J., Warner, D.O. and Rehder, K. (1992) Halothane changes the relationships between lung resistances and lung volume. *Anesthesiology* **76**, 229

Juno, P., Marsh, M., Knopp, T.J. and Rehder, K. (1978) Closing capacity in awake and anesthetized–paralyzed man. *J. appl. Physiol.* **44**, 238

Junod, A.F. (1985) 5-Hydroxytryptamine and other amines in the lung. *Handbk Physiol., section 3*, **1**, 337

Kaasik, A.E., Nilsson, L. and Siesjö, B.K. (1970a) The effect of asphyxia upon the lactate, pyruvate and bicarbonate concentrations of brain tissue and cisternal CSF, and upon the tissue concentrations of phosphocreatine and adenine nucleotides in anesthetized rats. *Acta physiol. scand.* **78**, 433

Kaasik, A.E., Nilsson, L. and Siesjö, B.K. (1970b) The effect of arterial hypotension upon the lactate, pyruvate and bicarbonate concentrations of brain tissue and cisternal CSF, and upon the tissue concentrations of phosphocreatine and adenine nucleotides in anesthetized rats. *Acta physiol. scand.* **78**, 448

Kagawa, S., Stafford, M.J., Waggener, T.B. and Severinghaus, J.W. (1982) No effect of naloxone on hypoxia-induced ventilatory depression in adults. *J. appl. Physiol.* **52**, 1030

Kain, M.L., Panday, J. and Nunn, J.F. (1969) The effect of intubation on the dead space during halothane anaesthesia. *Br. J. Anaesth.* **41**, 94

Kalia, M., Senapati, J.M., Parida, B. and Panda, A. (1972) Reflex increase in ventilation by muscle receptors with nonmedullated fibers (C fibers). *J. appl. Physiol.* **32**, 189

Kaneko, K., Milic-Emili, M.E., Dolovich, M.B., Dawson, A. and Bates, D.V. (1966) Regional distribution of ventilation and perfusion as a function of body position. *J. appl. Physiol.* **21**, 767

Kao, F.F. (1963) An experimental study of the pathways involved in exercise hyperpnoea employing cross-circulation techniques. In: *The Regulation of Human Respiration*, edited by D.J.C. Cunningham and B.B. Lloyd. Oxford: Blackwell Scientific

Kapp, J.R. (1981) Neurological response to hyperbaric oxygen – a criterion for cerebral revascularization. *Surg. Neurol.* **15**, 43

Katz, J.A., Laverne, R.G., Fairley, H.B. and Thomas, A.N. (1982) Pulmonary oxygen exchange during endobronchial anesthesia. *Anesthesiology* **56**, 164

Katz, S. and Horres, A.D. (1972) Medullary respiratory neuron response to pulmonary emboli and pneumothorax. *J. appl. Physiol.* **33**, 390

Kaul, S.U., Heath, J.R. and Nunn, J.F. (1973) Factors influencing the development of expiratory muscle activity during anaesthesia. *Br. J. Anaesth.* **45**, 1013

Kaye, G.W.C. and Laby, T.H. (1986) *Tables of Physical and Chemical Constants*, 15th edn. London: Longman

Kelman, G.R. (1966) Digital computer subroutine for the conversion of oxygen tension into saturation. *J. appl. Physiol.* **21**, 1375

Kelman, G.R. (1971) *Applied Cardiovascular Physiology*. London and Boston, Mass: Butterworths

Kelman, G.R. and Nunn, J.F. (1966a) Clinical recognition of hypoxaemia under fluorescent lamps. *Lancet* **1**, 1400

Kelman, G.R. and Nunn, J.F. (1966b) Nomograms for correction of blood Po_2, Pco_2, pH and base excess for time and temperature. *J. appl. Physiol.* **21**, 1484

Kelman, G.R. and Nunn, J.F. (1968) *Computer Produced Physiological Tables*. London and Boston, Mass: Butterworths

Kelman, G.R. and Prys-Roberts, C. (1967) Circulatory influences of artificial ventilation during nitrous oxide anaesthesia in man. I. Introduction and methods. *Br. J. Anaesth.* **39**, 523

Kelman, G.R., Coleman, A.J. and Nunn, J.F. (1966) Evaluation of a microtonometer used with a capillary glass pH electrode. *J. appl. Physiol.* **21**, 1103

Kelman, G.R., Nunn, J.F., Prys-Roberts, C. and Greenbaum, R. (1967) The influence of cardiac output on arterial oxygenation. *Br. J. Anaesth.* **39**, 450

Kelman, G.R., Swapp, G.H., Smith, I., Benzie, R.J. and Gordon, N.L.M. (1972) Cardiac output and arterial blood-gas tension during laparoscopy. *Br. J. Anaesth.* **44**, 1155

Kerr, J.H., Smith, A.C., Prys-Roberts, C., Melonche, R. and Foëx, P. (1974) Observations during endobronchial anaesthesia. II. Oxygenation. *Br. J. Anaesth.* **46**, 84

Kety, S.S. and Schmidt, C.F. (1948) The effects of altered arterial tensions of carbon dioxide and oxygen on cerebral blood flow and cerebral oxygen consumption of normal young men. *J. clin. Invest.* **27**, 500

Khanam, T. and Branthwaite, M.A. (1973) Arterial oxygenation during one-lung anaesthesia (2). *Anaesthesia* **28**, 280

Kilmartin, J.V. and Rossi-Bernardi, L. (1973) Interaction of hemoglobin with hydrogen ions, carbon dioxide, and organic phosphates. *Physiol. Rev.* **53**, 836

King, A.J., Cooke, N.J., Leitch, A.G. and Flenley, D.C. (1973) The effects of 30% oxygen on the respiratory response to treadmill exercise in chronic respiratory failure. *Clin. Sci.* **44**, 151

King, R.J. (1974) The surfactant system of the lung. *Fedn Proc.* **33**, 2238

King, R.J. and Clements, J.A. (1985) Lipid synthesis and surfactant turnover in the lungs. *Handbk Physiol., section 3,* **1**, 309

Kirby, R.R., Perry, J.C., Calderwood, H.W., Ruiz, B.C. and Lederman, D.S. (1975) Cardiorespiratory effects of high positive end-expiratory pressure. *Anesthesiology* **43**, 533

Klein, J., Trouwborst, A. and Salt, P.J. (1985) Endotoxin protection against oxygen toxicity and its reversal by acetylsalicylic acid. *Crit. Care Med.* **14**, 32

Klein, M.G. (1988) Neonatal ECMO. *Trans. Am. Soc. artif. intern. Organs* **34**, 39

Klocke, F.J. and Rahn, H. (1959) Breath holding after breathing of oxygen. *J. appl. Physiol.* **14**, 689

Klocke, F.J. and Rahn, H. (1961) The arterial–alveolar inert gas ('N₂') difference in normal and emphysematous subjects, as indicated by the analysis of urine. *J. clin. Invest.* **40**, 286

Klocke, R.A. (1991) Carbon dioxide. In: *The Lung: scientific foundations*, p. 1233, edited by R.G. Crystal and J.B. West. New York: Raven Press

Knill, R.L. and Clement, J.L. (1982) Variable effects of anaesthetics on the ventilatory response to hypoxaemia in man. *Can. Anaesth. Soc. J.* **29**, 93

Knill, R.L. and Clement, J.L. (1984) Site of selective action of halothane on the peripheral chemoreflex pathway in humans. *Anesthesiology* **61**, 121

Knill, R.L. and Clement, J.L. (1985) Ventilatory respones to acute metabolic acidemia in humans awake, sedated and anesthetized with halothane. *Anesthesiology* **62,** 745

Knill, R.L. and Gelb, A.W. (1978) Ventilatory responses to hypoxia and hypercapnia during halothane sedation and anesthesia in man. *Anesthesiology* **49,** 244

Knill, R.L., Moote, C.A., Skinner, M.I. and Rose, E.A. (1990) Anesthesia with abdominal surgery leads to intense REM sleep during the first postoperative week. *Anesthesiology* **73,** 52

Koizumi, M., Frank, L. and Massaro, D. (1985) Oxygen toxicity in rats: varied effect of dexamethasone treatment depending on duration of hyperoxia. *Am. Rev. resp. Dis.* **131,** 907

Kolton, M.A. (1984) A review of high-frequency oscillation. *Can. Anaesth. Soc. J.* **31,** 416

Kolton, M., Cathran, C.B., Kent, G., Volgyesi, G., Froese, A.B. and Bryan, A.C. (1982) Oxygenation during high frequency ventilation compared with conventional mechanical ventilation in two models of lung injury. *Anesth. Analg.* **61,** 323

Konno, K. and Mead, J. (1967) Measurement of the separate volume changes of rib cage and abdomen during breathing. *J. appl. Physiol.* **22,** 407

Korenaga, S., Takeda, K. and Ito, Y. (1984) Differential effects of halothane on airway nerves and muscle. *Anesthesiology* **60,** 309

Krahl, V.E. (1964) Anatomy of the mammalian lung. *Handbk Physiol., section 3,* **1,** 213

Kram, H.B. and Shoemaker, W.C. (1984) Method for intraoperative assessment of organ perfusion and viability using a miniature oxygen sensor. *Am. J. Surg.* **148,** 404

Kraus, W.A., Draper, E.A. Wagner, D.P. and Zimmerman, J.E. (1985) Apache II: a severity of disease classification. *Crit. Care Med.* **13,** 818

Krayer, S., Rehder, K., Beck, C.K., Cameron, P.D., Didier, E.P. and Hoffman, E.A. (1987) Quantification of thoracic volumes by three-dimensional imaging. *J. appl. Physiol.* **62,** 591

Krayer, S., Rehder, K., Vettermann, J., Didier, P. and Ritman, E.L. (1989) Position and motion of the human diaphragm during anesthesia-paralysis. *Anesthesiology* **70,** 891

Kuida, H., Hinshaw, L.B., Gilbert, B.P. and Vischer, M.B. (1958) Effect of Gram-negative endotoxin on pulmonary circulation. *Am. J. Physiol.* **192,** 335

Kumar, A., Pontoppidan, H., Falke, K.J. et al. (1973) Pulmonary barotrauma during mechanical ventilation. *Crit. Care Med.* **1,** 181

Kuna, S.T. and Smickley, J. (1988) Response of genioglossus muscle activity to nasal airway occlusion in normal sleeping adults. *J. appl. Physiol.* **64,** 347

Kuna, S.T., Insalco, G. and Woodson, G.E. (1988) Thyroarytenoid muscle activity during wakefulness and sleep in normal adults. *J. appl. Physiol.* **65,** 1332

Kusumi, F., Butts, W.C. and Ruff, W.L. (1973) Superior analytical performance by electrolytic cell analysis of blood oxygen content. *J. appl. Physiol.* **35,** 299

Lagercrantz, H., Milerad, J. and Walker, D. (1991) Control of ventilation in the neonate. In: *The Lung: scientific foundations,* p. 1711, edited by R.G. Crystal and J.B. West. New York: Raven Press

Lahiri, S. (1984) Respiratory control in Andean and Himalayan high-altitude natives. In: *High Altitude and Man,* edited by J.B. West and S. Lahiri. Bethesda, Md: American Physiological Society

Lahiri, S. (1991) Physiological responses: peripheral chemoreceptors. In: *The Lung: scientific foundations,* p. 1333, edited by R.G. Crystal and J.B. West. New York: Raven Press

Laine, G.A., Allen, S.J., Katz, J., Gabel, J.C. and Drake, R.E. (1986) Effect of systemic venous pressure elevation on lymph flow and lung edema formation. *J. appl. Physiol.* **61,** 1634

Lall, A., Graf, P.D., Nadel, J.A. and Edmunds, L.H. (1973) Adrenergic reinnervation of the reimplanted dog lung. *J. appl. Physiol.* **35,** 439

Lambert, M.W. (1955) Accessory bronchiole–alveolar communications. *J. Path. Bact.* **70,** 311

Lambertsen, C.J. (1963) Factors in the stimulation of respiration by carbon dioxide. In: *The Regulation of Human Respiration,* edited by D.J.C. Cunningham and B.B. Lloyd. Oxford: Blackwell Scientific

Lambertsen, C.J. (1965) Effects of oxygen at high partial pressure. *Handbk Physiol., section 3,* **2,** 1027

Landon, M.J., Matson, A.M., Royston, B.D., Hewlett, A.M., White, D.C. and Nunn, J.F. (1993) Components of the inspiratory/arterial isoflurane partial pressure difference. *Br. J. Anaesth.* **70,** 605

Lanphier, E.H. and Camporesi, E.M. (1982) Respiration and exercise. In: *The Physiology and Medicine of Diving,* edited by P.B. Bennett and D.H. Elliott. London: Baillière Tindall

Lanza, V., Mercadante, S. and Pignataro, A. (1988) Effects of halothane, enflurane, and nitrous oxide on hemoglobin affinity. *Anesthesiology* **68,** 591

Larrick, J.W. and Wright, S.C. (1990) Cytotoxic mechanism of tumor necrosis factor-α. *FASEB J.* **4,** 3215

Larson, C.P., Eger, E.I., Muallem, M., Buechel, D.R., Munson, E.S. and Eisele, J.H. (1969) The effects of diethyl ether and methoxyflurane on ventilation. *Anesthesiology* **30,** 174

Lassen, N.A. (1959) Cerebral blood flow and oxygen consumption in man. *Physiol. Rev.* **39,** 183

Lassen, N.A. (1966) The luxury perfusion syndrome and its possible relation to acute metabolic acidosis localized within the brain. *Lancet* **2,** 1113

Lassen, N.A. and Ingvar, D.H. (1961) The blood flow of the cerebral cortex determined by radioactive krypton-85. *Experientia* **17,** 42

Lassen, N.A. and Palvalgyi, R. (1968) Cerebral steal during hypercapnia and the inverse reaction during hypocapnia observed by the ^{133}Xe technique in man. *Scand. J. clin. Lab. Invest.* suppl. 102

Laurell, C.-B. and Eriksson, S. (1963) The electrophoretic α_1-globulin pattern of serum in α_1-antitrypsin deficiency. *Scand. J. clin. Lab. Invest.* **15,** 132

Laver, M.B. and Seifen, A. (1965) Measurement of blood oxygen tension in anesthesia. *Anesthesiology* **26,** 73

Lawler, P.G.P. and Nunn, J.F. (1984) A reassessment of the validity of the iso-shunt graph. *Br. J. Anaesth.* **56,** 1325

Laws, A.K. (1968) Effects of induction of anaesthesia and muscle paralysis on functional residual capacity of the lungs. *Can. Anaesth. Soc. J.* **15,** 325

Leake, C.D. and Waters, R.M. (1928) The anesthetic properties of carbon dioxide. *J. Pharmac. exp. Ther.* **33,** 280

Leblanc, P., Ruff, F. and Milic-Emili, J. (1970) Effects of age and body position on 'airway closure' in man. *J. appl. Physiol.* **28,** 448

Ledingham, I. McA. and Norman, J.N. (1965) Metabolic effects of combined hypothermia and hyperbaric oxygen in experimental total circulatory arrest. In: *Hyperbaric Oxygenation*, edited by I. Ledingham. Edinburgh and London: Churchill Livingstone

Lee, G. de J. and DuBois, A.B. (1955) Pulmonary capillary blood flow in man. *J. clin. Invest.* **34,** 1380

Legallois, C. (1812) *Experiences sur le Principe de la Vie*. Paris: d'Hautel

Lehane, J.R., Jordan, C. and Jones, J.G. (1980) Influence of halothane and enflurane on respiratory airflow resistance and specific conductance in anaesthetized man. *Br. J. Anaesth.* **52,** 773

Lehmann, H. and Huntsman, R.G. (1966) *Man's Haemoglobin*. Amsterdam: North Holland Publ.

Leigh, J.M. (1973) Variation in performance of oxygen therapy devices. *Ann. R. Coll. Surg.* **52,** 234

Lejeune, P., Vachiery, J.L., De Smet, J.M., Leeman, M., Brimioulle, S., Delcroix, M., Melot, C. and Naeije, R. (1991) PEEP inhibits hypoxic pulmonary vasoconstriction in dogs. *J. appl. Physiol.* **70,** 1867

Lenfant, C. and Howell, B.J. (1960) Cardiovascular adjustments in dogs during continuous pressure breathing. *J. appl. Physiol.* **15,** 425

Lenfant, C., Torrance, J., English, E., Finch, C.A., Reynafarje, C., Ramas, J. and Faura, J. (1968) Effect of altitude on oxygen binding by hemoglobin and on organic phosphate levels. *J. clin. Invest.* **47,** 2652

Leusen, I.R. (1950) Influence du pH du liquide cephalo-rachidien sur la respiration. *Experientia* **6,** 272

Leusen, I.R. (1954) Chemosensitivity of the respiratory center. *Am. J. Physiol.* **176,** 39

Liebow, A.A. (1962) Recent advances in pulmonary anatomy. In: *Pulmonary Structure and Function*, edited by A.V.S. de Reuck and M. O'Connor. Edinburgh and London: Churchill Livingstone

Light, R.B. (1988) Intrapulmonary oxygen consumption in experimental pneumococcal pneumonia. *J. appl. Physiol.* **64,** 2490

Linden, R.J., Ledsome, J.R. and Norman, J. (1965) Simple methods for the determination of the concentrations of carbon dioxide and oxygen in blood. *Br. J. Anaesth.* **37,** 77

Lindenberg, R. (1963) Patterns of CNS vulnerability in acute hypoxaemia including anaesthetic accidents. In: *Selective Vulnerability of the Brain in Hypoxaemia*, edited by J.P. Schade and W.H. McMenemy. Oxford: Blackwell Scientific

Llewellyn, M.A. and Swyer, P.R. (1975) Mechanical ventilation and continuous distending pressure. In: *The Intensive Care of the Newly Born*. Monographs in Paediatrics no. 6, edited by P.R. Sywer. Basel: Karger

Lloyd, B.B. and Cunningham, D.J.C. (1963) A quantitative approach to the regulation of human respiration. In: *The Regulation of Human Respirations*, edited by D.J.C. Cunningham and B.B. Lloyd. Oxford: Blackwell Scientific

Lloyd, B.B., Jukes, M.G.M. and Cunningham, D.J.C. (1958) The relation between alveolar oxygen pressure and the respiratory response to carbon dioxide in man. *J. exp. Physiol.* **43**, 214

Lloyd, J.E., Newman, J.H. and Brigham, K.L. (1984) Permeability pulmonary edema. *Archs intern. Med.* **144**, 143

Loeschcke, H.H. (1965) A concept of the role of intracranial chemosensitivity in respiratory control. In: *Cerebrospinal Fluid and the Regulation of Ventilation*, edited by C.McC. Brookes, F.F. Kao and B.B. Lloyd. Oxford: Blackwell Scientific

Loeschcke, H.H. (1983) Central chemoreceptors. In: *Control of Respiration*, edited by D.J. Pallot. London: Croom Helm

Loeschcke, H.H., Sweel, A., Kough, R.H. and Lambertsen, C.J. (1953) The effect of morphine and of meperidine (dolantin, demerol) upon the respiratory response of normal men to low concentrations of inspired carbon dioxide. *J. Pharmac. exp. Ther.* **108**, 376

Loewy, A. (1894) Ueber die Bestimmung der Gröse des 'schädlichen Luftraumes' im Thorax und der alveolaren Sauerstoffspannung. *Pflügers Arch. ges. Physiol.* **58**, 416

Logan, M.R. and Drummond, G.B. (1991) Cranio-caudal movement of the sternum on induction of anaesthesia. *Br. J. Anaesth.* **66**, 433

Longo, L.D. (1970) Carbon monoxide in the pregnant mother and fetus and its exchange across the placenta. *Ann. N.Y. Acad. Sci.* **174**, 313

Longo, L.D. (1991) Fetal gas exchange. In: *The Lung: scientific foundations*, p. 1699, edited by R.G. Crystal and J.B. West. New York: Raven Press

Lorius, C., Jouzel, J., Raynaud, D., Hansen, J. and Le Treut, H. (1990) The ice-core record: climate sensitivity and future greenhouse warming. *Nature* **347**, 139

Lovelock, J.E. (1979) *Gaia. A new look at life on earth*, p. 71. Oxford: Oxford University Press

Lowe, K.C. (1991) Synthetic oxygen transport fluids based on perfluorochemicals. *Vox Sang.* **60**, 129

Lucey, J.F. and Dangman, B. (1984) A reexamination of the role of oxygen in retrolental fibroplasia. *Pediatrics* **73**, 82

Lugaresi, E., Cirignotta, F., Coccagna, G. and Montagna, P. (1984) Clinical significance of snoring. In: *Sleep and Breathing*, edited by N.A. Saunders and C.E. Sullivan. New York: Marcel Dekker

Lumb, A.B., Petros, A.J. and Nunn, J.F. (1991) Rib cage contribution to resting and carbon dioxide stimulated ventilation during 1 MAC isoflurane anaesthesia. *Br. J. Anaesth.* **67**, 712

Lumb, A.B. and Nunn, J.F. (1991a) Respiratory function and ribcage contribution to ventilation in body positions commonly used during anesthesia. *Anesth. Analg.* **73**, 422

Lumb, A.B. and Nunn, J.F. (1991b) Ribcage contribution to CO_2 response during rebreathing and steady state methods. *Resp. Physiol.* **85**, 97

Lumsden, T. (1923a) Observations on the respiratory centres in the cat. *J. Physiol.* **57**, 153

Lumsden, T. (1923b) Observations on the respiratory centres. *J. Physiol.* **57**, 354

Lumsden, T. (1923c) The regulation of respiration. Part 1. *J. Physiol.* **58**, 81

Lumsden, T. (1923d) The regulation of respiration. Part 2. *J. Physiol.* **58**, 111

Lundgren, C.E.G. (1984) Respiratory function during simulated wet dives. *Undersea Biomed. Res.* **11**, 139

Lundgren, C. (1991) Diving. In: *The Lung: scientific foundations*, p. 2109, edited by R.G. Crystal and J.B. West. New York: Raven Press

Lundsgaard, C. and Van Slyke, D.D. (1923) *Cyanosis*. Baltimore: Williams & Wilkins

Lunn, J.N. and Mushin, W.W. (1982) *Mortality Associated with Anaesthesia*. London: Nuffield Provincial Hospitals Trust

Lurie, A.A., Jones, R.E., Linde, H.W., Price, M.L., Dripps, R.D. and Price, H.L. (1958) Cyclopropane anesthesia: cardiac rate and rhythm during steady levels of cyclopropane anesthesia in man at normal and elevated end-expiratory carbon dioxide tensions. *Anesthesiology* **19**, 457

Lynch, J.P., Mhyre, J.G. and Dantzker, D.R. (1979) Influence of cardiac output on intrapulmonary shunt. *J. appl. Physiol.* **46**, 315

Lynch, S., Brand, L. and Levy, A. (1959) Changes in lung thorax compliance during orthopedic surgery. *Anesthesiology* **20**, 278

McArdle, L. and Roddie, I.C. (1958) Vascular responses to carbon dioxide during anaesthesia in man. *Br. J. Anaesth.* **30,** 358

McConn, R. and Derrick, J.B. (1972) The respiratory function of blood: transfusion and blood storage. *Anesthesiology* **36,** 119

McCord, J.M. and Fridovich, I. (1968) The reduction of cytochrome c by milk xanthine oxidase. *J. biol. Chem.* **243,** 5753

McCord, J.M. and Roy, R.S. (1982) The pathophysiology of superoxide: roles in inflammation and ischaemia. *Can. J. Physiol. Pharmacol.* **60,** 1346

McDonald, D.M. (1981) Peripheral chemoreceptors. In: *Regulation of Breathing*, edited by T.F. Hornbein. New York: Marcel Dekker

McDonald, D.M. and Mitchell, R.A. (1975) The innervation of glomus cells, ganglion cells and blood vessels in the rat carotid body: a quantitative ultrastructural analysis. *J. Neurocytol.* **4,** 177

McDonald, R.J., Berger, E.M., White, C.W., White, J.G., Freeman, B.A. and Repine, J.E. (1985) Effect of superoxide dismutase encapsulated in liposomes or conjugated with polyethylene glycol on neutrophil bactericidal activity in vitro and bacterial clearance in vivo. *Am. Rev. resp. Dis.* **131,** 633

McDowall, D.G. (1967) The effects of clinical concentrations of halothane on the blood flow and oxygen uptake of the cerebral cortex. *Br. J. Anaesth.* **39,** 186

McEvoy, R.D. (1985) Recently developed alternatives to conventional mechanical ventilation. *Anaesth. Intens. Care* **13,** 178

McEvoy, J.D.S., Jones, N.L. and Campbell, E.J.M. (1974) Mixed venous and arterial P_{CO_2}. *Br. med. J.* **4,** 687

McHardy, G.J.R. (1972) Diffusing capacity and pulmonary gas exchange. *Br. J. Dis. Chest* **66,** 1

McIlroy, M.B., Eldridge, F.L., Thomas, J.P. and Christie, R.V. (1956) The effect of added elastic and non-elastic resistances on the pattern of breathing in normal subjects. *Clin. Sci.* **15,** 337

MacIntyre, N.R. (1986) Respiratory function during pressure support ventilation. *Chest* **89,** 667

MacIntyre, N., Nishimura, M., Usada, Y., Tokioka, H., Takezawa, J. and Shimada, Y. (1990) The Nagoya conference on system design and patient–ventilator interactions during pressure support ventilation. *Chest* **94,** 1463

Mackay, A.D., Baldwin, C.J. and Tattersfield, A.E. (1983) Action of intravenously administered aminophylline on normal airways. *Am. Rev. resp. Dis.* **127,** 609

McKenzie, D.K. and Gandevia, S.C. (1991) Skeletal muscle properties: diaphragm and chest wall. In: *The Lung: scientific foundations,* p. 649, edited by R.G. Crystal and J.B. West. New York: Raven Press

Mackie, I. (1979) Alcohol and aquatic disasters. *Practitioner* Special Report on Drowning, edited by M.G. Harries, page 9

Macklem, P.T. (1971) Airway obstruction and collateral ventilation. *Physiol. Rev.* **51,** 368

Macklem, P.T. and Mead, J. (1967) Resistance of central and peripheral airways measured by a retrograde catheter. *J. appl. Physiol.* **22,** 395

Macklem, P.T. and Wilson, N.J. (1965) Measurement of intrabronchial pressure in man. *J. appl. Physiol.* **20,** 653

Macklem, P.T., Fraser, R.G. and Bates, D.V. (1963) Bronchial pressures and dimensions in health and obstructive airway disease. *J. appl. Physiol.* **18,** 699

McNicholas, W.T, Coffey, M., McDonnell, T., O'Regan, R. and Fitzgerald, M.X. (1987) Upper airway obstruction during sleep in normal subjects after selective topical oropharyngeal anesthesia. *Am. Rev. resp. Dis.* **135,** 1316

McNicol, M.W. and Campbell, E.J.M. (1965) Severity of respiratory failure. *Lancet,* **1,** 336

McQueen, D.S. and Pallot, D.J. (1983) Peripheral arterial chemoreceptors. In: *Control of Respiration,* edited by D.J. Pallot. London: Croom Helm

Makita, K., Nunn, J.F. and Royston, B. (1990) Evaluation of metabolic measuring instruments for use in critically ill patients. *Crit. Care Med.* **18,** 638

Malik, A.B., Selig, W.M. and Burhop, K.E. (1985) Cellular and humoral mediators of pulmonary edema. *Lung* **163,** 193

Mandell, G. (1974) Bactericidal activity of aerobic and anaerobic polymorphonuclear neutrophils. *Infect. Immun.* **9,** 337

Mankikian, B., Cantineau, J.P., Sartene, R., Clergue, F. and Viars, P. (1986) Ventilatory pattern and chest wall mechanics during ketamine anesthesia in humans. *Anesthesiology* **65**, 492

Mansell, A., Bryan, A.C. and Levison, H. (1972) Airway closure in children. *J. appl. Physiol.* **33**, 711

Mapleson, W.W. (1954) The elimination of rebreathing in various anaesthetic systems. *Br. J. Anaesth.* **26**, 323

Marchand, P., Gilroy, J.C. and Wilson, V.H. (1950) An anatomical study of the bronchial vascular system and its variation in disease. *Thorax* **5**, 207

Marckwald, M. and Kronecker, H. (1880) Die Athembewegungen des Zwerchfells des Kaninchens. *Arch. Physiol. Leipzig*, p. 441

Maren, T.H. (1967) Carbonic anhydrase: chemistry, physiology, and inhibition. *Physiol. Rev.* **47**, 595

Marquez, J.M., Douglas, M.E., Downs, J.B., Wu, W.-H., Mantini, E.L., Kuck, E.J. and Calderwood, H.W. (1979) Renal function and cardiovascular responses during positive airway pressure. *Anesthesiology* **50**, 393

Marquez, J., Sladen, A., Gendell, H., Boehnke, M. and Medelow, H. (1981) Pardoxical cerebral air embolism without an intracardiac septal defect. *J. Neurosurg.* **55**, 997

Marrubini, M.G., Rossanda, M. and Tretola, L. (1964) The role of artificial hyperventilation in the control of brain tension during neurosurgical operations. *Br. J. Anaesth.* **36**, 415

Marsh, A.M., Nunn, J.F., Taylor, S.J. and Charlesworth, C.H. (1991) Airway obstruction associated with the use of the Guedel airway. *Br. J. Anaesth.* **67**, 517

Marshall, B.E. (1988) Pulmonary blood flow and oxygenation. In: *Anesthesia for Thoracic Procedures*, edited by B.E. Marshall, D.E. Longnecker and H.B. Fairley. Oxford: Blackwell Scientific

Marshall, B.E. (1990) Pulmonary vasoconstriction. *Acta anaesth. scand.* **34** suppl 94, 37

Marshall, B.E. and Marshall, C. (1985) Anesthesia and pulmonary circulation. In: *Effects of Anesthesia*, edited by B.G. Covino, H.A. Fozzard, K. Rehder and G. Strichartz. Bethesda, Md: American Physiological Society

Marshall, B.E. and Marshall, C. (1992) Pulmonary circulation during anaesthesia. In: *Anesthesia and the Lung*, p. 31, edited by T.H. Stanley and R.J. Sperry. Dordrecht: Kluwer

Marshall, B.E. and Whyche, M.Q. (1972) Hypoxemia during and after anesthesia. *Anesthesiology* **37**, 178

Marshall, B.E., Marshall, C. and Frasch, H.F. (1992) Control of the pulmonary circulation. In: *Anesthesia and the Lung*, p.9, edited by T.H. Stanley and R.J. Sperry. Dordrecht: Kluwer

Marshall, B.E., Cohen, P.J., Klingenmaier, C.H. and Aukberg, S. (1969) Pulmonary venous admixture before, during, and after halothane: oxygen anesthesia in man. *J. appl. Physiol.* **27**, 653

Marshall, B.E., Marshall, C., Benumof, J. and Saidman, L.J. (1981) Hypoxic pulmonary vasoconstriction in dogs: effects of lung segment size and oxygen tension. *J. appl. Physiol.* **51**, 1543

Marshall, B.E., Marshall, C., Magno, M., Lilagan, P. and Pietra, G.G. (1991) Influence of bronchial artery Po_2 on pulmonary vascular resistance. *J. appl. Physiol.* **70**, 405

Marshall, C. and Marshall, B. (1983) Site and sensitivity for stimulation of hypoxic pulmonary vasoconstriction. *J. appl. Physiol.* **55**, 711

Marshall, I., Rogers, M. and Drummond, G. (1961) Acoustic reflectometry for airway measurement. Principles, limitations and previous works. *Clin. Phys. Physiol. Meas.* **12**, 131

Marshall, R. (1957) The physical properties of the lungs in relation to the subdivisions of lung volume. *Clin. Sci.* **16**, 507

Marshall, R. and Widdicombe, J.G. (1958) The activity of pulmonary stretch receptors during congestion of the lung. *Q. Jl Physiol.* **43**, 320

Marshall, R. and Widdicombe, J.G. (1961) Stress relaxation in the human lung. *Clin. Sci.* **20**, 19

Mason, R.J. and Williams, M.C. (1991) Alveolar type II cells. In: *The Lung: scientific foundations*, p. 235, edited by R.G. Crystal and J.B. West. New York: Raven Press

Massaro, D. and Massaro, G.D. (1978) Biochemical and anatomical adaptation of the lung to oxgyen-induced injury. *Fedn Proc.* **37**, 2485

Mathew, O.P., Abu-Osba, Y.K. and Thach, B.T. (1982a) Influence of upper airway pressure changes on genioglossus muscle respiratory activity. *J. appl. Physiol.* **52**, 438

Mathew, O.P., Abu-Osba, Y.K. and Thach, B.T. (1982b) Genioglossus muscle responses to upper airway pressure changes: afferent pathways. *J. appl. Physiol.* **52**, 445

Mattson, S.B. and Carlens, E. (1955) Lobar ventilation and oxygen uptake in man: influence of body position. *J. thorac. Surg.* **30**, 676

Mead, J. (1961) Mechanical properties of lungs. *Physiol. Rev.* **41,** 281

Mead, J. and Agostoni, E. (1964) Dynamics of breathing. *Handbk Physiol., section 3,* **1,** 1

Meade, F. and Owen-Thomas, J.B. (1975) The estimation of carbon dioxide concentration in the presence of nitrous oxide using a Lloyd–Haldane apparatus. *Br. J. Anaesth.* **47,** 22

Meldrum, N.U. and Roughton, F.J.W. (1933) Carbonic anhydrase: its preparation and properties. *J. Physiol.* **80,** 833

Mendelson, C.L. (1946) Aspiration of stomach contents into the lungs during obstetric anesthesia. *Am. J. Obstet. Gynec.* **52,** 191

Merwarth, C.R. and Sieker, H.O. (1961) Acid–base changes in blood and cerebrospinal fluid during altered ventilation. *J. appl. Physiol.* **16,** 1016

Meyer, B.J., Meyer, A. and Guyton, A.C. (1968) Interstitial fluid pressure. V. Negative pressure in the lungs. *Circulation Res.* **22,** 263

Meyer, E.C. and Ottaviano, R. (1972) Pulmonary collateral lymph flow: detection using lymph oxygen tensions. *J. appl. Physiol.* **32,** 806

Michaelson, E.D., Grassman, E.D. and Peters, W.R. (1975) Pulmonary mechanics by spectral analysis of forced random noise. *J. clin. Invest.* **56,** 1210

Michel, C.C. and Milledge, J.S. (1963) Respiratory regulation in man during acclimatization to high altitude. *J. Physiol.* **168,** 631

Michels, D.B. and West, J.B. (1978) Distribution of pulmonary ventilation and perfusion during short periods of weightlessness. *J. appl. Physiol.* **45,** 987

Michels, D.B., Friedman, P.J. and West, J.B. (1979) Radiographic comparison of human lung shape during normal gravity and weightlessness. *J. appl. Physiol.* **47,** 851

Michenfelder, J.D., Fowler, W.S. and Theye, R.A. (1966) CO_2 levels and pulmonary shunting in anesthetized man. *J. appl. Physiol.* **21,** 1471

Miles, S. (1957) The effect of changes in barometric pressure on maximum breathing capacity *J. Physiol.* **137,** 85P

Milic-Emili, J. (1991) Work of breathing. In: *The Lung: scientific foundations,* p. 1065, edited by R.G. Crystal and J.B. West. New York: Raven Press

Milic-Emili, J. (1992) How to monitor intrinsic PEEP – and why. *J. Crit. Illness* **7,** 25

Milic-Emili, J., Robatto, F.M. and Bates, J.H.T. (1990) Respiratory mechanics in anaesthesia. *Br. J. Anaesth.* **65,** 4

Milic-Emili, J., Mead, J., Turner, J.M. and Glauser, E.M. (1964) Improved technique for estimating pleural pressure from esophageal balloons. *J. appl. Physiol.* **19,** 207

Millar, R.A. (1960) Plasma adrenaline and noradrenaline during diffusion respiration. *J. Physiol.* **150,** 79

Milar, R.A. and Gregory, I.C. (1972) Reduced oxygen content in equilibrated fresh heparinised and ACD-stored blood from cigarette smokers. *Br. J. Anaesth.* **44,** 1015

Millar, R.A., Beard, D.J. and Hulands, G.H. (1971) Oxyhaemoglobin dissociation curves *in vitro* with and without the anaesthetics halothane and cyclopropane. *Br. J. Anaesth.* **43,** 1003

Milledge, J.S. (1984) Renin–aldosterone system. In: *High Altitude and Man,* edited by J.B. West and S. Lahiri. Bethesda, Md: American Physiological Society

Milledge, J.S. (1985a) Acute mountain sickness: pulmonary and cerebral oedema of high altitude. *Intens. Care Med.* **11,** 110

Milledge, J.S. (1985b) The great oxygen secretion controversy. *Lancet* **2,** 1408

Milledge, J.S. and Nunn, J.F. (1975) Criteria of fitness for anaesthesia in patients with chronic obstructive lung disease. *Br. med. J.* **3,** 670

Milledge, J.S. and Stott, F.D. (1971) Inductive plethysmography – a new respiratory transducer. *J. Physiol.* **267,** 4P

Milledge, J.S., Minty, K.B. and Duncalf, D. (1974) On-line assessment of ventilatory response to carbon dioxide. *J. appl. Physiol.* **37,** 596

Miller, A.H. (1925) Ascending respiratory paralysis under general anesthesia. *J. Am. med. Assoc.* **84,** 201

Miller, S.L. (1953) A production of amino acids under possible primitive earth conditions. *Science* **117,** 528

Miller, W.C., Rice, D.L., Unger, K.M. and Bradley, B.L. (1981) Effect of PEEP on lung water content in experimental noncardiogenic pulmonary edema. *Crit. Care Med.* **9,** 7

Miller, W.S. (1947) *The Lung,* 2nd ed. Springfield, Ill: Thomas

Millman, R.P., Knight, H., Kline, L.R., Shore, E.T., Chung, D.C. and Pack, A.I. (1988) Changes in compartmental ventilation in association with eye movements during REM sleep. *J. appl. Physiol.* **65,** 1196

Mills, E. and Jöbsis, F.F. (1972) Mitochondrial respiratory chain of carotid body and chemoreceptor response to changes in oxygen tension. *J. Neurophysiol.* **35,** 405

Mills, F.J. and Harding, R.M. (1983a) Special forms of flight. III: Supersonic transport aircraft. *Br. med. J.* **287,** 411

Mills, F.J. and Harding, R.M. (1983b) Special forms of flight. IV: Manned spacecraft. *Br. med. J.* **287,** 478

Mills, J.E., Sellick, H. and Widdicombe, J.G. (1970) Epithelial irritant receptors in the lungs. In: *Breathing: Hering–Breuer Centenary Symposium*, p. 77, edited by R. Porter. Edinburgh and London: Churchill Livingstone

Mills, R.J., Cumming, G. and Harris, P. (1963) Frequency-dependent compliance at different levels of inspiration in normal adults. *J. appl. Physiol.* **18,** 1061

Minty, B.D. and Barrett, A.M. (1978) Accuracy of automated blood-gas analyser operated by untrained staff. *Br. J. Anaesth.* **50,** 1031

Minty, B.D. and Royston, D. (1985) Cigarette smoke induced changes in rat pulmonary clearance of ^{99m}Tc DTPA. A comparison of particulate and gas phases. *Am. Rev. resp. Dis.* **132,** 1170

Minty, B.D., Jordan, C. and Jones, J.G. (1981) Rapid improvement in abnormal pulmonary epithelial permeability after stopping cigarettes. *Br. med. J.* **282,** 83

Mitchell, R.A. (1966) Cerebrospinal fluid and the regulation of respiration. In: *Advances in Respiratory Physiology*, edited by C.G. Caro. London: Edward Arnold

Mitchell, R.A. and Berger, A.J. (1975) Neural regulation of respiration. *Am. Rev. resp. Dis.* **111,** 206

Mitchell, R.A. and Berger, A.J. (1981) Neural regulation of respiration. In: *Regulation of Breathing*, part I, edited by T.F. Hornbein. New York: Marcel Dekker

Mitchell, R.A. and Herbert, D.A. (1975) Potencies of doxapram and hypoxia in stimulating carotid-body chemoreceptors and ventilation in anesthetized cats. *Anesthesiology* **42,** 559

Mitchell, R.A., Loeschcke, H.H., Massion, W.H. and Severinghaus, J.W. (1963) Respiratory responses mediated through superficial chemosensitive areas on the medulla. *J. appl. Physiol.* **18,** 523

Mitchell, R.A., Bainton, C.R., Severinghaus, J.W. and Edelist, G. (1964) Respiratory response and CSF pH during disturbances in blood acid–base balance in awake dogs with denervated aortic and carotid bodies. *Physiologist* **7,** 208

Mitchell, R.A., Carman, C.T., Severinghaus, J.W., Richardson, B.W., Singer, M.M. and Snider, S. (1965) Stability of cerebrospinal fluid pH in chronic acid–base disturbances in blood. *J. appl. Physiol.* **20,** 443

Mitzner, W., Blosser, S., Yager, D. and Wagner, E. (1992) Effect of bronchial smooth muscle contraction on lung compliance. *J. appl. Physiol.* **72,** 158

Modell, J.H. (1984) Drowning. In: *Edema*, p. 679, edited by N.C. Staub and A.E. Taylor. New York: Raven Press

Modell, J.H. and Moya, F. (1966) Effects of volume of aspirated fluid during chlorinated water fresh water drowning. *Anesthesiology* **27,** 662

Modell, J.H. and Spohr, R.W. (1989) Drowning and near-drowning. In: *General Anaesthesia*, 5th edn, edited by J.F. Nunn, J.E. Utting and B.R. Brown. London: Butterworths

Modell, J.H., Graves, S.A. and Ketover, A. (1976) Clinical course of 91 consecutive near-drowning victims. *Chest* **70,** 231

Modell, J.H., Calderwood, H.W., Ruiz, B.C., Downs, J.B. and Chapman, R. (1974) Effects of ventilatory patterns on arterial oxygenation after near-drowning in sea water. *Anesthesiology* **40,** 376

Moller, J.T., Johannessen, N.W., Berg, H., Espersen, K. and Larsen, L.E. (1991) Hypoxaemia during anaesthesia – an observer study. *Br. J. Anaesth.* **66,** 437

Moncada, S., Palmer, R.M.J. and Higgs, E.A. (1991) Nitric oxide: physiology, pathophysiology, and pharmacology. *Pharmacol. Rev.* **43,** 109

Moore, L.G., McCullough, R.E. and Weil, J.V. (1987) Increased HVR in pregnancy: relationship to hormonal and metabolic changes. *J. appl. Physiol.* **62,** 158

Moote, C.A., Knill, R.L. and Clement, J. (1986) Ventilatory compensation for continuous inspiratory resistive and elastic loads during halothane anesthesia in humans. *Anesthesiology* **64**, 582

Morikawa, S., Safar, P. and DeCarlo, J. (1961) Influence of the head–jaw position upon upper airway patency. *Anesthesiology* **22**, 265

Morrell, N.W. and Seed, W.A. (1992) Diagnosing pulmonary embolism. *Br. med. J.* **304**, 1126

Morris, H.R., Taylor, G.W., Piper, P.J. and Tippins, J.R. (1980) Structure of slow reacting substance of anaphylaxis from guinea-pig lung. *Nature* **285**, 104

Morris, J.G. (1968) *A Biologist's Physical Chemistry*. London: Edward Arnold

Mortensen, J.D. and Berry, G. (1989) Conceptual and design features of a practical, clinically effective intravenous mechanical blood oxygen/carbon dioxide exchange device (Ivox). *Int. J. artif. Organs* **12**, 384

Moser, K.M. (1990) Venous thromboembolism. *Am. Rev. resp. Dis.* **141**, 235

Moser, K.M., Rhodes, P.G. and Kwaan, P.L. (1965) Post-hyperventilation apnea. *Fedn Proc.* **24**, 273

Mount, L.E (1955) The ventilation flow-resistance and compliance of rat lungs. *J. Physiol.* **127**, 157

Moxham, J. (1984) Failure of the respiratory muscle pump. In: *Effects of anesthesia and surgery on pulmonary mechanisms and gas exchange, International Anesthesiology Clinics*, vol. 22, no. 4, edited by J.G. Jones. Boston, Mass: Little, Brown

Moxham, J. (1990) Respiratory muscle fatigue; mechanisms, evaluation and therapy. *Br. J. Anaesth.* **65**, 43

Muller, N., Volgyesi, G., Becker, L., Bryan, M.H. and Bryan, A.C. (1979) Diaphragmatic muscle tone. *J. appl. Physiol.* **47**, 279

Munson, E.S. and Merrick, H.C. (1967) Effect of nitrous oxide on venous air embolism. *Anesthesiology* **27**, 783

Munson, E.S., Larson, C.P., Babad, A.A., Regan, M.J., Buechel, D.R. and Eger, E.I. (1966) The effects of halothane, fluroxene and cyclopropane on ventilation: a comparative study in man. *Anesthesiology* **27**, 716

Murciano, D., Aubier, M., Lecocque, Y. and Pariente, R. (1984) Effects of theophylline on diaphragmatic strength and fatigue in patients with chronic obstructive pulmonary disease. *New Engl. J. Med.* **311**, 349

Murray, T.R., Chen, L., Marshall, B.E. and Macarack, E.J. (1990) Hypoxic contraction of cultured pulmonary vascular smooth muscle cells. *Am. J. Resp. cell. mol. Biol.* **3**, 457

Murray, J.F., Matthay, M.A., Luce, J.M. and Flick, M.R. (1988) An expanded definition of the adult respiratory distress syndrome. *Am. Rev. resp. Dis.* **138**, 720

Murrell, G.A.C. (1992) An insight into Dupuytren's contracture. *Ann. R. Coll. Surg.* **74**, 156

Murrell, G.A.C., Francis, M.J.O. and Bromley, L. (1987) Free radicals and Dupuytren's contracture. *Br. med. J.* **295**, 1373

Nahas, G.C., Ligou, J.C. and Mehlman, B. (1960) Effects of pH changes on O_2 uptake and plasma catecholamine levels in the dog. *J. appl. Physiol.* **198**, 60

Naito, H. and Gillis, C.N. (1973) Effects of halothane and nitrous oxide on removal of norepinephrine from the pulmonary circulation. *Anesthesiology* **39**, 575

Nandi, P.R., Charlesworth, C.H., Taylor, S.J., Nunn, J.F. and Doré, C.J. (1991a) Effect of general anaesthesia on the pharynx. *Br. J. Anaesth.* **66**, 157

Nandi, P.R., Nunn, J.F., Charlesworth, C.H. and Taylor, S.J. (1991b) Radiological study of the laryngeal mask. *Eur. J. Anaesthesiol.* **4**, 33

Nash, G., Blennerhassett, J.B. and Pontoppidan, H. (1967) Pulmonary lesions associated with oxygen therapy and artificial ventilation. *New Engl. J. Med.* **276**, 368

Natelson, S. (1951) Routine use of ultramicro-methods in the clinical laboratory. *Am. J. clin. Path.* **21**, 1153

Nathan, P.W. and Sears, T.A. (1960) Effects of posterior root section on the activity of some muscles in man. *J. Neurol. Neurosurg. Psychiat.* **23**, 10

Navaratnarajah, M., Nunn, J.F., Lyons, D. and Milledge, J.S. (1984) Bronchiolectasis caused by positive end-expiratory pressure. *Crit. Care Med.* **12**, 1036

Naylor, B.A., Welch, M.H., Shafer, A.W. and Guenter, C.A. (1972) Blood affinity for oxygen in hemorrhagic shock. *J. appl. Physiol.* **32**, 829

Needham, C.D., Rogan, M.C. and McDonald, I. (1954) Normal standards for lung volumes, intrapulmonary gas-mixing, and maximum breathing capacity. *Thorax* **9**, 313

Needleman, P., Blaine, E.H., Greenwald, J.E., Michener, M.L., Saper, C.B., Stockman, P.T. and Tolunay, H.E. (1989) The biochemical pharmacology of atrial peptides. *A. Rev. Pharmacol. Toxicol.* **29**, 23

von Neergard, K. (1929) Neue Auffassungen über einen Grundbegriff der Atemmechanik. Die Retraktionskraft der Lunge, abhängig von der Oberflächenspannung in der Alveolen. *Z. ges. exp. Med.* **66**, 373

von Neergaard, K. and Wirz, K. (1927a) Ueber eine Methode zur Messung der Lungenelastizität am lebenden Menschen, inbesondere beim Emphysem. *Z. klin. Med.* **105**, 35

von Neergaard, K. and Wirz, K. (1927b) Die Messung der Strömungswiderstände in der Atemwege des Menschen inbesondere bei Asthma und Emphysem. *Z. klin. Med.* **105**, 51

Neil, E. and Joels, N. (1963) The carotid glomus sensory mechanism. In: *The Regulation of Human Respiration*, p. 163, edited by D.J.C. Cunningham and B.B. Lloyd. Oxford: Blackwell Scientific

Nelson, N.M. (1966) Neonatal lung function. *Pediat. Clins N. Am.* **13**, 769

Nemir, P., Stone, H.H., Mackrell, T.N. and Hawthorne, H.R. (1953) Studies on pulmonary function utilizing the method of controlled unilateral bronchovascular occlusion. *Surg. Forum* **4**, 234

Newberg, L.A. and Jones, J.G. (1974) A closing volume bolus method using SF_6 enhancement of the nitrogen glow discharge. *J. appl. Physiol.* **36**, 488

Newman, H.C., Campbell, E.J.M. and Dinnick, O.P. (1959) A simple method of measuring the compliance and the non-elastic resistance of the chest during anaesthesia. *Br. J. Anaesth.* **31**, 282

Newsom-Davis, J. (1974) Control of the muscles in breathing. In: *Respiratory Physiology*, p. 221. London: Butterworths

Newsom-Davis, J. and Plum, F. (1972) Separation of descending spinal pathways to respiratory motoneurones. *Expl Neuronol.* **34**, 78

Ng, K.K.F. and Vane, J.R. (1967) Conversion of angiotensin I to angiotensin II. *Nature* **216**, 762

Ngai, S.H., Katz, R.L. and Farhi, S.E. (1965) Respiratory effects of trichlorethylene, halothane and methoxyflurane in the cat. *J. Pharmac. exp. Ther.* **148**, 123

Niden, A.H. and Aviado, D.M. (1956) Effects of pulmonary embolus on the pulmonary circulation with special reference to arteriovenous shunts in the lung. *Circulation Res.* **6**, 67

Nielsen, H. (1932) En oplivningsmetode. *Ugeskr. Laeg.* **94**, 1201

Nims, R.G., Connor, E.H. and Comroe, J.H. (1955) Compliance of the human thorax in anesthetized patients. *J. clin. Invest.* **34**, 744

Nishino, T., Honda, Y., Kohchi, T., Shirahata, M. and Yonezawa, T. (1984) Comparison of changes in the hypoglossal and phrenic nerve activity in response to increasing depth of anesthesia in cats. *Anesthesiology* **70**, 812

Nishino, T., Honda, Y., Kohchi, T., Shirahata, M. and Yonezawa, T. (1985) Effects of increasing depth of anaesthesia on phrenic nerve and hypoglossal nerve activity during the swallowing reflex in cats. *Br. J. Anaesth.* **57**, 208

Noble, M.I.M., Eisele, J.H., Frankel, H.L., Else, W. and Guz, A. (1971) The role of the diaphragm in the sensation of holding the breath. *Clin. Sci.* **41**, 275

Nørregaard, O., Schultz, P. Østergaard, A. and Dahl, R. (1989) Lung function and postural changes during pregnancy. *Resp. Med.* **83**, 467

Norton, P.G. and Dunn, E.V. (1985) Snoring as a risk factor for disease: an epidemiological survey. *Br. med. J.* **291**, 630

Nunn, J.F. (1956) A new method of spirometry applicable to routine anaesthesia. *Br. J. Anaesth.* **28**, 440

Nunn, J.F. (1958a) Ventilation and end-tidal carbon dioxide tension. *Anaesthesia* **13**, 124

Nunn, J.F. (1958b) Respiratory measurements in the presence of nitrous oxide. *Br. J. Anaesth.* **30**, 254

Nunn, J.F. (1960a) Prediction of carbon dioxide tension during anaesthesia. *Anaesthesia* **15**, 123

Nunn, J.F. (1960b) The solubility of volatile anaesthetics in oil. *Br. J. Anaesth.* **32**, 346

Nunn, J.F. (1961a) The distribution of inspired gas during thoracic surgery. *Ann. R. Coll. Surg.* **28**, 223

Nunn, J.F. (1961b) Portable anaesthetic apparatus for use in the Antarctic. *Br. med. J.* **1**, 1139

Nunn, J.F. (1962a) Measurement of blood oxygen tension: handling of samples. *Br. J. Anaesth.* **34**, 621

Nunn, J.F. (1962b) The effects of hypercapnia. In: *Modern Trends in Anaesthesia – 2*, edited by F.T. Evans and T.C. Gray. London and Boston, Mass: Butterworths

Nunn, J.F. (1963) Indirect determination of the ideal alveolar oxygen tension during and after nitrous oxide anaesthesia. *Br. J. Anaesth.* **35,** 8

Nunn, J.F. (1964) Factors influencing the arterial oxygen tension during halothane anaesthesia with spontaneous respiration. *Br. J. Anaesth.* **36,** 327

Nunn, J.F. (1968) The evolution of atmospheric oxygen. *Ann. R. Coll. Surg.* **43,** 200

Nunn, J.F. (1972) Nomograms for calculation of oxygen consumption and respiratory exchange ratio. *Br. med. J.* **4,** 18

Nunn, J.F. (1978) Measurement of closing volume. *Acta anaesth. scand.* suppl. 70, 154

Nunn, J.F. (1983) Mandatory minute volume. *Jap. J. clin. Anaesth.* **31,** 1063

Nunn, J.F. (1984) Positive end-expiratory pressure. In: *Effects of anesthesia and surgery on pulmonary mechanisms and gas exchange, International Anesthesiology Clinics*, vol. 224, no. 4, edited by J.G. Jones. Boston, Mass: Little, Brown

Nunn, J.F. (1985a) Oxygen – friend or foe. *Jl R. Soc.Med.* **78,** 618

Nunn, J.F. (1985b) Anesthesia and pulmonary gas exchange. In: *Effects of Anesthesia*, edited by B.G. Covino, H.A. Fazzard, K. Rehder and G. Strichartz. Bethesda, Md: American Physiological Society

Nunn, J.F. (1989) In: *High Altitude Medicine and Physiology*, p. 481, edited by M.P. Ward, J.S. Milledge and J.B. West. London: Chapman & Hall

Nunn, J.F. (1990) Effects of anaesthesia on respiration. *Br. J. Anaesth.* **65,** 54

Nunn, J.F. and Bergman, N.A. (1964) The effect of atropine on pulmonary gas exchange. *Br. J. Anaesth.* **36,** 68

Nunn, J.F. and Ezi-Ashi, T.I. (1961) The respiratory effects of resistance to breathing in anesthetized man. *Anesthesiology* **22,** 174

Nunn, J.F. and Ezi-Ashi, T.I. (1962) The accuracy of the respirometer and ventigrator. *Br. J. Anaesth.* **34,** 422

Nunn, J.F. and Freeman, J. (1964) Problems of oxygenation and oxygen transport during haemorrhage. *Anaesthesia* **19,** 206

Nunn, J.F. and Hill, D.W. (1960) Respiratory dead space and arterial to end-tidal CO_2 tension difference in anesthetized man. *J. appl. Physiol.* **15,** 383

Nunn, J.F. and Lyle, D.J.R. (1986) The Ohmeda CPU-1 Ventilator. *Br. J. Anaesth.* **58,** 653

Nunn, J.F. and Matthews, R.L. (1959) Gaseous exchange during halothane anaesthesia: the steady respiratory state. *Br. J. Anaesth.* **31,** 330

Nunn, J.F. and Newman, H.C. (1964) Inspired gas, rebreathing and apparatus dead space. *Br. J. Anaesth.* **36,** 5

Nunn, J.F. and Payne, J.P. (1962) Hypoxaemia after general anaesthesia. *Lancet* **2,** 631

Nunn, J.F. and Pouliot, J.C. (1962) The measurement of gaseous exchange during nitrous oxide anaesthesia. *Br. J. Anaesth.* **34,** 752

Nunn, J.F., Bergman, N.A. and Coleman, A.J. (1965) Factors influencing the arterial oxygen tension during anaesthesia with artificial ventilation. *Br. J. Anaesth.* **37,** 898

Nunn, J.F., Campbell, E.J.M. and Peckett, B.W. (1959) Anatomical subdivisions of the volume of respiratory dead space and effect of position of the jaw. *J. appl. Physiol.* **14,** 174

Nunn, J.F., Makita, K. and Royston, B. (1989) Validation of oxygen consumption measurements during artificial ventilation. *J. appl. Physiol.* **67,** 2129

Nunn, J.F., Milledge, J.S. and Sigaraya, J. (1979) Survival of patients ventilated in an intensive care unit. *Br. med. J.* **1,** 1525

Nunn, J.F., Bergman, N.A., Coleman, A.J. and Casselle, D.C. (1964) Evaluation of the Servomex paramagnetic analyser. *Br. J. Anaesth.* **36,** 666

Nunn, J.F., Bergman, N.A., Bunatyan, A. and Coleman, A.J. (1965a) Temperature coefficients of P_{CO_2} and P_{O_2} of blood *in vitro*. *J. appl. Physiol.* **20,** 23

Nunn, J.F., Coleman, A.J., Sachithanandan, T., Bergman, N.A. and Laws, J.W. (1965b) Hypoxaemia and atelectasis produced by forced expiration. *Br. J. Anaesth.* **37,** 3

Nunn, J.F., Sturrock, J.E., Willis, E.J., Richmond, J.E. and McPherson, C.K. (1974) The effect of inhalational anaesthetics on the swimming velocity of *Tetrahymena pyriformis*. *J. Cell Sci.* **15,** 537

Nunn, J.F., Williams, I.P., Jones, J.G., Hewlett, A.M., Hulands, G.H. and Minty, B.D. (1978) Detection and reversal of pulmonary absorption collapse. *Br. J. Anaesth.* **50,** 91

Nunn, J.F., Sturrock, J.E., Jones, A.J., O'Morain, C., Segal, A.W., Coade, S.B., Dorling, J. and

Walker, D. (1979) Halothane does not inhibit human neutrophil function in vitro. *Br. J. Anaesth.* **51**, 1101

Nunn, J.F., Milledge, J.S., Chen, D. and Doré, C. (1988) Respiratory criteria of fitness for surgery and anaesthesia. *Anaesthesia* **43**, 543

Ochiai, R., Guthrie, R.D. and Motoyama, E.K. (1989) Effects of varying concentrations of halothane on the activity of the genioglossus, intercostals, and diaphragm in cats: an electromyographic study. *Anesthesiology* **70**, 812

Ogilvie, C.M., Forster, R.E., Blakemore, W.S. and Morton, J.W. (1957) A standardized breath holding technique for the clinical measurement of the diffusing capacity of the lung for carbon monoxide. *J. clin. Invest.* **36**, 1

Otis, A.B. (1954) The work of breathing. *Physiol. Rev.* **34**, 449

Otis, A.B. (1964) The work of breathing. *Handbk Physiol., section 3*, **1**, 463

Otis, A.B., Fenn, W.O. and Rahn, H. (1950) Mechanics of breathing in man. *J. appl. Physiol.* **2**, 592

Otis, A.B., Rahn, H. and Fenn, W.O. (1948) Alveolar gas changes during breath holding. *Am. J. Physiol.* **152,** 674

Otis, A.B., McKerrow, C.B., Bartlett, R.A., Mead, J., McIlroy, M.B., Selverstone, N.J. and Radford, E.P. (1956) Mechanical factors in distribution of pulmonary ventilation. *J. appl. Physiol.* **8**, 427

Ozanam, C. (1862) De l'acide carbonique en inhalations comme agent anesthésique efficace et sans danger pendant les operations chirurgicales. *C.r. Acad. Sci.* **54**, 1154

Padmanabhan, R.V., Gudapaty, R., Liener, I.E., Schwartz, B.A. and Hoidal, J.R. (1985) Protection against pulmonary oxygen toxicity in rats by the intratracheal administration of liposome-encapsulated superoxide dismutase or catalase. *Am. Rev. resp. Dis.* **132**, 164

Padmore, G.R.A. and Nunn, J.F. (1974) SI units in relation to anaesthesia. *Br. J. Anaesth.* **46**, 236

Pain, M.C.F. (1964) Digital clubbing in chronic obstructive lung disease. *Australas Ann. Med.* **13**, 167

Paintal, A.S. (1983) Lung and airway receptors. In: *Control of Respiration*, edited by D.J. Pallot. London: Croom Helm

Paiva, M., Estenne, M. and Engel, L.A. (1989) Lung volumes, chest wall configuration, and pattern of breathing in microgravity. *J. appl. Physiol.* **67**, 1542

Palmer, K.N.V. and Diament, M.L. (1967) Effect of aerosol isoprenaline on blood-gas tensions in severe bronchial asthma. *Lancet* **2**, 1232

Palmer, R.M.J., Ferrige, A.G. and Moncada, S. (1987) Nitric oxide release accounts for the biological activity of endothelium-derived relaxing factor. *Nature* **327**, 524

Panday, J. and Nunn, J.F. (1968) Failure to demonstrate progressive falls of arterial Po_2 during anaesthesia. *Anaesthesia* **23**, 38

Pappenheimer, J.R., Comroe, J.H., Cournand, A. et al. (1950) Standardization of definitions and symbols in respiratory physiology. *Fedn Proc.* **9**, 602

Pare, P.D., Warriner, B., Baile, E.M. and Hogg, J.C. (1983) Redistribution of extravascular water with positive end-expiratory pressure in canine pulmonary edema. *Am. Rev. resp. Dis.* **127**, 590

Parisi, R.A., Santiago, T.V. and Edelman, N.H. (1988) Genioglossal and diaphragmatic EMG responses to hypoxia during sleep. *Am. Rev. resp. Dis.* **138**, 610

Parks, D.A., Bulkley, G.B. and Granger, D.N. (1983) Role of oxygen free radicals in shock, ischaemia and organ preservation. *Surgery* **94**, 428

Passavant, G. (1869) Ueber die Verschliessung des Schlundes beim Sprechen. *Arch. path. Anat. Physiol. klin. Med.* **46**, 1

Pattle, R.E. (1955) Properties, function and origin of the alveolar lining fluid. *Nature* **175**, 1125

Pattle, R.E., Schock, C. and Battensby, J. (1972) Some effects of anaesthetics on lung surfactant. *Br. J. Anaesth.* **44**, 1119

Pattle, R.E., Claireaux, A.E., Davies, P.A. and Cameron, A.H. (1962) Inability to form a lung lining film as a cause of the respiratory distress syndrome in newborn. *Lancet* **2**, 469

Pauling, L., Wood, R.E. and Sturdivant, J.H. (1946) Instrument for determining partial pressure of oxygen in gas. *J. Am. chem. Soc.* **68**, 795

Pavlin, E.G. and Hornbein, T.F. (1975a) Distribution of H^+ and HCO_3^- between CSF and blood during metabolic acidosis in dogs. *J. Physiol.* **228**, 1134

Pavlin, E.G. and Hornbein, T.F. (1975b) Distribution of H^+ and HCO_3^- between CSF and blood during metabolic alkalosis in dogs. *J. Physiol.* **228**, 1141

Pavlin, E.G. and Hornbein, T.F. (1975c) Distribution of H$^+$ and HCO$_3^-$ between CSF and blood during respiratory acidosis in dogs. *J. Physiol.* **228**, 1145

Pavlin, E.G. and Hornbein, T.F. (1986) Anesthesia and the control of ventilation. *Handbk Physiol.*, section II, **3**, part 2, 793

Pavlin, D.J., Nessly, M.L. and Cheney, F.W. (1981) Increased pulmonary vascular permeability as a cause of re-expansion edema in rabbits. *Am. Rev. resp. Dis.* **124**, 422

Payne, J.P. (1958) Hypotensive response to carbon dioxide. *Anaesthesia* **13**, 279

Payne, J.P. (1962) Apnoeic oxygenation in anaesthetized man. *Acta anaesth. scand.* **6**, 129

Peacock, A.J., Morgan, M.D.L., Turton, C., Gourlay, A.R. and Denison, D.M. (1984) Optical mapping of the thoraco-abdominal wall. *Thorax* **39**, 93

Pearce, A.C. and Jones, R.M. (1984) Smoking and anesthesia: preoperative abstinence and perioperative morbidity. *Anesthesiology* **61**, 576

Pearn, J. (1985) The management of near-drowning, *Br. med. J.* **291**, 1447

Pepe, P.E., Hudson, L.D. and Carrico, C.J. (1984) Early application of positive end-expiratory pressure in patients at risk for the adult respiratory distress syndrome. *New Engl. J. Med.* **311**, 281

Pepe, P.E., Potkin, R.T., Reus, D.H., Hudson, L.D. and Carrico, C.J. (1982) Clinical predictors of the adult respiratory distress syndrome. *Am. J. Surg.* **144**, 124

Perez-Chada, R.D., Gardaz, J.-P., Madgwick, R.G. and Sykes, M.K. (1983) Cardiorespiratory effects of an inspiratory hold and continuous positive pressure ventilation in goats. *Intens. Care Med.* **9**, 263

Perkins, K.A. (1992) Metabolic effects of cigarette smoking. *J. appl. Physiol.* **72**, 401

Perkins, N.A.K. and Bedford, R.F. (1984) Hemodynamic consequences of PEEP in seated neurological patients – implications for paradoxical air embolism. *Anesth. Analg.* **63**, 429

Perkins-Pearson, N.A.K., Marshall, W.K. and Bedford, R.F. (1982) Atrial pressures in the seated position. *Anesthesiology* **57**, 493

Permutt, S. and Riley, R.L. (1963) Hemodynamics of collapsible vessels with tone: the vascular waterfall. *J. appl. Physiol.* **18**, 924

Pernoll, M.L., Metcalfe, J., Schlenker, T.L., Welch, J.E. and Matsumoto, J.A. (1975) Oxygen consumption at rest and during exercise in pregnancy. *Resp. Physiol.* **25**, 285

Perutz, M.F. (1969) The haemoglobin molecule. *Proc. R. Soc. B* **173**, 113

Pesenti, A., Pelizzola, A., Mascheroni, D. et al. (1981) Low frequency positive pressure ventilation with extracorporeal CO$_2$ removal (LFPPV-ECCO$_2$R) in acute respiratory failure (ARF): technique. *Trans. Am. Soc. artif. intern. Organs* **27**, 263

Pesenti, A., Pelosi, P., Rossi, N., Virtuani, A., Brazzi, L. and Rossi, A. (1991) The effects of positive end-expiratory pressure on respiratory resistance in patients with the adult respiratory distress syndrome and in normal anesthetized subjects. *Am. Rev. resp. Dis.* **144**, 101

Petheram, I.S. and Branthwaite, M.A. (1980) Mechanical ventilation for pulmonary disease. *Anaesthesia* **35**, 467

Petros, A.J., Doré, C.J. and Nunn, J.F. (1993) Modification of the iso-shunt lines for low inspired oxygen concentrations. *Br. J. Anaesth.* **71**, in press

Petty, T.L. and Ashbaugh, D.G. (1971) The adult respiratory distress syndrome. *Chest* **60**, 233

Pflüger, E. (1866) Zur gasometrie des Blutes. *Zbl. med. Wiss.* **4**, 305

Pflüger, E. (1868) Ueber die Urasche der Athembewegungen, sowie der Dyspnoë und Apnoë. *Arch. ges. Physiol.* **1**, 61

Phillipson, E.A. (1977) Regulation of breathing during sleep. *Am. Rev. resp. Dis.* **155**, 217

Philpot, R.M., Anderson, M.W. and Eling, T.E. (1977) Uptake, accumulation and metabolism of chemicals by the lung. In: *Metabolic Functions of the Lung*, edited by Y.S. Bakhle and J.R. Vane. New York: Marcel Dekker

Pierce, E.C., Lambertsen, C.J., Deutsch, S., Chase, P.E., Linde, H.W., Dripps, R.D. and Price, H.L. (1962) Cerebral circulation and metabolism during thiopental anesthesia and hyperventilation in man. *J. clin. Invest.* **41**, 1664

Pietak, S., Weening, C.S., Hickey, R.F. and Fairley, H.B. (1975) Anesthetic effects on ventilation in patients with chronic obstructive pulmonary disease. *Anesthesiology* **42**, 160

Piiper, J. (1961) Variations of ventilation and diffusing capacity to perfusion determining the alveolar–arterial O$_2$ difference: theory. *J. appl. Physiol.* **16**, 507

Piiper, J., Haab, P. and Rahn, H. (1961) Unequal distribution of pulmonary diffusing capacity in the anesthetized dog. *J. appl. Physiol.* **16**, 499

The PIOPED Investigators. (1990) Value of the ventilation/perfusion scan in acute pulmonary embolism: results of the Prospective Investigation of Pulmonary Embolism Diagnosis (PIOPED). *J. Am. med. Assoc.* **263**, 2753

Piper, P.J., Samhoun, M.N., Tippins, J.R., Williams, T.J., Palmer, M.A. and Peck, M.J. (1981) Pharmacological studies on pure SRS-A and synthetic leukotrienes C_4 and D_4. In: *SRS-A and Leukotrienes*, edited by P.J. Piper. New York: Wiley

Pitts, R.F. (1946) Organization of the respiratory center. *Physiol. Rev.* **26**, 609

Pitts, R.F., Magoun, H.W. and Ranson, S.W. (1939a) Localization of the medullary respiratory centers in the cat. *Am. J. Physiol.* **126**, 673

Pitts, R.F., Magoun, H.W. and Ranson, S.W. (1939b) Interrelations of the respiratory centers in the cat. *Am. J. Physiol.* **126**, 689

Pitts, R.F., Magoun, H.W. and Ranson, S.W. (1939c) The origin of respiratory rhythmicity. *Am. J. Physiol* **127**, 654

Plopper, C.G., Hyde, D.M. and Buckpitt, A.R. (1991) Clara cells. In: *The Lung: scientific foundationss*, p. 215, edited by R.G. Crystal and J.B. West. New York: Raven Press

Ponte, J. and Purves, M.J. (1974) Frequency response of carotid body chemoreceptors in the cat to changes of Pa_{O_2}, Pa_{CO_2} and pH. *J. appl. Physiol.* **37**, 635

Pontoppidan, H., Geffin, B. and Lowenstein, E. (1972) Acute respiratory failure in the adult. *New Engl. J. Med.* **287**, 690, 743 and 799

Potgieter, S.V. (1959) Atelectasis: its evolution during upper urinary tract surgery. *Br. J. Anaesth.* **31**, 472

Price, H.L. (1960) Effects of carbon dioxide on the cardiovascular system. *Anesthesiology* **21**, 652

Price, H.L. and Widdicombe, J. (1962) Actions of cyclopropane on carotid sinus baroreceptors and carotid body chemoreceptors. *J. Pharmac. exp. Ther.* **135**, 233

Price, H.L., Lurie, A.A., Jones, R.E. and Linde, H.W. (1958) Role of catecholamines in the initiation of arrhythmic cardiac contraction by carbon dioxide inhalation in anesthetized man. *J. Pharmac. exp. Ther.* **122**, 63A

Price, H.L., Lurie, A.A., Black, G.W., Sechzer, P.H., Linde, H.W. and Price, M.L. (1960) Modification by general anesthetics (cyclopropane and halothane) of circulatory and sympatho-adrenal responses to respiratory acidosis. *Ann. Surg.* **152**, 1071

Price, H.L., Cooperman, L.H., Warden, J.C., Morris, J.J. and Smith, T.C. (1969) Pulmonary hemodynamics during general anesthesia in man. *Anesthesiology* **30**, 629

Prisk, G.K., Guy, H.J.B., Elliott, A.R. and West, J.B. (1992) Diffusing capacity and its subdivisions during sustained microgravity on Spacelab SLS–1. *FASEB J.* **6**, A1772

Prutow, R.J., Dueck, R., Davies, N.J.H. and Clausen, J. (1982) Shunt development in young adult surgical patients due to inhalational anesthesia. *Anesthesiology* **57**, A477

Prys-Roberts, C. (1980) Hypercapnia. In: *General Anaesthesia*, 4th edn., edited by T.C. Gray, J.F. Nunn and J.E. Utting. London: Butterworths

Prys-Roberts, C., Kelman, G.R. and Nunn, J.F. (1966) Determination of the *in vivo* carbon dioxide titration curve of anaesthetized man. *Br. J. Anaesth.* **38**, 500

Prys-Roberts, C., Smith, W.D.A. and Nunn, J.F. (1967) Accidental severe hypercapnia during anaesthesia. *Br. J. Anaesth.* **39**, 257

Prys-Roberts, C., Kelman, G.R., Greenbaum, R. and Robinson, R.H. (1967) Circulatory influences of artificial ventilation during nitrous oxide anaesthesia in man. II. Results: the relative influence of mean intrathoracic pressure and arterial carbon dioxide tension. *Br. J. Anaesth.* **39**, 533

Prys-Roberts, C., Greenbaum, R., Nunn, J.F. and Kelman, G.R. (1970) Disturbances of pulmonary function in patients with fat embolism. *J. clin. Path.* **23**, suppl. (Roy. Coll. Path.) **4**, 143

Pugh, L.G.C.E. (1962) Physiological and medical aspects of the Himalayan Scientific and Mountain-eering Expedition, 1960–61. *Br. med. J.* **2**, 621

Pugh, L.G.C.E. (1964) Cardiac output in muscular exercise at 5,800 m (19,000 ft). *J. appl. Physiol.* **19**, 441

Pugh, L.G.C.E., Gill, M.B., Lahiri, S., Milledge, J.S., Ward, M.P. and West, J.B. (1964) Muscular exercise at great altitudes. *J. appl. Physiol.* **19**, 431

Qvist, J., Hill, R.D., Schneider, R.C., Falke, K.J., Liggins, G.C., Guppy, M. et al. (1986) Hemoglobin concentrations and blood gas tensions of free-diving Weddell seals. *J. appl. Physiol.* **61**, 1560

Radford, E.P. (1955) Ventilation standards for use in artificial respiration. *J. appl. Physiol.* **7**, 451

Rahn, H. (1964) Oxygen stores of man. In: *Oxygen in the Animal Organism*, edited by F. Dickens and E. Neil. Oxford: Pergamon

Rahn, H. and Farhi, L.E. (1964) Ventilation, perfusion, and gas exchange – the $\dot{V}_A/\dot{Q}$ concept. *Handbk Physiol., section 3*, **1**, 735

Rahn, H. and Otis, A.B. (1949) Man's respiratory response during and after acclimatization to high altitude. *Am. J. Physiol.* **157**, 445

Rahn, H., Mohney, J., Otis, A.B. and Fenn, W.O. (1946) A method for the continuous analysis of alveolar air. *A. Aviat. Med.* **17**, 173

Raine, J.M. and Bishop, J.M. (1963) A–a difference in O_2 tension and physiological dead space in normal man. *J. appl. Physiol.* **18**, 284

Ramon y Cajal, S. (1909) *Histologia du systeme Nerveux de l'Homme et des Vertebres.* Paris: Moloine

Ramwell, P.W. (1958) An investigation into the changes in blood gases during anaesthesia. *PhD Thesis*, University of Leeds

Ranieri, V.M., Eissa, N.T., Corbeil, C., Chassé, M., Braidy, J., Matar, N. and Milic-Emili, J. (1991) Effects of positive end-expiratory pressure on alveolar recruitment and gas exchange in patients with the adult respiratory distress syndrome. *Am. Rev. resp. Dis.* **144**, 544

Rapace, J.L. and Lowrey, A.H. (1982) Tobacco smoke, ventilation and indoor air quality. *Am. Soc. Heating, Refrigerating and Air-conditioning Engineers, Inc. Trans.* **88**, 895

Räsänen, J., Heikkilä, J., Downs, J., Nikki, P., Väisänen, I. and Viitanen, A. (1985) Continuous positive airway pressure by face mask in acute cardiogenic pulmonary edema. *Am. J. Cardiol.* **55**, 296

Ravin, M.G., Epstein, R.M. and Malm, J.R. (1965) Contribution of thebesian veins to the physiologic shunt in anesthetized man. *J. appl. Physiol.* **20**, 1148

Raymond, L.W. and Standaert, F.G. (1967) The respiratory effects of carbon dioxide in the cat. *Anesthesiology* **28**, 974

Read, D.J.C. (1967). A clinical method for assessing the ventilatory response to carbon dioxide. *Australas. Ann. Med.* **16**, 20

Rebuck, A.S. and Campbell, E.J.M. (1974) A clinical method for assessing the ventilatory response to hypoxia. *Am. Rev. resp. Dis.* **109**, 345

Rebuck, A.S. and Slutsky, A.S. (1981) Measurement of ventilatory responses to hypercapnia and hypoxia. In: *Regulation of Breathing*, part II, edited by T.F. Hornbein. New York: Marcel Dekker

Reeder, M.K., Muir, A.D., Foëx, P., Goldman, M.D., Loh, L. and Smart, D. (1991) Postoperative myocardial ischaemia: temperal association with nocturnal hypoxaemia. *Br. J. Anaesth.* **67**, 626

Reeder, M.K., Goldman, M.D., Loh, L., Muir, A.D., Foëx, P., Casey, K.R. and McKenzie, P.J. (1992) Postoperative hypoxaemia after major abdominal vascular surgery. *Br. J. Anaesth.* **68**, 23

Rees, G.J. (1980) Neonatal physiology. In: *General Anaesthesia*, 4th edition, vol. 2, edited by T.C. Gray, J.F. Nunn and J.E. Utting. London: Butterworths

Refsum, H.E. (1963) Relationship between state of consciousness and arterial hypoxaemia and hypercapnia in patients with pulmonary insufficiency, breathing air. *Clin. Sci.* **25**, 361

Register, S.D., Downs, J.B., Stock, M.C. and Kirby, R.R. (1987) Is 50% oxygen harmful? *Crit. Care Med.* **15**, 598

Rehder, K. (1985) Anesthesia and the mechanics of respiration. In: *Effects of Anesthesia*, edited by B.G. Covino, H.A. Fozzard, K. Rehder and G. Strichartz. Bethesda, Md: American Physiological Society

Rehder, K. and Marsh, H.M. (1986) Respiratory mechanics during anesthesia and mechanical ventilation. *Handbk Physiol. section 3*, **3**, part 2, 737

Rehder, K. and Sessler, A.D. (1973) Function of each lung in spontaneously breathing man anesthetized with thiopentalmeperidine. *Anesthesiology* **38**, 320

Rehder, K., Schmid, E.R. and Knopp, T.J. (1983) Long-term high-frequency ventilation in dogs. *Am. Rev. resp. Dis.* **126**, 476

Rehder, K., Sessler, A.D. and Marsh, H.M. (1975) General anesthesia and the lung. *Am. Rev. resp. Dis.* **112**, 541

Rehder, K., Theye, R.A. and Fowler, W.S. (1961) Effect of position and thoracotomy on distribution of air and blood to each lung during intermittent positive pressure breathing. *Physiologist* **4**, 93

Rehder, K., Hatch, D.J., Sessler, A.D., Marsh, H.M. and Fowler, W.S. (1971) Effects of general anesthesia, muscle paralysis, and mechanical ventilation on pulmonary nitrogen clearance. *Anesthesiology* **35**, 591

Rehder, K., Hatch, D.J., Sessler, A.D. and Fowler, W.S. (1972) The function of each lung of anesthetized and paralyzed man during mechanical ventilation. *Anesthesiology* **37**, 16

Rehder, K., Knopp, T.J., Sessler, A.D. and Didier, E.P. (1979) Ventilation–perfusion relationship in young healthy awake and anesthetized–paralyzed man. *J. appl. Physiol.* **47**, 745

Reinhardt, D. (1989) Adrenoreceptors and the lung: their role in health and disease. *Eur. J. Pediatr.* **148**, 286

Reivich, M. (1964) Arterial P_{CO_2} and cerebral hemodynamics. *Am. J. Physiol.* **206**, 25

Remmers, J.E., deGroot, W.J., Sauerland, E.K. and Anch, A.M. (1978) Pathogenesis of upper airway occlusion during sleep. *J. appl. Physiol.* **44**, 931

Report of the Surgeon General (1981) *The Health Consequences of Smoking. The Changing Cigarette.* Washington DC: US Department of Health and Human Services

Report of the Surgeon General (1984) *The Health Consequences of Smoking. Chronic Obstructive Lung Disease.* Washington DC: US Department of Health and Human Services

Richardson, F.J., Chinn, S. and Nunn, J.F. (1976) Performance and application of the Quantiflex air/oxygen mixer. *Br. J. Anaesth.* **48**, 1057

Richardson, T.Q. and Guyton, A.C. (1959) Effects of polycythemia and anemia on cardiac output and other circulatory factors. *Am. J. Physiol.* **197**, 1167

Riley, R.L., Campbell, E.J.M. and Shepard, R.H. (1957) A bubble method for estimation of P_{CO_2} and P_{O_2} in whole blood. *J. appl. Physiol.* **11**, 245

Riley, R.L., Lilienthal, J.L., Proemmel, D.D. and Franke, R.E. (1946) On the determination of the physiologically effective pressures of oxygen and carbon dioxide in alveolar air. *Am. J. Physiol.* **147**, 191

Riley, R.L., Shepard, R.H., Cohn, J.E., Carroll, D.G. and Armstrong, B.W. (1954) Maximal diffusing capacity of lungs. *J. appl. Physiol.* **6**, 573

Rinaldo, J.E. and Rogers, R.M. (1982) Adult respiratory-distress syndrome: changing concepts of lung injury and repair. *New Engl. J. Med.* **306**, 900

Rippe, B. and Crone, C. (1991) Pores and intercellular junctions. In: *The Lung: scientific foundations*, p. 349, edited by R.G. Crystal and J.B. West. New York: Raven Press

Rizk, N.W. and Murray, J.F. (1982) PEEP and pulmonary edema. *Am. J. Med.* **72**, 381

Rizk, N.W., Luce, J.M., Hoeffel, J.M., Price, D.C. and Murray, J.F. (1984) Site of deposition and factors affecting clearance of aerosolized solute from canine lungs. *J. appl. Physiol.* **56**, 723

Robertson, J.D. and Reid, D.D. (1952) Standards for the basal metabolism of normal people in Britain. *Lancet* **1**, 940

Robertson, J.D., Swan, A.A.B. and Whitteridge, D. (1956) Effect of anaesthetics on systemic baroreceptors. *J. Physiol.* **131**, 463

Robin, E.D., Theodore, J., Burke, C.M., Oesterle, S.N., Fowler, M.B., Jamieson, S.W. et al. (1987) Hypoxic pulmonary vasoconstriction persists in the human transplanted lung. *Clin. Sci.* **72**, 283

Robinson, C. and Holgate, S.T. (1985) Mast cell-dependent inflammatory mediators and their putative role in bronchial asthma. *Clin. Sci.* **68**, 103

Robson, J.G. (1967) The respiratory centres and their responses. In: *Modern Trends in Anaesthesia – 3*, edited by F.T. Evans and T.C. Gray. London and Boston, Mass: Butterworths

Rodenstein, D.O. and Stanescu, D.C. (1986) The soft palate and breathing. *Am. Rev. resp. Dis.* **134**, 311

Rodman, D.M., Yamaguchi, T., Hasunuma, K., O'Brien, R.F. and McMurtry, I.F. (1990) Effects of hypoxia on endothelium-dependent relaxation of rat pulmonary artery. *Am. J. Physiol.* **258**, L205

Rohrer, F. (1915) Der Strömungswiderstand in den menschlichen Atemwegen. *Plügers Arch. ges. Physiol.* **162**, 225

Romaldini, H., Rodriguez-Roisin, R., Wagner, P.D. and West, J.B. (1983) Enhancement of hypoxic pulmonary vasoconstriction by almitrine in the dog. *Am. Rev. resp. Dis.* **128**, 288

Rossaint, R., Falke, K.J., López, F., Slama, K., Pison, U. and Zapol, W.M. (1993) Inhaled nitric oxide for the adult respiratory distress syndrome. *New Engl. J. Med.* **328**, 399

Rossier, P.H. and Méan, H. (1943) L'insuffisance pulmonaire: ses diverses formes. *J. suisse Med.* **11**, 327

Rossing, T.H., Slutsky, A.S., Lehr, J.L., Drinker, P.A., Kamm, R. and Drazen, J.M. (1981) Tidal volume and frequency dependence on carbon dioxide elimination by high frequency ventilation. *New Engl. J. Med.* **305**, 1375

Roughton, F.J.W. (1964) Transport of oxygen and carbon dioxide. *Handbk Physiol., section 3*, **1**, 767

Roughton, F.J.W. and Darling, R.C. (1944) The effect of carbon monoxide on the oxyhemoglobin dissociation curve. *Am. J. Physiol.* **141**, 17

Roughton, F.J.W. and Forster, R.E. (1957) Relative importance of diffusion and chemical reaction rates in determining rate of exchange of gas in the human lung. *J. appl. Physiol.* **11**, 290

Roughton, F.J.W. and Severinghaus, J.W. (1973) Accurate determination of O_2 dissociation curve of human blood above 98.7% saturation with data on O_2 solubility in unmodified human blood from 0°C to 37°C. *J. appl. Physiol.* **35**, 861

Roussos, C. and Macklem, P.T. (1977) Diaphragmatic fatigue in man. *J. appl. Physiol.* **43**, 189

Roussos, C. and Macklem, P.T. (1983) The respiratory muscles. *Intens. Care Dig.* **2**, 3

Roy, R., Powers, S.R., Fuestel, P.J. and Dutton, R.E. (1977) Pulmonary wedge catheterization during positive end-expiratory pressure ventilation in the dog. *Anesthesiology* **46**, 385

Royston, D. (1988) Free radicals. *Anaesthesia* **43**, 315

Russell, J.A., Ronco, J.J., Lockhat, D., Belzberg, A., Keiss, M. and Dodek, P.M. (1990) Oxygen delivery and consumption and ventricular preload are greater in survivors than in nonsurvivors of the adult respiratory distress syndrome. *Am. Rev. resp. Dis.* **141**, 659

Russell, M.A.H., Wilson, C., Patel, U.A., Cole, P.V. and Feyeraband, C. (1975) Plasma nicotine levels after smoking cigarettes with high, medium and low nicotine yields. *Br. med. J.* **2**, 414

Ryan, U.S. (1982) Structural bases for metabolic activity. *A. Rev. Physiol.* **44**, 223

Ryan, U.S. (1985) Processing of angiotensin and other peptides by the lungs. *Handbk Physiol., section 3*, **1**, 351

Ryan, U.S. and Ryan, J.W. (1977) Correlations between the fine structure of the alveolar–capillary unit and its metabolic activities. In: *Metabolic Functions of the Lung*, edited by Y.S. Bakhle and J.R. Vane. New York: Marcel Dekker

Safar, P. (1959) Failure of manual respiration. *J. appl. Physiol.* **14**, 84

Safar, P., Escarraga, L.A. and Chang, F. (1959) Upper airway obstruction in the unconscious patient. *J. appl. Physiol.* **14**, 760

Sahn, S.A. (1988) The pleura. *Am. Rev. resp. Dis* **138**, 1

Said, S.I. (1982) Metabolic functions of the pulmonary circulation. *Circulation Res.* **50**, 325

St John, W.M., Glasser, R.L. and King, R.A. (1972) Rhythmic respiration in awake vagotomized cats with chronic pneumotaxic area lesions. *Resp. Physiol.* **15**, 233

Salmoiraghi, G.C. (1963) Functional organization of brain stem respiratory neurones. *Ann. N.Y. Acad. Sci.* **109**, 571

Salmoiraghi, G.C. and Burns, B.D. (1960) Localization and patterns of discharge of respiratory neurones in brain stem of cat. *J. Neurophysiol.* **23**, 2

Salzano, J.V., Camporesi, E.M., Stolp, B.W. and Moon, R.E. (1984) Physiological responses to exercise at 47 and 66 ATA. *J. appl. Physiol.* **57**, 1055

Samet, J.M. (1990) The 1990 Report of the Surgeon General: The health benefits of smoking cessation. *Am. Rev. resp. Dis.* **142**, 993

Sanders, R.D. (1967) Two ventilating attachments for bronchoscopes. *Delaware St. med. J.* **39**, 170

Sant'Ambrogio, G. and Sant'Ambrogio, F.B. (1991) Reflexes from the airway, lung, chest wall and limbs. In: *The Lung: scientific foundations*, p. 1383, edited by R.G. Crystal and J.B. West. New York: Raven Press

Sato, M., Severinghaus, J.W. and Basbaum, A.I. (1991) Medullary CO_2 chemoreceptor neuron identification by c-fos immunochemistry. *FASEB J.* **5**, A1120

Sauerland, E.K., Sauerland, B.A.T., Orr, W.C. and Hairston, L.E. (1981) Non-invasive electromyography of human genioglossal (tongue) activity. *Electromyogr. clin. Neurophysiol.* **21**, 279

Saugstad, O.D., Hallman, M., Abraham, J.L., Epstein, B., Cochrane, C. and Gluck, L. (1984) Hypoxanthine and oxygen induced lung injury: a possible basic mechanism of tissue damage? *Pediat.*

Res. **18,** 501

Schafer, E.A. (1904) Description of a simple and efficient method of performing artificial respiration in the human subject. *Trans. R. med. chir. Soc. London* **87,** 609

Scheidt, M., Hyatt, R.E. and Rehder, K. (1981) Effects of rib cage or abdominal restriction on lung mechanics. *J. appl. Physiol.* **51,** 1115

Schläfke, M.E., Pokorski, M., See, W.R., Prill, R.K. and Loeschcke, H.H. (1975) Chemosensitive neurons on the ventral medullary surface. *Bull. Physio-Pathol. Resp.* **11,** 277

Schmidt, E.R. and Rehder, K. (1981) General anesthesia and the chest wall. *Anesthesiology* **55,** 668

Schmidt, G.B., O'Neill, W.W., Koth, K., Hwang, K.K., Bennett, E.J. and Bombeck, C.T. (1976) Continuous positive airway pressure in the prophylaxis of the adult respiratory distress syndrome. *Surg. Gynec. Obst.* **143,** 613

Schneeberger, E.E. (1991) Alveolar type I cells. In: *The Lung: scientific foundations,* p. 229, edited by R.G. Crystal and J.B. West. New York: Raven Press

Schofield, E.J. and Williams, N.E. (1974) Prediction of arterial carbon dioxide tension using a circle system without carbon dioxide absorption. *Br. J. Anaesth.* **46,** 442

Scholander, P.F. (1947) Analyzer for accurate estimation of respiratory gases in one-half cubic centimeter samples. *J. biol. Chem.* **167,** 235

Schraufnagel, D.E. and Patel, K.R. (1990) Sphincters in pulmonary veins. *Am. Rev. resp. Dis.* **141,** 721

Schwartz, A.R., Smith, P.L., Wise, R.A., Gold, A.R. and Permutt, S. (1988) Induction of upper airway occlusion in sleeping individuals with subatmospheric pressure. *J. appl. Physiol.* **64,** 535

Scott, D.B., Stephen, G.W. and Davie, I.T. (1972) Haemodynamic effects of a negative (subatmospheric) pressure expiratory phase during artificial ventilation. *Br. J. Anaesth.* **44,** 171

Scott, J. (1847) Etherisation and asphyxia. *Lancet* **1,** 355

Sechzer, P.H., Egbert, L.D., Linde, H.W., Cooper, D.Y., Dripps, R.D. and Price, H.L. (1960) Effect of CO_2 inhalation on arterial pressure ECG and plasma catecholamines and 17-OH corticosteroids in normal man. *J. appl. Physiol.* **15,** 454

Seebohm, P.M. and Hamilton, W.K. (1958) A method for measuring nasal resistance without intranasal instrumentation. *J. Allergy* **29,** 56

Seeger, W., Stohr, G., Wolf, H.R.D. and Neufof, H. (1985) Alteration of surfactant function due to protein leakage. *J. appl. Physiol.* **58,** 326

Selman, B.J., White, Y.S. and Tait, A.R. (1975) An evaluation of the Lex-O_2-Con oxygen content analyser. *Anaesthesia* **30,** 206

Semple, S.J.G. (1965) Respiration and the cerebrospinal fluid. *Br. J. Anaesth.* **37,** 262

Senior, R.M., Griffen, G.L. and Mecham, R.P. (1980) Chemotactic activity of elastin-derived peptides. *J. clin. Invest.* **66,** 859

Servetus, M. (1553) *Christianismi Restitutio.* Vienne

Severinghaus, J.W. (1963) High temperature operation of the oxygen electrode giving fast response for respiratory gas sampling. *Clin. Chem.* **9,** 727

Severinghaus, J.W. (1965) Blood gas concentrations. *Handbk Physiol., section 3,* **2,** 1475

Severinghaus, J.W. (1966) Blood gas calculator. *J. appl. Physiol.* **21,** 1108

Severinghaus, J.W. (1976) Proposed standard determination of ventilatory responses to hypoxia and hypercapnia in man. *Chest* **70,** 129S

Severinghaus, J.W. (1981) A combined transcutaneous Po_2–Pco_2 electrode with electrochemical HCO_3^- stabilization. *J. appl. Physiol.* **51,** 1027

Severinghaus, J.W. (1992) Respiratory control related to altitude and anesthesia. In: *Anesthesia and the Lung,* p. 97, edited by T.H. Stanley and R.J. Sperry. Dordrecht: Kluwer

Severinghaus, J.W. and Astrup, P.B. (1986) History of blood gas analysis. III. Carbon dioxide tension. *J. clin. Monitor.* **2,** 60

Severinghaus, J.W. and Bradley, A.F. (1958) Electrodes for blood Po_2 and Pco_2 determination. *J. appl. Physiol.* **13,** 515

Severinghaus, J.W. and Kelleher (1992) Recent developments in pulse oximetry. *Anesthesiology* **76,** 1018

Severinghaus, J.W. and Koh, S.O. (1990) Effect of anemia on pulse oximeter accuracy at low saturation. *J. clin. Monitor.* **6,** 85

Severinghaus, J.W. and Mitchell, R.A. (1962) Ondine's curse: failure of respiratory center automaticity while awake. *Clin. Res.* **10,** 122

Severinghaus, J.W. and Spellman, M.J. (1990) Pulse oximeter failure thresholds in hypotension and vasoconstriction. *Anesthesiology* **73,** 532

Severinghaus, J.W. and Stupfel, M. (1955) Respiratory dead space increase following atropine in man, and atropine, vagal or ganglionic blockade and hypothermia in dogs. *J. appl. Physiol.* **8,** 81

Severinghaus, J.W. and Stupfel, M. (1957) Alveolar dead space as an index of distribution of blood flow in pulmonary capillaries. *J. appl. Physiol.* **10,** 335

Severinghaus, J.W., Stafford, M. and Thunstrom, A.M. (1978) Estimation of skin metabolism and blood flow with $tcPO_2$ and $tcPCO_2$ electrodes by cuff occlusion of the circulation. *Acta anaesth. scand.* **68,** 9

Severinghaus, J.W., Stupfel, M. and Bradley, A.F. (1956a) Accuracy of blood pH and P_{CO_2} determinations. *J. appl. Physiol.* **9,** 189

Severinghaus, J.W., Stupfel, M. and Bradley, A.F. (1956b) Variations of serum carbonic acid pK' with pH and temperature. *J. appl. Physiol.* **9,** 197

Severinghaus, J.W., Mitchell, R.A., Richardson, B.W. and Singer, M.M. (1963) Respiratory control at high altitude suggesting active transport regulation of CSF pH. *J. appl. Physiol.* **18,** 1153

Severinghaus, J.W., Sato, M., Powell, F., Jensen, J.B., Sperling, B. and Lassen, N.A. (1991) Altitude acclimatization slowly augments hypoxic responses of ventilation and cerebral circulation. *Clin. Res.* **39,** 387A

Shafer, A.W., Tague, L.L., Welch, M.H. and Guenter, C.A. (1971) 2,3-Diphosphoglycerate in red cells stored in acid–citrate–dextrose and citrate–phosphate–dextrose. *J. Lab. clin. Med.* **77,** 430

Shammea, M.H., Nasrallah, S.M. and Al-Khalidi, U.A.S. (1973) Serum xanthine oxidase. *Dig. Dis.* **18,** 15

Shappell, S.D. and Lenfant, C.J.M. (1972) Adaptive, genetic and iatrogenic alterations of the oxyhemoglobin-dissociation curve. *Anesthesiology* **37,** 127

Sharp, G.R., Ledingham, I. McA. and Norman, J.N. (1962) The application of oxygen at 2 atmospheres pressure in the treatment of acute anoxia. *Anaesthesia* **17,** 136

Sharpey-Schafer, E.P. (1953) Effects of coughing on intra-thoracic pressure, arterial pressure and peripheral blood flow. *J. Physiol.* **122,** 351

Shaw, I.H., Kirk, A.J.B. and Conacher, I.D. (1991) Anaesthesia for patients with transplanted hearts and lungs undergoing non-cardiac surgery. *Br. J. Anaesth.* **67,** 772

Shaw, L.A. and Messer, A.C. (1932) The transfer of bicarbonate ion between the blood and tissues caused by alterations of the carbon dioxide concentrations in the lungs. *Am. J. Physiol.* **100,** 122

Shenkin, H.A. and Bouzarth, W.F. (1970) Clinical methods of reducing intracranial pressure. *New Engl. J. Med.* **282,** 1465

Shepard, R.H., Campbell, E.J.M., Martin, H.B. and Enns, T. (1957) Factors affecting the pulmonary dead space as determined by single breath analysis. *J. appl. Physiol.* **11,** 241

Shephard, R.J. (1967) The maximum sustained voluntary ventilation in exercise. *Clin. Sci.* **32,** 167

Shigeoka, J.W., Colice, G.L. and Ramirez, G. (1985) Effect of normoxemic and hypoxemic exercise on renin and aldosterone. *J. appl. Physiol.* **59,** 142

Shoemaker, W.C., Bland, R.D. and Appel, P.L. (1985) Therapy of critically ill postoperative patients based on outcome prediction and prospective clinical trials. *Surg. Clins N. Am.* **65,** 811

Sibbald, W.I. and Dredger, A.A. (1983) Right ventricular function in acute disease states. *Crit. Care Med.* **11,** 339

Sibbald, W.J., Anderson, R.R., Reid, B., Holliday, R.L. and Driedger, A.A. (1981) Alveolocapillary permeability in human septic ARDS. *Chest* **79,** 133

Siesjö, B.K. and Nilsson, L. (1971) The influence of arterial hypoxaemia upon labile phosphates and upon extracellular and intracellular lactate and pyruvate concentrations in the rat brain. *Scand. J. clin. Lab. Invest.* **27,** 83

Siggaard-Andersen, O. (1962) The pH, log pCO_2 blood acid–base nomogram revised. *Scand. J. clin. Lab. Invest.* **14,** 598

Siggaard-Andersen, O. (1964) *The Acid–Base Status of Blood.* Copenhagen: Munksgaard

Siggaard-Andersen, O., Engel, K., Jorgensen, K. and Astrup, P. (1960) A micro-method for determination of pH, carbon dioxide tension, base excess and standard bicarbonate in capillary blood. *Scand. J. clin. Lab. Invest.* **12,** 172

Silvester, H.R. (1857) The natural method of treating asphyxia. *Med. Times Gaz.* **11**, 485

Simani, A.S., Inoue, S. and Hogg, J.C. (1974) Penetration of the respiratory epithelium of guinea pigs following exposure to cigarette smoke. *Lab. Invest.* **31**, 75

Simcock, A.D. (1986) Treatment of near drowning – a review of 130 cases. *Anaesthesia* **41**, 643

Simionescu, M. (1980) Ultrastructural organization of the alveolar–capillary unit. In: *Metabolic Activities of the Lung.* Ciba Foundation Symposium no. 78. Amsterdam: Excerpta Medica

Simionescu, M. (1991) Lung endothelium: structure–function correlates. In: *The Lung: scientific foundations*, p. 301, edited by R.G. Crystal and J.B. West. New York: Raven Press

Singer, M.M., Wright, F., Stanley, L.K., Roe, B.B. and Hamilton, W.K. (1970) Oxygen toxicity in man. A prospective study in patients after open-heart surgery. *New Engl. J. Med.* **283**, 1473

Singhal, S., Henderson, R., Horsfield, K., Harding, K. and Cumming, G. (1973) Morphometry of the human pulmonary arterial tree. *Circulation Res.* **33**, 190

Sjöstrand, U. (1980) High-frequency positive-pressure ventilation (HFPPV): a review. *Crit. Care Med.* **8**, 345

Skootsky, S.A. and Abraham, E. (1988) Continuous oxygen consumption measurement during initial emergency department resuscitation of critically ill patients. *Crit. Care Med.* **16**, 706

Slavin, G., Nunn, J.F., Crow, J. and Dore, C.J. (1982) Bronchiolectasis – a complication of artificial ventilation. *Br. med. J.* **285**, 931

Slome, D. (1965) Physiology of respiration. In: *General Anaesthesia*, vol. 1, 2nd edn, edited by F.T. Evans and T.C. Gray. London and Boston, Mass: Butterworths

Slutsky, A.S. (1988) Nonconventional methods of ventilation. *Am. Rev. resp. Dis.* **138**, 175

Smith, A.L. and Wollman, H. (1972) Cerebral blood flow and metabolism. *Anesthesiology* **36**, 378

Smith, B.E. (1990) High frequency ventilation: past, present and future? *Br. J. Anaesth.* **65**, 130

Smith, B.E.. and Hanning, C.D. (1986) Advances in respiratory support. *Br. J. Anaesth.* **58**, 138

Smith, G. and Lawson, D.A. (1958) Experimental coronary arterial occlusion: effects of the administration of oxygen under pressure. *Scott. med. J.* **3**, 346

Smith, G., Stevens, J., Griffiths, J.C. and Ledingham, I.McA. (1961) Near avulsion of foot treated by replacement and subsequent prolonged exposure of patient to oxygen at two atmospheres pressure. *Lancet* **2**, 1122

Smith, H. and Pask, E.A. (1959) Method for the estimation of oxygen in gas mixtures containing nitrous oxide. *Br. J. Anaesth.* **31**, 440

Smith, W.D.A. (1964) The measurement of uptake of nitrous oxide by pneumotachography. I. Apparatus, methods and accuracy. *Br. J. Anaesth.* **36**, 363

Smithies, M.N., Royston, K., Makita, K., Konieczko, K. and Nunn, J.F. (1991) Comparison of oxygen consumption measurements: indirect calorimetry versus the reversed Fick method. *Crit. Care Med.* **19**, 1401

Snow, J. (1858) *On Chloroform and other Anaesthetics; their action and administration.* London: John Churchill

Sobin, S.S., Fung, Y.C., Tremer, H.M. and Rosenquist, T.H. (1972) Elasticity of the pulmonary alveolar microvascular sheet in the cat. *Circulation Res.* **30**, 440

Sole, M.J., Dobrac, M., Schwartz, L., Hussain, M.N. and Vaughan-Neil, E.F. (1979) The extraction of circulating catecholamines by the lungs in normal man and in patients with pulmonary hypertension. *Circulation* **60**, 160

Southall, D.P. and Samuels, M.P. (1992) Reducing risks in the sudden infant death syndrome. *Br. med. J.* **304**, 265

Southall, D.P., Talbert, D.G., Johnson, P., Morley, C.J., Salmons, S., Miller, J. and Helms, P.J. (1985) Prolonged expiratory apnoea: a disorder resulting in episodes of severe arterial hypoxaemia in infants and young children. *Lancet* **2**, 571

Speck, D.F. and Beck, E.R. (1989) Respiratory rhythmicity after extensive lesions of the dorsal and ventral respiratory groups in the decerebrate cat. *Brain Res.* **482**, 387

Spence, A.A. and Ellis, F.R. (1971) A critical evaluation of a nitrogen rebreathing method for the estimation of $P\bar{v}_{O_2}$. *Resp. Physiol.* **10**, 313

Staněk, V., Widimisky, J., Kasalicky, J., Navratil, M., Daum, S. and Levinsky, L. (1967) The pulmonary gas exchange during exercise in patients with pulmonary fibrosis. *Scand. J. resp. Dis.* **48**, 11

Stanley, T.H., Zikria, B.A. and Sullivan, S.F. (1972) The surface tension of tracheobronchial secretions during general anesthesia. *Anesthesiology* **37**, 445

Stark, D.C.C. and Smith, H. (1960) Pulmonary vascular changes during anesthesia. *Br. J. Anaesth.* **32**, 460

Starling, E.H. and Verney, E.B. (1925) The secretion of urine as studied in the isolated kidney. *Proc. R. Soc. B* **97**, 321

Staub, N.C. (1963a) Alveolar–arterial oxygen tension gradient due to diffusion. *J. appl. Physiol.* **18**, 673

Staub, N.C. (1963b) The interdependence of pulmonary structure and function. *Anesthesiology* **24**, 831

Staub, N.C. (1974) Pulmonary edema. *Physiol. Rev.* **54**, 679

Staub, N.A. (1983) Alveolar flooding and clearance. *Am. Rev. resp. Dis.* **127**, S44

Staub, N.A. (1984) Pathophysiology of pulmonary edema. In: *Edema*, edited by N.A. Staub and A.E. Taylor. New York: Raven Press

Staub, N.C., Bishop, J.M. and Forster, R.E. (1961) Importance of diffusion and chemical blood cells. *J. appl. Physiol.* **16**, 511

Staub, N.C., Bishop, J.M. and Forster, R.E. (1962) Importance of diffusion and chemical reaction rates in O_2 uptake in the lung. *J. appl. Physiol.* **17**, 21

Stein, M., Forkner, C.E., Robin, E.D. and Wessler, S. (1961) Gas exchange after autologous pulmonary embolism in dogs. *J. appl. Physiol.* **16**, 488

Stephenson, J.A.E. and Scourfield, M.W.J. (1991) Importance of energetic solar protons in ozone depletion. *Nature* **352**, 137

Stevens, J.H. and Raffin, T.A. (1984) Adult respiratory distress syndrome – 1. Aetiology and mechanisms. *Postgrad. med. J.* **60**, 505

Stock, M.C., Downs, J.B., McDonald, J.S., Silver, M.J., McSweeney, T.D. and Fairley, D.S. (1988) The carbon dioxide rate of rise in awake apneic humans. *J. clin. Anesth.* **1**, 96

Strang, L.B. (1959) The ventilatory capacity of normal children. *Thorax* **14**, 305

Strang, L.B. (1965) The lungs at birth. *Archs Dis. Childh.* **40**, 575

Sturrock, J.E. and Hulands, G.H. (1980) Protective effect of steroids on cultured cells damaged by high concentrations of oxygen. *Br. J. Anaesth.* **52**, 567

Sturrock, J.E. and Nunn, J.F. (1978) Chromosomal damage and mutations after exposure of Chinese hamster cells to high concentrations of oxygen. *Mutation Res.* **57**, 27

Suggett, A.J., Barer, G.R., Mohammed, F.H. and Gill, G.W. (1982) The effects of localized hypoventilation on ventilation/perfusion ratios and gas exchange in the dog lung. *Clin. Sci.* **63**, 497

Sugihara, T., Hildebrandt, J. and Martin, C.J. (1972) Viscoelastic properties of alveolar wall. *J. appl. Physiol.* **33**, 93

Sullivan, C.E., Berton-Jones, M. and Issa, F.G. (1983) Remission of severe obesity hypoventilation syndrome following short-term treatment during sleep with nasal continuous positive airway pressure. *Am. Rev. resp. Dis.* **128**, 177

Surratt, P.M., Turner, B.L. and Wilhoit, S.C. (1986) Effect of intranasal obstruction on breathing during sleep. *Chest* **90**, 325

Suter, P.M., Fairley, H.B. and Isenberg, M.D. (1975) Optimum end-expiratory airway pressure in patients with acute pulmonary failure. *New Engl. J. Med.* **292**, 284

Sutton, J.T., Reeves, J.T., Wagner, P.D., Groves, B.M., Cymerman, A., Malconian, M.K. et al. (1988) Operation Everest II: oxygen transport during exercise at extreme simulated altitude. *J. appl. Physiol.* **64**, 1309

Svanberg, L. (1957) Influence of posture on lung volumes, ventilation and circulation in normals. *Scand. J. clin. Lab. Invest.* **9**, suppl. 25

Svensson, K.L., Sonander, H.G. and Stenqvist, O. (1990) Validation of a system for measurement of metabolic gas exchange during anaesthesia with controlled ventilation in an oxygen consuming lung model. *Br. J. Anaesth.* **64**, 311

de Sweit, M. (1980) The respiratory system. In: *Clinical Physiology in Obstetrics*, p. 79, edited by F. Hytten. Oxford: Blackwell Scientific

Swyer, P.R. (1975) (ed.) *The Intensive Care of the Newly Born*. Monographs in Paediatrics no. 6. Basel: Karger

Sykes, M.K. (1960) Observations on a rebreathing technique for the determination of arterial P_{CO_2} in the apnoeic patient. *Br. J. Anaesth.* **32**, 256

Sykes, M.K. (1986) Effects of anesthetics and drugs used during anesthesia on the pulmonary circulation. In: *Cardiovascular Actions of Anesthetics*, edited by B.M. Altura and S. Halevy. Basel: Karger

Sykes, M.K. and Lumley, J. (1969) The effect of varying inspiratory:expiratory ratios during anaesthesia for open-heart surgery. *Br. J. Anaesth.* **41**, 374

Sykes, M.K., Adams, A.P., Finlay, W.E.I., McCormick, P.W. and Economider, A. (1970) The effect of variations in end-expiratory inflation pressure on cardiorespiratory function in normo-, hypo-, and hyper-volaemic dogs. *Br. J. Anaesth.* **42**, 669

Sykes, M.K., Loh, L., Seed, R.F., Kafer, E.R. and Chakrabarti, M.K. (1972) The effect of inhalational anaesthetics on hypoxic pulmonary vasoconstriction and pulmonary vascular resistance in the perfused lungs of the dog and cat. *Br. J. Anaesth.* **44**, 776

Taghizadeh, A. and Reynolds, E.O.R. (1976) Pathogenesis of bronchopulmonary dysplasia following hyaline membrane disease. *Am. J. Pathol.* **82** (2), 241

Takala, J., Keinanen, O., Vaisanen, P. and Kari, A. (1989) Measurement of gas exchange in intensive care: laboratory and clinical validation of a new device. *Crit. Care Med.* **17**, 1041

Tangel, D.J., Mezzanotte, W.S. and White, D.P. (1991) Influence of sleep on tensor palatini EMG and upper airway resistance in normal men. *J. appl. Physiol.* **70**, 2574

Tantucci, C., Corbeil, C., Chassé, M., Robatto, F.M., Nava, S., Braidy, J., Matar, N. and Milic-Emili, J. (1992) Flow and volume dependence of respiratory system flow resistance in patients with the adult respiratory distress syndrome. *Am. Rev. resp. Dis.* **145**, 355

Tate, R.M. and Repine, J.E. (1983) Neutrophils and the adult respiratory distress syndrome. *Am. Rev. resp. Dis.* **127**, 552

Taylor, S.H., Scott, D.B. and Donald, K.W. (1964) Respiratory effect of general anaesthesia. *Lancet* **1**, 841

Tennenberg, S.D., Jacobs, M.P., Solomkin, J.S. and Ehlers, N.A. (1987) Increased pulmonary alveolar–capillary permeability in patients at risk for ARDS. *Crit. Care Med.* **15**, 409

Tenney, S.M. (1956) Sympatho-adrenal stimulation by carbon dioxide and the inhibitory effect of carbonic acid on epinephrine response. *Am. J. Physiol.* **187**, 341

Tenney, S.M. (1960) The effect of carbon dioxide on neurohumoral and endocrine mechanisms. *Anesthesiology* **21**, 674

Tenney, S.M. and Lamb, T.W. (1965) Physiological consequences of hypoventilation and hyperventilation. *Handbk Physiol.*, section 3, **2**, 979

Thews, G. (1961) In: *Bad Oeynhausener Gespräche*, IV, edited by H. Bartels and E. Witzleb, Berlin: Springer

Theye, R.A. and Tuohy, G.F. (1964a) Oxygen uptake during light halothane anesthesia in man. *Anesthesiology* **25**, 627

Theye, R.A. and Tuohy, G.F. (1964b) Considerations in the determination of oxygen uptake and ventilatory performance during methoxyflurane anesthesia in man. *Curr. Res. Anesth. Analg.* **43**, 306

Thilenius, O.G. (1966) Effect of anesthesia on response of pulmonary circulation of dogs to acute hypoxia. *J. appl. Physiol.* **21**, 901

Thom, S.R. (1989) Hyperbaric oxygen therapy. *J. int. Care Med.* **4**, 58

Thomas, D.P. and Vane, J.R. (1967) 5-Hydroxytryptamine in the circulation of the dog. *Nature* **216**, 335

Thompson, S.P. (1965) *Calculus Made Easy.* London: Macmillan

Thoning, K.W., Tans, P.P. and Komhyr, W.D. (1989) Atmospheric carbon dioxide at Mauna Loa observatory. *J. geophys. Res.* **94**, 8549

Thornton, J.A. (1960) Physiological dead space: changes during general anaesthesia. *Anaesthesia* **15**, 381

Thornton, J.A. and Nunn, J.F. (1960) Accuracy of determination of P_{CO_2} by the indirect method. *Guy's Hosp. Rep.* **109**, 203

Tibes, U. (1977) Reflex inputs to the cardiovascular and respiratory centers from dynamically working canine muscles. *Circulation Res.* **41**, 332

Tierney, D.F. and Young, S.L. (1985) Glucose and intermediary metabolism of the lungs. *Handbk Physiol.* section 3, **1**, 255

Timms, R.M., Khaja, F.U. and Williams, G.W. (1985) Hemodynamic response to oxygen therapy in chronic obstructive pulmonary disease. *Ann. intern. Med.* **102**, 29

Tobin, C.E. and Zariquiey, M.O. (1950) Arteriovenous shunts in the human lung. *Proc. Soc. exp. Biol. Med.* **75,** 827

Tockman, M., Menkes, H., Cohen, B., Permutt, S., Benjamin, J., Ball, W.C. and Tonascia, J. (1976) A comparison of pulmonary function in male smokers and non-smokers. *Am. Rev. resp. Dis.* **114,** 711

Tod, M.L. and Cassin, S. (1991) Fetal and neonatal pulmonary circulation. In: *The Lung: scientific foundations*, p. 1687, edited by R.G. Crystal and J.B. West. New York: Raven Press

Tokics, L., Hedenstierna, G., Brismar, B., Lundquist, H. and Hedenstierna, G. (1987) Lung collapse and gas exchange during general anaesthesia. *Anesthesiology* **66,** 157

The Toronto Lung Transplant Group. (1988) Experience with single lung transplantation for pulmonary fibrosis. *J. Am. med. Assoc.* **259,** 2258

Torrance, J., Jacobs, P., Restrepo, A., Eschbach, J., Lenfant, C. and Finch, C.A. (1970) Intraerythrocytic adaptation to anemia. *New Engl. J. Med.* **283,** 165

Traystman, R.J., Kirsch, J.R. and Koehler, R.C. (1991) Oxygen radical mechanisms of brain injury following ischaemia and reperfusion. *J. appl. Physiol.* **71,** 1185

Trichet, B., Falke, K., Togut, A. and Laver, M.B. (1975). The effect of pre-existing pulmonary vascular disease on the response to mechanical ventilation with PEEP following open-heart surgery. *Anesthesiology* **42,** 56

Trinkle, J.K., Richardson, J.D., Franz, J.L., Grover, F.L., Aron, K.V. and Holmstrom, F.M.G. (1975) Management of flail chest without mechanical ventilation. *Ann. thorac. Sug.* **19,** 355

Tsukimoto, K., Mathieu-Costello, O., Prediletto, R., Elliott, A.R. and West, J.B. (1991) Ultrastructural appearances of pulmonary capillaries at high transmural pressures. *J. appl. Physiol.* **71,** 573

Turner, J.E., Lambertsen, C.J., Owen, S.G., Wendel, H. and Chiodi, H. (1957) Effects of 0.08 and 0.8 atmospheres of inspired P_{O_2} upon cerebral hemodynamics at a 'constant' alveolar P_{CO_2} of 43 mm Hg. *Fedn Proc.* **16,** 130

Turrens, J.F., Crapo, J.D. and Freeman, B.A. (1984) Protection against oxygen toxicity by intravenous injection of liposome-entrapped catalase and superoxide dismutase. *J. clin. Invest.* **73,** 87

Tusiewicz, K., Bryan, A.C. and Froese, A.B. (1977) Contributions of changing rib cage–diaphragm interactions to the ventilatory depression of halothane anesthesia. *Anesthesiology* **47,** 327

Tyler, S.A. and Barghoorn, E.S. (1954) Occurrence of structurally preserved plants in pre-Cambrian rocks of the Canadian shield. *Science* **119,** 606

Ullman, E. (1970) About Hering and Breuer. In: *Breathing: Hering–Breuer Centenary Symposium*, p. 3, edited by R. Porter. Edinburgh and London: Churchill Livingstone

Urbaniak, S.J. (1991) Artificial blood. *Br. med. J.* **303,** 1348

Utting, J.E. (1980) Hypocapnia. In: *General Anaesthesia*, 4th edn, vol. 1, edited by T.C. Gray, J.F. Nunn and J.E. Utting. London: Butterworths

Valentine, D.D., Hammond, M.D., Downs, J.B., Sears, N.J. and Sims, W.R. (1991) Distribution of ventilation and perfusion with different modes of mechanical ventilation. *Am. Rev. resp. Dis.* **143,** 1262

Valeri, C.R. (1975) Blood components in the treatment of acute blood loss, use of freeze-preserved red cells, platelets, and the plasma proteins. *Anesth. Analg.* **54,** 1

Vanhoutte, P.M. (1988) Epithelium-derived relaxing factor(s) and bronchial reactivity. *Am. Rev. resp. Dis.* **138,** S24

Van Slyke, D.D. and Neill, J.M. (1924) The determination of gases in blood and other solutions by vacuum extraction and monometric measurement. *J. biol. Chem.* **61,** 523

Vance, J.P., Brown, D.M. and Smith, G. (1973) The effects of hypocapnia on myocardial blood flow and metabolism. *Br. J. Anaesth.* **45,** 455

Vane, J.R. (1969) The release and fate of vaso-active hormones in the circulation. *Br. J. Pharmac.* **35,** 209

Vann, R.D. (1982) Decompression theory and application. In: *The Physiology and Medicine of Diving*, edited by P.B. Bennett and D.H. Elliott. London: Baillière Tindall

Velasquez, T. and Farhi, L.E. (1964) Effect of negative pressure breathing on lung mechanics and venous admixture. *J. appl. Physiol.* **19,** 665

Vellody, V.P.S., Nassery, M., Balasaraswathi, K., Goldberg, N.G. and Sharp, J.T. (1978) Compliances of human rib cage and diaphragm–abdomen pathways in relaxed versus paralyzed states. *Am. Rev. resp. Dis.* **118,** 479

Verloop, M.C. (1948) The arteriae bronchiales and their anastomoses with the arteria pulmonalis in the human lung: a micro-anatomical study. *Acta anat.* **5,** 171

Virgil, Publius Vergilus Marto (19 BC) *The Aeneid,* Book II, p. 1

Viteri, F.E. and Torún, B. (1974) Anaemia and physical work capacity. In: *Clinics in Hematology,* vol. 3, pp. 609–26, edited by L. Garby. London: W. B. Saunders

Wade, J.G., Larson, C.P., Hickey, R.F., Ehrenfeld, W.K. and Severinghaus, J.W. (1970) Effect of carotid endarterectomy on carotid chemoreceptor and baroreceptor function in man. *New Engl. J. Med.* **282,** 823

Wade, O.L. and Gilson, J.C. (1951) The effect of posture on diaphragmatic movement and vital capacity in normal subjects. *Thorax* **6,** 103

Wagner, P.D., Naumann, P.F. and Laravuso, R.B. (1974) Simultaneous measurements of eight foreign gases in blood by gas chromatography. *J. appl. Physiol.* **36,** 600

Wagner, P.D., Saltzman, H.A. and West, J.B. (1974) Measurement of continuous distribution of ventilation–perfusion ratios: theory. *J. appl. Physiol.* **36,** 588

Wagner, P.D., Laravuso, R.B., Uhl, R.R. and West, J.B. (1974) Continuous distributions of ventilation–perfusion ratios in normal subjects breathing air and 100% O_2. *J. clin. Invest.* **54,** 54

Wagner, P.D., Laravuso, R.B., Goldzimmer, E., Naumann, P.F. and West, J.B. (1975) Distribution of ventilation–perfusion ratios in dogs in normal and abnormal lungs. *J. appl. Physiol.* **38,** 1099

Wagner, P.D., Sutton, J.T., Reeves, J.T., Cymerman, A., Groves, B.M. and Malconian, M.K. (1987) Operation Everest II: pulmonary gas exchange during a simulated ascent of Mt Everest. *J. appl. Physiol.* **63,** 2348

Wahba, R.W.M. (1990) Pressure support ventilation. *J. cardiothor. Anesth.* **4,** 624

Wahba, R.W.M. (1991) Perioperative functional residual capacity. *Can. J. Anaesth.* **38,** 384

Walder, D.N. (1982) The compressed air environment. In: *The Physiology and Medicine of Diving,* edited by P.B. Bennett and D.H. Elliott. London: Baillière Tindall

Walter, M.R., Buick, R. and Dunlop, J.S.R. (1980) Stromatolites 3,400–3,500 Myr old from the North Pole area, Western Australia. *Nature* **284,** 443

Wang, S.C., Ngai, S.H. and Frumin, M.J. (1957) Organization of central respiratory mechanisms in the brain stem of the cat: genesis of normal respiratory rhythmicity. *Am. J. Physiol.* **190,** 333

Ward, M.P., Milledge, J.S. and West, J.B. (1989) *High Altitude Medicine and Physiology.* London: Chapman & Hall

Warrell, D.A., Evans, J.W., Clarke, R.O., Kingaby, G.P. and West, J.B. (1972) Pattern of filling in the pulmonary capillary bed. *J. appl. Physiol.* **32,** 346

Warren, B.A. (1963) Fibrinolytic properties of vascular endothelium. *Br. J. exp. Path.* **44,** 365

Warren, J.B., Maltby, N.H., MacCormack, D. and Barnes, P.J. (1989) Pulmonary endothelium-derived relaxing factor is impaired in hypoxia. *Clin. Sci.* **77,** 671.

Wasserman, K. (1978) Breathing during exercise. *New Engl. J. Med.* **298,** 780

Watson, W.E. (1962a) Some observations on dynamic lung compliance during intermittent positive pressure respiration. *Br. J. Anaesth.* **34,** 153

Watson, W.E. (1962b) Observations on physiological dead space during intermittent positive pressure respiration. *Br. J. Anaesth.* **34,** 502

Wayne, D.J. and Chamney, A.R. (1969) Oxygen tents. *Anaesthesia* **24,** 591

Weatherall, D.J., Ledingham, J.G.G. and Warrell, D.A. (1983) (eds) *Oxford Textbook of Medicine.* Oxford: Oxford University Press

Webb, S.J.S. and Nunn, J.F. (1967) A comparison between the effect of nitrous oxide and nitrogen on arterial P_{O_2}. *Anaesthesia* **22,** 69

Webb, W.R. (1984) Metabolic effects of fructose diphosphate in hypoxic and ischaemic states. *Thorac. Cardiovasc. Surg.* **88,** 863

Webster, N.R. and Nunn, J.F. (1988) Molecular structure of free radicals and their importance in biological reactions. *Br. J. Anaesth.* **60,** 98

Webster, N.R., Cohen, A.T. and Nunn, J.F. (1988) Adult respiratory distress syndrome – how many cases in the UK? *Anaesthesia* **43,** 923

Weibel, E.R. (1962) Morphometrische Bestimmung von Zahl, Volumen und Oberfläche der Alveolen und Kapillaren der menschlichen Lunge. *Z. Zellforsch. mikrosk. Anat.* **57,** 648

Weibel, E.R. (1963) *Morphometry of the Human Lung.* Berlin: Springer

Weibel, E.R. (1964) Morphometrics of the lung. *Handbk Physiol., section 3*, **1**, 285

Weibel, E.R. (1971) Oxygen effect on lung cells. *Archs intern. Med.* **128**, 54

Weibel, E.R. (1973) Morphological basis of alveolar–capillary gas exchange. *Physiol. Rev.* **53**, 419

Weibel, E.R. (1983) How does lung structure affect gas exchange. *Chest* **83**, 657

Weibel, E.R. (1984) *The Pathway for Oxygen*. Cambridge, Mass: Harvard University Press

Weibel, E.R. (1985) Lung cell biology. *Handbk Physiol., section 3*, **1**, 47

Weibel, E.R. (1991a) Design of airways and blood vessels considered as branching trees. In: *The Lung: scientific foundations*, p. 711, edited by R.G. Crystal and J.B. West. New York: Raven Press

Weibel. E.R. (1991b) Design and morphometry of the pulmonary gas exchanger. In: *The Lung: scientific foundations*, p. 795, edited by R.G. Crystal and J.B. West. New York: Raven Press

Weibel, E.R. and Bachofen, H. (1991) The fiber scaffold of lung parynchyma. In: *The Lung: scientific foundations*, p. 787, edited by R.G. Crystal and J.B. West. New York: Raven Press

Weibel, E.R. and Gil, J. (1968) Electron microscopic demonstration of an extracellular duplex lining layer of alveoli. *Resp. Physiol.* **4**, 42

Weibel, E.R. and Gomez, D.M. (1962) Architecture of the human lung. *Science* **137**, 577

Weigelt, J.A., Norcross, J.F., Borman, K.R. and Snyder, W.H. (1985) Early steroid therapy for respiratory failure. *Archs Surg.* **120**, 536

Weil, J.V., Byrne-Quinn, E., Sodal, I.D., Friessen, W.O., Underhill, B., Filley, G.F. and Grover, R.F. (1970) Hypoxic ventilatory drive in normal man. *J. clin. Invest.* **49**, 1061

Weil, J.V.W., Byrne-Quinn, E., Sodal, I.E., Filley, G.F. and Grover, R.F. (1971) Acquired attenuation of chemoreceptor function in chronically hypoxic man at high altitude. *J. clin. Invest.* **50**, 186

Weil, J.V., Byrne-Quinn, E., Sodal, I.E., Kline, J.S., McCullough, R.E. and Filley, G.F. (1972) Augmentation of chemosensitivity during mild exercise in normal man. *J. appl. Physiol.* **33**, 813

Weiland, J.E., Davis, W.B., Holter, J.F., Mohammed, J.R., Dorinsky, P.M and Gadek, J.E. (1986) Lung neutrophils in the adult respiratory distress syndrome. *Am. Rev. resp. Dis.* **133**, 218

Weiner-Kronish, J.P., Gropper, M.A. and Matthay, M.A. (1990) The adult respiratory distress syndrome: definition and prognosis, pathogenesis and treatment. *Br. J. Anaesth.* **65**, 107

Weiskopf, R.B. and Severinghaus, J.W. (1972) Lack of effect of high altitude on hemoglobin oxygen affinity. *J. appl. Physiol.* **33**, 276

Weiskopf, R.B., Nishimura, M. and Severinghaus, J.W. (1971) The absence of an effect of halothane on blood hemoglobin O_2 equilibrium *in vitro*. *Anesthesiology* **35**, 579

Weiskopf, R.B., Raymond, L.W. and Severinghaus, J.W. (1974) Effects of halothane on canine respiratory responses to hypoxia with and without hypercarbia. *Anesthesiology* **41**, 350

Weisman, I.M., Rinaldo, J.E., Rogers, R.M. and Sanders, M.H. (1983) Intermittent mandatory ventilation. *Am. Rev. resp. Dis.* **127**, 641

West, J.B. (1962) Regional differences in gas exchange in the lung of erect man. *J. appl. Physiol.* **17**, 893

West, J.B. (1963) Distribution of gas and blood in the normal lung. *Br. med. Bull.* **19**, 53

West, J.B. (1974) Blood flow to the lung and gas exchange. *Anesthesiology* **41**, 124

West, J.B. (1986) Highest inhabitants in the world. *Nature* **324**, 517

West, J.B. (1990) *Ventilation: Blood Flow and Gas Exchange*, 5th edn. Oxford: Blackwell Scientific

West, J.B. (1991) Space. In: *The Lung: scientific foundations*, p. 2133, edited by R.G. Crystal and J.B. West. New York: Raven Press

West, J.B. (1992a) Gravity and the lung: lessons from space. In: *Anesthesia and the Lung*, p. 1, edited by T.H. Standley and R.J. Sperry. Dordrecht: Kluwer

West, J.B. (1992b) Severe hypoxia: insights from extreme altitude. In: *Anesthesia and the Lung*, p. 97, edited by T.H. Standley and R.J. Sperry. Dordrecht: Kluwer

West, J.B. (1992c) Life in space. *J. appl. Physiol.* **72**, 1623

West, J.B. and Dollery, C.T. (1965) Distribution of blood flow and the pressure–flow relations of the whole lung. *J. appl. Physiol.* **20**, 175

West, J.B., Dollery, C.T. and Naimark, A. (1964) Distribution of blood flow in isolated lung: relation to vascular and alveolar pressures. *J. appl. Physiol.* **19**, 713

West, J.W., Lahiri, S., Gill, M.B., Milledge, J.S., Pugh, L.G.C.E. and Ward, M.P. (1962) Arterial oxygen saturation during exercise at high altitude. *J. appl. Physiol.* **17**, 617

West, J.B., Boyer, S.J., Graber, D.J. et al. (1983a) Maximal exercise at extreme altitudes on Mount

642 References and further reading

Everest. *J. appl. Physiol.* **55,** 688

West, J.B., Hackett, P.H., Maret, K.H. et al. (1983b) Pulmonary gas exchange on the summit of Mount Everest. *J. appl. Physiol.* **55,** 678

West, J.B., Peters, R.M., Aksnes, G., Maret, K.H., Milledge, J.S. and Schoene, R.B. (1986) Nocturnal periodic breathing at altitudes of 6300 and 8050 metres. *J. appl. Physiol.* **61**

West, J.B., Tsukimoto, K., Mathieu-Costello, O. and Prediletto, R. (1991) Stress failure in pulmonary capillaries. *J. appl. Physiol.* **70,** 1731

Westbrook, P.R., Stubbs, S.E., Sessler, A.D., Rehder, K. and Hyatt, R.E. (1973) Effects of anesthesia and muscle paralysis on respiratory mechanics in normal man. *J. appl. Physiol.* **34,** 81

Western, P.J. and Patrick, J.M. (1988) Effects of focussing attention on breathing with and without apparatus on the face. *Resp. Physiol.* **72,** 123

Westlake, E.K., Simpson, T. and Kaye, M. (1955) Carbon dioxide narcosis in emphysema. *Q. Jl Med.* **24,** 155

Wheatley, J.R., Kelley, W.T., Tully, A. and Engel, L.A. (1991) Pressure–diameter relationships in the upper airway in awake supine subjects. *J. appl. Physiol.* **70,** 2242

Whillis, J. (1930) A note on the muscles of the palate and the superior constrictor. *J. Anat.* **65,** 92

Whipp, B.J. (1981) The control of exercise hyperpnea. In: *Regulation of Breathing*, edited by T.F. Hornbein. New York: Marcel Dekker

Whitelaw, W.A., Derenne, J.-P. and Milic-Emilli, J. (1975) Occlusion pressure as a measure of respiratory center output in conscious man. *Resp. Physiol.* **23,** 181

Whitfield, A.G.W., Waterhouse, J.A.H. and Arnott, W.M. (1950) The total lung volume and its subdivisions. *Br. J. soc. Med.* **4,** 1

Whitsett, J.A. (1991) Pulmonary surfactant and respiratory distress syndrome in the premature infant. In: *The Lung: scientific foundations*, p. 1723, edited by R.G. Crystal and J.B. West. New York: Raven Press

Whitteridge, D. and Bulbring, E. (1944) Changes in activity of pulmonary receptors in anaesthesia and the influence of respiratory behaviour. *J. Pharmac. exp. Ther.* **81,** 340

Whitwam, J.G., Chakrabarti, M.K., Konarzewski, W.H. and Askitopoulou, H. (1983) A new valveless all-purpose ventilator. *Br. J. Anaesth.* **55,** 1017

Widdicombe, J.G. (1961) Respiratory reflexes in man and other mammalian species. *Clin. Sci.* **21,** 163

Widdicombe, J.G. (1964) Respiratory reflexes. *Handbk Physiol., section 3,* **1,** 585

Widdicombe, J.G. (1981) Nervous receptors in the respiratory tract. In: *Regulation of Breathing*, part I, edited by T.F. Hornbein. New York: Marcel Dekker

Wiegand, D.A., Zwillich, C.W. and White, D.P. (1989) Collapsibility of the human upper airway during normal sleep. *J. appl. Physiol.* **66,** 1800

Wiegand, D.A., Zwillich, C.W., Latz, B. and Wiegand, L. (1989) The influence of sleep on geniohyoid muscle activity and supraglottic airway resistance. *Am. Rev. resp. Dis.* **139,** A447

Wigfield, R.E., Fleming, P.J., Berry, P.J., Rudd, P.T. and Golding, J. (1992) Can the fall in Avon's sudden infant death rate be explained by changes in sleeping position? *Br. med. J.* **304,** 282

Wiles, C.M., Clarke, C.R.A., Irwin, H.P., Edgar, E.F. and Swan, A.V. (1986) Hyperbaric oxygen in multiple sclerosis: a double blind trial. *Br. med. J.* **292,** 367

Williams, K.G. and Hopkinson, W.I. (1965) Small chamber techniques in hyperbaric oxygen therapy. In: *Hyperbaric Oxygenation*, edited by I. Ledingham. Edinburgh and London: Churchill Livingstone

Windebank, W.J., Boyd, G. and Moran, F. (1973) Pulmonary thromboembolism presenting as asthma. *Br. med. J.* **1,** 90

Winterstein, H. (1911) Die Regulierung der Athmung durch das Blut. *Pflügers Arch. ges. Physiol.* **138,** 167

Wolf, Y.G., Cotev, S., Perel, A. and Manny, J. (1987) Dependence of oxygen consumption on cardiac output in sepsis. *Crit. Care Med.* **15,** 198

Woo, S.W., Berlin, D. and Hedley-Whyte, J. (1969) Surfactant function and anesthetic agents. *J. appl. Physiol.* **26,** 571

Wood, J.D. and Watson, W.J. (1963) Gamma-aminobutyric acid levels in the brain of rats exposed to oxygen at high pressure. *Can. J. Biochem. Physiol.* **41,** 1907

Wood, J.D., Watson, W.J. and Murray, G.W. (1969) Correlation between decreases in brain gamma-aminobutyric acid levels and susceptibility to convulsions induced by hyperbaric oxygen. *J. Neurochem.* **16,** 281

Woodbury, D.M. and Karler, R. (1960) The role of carbon dioxide in the nervous system. *Anesthesiology* **21,** 686

Woodson, R.D., Wills, R.E. and Lenfant, C. (1978) Effect of acute and established anemia on O_2 transport at rest, submaximal and maximal work. *J. appl. Physiol.* **44,** 36

Woolcock, A.J., Vincent, N.J. and Macklem, P.T. (1969) Frequency dependence of compliance as a test for obstruction in the small airways. *J. clin. Invest.* **48,** 1097

Wright, B.M. (1955) A respiratory anemometer. *J. Physiol.* **127,** 25P

Wright, B.M. and McKerrow, C.B. (1959) Maximum forced expiratory flow rate as a measure of ventilatory capacity. *Br. med. J.* **2,** 1041

Wulf, R. J. and Featherstone, R.M. (1957) A correlation of Van der Waals constants with anesthetic potency. *Anesthesiology* **18,** 97

Wynne, J.W. (1984) Gas exchange during sleep in patients with chronic airway obstruction. In: *Sleep and Breathing*, edited by N.A. Saunders and C.E. Sullivan. New York: Marcel Dekker

Yildrim, N., Fitzpatrick, M.F., Whyte, K.F., Jalleh, R., Wightman, A.J.A. and Douglas, N.J. (1991) The effect of posture on upper airway dimensions in normal subjects and in patients with the sleep apnea/hypopnea syndrome. *Am. Rev. resp. Dis.* **144,** 845

Zahn, W.-Z. and Sieck, G.C. (1992) Adaptations of diaphragm and medial gastroenemius muscles to inactivity. *J. appl. Physiol.* **72,** 1445

Zamel, N., Jones, J.G., Bach, S.M. and Newberg, L. (1974) Analog computation of alveolar pressure and airway resistance during maximum expiratory flow. *J. appl. Physiol.* **36,** 240

Zandstra, D.F. (1989) Differential lung ventilation in the critically ill. *Thesis*, University of Groningen.

Zapol, W.M. (1987) Diving adaptations of the Weddell seal. *Sci. Am.* **255,** 100

Zapol, W.M. and Kolobow, T. (1991) Extracorporeal membrane lung gas exchange. In: *The Lung: scientific foundations*, p. 2197, edited by R.G. Crystal and J.B. West. New York: Raven Press

Zapol, W.M., Snider, M.T., Hill, J.D. et al. (1979) Extracorporeal membrane oxygenation in severe acute respiratory failure. *J. Am. med. Assoc.* **242,** 2193

Zechman, F., Hall, F.G. and Hull, W.E. (1957) Effects of graded resistance to tracheal air flow in man. *J. appl. Physiol.* **10,** 356

Zeigler, E.J., Fisher, C.J., Sprung, C.L., Straube, R.C., Sadoff, J.C., Foulke, G.E. et al. (1991) Treatment of gram-negative bacteraemia and septic shock with HA−1A human monoclonal antibody against antitoxin. *New Engl. J. Med.* **324,** 429

Zidulka, A., Gross, D., Minami, H., Vartian, V. and Chang, H.K. (1983) Ventilation by high frequency chest wall compression in dogs with normal lungs. *Am. Rev. resp. Dis.* **127,** 709

Zijlstra, W.G. (1958) *A Manual of Reflection Oximetry.* Assen, Netherlands: van Gorcum's Medical Library

Zuntz, N. (1882) Physiologie der Blutgase und des respiratorischen Gaswechsels. *Hermann's Handbuch Physiol.* **4,** 1

Index